EMERGENCY ORTHOPEDICS

──The Extremities──

Fourth Edition

NOTICE

EMERGENCY ORTHOPEDICS

——The Extremities——

Fourth Edition

Robert R. Simon, MD
Professor and Chairman
Department of Emergency Medicine
Cook County Hospital and Provident Hospital
Rush Medical College
Chicago, Illinois

Steven J. Koenigsknecht, MD
Director, Department of Emergency Medicine
St. Mary's Hospital
Racine, Wisconsin
Former Assistant Professor and Residency Director
Department of Emergency Medicine
University of Chicago
Chicago, Illinois

With illustrations by Susan Gilbert and Anthony Jones

McGraw-Hill
Medical Publishing Division

New York   St. Louis   San Francisco   Auckland   Bogotá   Caracas   Lisbon   London
Madrid   Mexico City   Milan   Montreal   New Delhi   San Juan   Singapore   Sydney   Tokyo   Toronto

McGraw-Hill

A Division of The **McGraw·Hill** *Companies*

EMERGENCY ORTHOPEDICS
The Extremities, Fourth Edition

4567890 KGPKGP   4567890

ISBN 0-8385-2210-6 (domestic)
ISBN 0-07-112015-7 (international)

Exclusive rights by The McGraw-Hill Companies, Inc., for manufacture and export. This book cannot be re-exported from the country to which it is consigned by McGraw-Hill.

This book was set in 10/12 - Times Roman by Progressive Information Technologies, Inc.
The editors were Michael Medina, Susan Noujaim, and Barbara Holton.
The production supervisor was Catherine Saggese.
The cover designer was Mary Skudlarek.
The index was prepared by Kathrin Unger.
Quebecor Printing/Kingsport was printer and binder.
This book is printed on acid-free paper.

Library of Congress Cataloging-in Publication-Data

Simon, Robert R. (Robert Rutha)
    Emergency orthopedics: the extremities / Robert R. Simon, Steven J. Koenigsknecht.--
4th ed.
      p. ; cm.
    Includes bibliographical references and index.
    ISBN 0-8385-2210-6 (alk. paper)
    1. Extremities (Anatomy)--Fractures. 2. Extremities (Anatomy)--Dislocations. 3.
  Orthopedic emergencies.   I. Koenigsknecht, Steven J. II. Title.
    [DNLM: 1. Extremities--injuries. 2. Emergency Medicine--methods. 3.
  Orthopedics--methods. 4. Wounds and Injuries--therapy. WE 800 S596e 2001]
  RD551 .S545 2001
  617.5′80446--dc21   00-020715

To my wife, Marilynn, and my sons, Adam, Timothy, and Jeremy, who give purpose and meaning to my life, and my mother, Fatme, who while being illiterate has taught me more than any literate "teacher" I know.

R.R. Simon

To my parents, Frank and Joann, and my wife, Gail, who by their support and encouragement transformed ideas and ideals into reality.

S.J. Koenigsknecht

CONTENTS

ACKNOWLEDGMENTS

I would like to acknowledge a partner and a friend in all of the work that I have done over the past several years who has helped me in every aspect of my professional life as an advisor and friend, and has assisted in the creation of every piece of work that has come out of this office—including this book, Mishelle Taylor.

PREFACE

A multitude of texts and publications currently exist directed at the "ER doc." The "ER doc" is rapidly being replaced by a new physician who practices only emergency medicine. No current orthopedics text is directed at this physician. As emergency medicine grows, there must evolve a cooperative relationship between the orthopedic surgeon and the emergentologist based on acknowledging the experience and expertise of one another to make prudent decisions and to recognize areas beyond their limitations. It is this spirit that permeates this text.

Currently available publications can be divided into two groups: those that are directed to the orthopedic surgeon and those that, although supposedly directed toward a more advanced audience, are in reality directed to the junior medical student. When one considers that disorders and injuries to the "extremities" compose over 50 percent of what the emergentologist will see and that he or she will see more acute injuries initially than will the orthopedic surgeon, can it be acceptable to give only bits of information rather than the full range of mechanism of injury, treatment, associated injuries, and complications of a particular fracture or injury? Current fracture classifications are directed more toward the orthopedic surgeon and are not presented in a format that the nonspecialist can use quickly and easily. This text categorizes fractures according to degree of complexity, treatment modality, and prognosis—a system much more relevant to the emergency physician.

The fourth edition is a *major rewriting of the text* with the addition of many x-rays placed at appropriate locations throughout. There are new figures for added clarity, and the therapies have been updated to include the latest procedures. A major chapter on Rheumatology has been added which gives all the information needed by the emergentologist to make informed decisions.

This text is divided into three parts:

Part I includes chapters on biomechanics and clinical features of fractures, treatment procedures including basic casting techniques, emergency splinting, the selection of definitive treatment, and indications for operative treatment. In addition, the repair of tendons and ligaments are discussed as well as disorders of the muscles and joints, and complications such as Volkmann's ischemic contracture, gas gangrene, and posttraumatic reflex dystrophy. The chapter on joint disorders has been entirely rewritten, and a new chapter on current radiographic techniques has been expanded.

Part II, in two sections, is a bone-by-bone discussion of every type of fracture followed by a chapter on the soft tissue disorders of that anatomic region. Section One deals with the upper extremities and Section Two with the lower extremities. Each chapter begins with illustrations classifying all possible types of fractures for that site—an illustrated "summary" useful for quick reference. Page cross references to the in-depth textual discussion are included. A brief but complete discussion of functional anatomy follows. We then present a detailed discussion of each type of fracture including, where appropriate, mechanism of injury, associated injuries, pathogenesis, clinical picture, and x-ray presentation. Illustrations of the fracture site are repeated for utility; additional illustrations are often included. The indepth discussions are arranged by the classification system at the front of the chapter which is a compilation of currently existing classification systems, but geared toward emergency medicine. In orthopedics, many classification systems exist for fractures of an individual bone or fractures in a particular region of the body. It is not the intention of the authors to develop a separate and new classification system, but rather to use existing systems whenever possible and organize them in a fashion useful to the emergency physician.

Part III is the Appendix which describes and illustrates in detail the steps involved in placing a particular type of splint or cast. Major revisions with many more detailed step-by-step illustrations have been added to the fourth edition. References are made to the Appendix throughout the text.

The terms *urgent* and *emergent* are used. *Urgent* refers to immediate intervention whereas *emergent* indicates that intervention must take place within the first 24 hours. Although these terms are used throughout emergency medicine, they may not be familiar to everyone reading the text.

In addition, the reader will find *axioms*—major statements that serve as guidelines to prevent the misdiagnosis of a particular problem. These axioms carry the weight of a "pathognomonic" statement. Although the axioms are not truly pathognomonic in dealing with a particular entity, they should be regarded as laws by which the emergency physician should practice

There are a number of areas in orthopedics where treatment programs differ and legitimate controversy over some therapeutic modalities exists. In most cases, the authors have tried to present the various types of treatment for a particular injury. The author's preferred method of treatment is presented, however, to facilitate a plan of action for the patient. In cases where significant controversy exists, the authors advise referral or consultation with the orthopedic surgeon.

It is our hope that this text will be useful to the senior medical student, general practitioner, the junior orthopedic resident as well as the emergency physician.

PART I

ORTHOPEDIC PRINCIPLES AND MANAGEMENT

FRACTURE PRINCIPLES

TERMINOLOGY AND CLASSIFICATION OF FRACTURES

There are a number of ways in which fractures can be described, categorized, and presented. No one system of classification is all-encompassing, and physicians dealing with fractures on a day-to-day basis must be aware of the terminology used to better understand and convey exactly to colleagues what they are dealing with. There are five general divisions of terms that can be used to describe a fracture. Each fracture should be described and categorized by one of the terms from each group. The five groups are as follows:

1. *Anatomic location:* Fractures are usually categorized as being in either the proximal, middle, or distal thirds of a long bone. Other anatomic terms used to describe the location of a fracture are head, shaft, and base (eg, metacarpal and metatarsal fractures).

2. *Direction of fracture lines* (Figure 1–1):
   Transverse: Figure 1–1A shows a transverse fracture, running perpendicular to the bone.
   Oblique: Oblique fractures are similar to transverse in that there is no torsional appearance to the fracture. The fracture line usually runs across the bone at an angle of 45 to 60 degrees, as shown in Figure 1–1B.
   Spiral: A spiral fracture has a torsional component to it as shown in Figure 1–1C.
   Comminuted: A comminuted fracture is any fracture in which there are more than two fragments noted (Fig. 1–1D). Other examples of comminuted fractures are the segmental and butterfly fractures shown in Figures 1–1E and 1–1F.
   Impacted: An impacted fracture is one where the fractured ends are compressed together. These are usually very stable fractures (Fig. 1–1G).

3. *Relationship of the fracture fragments to each other:*
   Alignment: This is the relationship of the axes of the fragments of a long bone to one another. Alignment is described in degrees of angulation, of the *distal fragment* in relation to the *proximal* fragment (Fig. 1–2).
   Apposition: Apposition describes the contact of the fracture surfaces which may be partial (Fig. 1–3A). If the fragments are not only displaced but also overlapping the term commonly used is *bayonette apposition*, frequently seen in femoral shaft fractures (Fig. 1–3B). When the displacement is in the longitudinal axis of the bone, the term *distraction* is used (Fig. 1–3C).

4. *Stability:*
   Stable fracture: A fracture that does not have a tendency to displace after reduction.
   Unstable fracture: A fracture that tends to displace after reduction.

5. *Associated soft tissue injury:*
   Simple (closed): A fracture in which the overlying skin remains intact.
   Compound (open): A fracture in which the overlying skin is broken.
   Complicated: A fracture that is associated with either neurovascular, visceral, ligamentous, or muscular damage. Intra-articular fractures are also complicated.
   Uncomplicated: A fracture that has only a minimal amount of soft tissue injury.

Another method of discussing fractures is by the *mechanism* of injury. Mechanisms by which fractures occur are divided into the following two categories: direct and indirect. A *direct* force causing a fracture will usually result in a transverse, an oblique, or a commin-

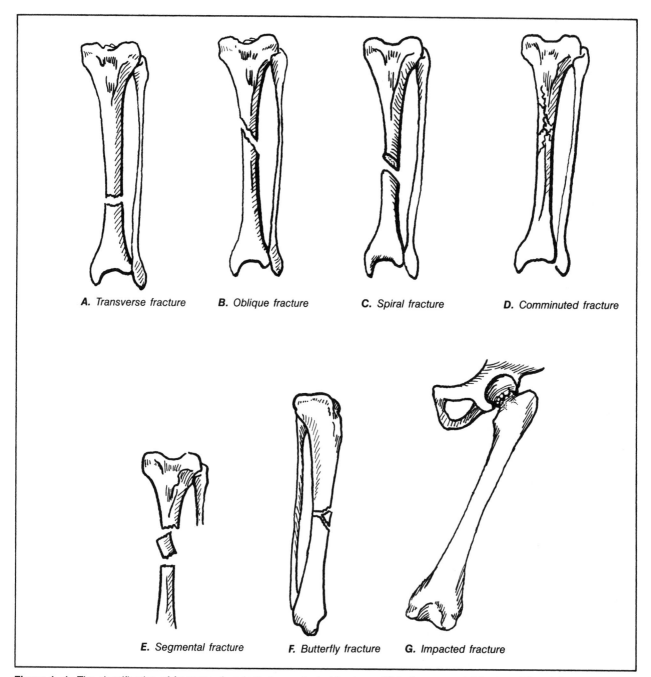

A. *Transverse fracture*   **B.** *Oblique fracture*   **C.** *Spiral fracture*   **D.** *Comminuted fracture*

E. *Segmental fracture*   **F.** *Butterfly fracture*   **G.** *Impacted fracture*

Figure 1–1. The classification of fractures. A variant of comminuted fractures *(D)* is the segmental fracture *(E)* and the butterfly fracture *(F)*.

uted fracture exemplified by the nightstick fracture caused by a blow to the ulna. A comminuted fracture resulting from a crush injury or a fracture from a high velocity bullet is also caused by direct impact.

Fractures also may be caused by *indirect* forces transmitting energy to the fracture site. Traction on a ligament attached to a bone can result in an avulsion fracture as shown in Figure 1–4A. An angulatory force, such as a valgus stress at the knee, can result in a compression or depression fracture of the tibial condyle

(Fig. 1–4B and C). A rotational force applied along the long axis of a bone can result in a spiral fracture. A stress fracture results from repeated stress applied to a bone, often referred to as a fatigue fracture; however, some stress fractures are caused by repeated direct trauma.

Dislocation, Subluxation, and Diastasis
Joint injuries are commonly seen in the emergency center. Joint dissociations can be categorized into three groups

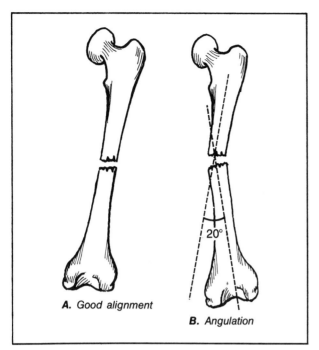

Figure 1–2. The description of fractures is according to the relationship of the distal segment to the proximal. Angulation is measured by drawing an imaginary line through the normal axis of the bone and then another line through the axis of the fractured distal segment and measuring the angle between them. **A.** There is no angulation and this is referred to as good alignment of the fractured ends. **B.** There is an angulatory deformity of the distal segment of 20 degrees.

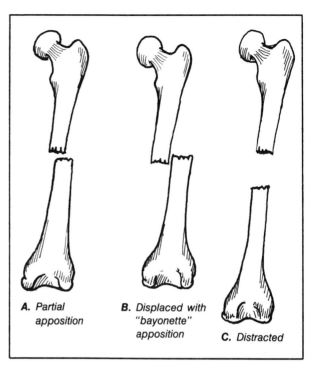

Figure 1–3. Another descriptive method of telling the relationship of the fractured ends to one another is by apposition. **A.** A partially apposed fracture is shown here. **B.** A displaced fracture occurs when the two ends are not in contact with one another. A special type of displaced fracture in which the two ends are not only displaced from one another but also there is overlap with shortening of the normal length of the bone is called bayonette apposition. **C.** Distraction occurs when fracture ends are displaced but rather than being separated in a side-to-side fashion they are "pulled apart" from one another.

depending on degree and type of joint involved. A *dislocation* is a total disruption of the joint surfaces with loss of normal contact between the two bony ends (Fig. 1–5A). A *subluxation* is a partial disruption of a joint with partial contact remaining between the two bones that make up the joint (Fig. 1–5B). Certain bones come together in what is called a *syndesmotic articulation* in which there is little motion. These joints are interconnected by an interosseous membrane that traverses the area between the two bones. Two syndesmotic joints occur in humans between the radius and ulna and between the fibula and tibia. A disruption of the interosseous membrane connecting these two joints is called a *diastasis* (Fig. 1–5C).

BIOMECHANICS OF FRACTURES

There are a number of extrinsic factors that directly relate to the kind of fracture: magnitude of a force, its duration and direction, and the rate at which it acts. A fracture occurs when the stress applied exceeds the plastic strain of the bone and goes beyond its yield point. When a bone is subjected to repeated stresses, the bone may ultimately fracture even though the magnitude of

one individual stress is much lower than the ultimate tensile strength of the bone. The strength of a bone is related directly to its density, which is reduced by osteoporosis or any condition in which the osseous structure is changed, thus lowering its resistance to stress.

FRACTURE HEALING

Fracture healing can be divided into several phases. Initially, after a fracture occurs, the periosteum is torn, usually on one side only. A hematoma forms rapidly at the site between the fracture ends. The hematoma rapidly organizes to form a clot, and the osteocytes at the ends are deprived of their nutrition and die, leaving the ends of the fracture virtually dead. With this necrotic tissue an intense inflammatory response results, accompanied by vasodilatation and leading to edema formation and the exudation of inflammatory cells. These cells migrate to the area along with polymorphonuclear leukocytes and are followed by macrophages. This stage is referred to as the *inflammatory phase* of fracture healing (Fig. 1–6A).

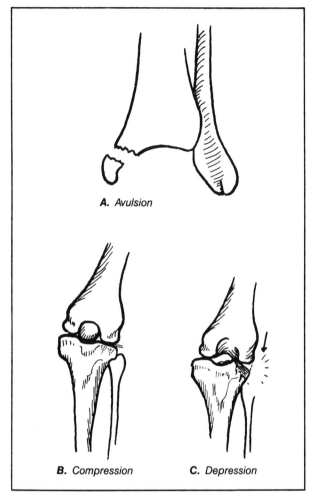

Figure 1–4. The mechanism of injury is often incorporated in fracture descriptions. **A.** An avulsed fracture in this case due to the deltoid ligament pulling the medial malleolus off as would occur with an eversion stress. **B.** A compression fracture caused by the femoral condyle compressing the tibial condyle due to a valgus stress on the lower leg. This is a type of impaction fracture, but the term compression not only tells one it is an impaction fracture but also the mechanism by which it occurred. **C.** Here more force has caused depression of the condyle.

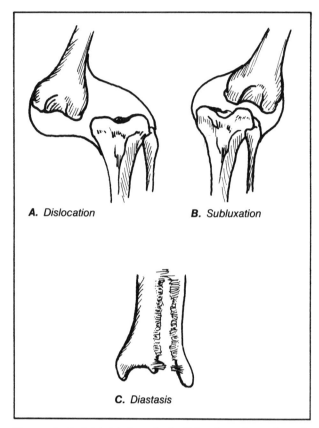

Figure 1–5. Joint injuries. **A.** A dislocation shown here is complete separation of the two bones that make up the joint. **B.** Subluxation indicates partial displacement of the bone ends. **C.** Diastasis is separation at a syndesmotic joint.

As the hematoma organizes, mesenchymal cells invade from the periosteum and form the earliest bone. Endosteal cells also form bone, which enters the fracture along with the granulation tissue. The granulation tissue invades from surrounding vessels. Most healing occurs around the capillary buds that invade the fracture site. Healing with new bone formation occurs primarily at the subperiosteal region; cartilage formation occurs in most other areas.

The initial step in bone formation is the formation of osteoblasts that move from the inside toward the outer surface. Collagen formation is followed by mineral deposition of calcium hydroxyapatite crystals. At this stage, called the *reparative phase*, there is callus formation, and the first signs of clinical union are noted (Fig. 1–6B). As the process of healing continues, the bone organizes into trabeculae. Osteoclastic activity is firs t seen resorbing poorly formed trabeculae and permitting the laying down of new bone corresponding to the lines of force or stress. This is called the *remodeling phase* (Fig. 1–6C).

Many conditions affect the rate of fracture healing. Cortical bone heals at a slower rate than does cancellous bone, which has many points of bony contact and a rich blood supply. The amount of apposition and distraction of the bony ends, and any associated soft tissue injuries adversely affect the rate of healing. Fractures that are inadequately immobilized heal poorly, thus leading to *delayed union* or *nonunion*. Fractures through pathologic bone lesions also heal slowly as do intra-articular fractures. The synovial fluid contains fibrinolysins that retard the initial stage of fracture healing due to lysis of the clot. Certain drugs, such as corticosteroids, inhibit the rate of healing as does excessive thyroid hormone. It is suspected that healing does not occur normally under conditions of chronic hypoxia, and this has been confirmed in hypoxic animals where a significant delay occurs in fracture healing. Exercise increases the rate of

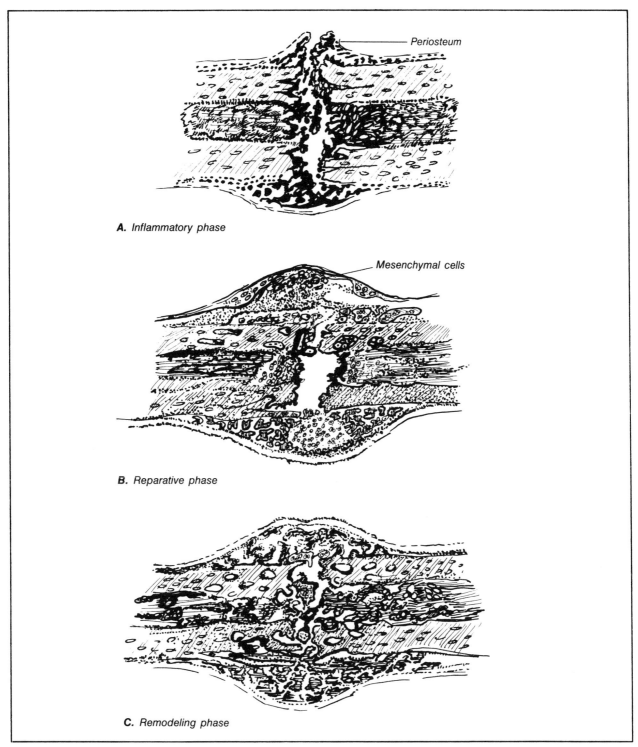

Periosteum

A. *Inflammatory phase*

Mesenchymal cells

B. *Reparative phase*

C. *Remodeling phase*

Figure 1–6. Phases of fracture healing.

repair and this should be encouraged, particularly isometric exercises around an immobilized joint.

Many terms are used in describing fracture healing. *Union* refers to the healing of a fracture. Clinical union permits the resumption of motion of a limb and occurs earlier than radiologic union. *Malunion* is the healing of a fracture with a residual deformity. Healing that takes a longer time than is usual for the particular bone or fracture is referred to as *delayed union*. Failure of the fracture to unite is called a *nonunion. Pseudoarthrosis* results from a nonunion with a false joint appearing between the fracture ends.

CLINICAL FEATURES OF FRACTURES

Pain and tenderness are the most common presenting complaints of a fracture. These symptoms will usually be well localized to the fracture site but can appear to be somewhat more generalized or diffuse if there is significant associated soft tissue injury. Loss of normal function may be noted, but in patients with incomplete fractures (stress fracture) the functional impairment may be minimal. When the fractured ends are in poor apposition, usually abnormal mobility and crepitation may be elicited. This should not be sought for, however, as it increases the chance of further soft tissue damage. Those patients with gross deformity or crepitation should be splinted immediately before they are moved or any radiographs are taken. Point tenderness should be looked for. A stress fracture may be tentatively diagnosed or suspected on the basis of bony tenderness even though a fracture might not be seen on X ray for 10 to 14 days. Radiographs should include the joint above and below the fracture to detect any associated fractures. No examination of a patient with a suspected fracture is complete without a neurovascular examination.

There are a number of common pitfalls in the diagnosis and therapy of fractures that should be pointed out:

1. Always consider an osteochondral fracture when treating a joint injury.
2. Avoid treating accessory ossicles as fractures by looking for the smooth border, and when doubt exists obtain comparison views.
3. Do not confuse epiphyseal injury with a ligamentous injury in a child. Remember that the epiphysis is the weakest point and the region most likely to be injured when an abnormal stress is applied across a joint, especially at the knee.

Bleeding is a common problem with most fractures. The amount of bleeding is often not appreciated. Table 1–1 shows the amount of bleeding that occurs around commonly seen fractures. A patient with multiple fractures can experience shock from blood loss. This is especially true in the elderly who are less able to vasoconstrict to support their pressure. Pelvic fractures bleed extensively and can result in exsanguinating hemorrhage.

TABLE 1–1. AVERAGE BLOOD LOSS WITH A CLOSED FRACTURE

Fracture Site	Amount (mL)
Radius and ulna	150-250
Humerus	250
Pelvis	1500-3000
Femur	1000
Tibia and fibula	500

Stress Fractures

A stress fracture is a common injury seen by health care professionals, particularly those who care for athletes. These fractures result from repetitive, cyclic loading of the bone that overwhelms the reparative ability of the skeletal system. Three events may lead to stress fracture. First, the applied load can be increased. Second, the number of applied stresses can increase. Finally, the surface area over which the load is applied can be decreased. The diagnosis requires a thorough clinical examination with a high index of suspicion.[3] The history must focus on examining the athlete's training regimen, especially changes that occur. Initially, plain X rays may be normal, especially early in the course of the fracture. Repeating the plain X rays, bone scintigraphy, magnetic resonance imaging (MRI), and computed tomography (CT) are all possible options for diagnosing a stress fracture.

Clinical Presentation

There are a number of possible factors that may predispose to stress fractures. The type of surface (ie, hard surface) may cause stress factors as could a change in the intensity and speed or distance at which a patient is doing exercise. Inappropriate shoes can result in stress fractures. Other factors include mechanical problems such as a leg length discrepancy that the athlete may not even be aware of, increased knee valgus, foot disorders, or decreased tibial bone width.

The common sites where stress fractures occur are shown in (see Fig. 1–23).[12] The patient presents with a complaint of pain and discomfort, describing an initial aching after exercise that progresses to pain localized to the site of the fracture. Pain progresses in severity during the activity to the extent that the exercise is discontinued. The time the patient presents is variable, resulting in a delay in diagnosis that may be several weeks later in some cases.[14]

The physical examination will vary depending on the location of the stress fracture. A stress fracture of the proximal femur will reveal minimal clinical findings; however, the Hop test is positive.[14] X rays are frequently normal in the initial evaluation of stress fractures. Bone scan is an imaging technique that utilizes technetium 99 m injected intravenously. This technetium is taken up rapidly by regenerating bone. This test is more sensitive than X rays in detecting new stress fractures. It should be noted, however, that a positive bone scan is a nonspecific finding and can occur in osteomyelitis, osteoid, osteoma, and other tumors.

Treatment

The treatment of stress fractures is variable depending on the location of the fracture. Abstinence or limitation of the activity causing the symptoms is a keystone to any treatment regimen. The vast majority of stress fractures will be treated with rest and cessation of the precipitating activity for a minimum of 4 to 6 weeks. Crutches may be used initially to allow non-weight-bearing in weight-bearing areas. One must remember that stress fractures occur more frequently in female athletes than in male athletes. One must look for the relationship between these fractures and eating disorders, amenorrhea, or osteoporosis.[13, 14]

TREATMENT OF FRACTURES

Initial Management
The initial assessment of a fracture must answer a number of important questions. Is the fracture stable or unstable? An unstable fracture must be stabilized by some form of external splinting or traction before any movement or transport of the patient. The second question that one must address is whether or not there are any associated injuries to surrounding vessels, viscera, skin, or nerves. A well-documented neurovascular examination must be performed before any further assessment can be made of the patient with a suspected or clinically obvious fracture.

Emergency Splinting
The purposes of emergency splinting are threefold: to prevent further soft tissue injury by the fracture fragments, for pain relief, and to lower the incidence of clinical fat embolism.

Perhaps the most commonly known splint used in the past was the *Thomas splint*, which is a half-ring splint used for femoral fractures. Modifications of this splint are the *Hare traction splint* based on the same principles of applying continuous traction to the fracture to stabilize it and prevent further soft tissue injury (Fig. 1–7A and B). These splints are practical and safe to use and provide good support for the patient in transport. The splint should not be removed before X ray evaluation.

The new *Sager traction splint* (Minto Research and Development, Inc.) is the authors' preference for emergency splinting of all proximal femoral and femoral shaft fractures in both the pediatric and adult age group. The splint is shown in Figures 1–7C and D. It can be applied to the outer side of the leg or the inner side as shown. The splint does not have a half-ring posteriorly, which eliminates any pressure on the sciatic nerve and most importantly eliminates the angulation of the fracture site, which occurs with half-ring splints. The advantages of this splint over half-ring splints currently in use are detailed.

1. No sciatic nerve compression, which may occur with half-ring splint devices.
2. No flexion of the midshaft or proximal femoral segment, as occurs with half-ring splint devices, thus resulting in a more acceptable alignment.

3. Overtraction, a common problem with half-ring devices resulting in knee edema and injury to epiphyseal growth centers in children, is eliminated because the precise weight of traction can be applied based on 10 percent of the patient's body weight. The traction is shown on a circular meter at the ankle portion of the splint. Traction should never exceed 22 pounds.
4. The same splint can be used for children and adults.
5. The splint can be used with trousers in place.
6. The splint can be used in patients with groin injuries by strapping it to the outer side of the hip.
7. The splint can be used in patients with pelvic fractures.
8. The ankle straps are placed so that one can monitor the dorsalis pedis pulse with the splint in place.
9. The splint includes a cross bar that permits splinting of bilateral femoral fractures with one splint between the legs.
10. Splinting of the fracture is done in a more anatomic position resulting in less outward rotation of the proximal fragment.

Inflatable splints made of a double-walled polyvinyl jacket with a zipper fastener placed around the injured limb are quite popular at present. Although they afford the advantages of easy application and control of swelling even after their removal, their disadvantages must be recognized.[11] They are useful only for fractures of the forearm, wrist, and ankle. When inflated to pressures of 40 mm Hg they reduce the blood flow to the limb markedly and may even cause complete cessation of blood flow in some patients. Thus, they can cause circulatory embarrassment when at high pressures and are ineffective at lower pressures. These splints should not be applied over clothing as they can cause skin blisters. The method of application is as shown in Figure 1–8.

Other alternative splints that can be used in the field stabilization of a fracture are the *pillow splint* (Fig. 1–9A), which is fashioned by wrapping an ordinary pillow tightly around a lower extremity fracture and securing it with safety pins as shown. A splint can be made from towels wrapped around the limb and supported on either side by wood splints as shown in Figure 1–9B. The same type of splint can be used in the upper extremity; the only additional support needed is a sling to support the forearm while such a splint is in place.

Patients who present with open fractures should be splinted in a similar manner; however, the site of skin puncture should be covered with a sterile dressing, and one should be careful not to replace any exposed bone fragment back into the wound to avoid further contamination.

Selection of Definitive Treatment
The selection of the definitive treatment of a fracture is a combined decision between the emergency physician

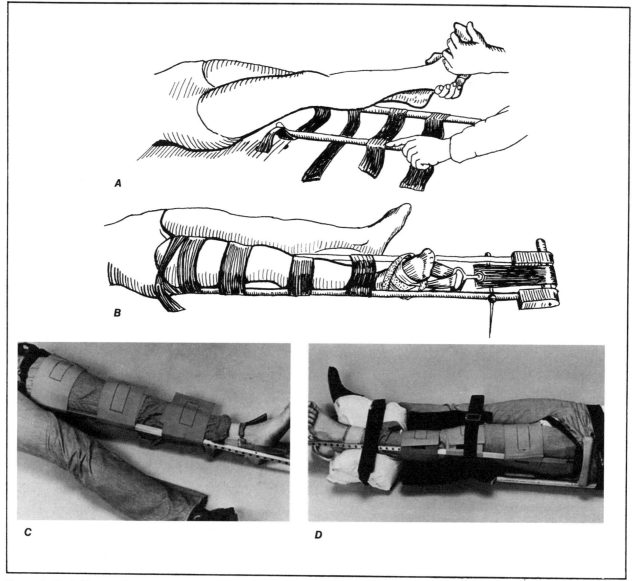

Figure 1–7. A. Hare traction is applied as shown by applying traction to the lower limb and elevating it with the knee held in extension. **B.** The splint is then inserted under the limb and the foot secured in the traction apparatus. **C.** The Sager traction splint. The gauged meter distally tells the amount of weight being applied to the ankle straps for distraction. **D.** The splint can be applied to the outer side of the leg in patients with groin injuries or pelvic fractures who also have a femoral fracture.

and the referral doctor. Some fractures can be treated safely and followed by the emergency physician whereas others require an emergent consultation for operative intervention. Those fractures requiring operative intervention are discussed in their individual sections. Closed manipulative reductions should be performed within 6 to 12 hours of the time of injury as swelling rapidly ensues making reduction more difficult. A displaced fracture usually leaves the periosteum intact on one side. Without this intact periosteal bridge, reduction would be difficult to maintain (Fig. 1–10A). To reduce a fracture one must apply traction in the long axis of the bone and reverse

the mechanism that produced the fracture (Fig. 1–10B and C). The fragment that can be controlled should be aligned with the one that cannot. An intact periosteal bridge will assist in not only the reduction but the maintenance of the reduction. Tissue interposition or a large hematoma may make reduction by closed means impossible. Once reduction is accomplished, immobilization with plaster or continuous traction or some form of splint is required to hold the position.

Traction is a good means for immobilization of some fractures. Skin traction should be used primarily in children and is usually temporary. Skin traction in adults

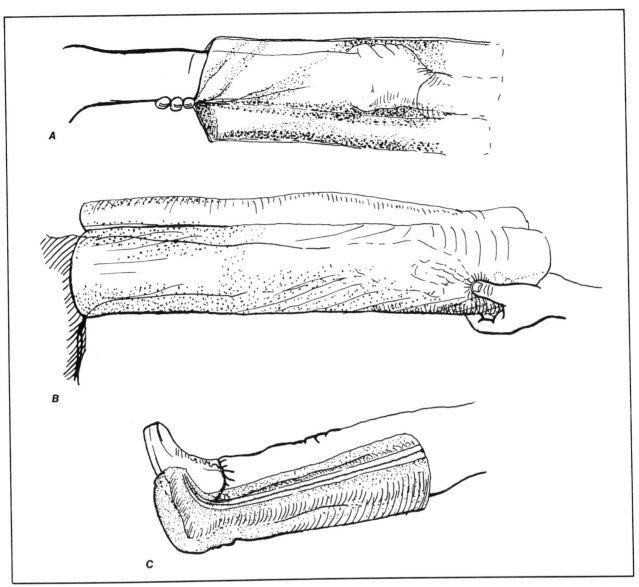

Figure 1–8. Inflatable splints are used in fractures of the wrist, forearm, and ankle. **A.** The limb is held as shown with one hand and a distracting force is applied with the limb held in extension. **B.** The inflatable splint is then applied over the fractured extremity either directly or by slipping it over the examiner's arm and onto the patient. It is then inflated. **C.** A similar technique is used for splints applied to the lower limb.

should always be temporary and one should never use adhesive tape on the skin but rather moleskin tape (Fig. 1–11). One must be careful to protect all bony prominences. Skeletal traction applied with a pin passed through a bony prominence distal to the fracture site is a good form of immobilization, especially in comminuted fractures that cannot be held by plaster fixation. Skeletal traction is used most frequently in fractures of the femur and also in some humeral fractures.

Fractures through the metaphysis of a long bone have a good blood supply and heal well as a general rule, whereas diaphyseal fractures heal more slowly and need more attention because of the poor blood supply in this portion of the bone.

Indications for Operative Treatment of Fractures

The emergency physician must be aware of the indications for operative intervention in managing fractures. These are discussed in the individual sections but some general guidelines can be stated here. Operative intervention is indicated in the following circumstances:

1. Displaced intra-articular fractures
2. Associated arterial injury
3. When experience shows that open treatment yields better results
4. When closed methods fail
5. Where the fracture is through a metastatic lesion
6. In patients in whom continued confinement in bed would be undesirable

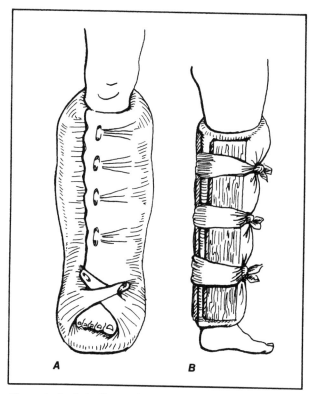

Figure 1–9. **A.** A pillow makes an excellent temporary splint for the prehospital management of a fracture to the ankle, foot, or distal tibia. **B.** A fracture of the lower leg can be stablized alternately by wrapping towels securely around the limb and then applying two splints of wood on either side and securing them to the extremity as shown.

CASTING

The presence of a fracture should not be equated with the need for casting. Casts are used for three reasons: to immobilize a fracture to permit healing, to relieve pain by rest, and to stabilize an unstable fracture.

The plaster rolls or slabs used in casting are muslin stiffened by dextrose or starch and impregnated with a hemihydrate of calcium sulfate. When water is added to the calcium sulfate a reaction occurs that liberates heat, which is noted by both the patient and the physician applying the cast.

$$CaSO_4 \cdot H_2O + H_2O \rightarrow CaSO_4 \cdot H_2O + Heat$$

Accelerator substances are added to the bandages that allow them to set at differing rates. Common table salt can be used to retard the setting of the plaster; if this is desired, simply add salt to the water. Acceleration of the setting occurs by increasing the temperature of the water or by adding alum to the water. The colder the water temperature, the longer the plaster takes to set. After placing a plaster roll in water squeeze the ends together (Fig. 1–12) in order to squeeze out excess water while retaining the plaster in the roll.

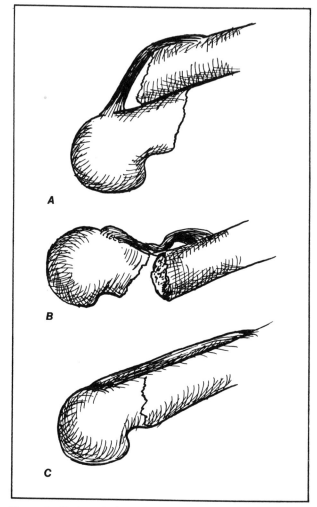

Figure 1–10. In reducing a fracture three maneuvers are basically used in sequence. These may be augmented by other steps but the basic principles apply. **A.** An intact periosteal bridge is usually present on one side and acts as a support on which the physician can rely to internally stabilize the fracture after reduction. **B.** Traction is applied first in the line of the deformity and this is followed by reproducing the same mechanism that caused the fracture, thus using the intact periosteal bridge. **C.** The ends are then reapposed and the fracture is reduced.

There are several methods of applying plaster. *Skin-tight* casts applied directly over the skin, although advocated by some in the past, are no longer used due to the complications of pressure sores and the circulatory embarrassment that ensues. Most commonly used today is stockinette applied at the ends of the cast (Fig. 1–13A), followed by sheet wadding that is applied from distal to the proximal end of the limb (Fig. 1–13B). Too much padding reduces the efficacy of the cast and permits excessive motion. Generally, the more padding used, the more plaster needed. The cotton wool interposed between the skin and the plaster provides elastic pressure and enhances the fixation of the limb by compensating for slight shrinkage of the tissues after

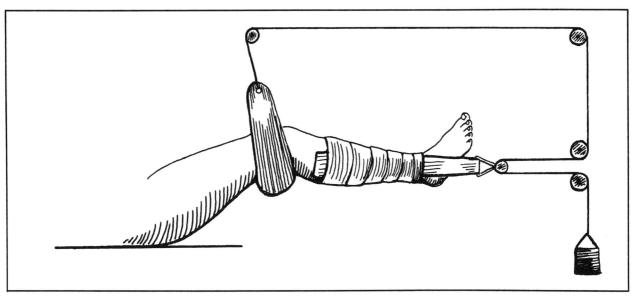

Figure 1–11. Skin traction can be used to temporarily distract a displaced fracture of the femur until the patient can be definitively managed the following day. Similar traction can be used in the upper extremity.

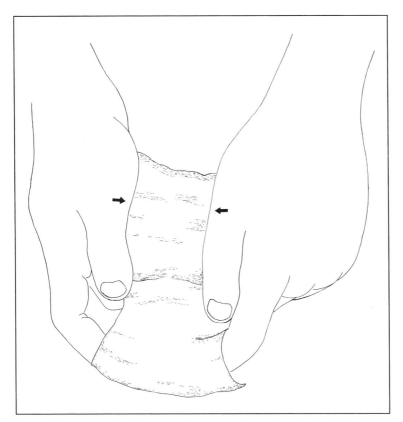

Figure 1–12. After placing a roll of plaster in water, lift the plaster out of the water and squeeze the ends together. Make certain that the free edge is separated from the plaster roll as shown so that one does not lose the end when trying to apply the roll to the extremity. Using this technique of squeezing the ends together one removes the excess water yet retains the plaster within the roll.

application of the cast. The plaster bandage should be rolled in the same direction as the cotton wadding, and each turn should overlap the preceding one by half. It should always be laid on transversely with the roll of bandage in contact with the surface of the limb almost continuously. The roll should be lightly guided around the limb, and pressure should be applied by the thenar eminence to mold the plaster. Each turn should be smoothed with the thenar eminence of the right hand as the left hand guides the roll around the limb. As the limb tapers, the bandage is made to lie evenly by small tucks made with the index finger and thumb of the right hand

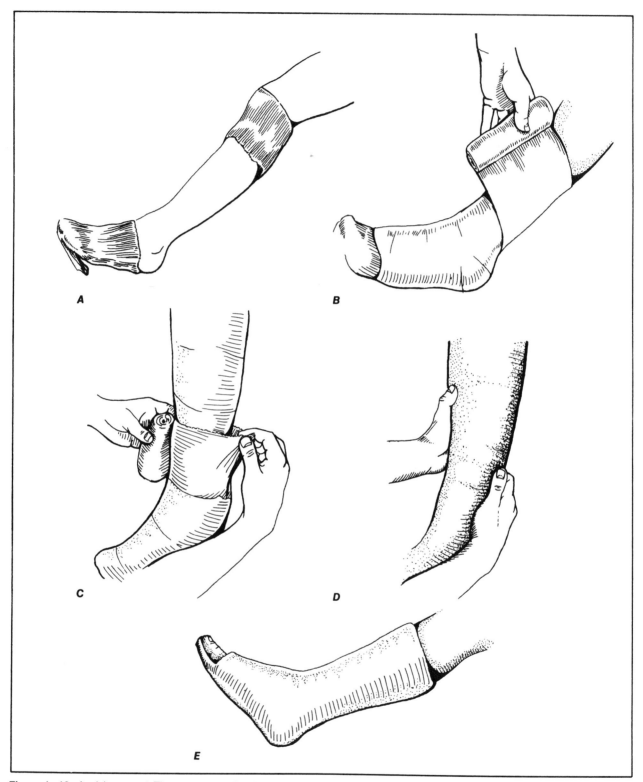

Figure 1–13. Applying a cast. The same general technique is used whether one is applying a cast to the upper or lower extremity. **A.** Stockinette is used to cover the proximal and distal ends of the area to be casted. **B.** Webril or another soft cotton-batting material is used under the plaster roll. **C.** The plaster is applied as shown with the roll held against the limb by the left hand. The right hand is used to smooth out the plaster and to pull and fold back the top corners, which are produced by the changing circumference of the limb. **D.** The plaster roll once applied is smoothed with the thenar eminence and palms of both hands to seal the interstices and give added support. **E.** The final step is to fold back the stockinette and apply your last roll of plaster after trimming the cast to the desired shape.

before each turn is smoothed into position (Fig. 1–13C). As the bandage is applied, it is smoothed by the palms of both hands and the thenar eminences (Fig. 1–13D). The technique of how to uplift the plaster roll during application and tucking the point as one encircles a tapering limb is demonstrated in Figure 1–14. Remember that the durability and strength of the cast depends on welding together of each individual layer by the smoothing movements of both hands (Fig. 1–13E). One should concentrate on making the two ends of the cast of adequate thickness because it is easy to make the center too thick, which provides no additional support at the fracture site (Fig. 1–15A and B). A common mistake is to use many narrow bandages, rather than fewer wider rolls creating a lumpy appearance to the cast. Bandages of widths of 4, 6, and 8 inches are most commonly used for casting. Another common mistake in bandaging is not applying the plaster snugly enough, especially over the proximal fleshy portion of the limb. A better fit is needed here than at the distal bony parts.

If one needs to reinforce the cast, as in an obese patient with a walking cast, this should be done by adding a fin to the front, *not* by adding excessive posterior splints to the back as this only adds weight to the cast and does not make it stronger. Plaster boots are available and preferred to walking heels by many orthopedists (Fig. 1–16), although a walking heel remains a commonly applied device for ambulation (Fig. 1–17).

The application of a walking heel should be under the center of the foot. The heel should be centered midway between the posterior tip of the calcaneous and the distal end of the "ball" of the foot.

When applying a cast to the upper extremity, one should leave the hand free by stopping the cast at the

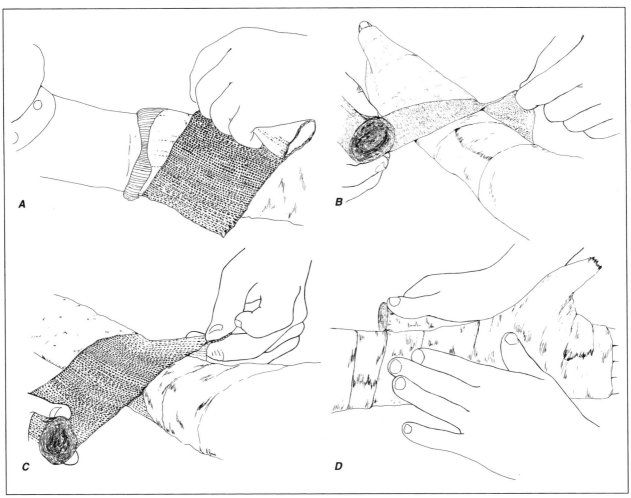

Figure 1–14. This demonstrates the method of rolling plaster around a tapering extremity **A.** As the roll is being applied one ends up with excess slack on one edge creating a "tent." **B.** The tent is uplifted by the index finger and is folded over to "absorb" the excess slack (C). This should be smoothed out with the palm of the hand, thus molding it into the remainder of the roll (D).

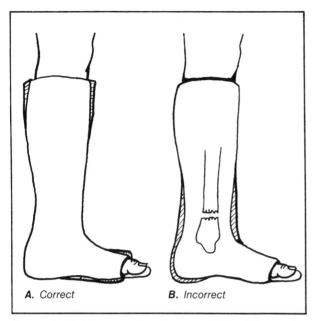

Figure 1–15. The correct way to apply plaster is to use the same thickness throughout. **A.** For added support one may add extra thickness at the proximal and distal ends. **B.** A common mistake is for physicians to think that one gains strength by adding thickness at the fracture site.

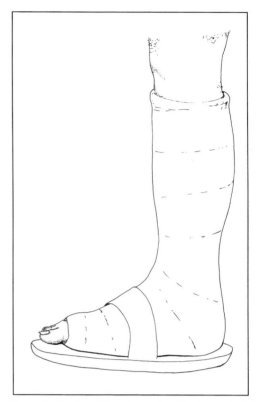

Figure 1–16. A walking shoe or boot is demonstrated.

metacarpal heads dorsally and the proximal flexor crease of the palm volarly to permit normal finger motion (Fig. 1–18).

A window may be placed in a cast when a fracture is accompanied by a laceration or any skin lesions that need care while treating the fracture. Windows are best made by covering the wound with a bulky piece of sterile gauze (Fig. 1–19A) and then applying the cast over the dressing in the normal manner (Fig. 1–19B). After completing the cast, a window is cut out in the cast over the "bulge" created by the gauze dressing (Fig. 1–19C). The defect should always be covered with a dressing and a piece of sponge rubber or felt snugly held in place with an ace bandage. Herniation of the soft tissue will be prevented, and subsequent swelling and skin ulceration is thus avoided.

There are many types of casts such as spica casts, patellar tendon bearing casts, and cast braces. These are not used by the emergency physician, however, and will not be discussed here.

Splints can also be used as casts. Most frequently used are the posterior splints of the lower extremity for ankle and foot injuries and similar splints to the upper extremity (Fig. 1–20). Splints offer the advantage of permitting soft tissue swelling to occur without compromising the circulation. Ice packs can be applied to the site of injury as the splint will permit penetration of the ice to maximize its effect. For these reasons and because of the ease of application, splints are frequently used for the emergent and temporary immobilization of fractures. Various splints are shown and discussed throughout the text as well as in

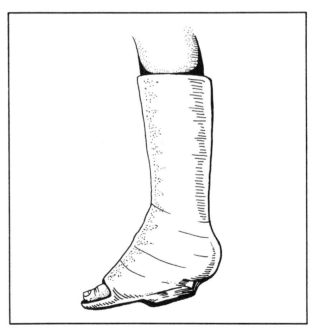

Figure 1–17. A walking cast.

the Appendix. Splints permit excessive motion, however, and provide little stability for a reduced fracture that needs to be maintained in a fixed position.

Lightweight fiberglass casts have been introduced that are long-wearing and radiolucent. They can become

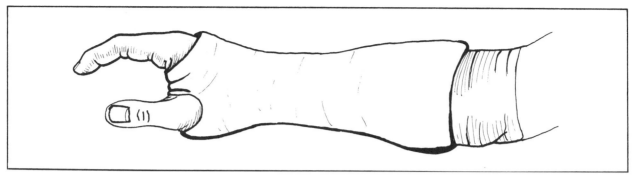

Figure 1–18. A short arm cast with the wrist in 15 to 20 degrees of extension and the fingers free at the metacarpophalangeal joint.

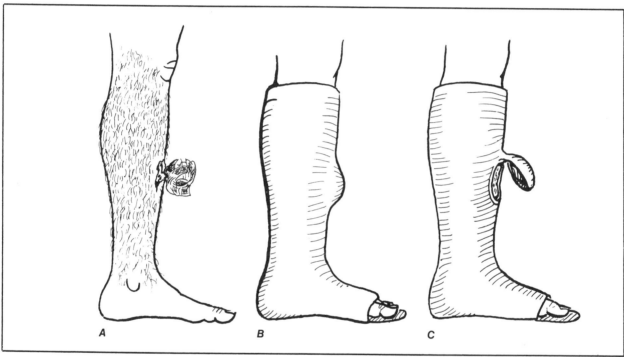

Figure 1–19. When an open wound requires care and is associated with a fracture to the extremity that must be casted, the following is a good technique for knowing where to cut a window in the cast for wound care and observation: **A.** The wound is covered with sterile dressings, which are wadded up in a ball over the wound. **B.** The cast is then applied in the routine fashion over the dressed wound. **C.** A window is cut out over the "bulge" produced in the cast.

wet without being softened or damaged. These have limited applications to fresh fractures but are commonly used as a second or subsequent cast. They are especially useful for open fractures because the patient can use whirlpool or other forms of wet therapy while in the cast. They are more difficult to apply, however, and a snug fit is more difficult to achieve.

Sores are complications of plaster that can occur from excessive pressure. Patients may complain of burning pain or discomfort. This can be avoided by eliminating sharp ends and indented spots in the cast. Felt pads placed between the layers of wadding in the cast padding tend to migrate and may result in pressure sores.

Checking Casts

Any patient with a circumferential cast should receive written instructions describing the symptoms of ischemia from a tight cast. Increasing pain, swelling, coolness, or change in skin color of the distal portions of the extremity are signs of a cast being too tight. The patient should be checked immediately; he or she must be made aware of the dangers of ignoring such problems. As a general rule, the authors would recommend that any circumferential cast be checked the following day for signs of circulatory compromise. The patient must be instructed to elevate the limb to avoid problems.

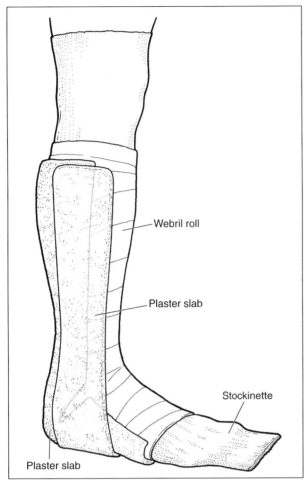

Webril roll

Plaster slab

Stockinette

Plaster slab

Figure 1–20. A posterior splint made by application of stockinette followed by a cotton bandage. Finally, a posterior slab of plaster is applied. Commercially available materials, which incorporate the cotton roll and plaster in one piece, are readily purchased. An elastic bandage is applied to secure the splint to the limb.

If the cast is too tight one must remember to split not only the plaster casting but also the inner wadding to significantly reduce the pressure. This was well demonstrated in a recent study that showed that no significant reduction in pressure occurred when only the plaster was opened. Splitting the plaster and the wadding did result in a significant reduction in the pressure.[1]

Anesthesia for Fractures

There are many forms of anesthesia that can be used in fracture reduction. Many fractures require general anesthesia, particularly those in small children. One must weigh the risk of general anesthesia against the advantages of regional blocks that can be used satisfactorily in many of the common reductions performed in the emergency center.

A *Bier block* is an excellent form of anesthesia for leg, foot, forearm, and hand fractures. The technique is quite simple, and complications of a properly performed block are few. A needle is inserted into a superficial vein in the arm or leg. The limb is then elevated and exsanguinated by wrapping the extremity distally to proximally with an elastic bandage. A pneumatic tourniquet is then inflated to 250 mm Hg in the upper extremity and to 400 mm Hg in the lower extremity. The bandage is then removed and 20 to 40 mL of 0.5 percent lidocaine is injected into the vein for the upper extremity and 40 to 80 mL for the lower extremity. Anesthesia is usually produced in 5 minutes. A second tourniquet is inflated distal to the first and the original tourniquet is then deflated as this is now over unanesthetized skin. This block provides excellent anesthesia. Caution must be exercised to be certain that the tourniquet does not deflate as this may result in a toxic dose of lidocaine being introduced into the central circulation.

A *regional block* is another good form of anesthesia for upper extremity reductions. This can be accomplished by a supraclavicular block or by an axillary block of the brachial plexus. Because of the higher incidence of pneumothorax associated with the supraclavicular approach, the authors advocate the axillary route. The patient should be supine with the arm abducted and the hand placed behind the head and the elbow flexed to 90 degrees. The skin of the axilla should be prepped and the axillary artery palpated. Use a 10mL syringe and a 5/8-inch, 25-gauge needle to raise a skin weal as high in the axilla as possible. The needle is then inserted into the neurovascular sheath and a distinct sensation is felt as the sheath is pierced and the needle pulsates. The physician should check for paresthesias, which confirm the sheath has been entered. Excellent anesthesia for most hand and forearm fractures occurs with 20mL of 1 percent lidocaine. One must wait 15 to 30 minutes to permit good analgesia to occur.

SPECIAL CONSIDERATIONS IN FRACTURE MANAGEMENT

Open Fractures

Gustilo and Anderson have classified open fractures by the severity of associated soft tissue damage. **Grade I** describes an open wound which is less than 1cm long and shows no evidence of contamination.[6] The fractures in Grade I wounds are usually simple, transverse, or short oblique with minimal comminution. **Grade II** wounds occur via a slight crushing injury with a moderate comminution of the fracture and moderate degree of contamination.[15] This category is characterized by a wound of greater than 1cm with no soft tissue stripped from the bone. The final category of open fractures is further divided into three subgroups:

- **Grade IIIA** a large wound with adequate soft tissue coverage of the bone,
- **Grade IIIB** a large wound with periosteal stripping and exposed bone. There is massive contamination and a severe comminution fracture in this subclass.[15]
- **Grade IIIC** a large wound with significant arterial injury.[7]

Thus, open fractures provide a significant challenge to the physician. One must check the skin around the wound and note what contaminants may be in the wound. There should be no attempt to explore the wound digitally in the emergency center as little information will be provided and an increased risk of infection will result. Local debridement is indicated in all cases and should be repeated in 48 to 72 hours to establish a viable environment for soft tissue coverage.[6] If a question arises when a small wound is noted on the skin that overlies a fracture as to whether or not it communicates with the fracture, one can safely check the wound with a sterile blunt probe to see if bone is touched. If a question still remains, the prudent management would dictate to simply treat it as if it were open and debride the wound in the operating room. The wound should be dressed with a sterile dressing and the extremity should be splinted. Note that keeping an open wound moist will increase the surface humidity, an important factor in healing. Also, occlusive dressings will facilitate local healing by raising the wound temperature.[2] One must always examine the blood supply to the limb by checking the peripheral pulses and the capillary blush as this may be compromised significantly.

The wound should be swabbed and a culture taken; the patient should be given broad-spectrum antibiotics. Broad-spectrum antibiotics are recommended for use in open fractures against both gram-positive and gram-negative organisms. The most common organism producing infection is *Staphylococcus aureus*. The open fracture wound most susceptible to secondary infection is the close range shotgun wound. Recommended antibiotics for these injuries include methicillin and kanamycin 1g IV every 6 hours and 0.5g IM every 12 hours, respectively. Cephalosporins are now more commonly used. The recommended doses here are 2g IV every 6 hours for cephalothin, 1g IV or IM every 6 to 8 hours for cefazolin, or 0.5g every 6 hours for cephalexin.

There are many key things the emergency physician should do with an open fracture. The wound should be cleaned, and a sterile dressing applied. A splint should be applied and appropriate radiographs ordered. Always check the X ray for radiopaque material that can easily be mistaken for a fracture fragment. The physician should assess and document the circulatory status and do a thorough neurologic examination. These patients should be started on antibiotics as indicated at the earliest possible time to attain maximum tissue levels. In addition, tetanus prophylaxis must be administered. All patients with open fractures must have their debridement performed in the operating room.

Pathologic Fracture

A pathologic fracture is a fracture that occurs in a bone with pre-existing disease causing structural weakness (Fig. 1–21). This may be due to osteoporosis or other causes such as an enchondroma, solitary cyst in a long bone, giant cell tumors, or metastatic lesions. Enchondromas occur commonly in the metacarpals and phalanges (Fig. 1–22). The lesions are well circumscribed by a zone of reactive bone and are treated by curettage and immobilization for 3 weeks.

Clinical Manifestations

Any fracture that occurs from trivial trauma must be considered a pathologic fracture. The patient may complain of pain that has existed in the area for a long time before the fracture. On the radiograph, one must look for rarefaction compared with other bones and changes in the trabecular pattern around the fracture site. Patients may note generalized bone pain or even painless swelling over the site of the pathologic fracture. The incidental finding of a fracture noted on a routine radiograph taken in a patient complaining of swelling is not uncommon.

Gunshot Wounds Associated with Fractures

Gunshot wounds are commonplace in our society and many patients with these injuries present to the emergency center with associated fractures. The examining physician should attempt to determine the caliber of the bullet and the type of weapon used and from this information determine if it is a high- or low-velocity bullet. High-velocity bullets have a muzzle or impact velocity of 2000 to 2500 feet per second and always need to be debrided. Most civilian injuries are caused by low-velocity bullets and can be treated without extensive debridement. Treatment consists of tetanus prophylaxis, IV antibiotics, cleansing of the skin adjacent to the wound, and local skin debridement of the wound edges in the operating room. Irrigation of the wound is followed by the application of a sterile dressing; the wound is left open and the fracture immobilized appropriately.

High-velocity bullets that cause a fracture are usually associated with a significant degree of comminution of the fracture, and this results in a gaping exit wound that requires debridement in the operating room. If the bullet enters a joint, debridement in the operating room is required in all cases. A shotgun wound requires extensive debridement in the operating room. If the bullet passes close to a vessel, an arteriogram is almost always

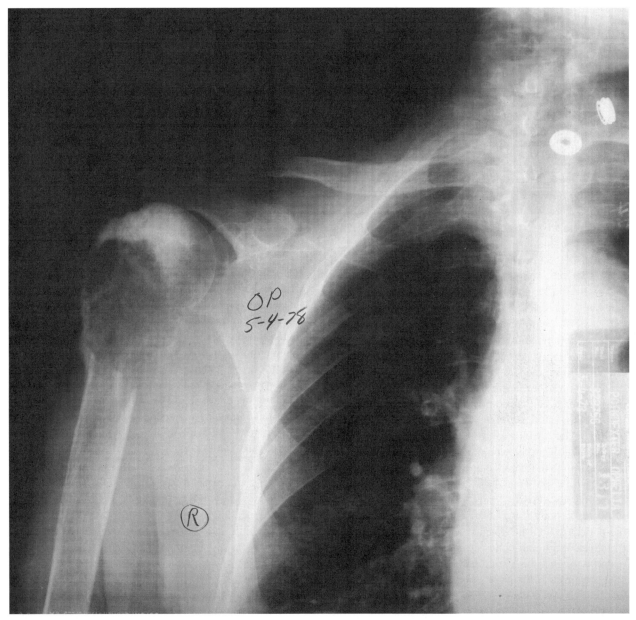

Figure 1–21. Lytic lesion of the humerus, pathologic fracture of the humerus. *(Courtesy of J. Wanggaard, NP.)*

indicated because there can be associated vascular damage even if the bullet has not actually penetrated the vessel wall.[6, 7]

Diagnosis of Occult Fractures and Dislocations

There are many areas where a fracture may occur and not be radiographically evident for 2 weeks postinjury. If there is significant trauma and the extremity is painful and one clinically suspects a fracture, it may only become radiographically visible on a later X ray. There are some regions where occult fractures occur quite commonly and are frequently missed to such an extent that it is commonplace to cast the patient for the mere suspicion of such a fracture even though it is not radiographi-

cally visible (Fig. 1–23). The scaphoid is notorious for displaying occult fractures that are not radiographically visible for 1 or 2 weeks after injury.

If acute trauma is not a feature of a painful extremity, X rays may show a stress fracture.[9] Occult fractures may occur at the midtarsal area or the talus. A fracture should be suspected if there is a history of forced abduction of the forefoot associated with pain and tenderness of the midtarsal joints.[5] Whenever a fracture is suspected but radiographically invisible, particularly in the carpal and tarsal regions, the patient should be splinted and reassessed at a later time. Epiphyseal injuries in which spontaneous reduction has occurred are accompanied by periosteal new bone formation a few weeks after the injury.

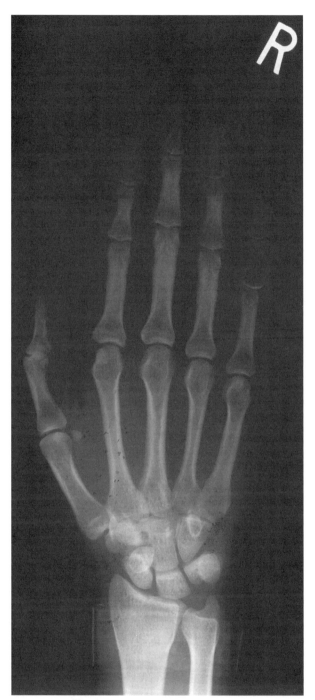

Figure 1–22. Enchondroma, fifth digit. *(Courtesy of Dr. Fitz-patrick.)*

LIGAMENTOUS INJURY AND REPAIR

Ligamentous injuries are divided into first-, second-, and third-degree disruptions. A *first-degree* disruption is a tear of only a few fibers and is characterized by minimal swelling, no functional disability, and normal joint motion. A *second-degree* injury varies in its amount of fiber disruption as well as symptoms and signs. Second-degree sprains may involve anywhere from a third of the

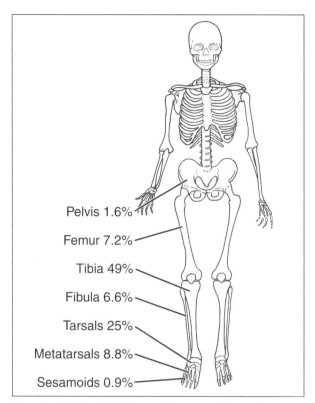

Figure 1–23. The distribution and frequency of stress fractures.

fibers being disrupted to only a few fibers remaining intact. Second-degree sprains present with swelling, tenderness, and functional disability; however, there is generally normal joint motion with no abnormal motion noted. In *third-degree* sprains, there is complete disruption of the ligament characterized by abnormal motion, significant swelling occurring shortly after injury, and functional disability.

A method of testing for the differentiation of second-and third-degree sprains is described.[4] Stress tests perpendicular to the normal plane of joint motion distinguish second- from third-degree injuries by significant opening in third-degree injuries. In patients undergoing stress tests of a ligament with no pain noted, gross ligament instability can often be demonstrated and operative treatment may be indicated. Severe pain is caused by stretching the partially damaged ligament, which remains intact, whereas the remaining fibers are stressed and painful. Subsequent healing occurs provided the joint is immobilized and protected from damaging mechanical stresses for approximately 6 weeks.

It is believed that direct apposition of the two severed ends of a ligament will result in a better outcome with minimal scar tissue than if the ligament ends have not been sutured. Apposition of the ligament ends hastens collagenization and restores normal ligament tissue. Ligaments divided and not immobilized heal with a gap. Testing under tension of the sutured ligaments compared with those not sutured showed the sutured ligaments to be stronger. The nonsutured ligaments failed at the scar. For these reasons, the authors would advocate repair of most third-degree (complete) disruptions of major supporting ligaments around weight-bearing joints within the first week after injury.

REPAIR OF TENDONS

Tendons heal more by paratendinous healing than from the tendon itself. Early mobilization of a ruptured tendon does not reduce the adhesions but instead may result in hypertrophy during the healing process. For many years it was believed that a tendon was an inert and nearly avascular structure. It has been demonstrated, however, that primary tendon healing of the two divided ends of the tendon brought into apposition by sutures occurs both from within and without the tendon. A suture can constrict the microcirculation of the tendon. Irrespective of what suture technique is used, tension on the tendon in the area of the repair can constrict the microcirculation to that tendon and result in an impairment in healing. The commonly used Bunnell crisscross suture technique is particularly invasive as shown by Bergljung.[8]

NERVE INJURY AND REPAIR

There are three types of nerve injuries. A simple contusion of a nerve is called a *neuropraxia* and is treated by simple observation; a return to normal function is noted over the ensuing several weeks or months. An *axonotmesis* is a more significant disruption that is followed by degeneration. The healing of these injuries takes a prolonged time. Complete division of a nerve is called a *neurotmesis*, which typically requires surgical repair.

USE OF THERAPEUTIC HEAT AND COLD

There are identifiable and measurable physiologic effects produced by heat and cold that are therapeutically desirable. There are many forms of heat therapy and the emergency physician should be aware of the indication for some of the commonly used forms. The differences and similarities of heat and cold application are that heat increases the blood flow and cold decreases it. Heat produces an inflammatory response that may be beneficial at some stages of a disease process, whereas cold applications decrease inflammation.[10] Heat increases the production of edema and cold decreases edema formation. It is well known that heat increases the amount of hemorrhage especially after trauma, whereas cold application decreases it. Of interest is that both heat and cold

have been demonstrated to reduce muscle spasm and decrease pain.[10]

With the combined application of heat and passive range of motion, significant changes are seen in the range of motion of patients with hip and shoulder problems. A residual elongation of the therapeutic benefit can be obtained only if heat is used in conjunction with stretch. If heat is used alone, there is no significant difference between the treated region and the control. For penetration to occur with either heat or cold, the application must be left in place for 20 minutes.[10] In degenerative joint disease, heat is used to relieve pain from secondary spasm. If the joint is covered by a significant amount of soft tissue, ultrasound is the only effective modality. However, diathermy and ultrasound may aggravate the symptoms experienced by patients with panarthritis of the shoulder, especially in the acute phase when tightness of capsular tissue, tenderness, and acute shoulder pain occur. In the acute phase after injury, pain relief is best obtained with ice packs or ice massage.[10] In the subacute stage, mild superficial heat is acceptable as an alternative when applied with either a heat lamp or hot packs. In the subacute stage, microwave or ultrasound are the methods of choice. Similarly, in patients with bursitis, the acute inflammation and pressure within the bursa produces pain contraindicating the use of heat. Cold application is recommended with superficial heat the preferred treatment when the inflammatory stage is resolved.

Joint trauma should be treated initially with ice packs to reduce the edema and bleeding. Later, heat is best employed by the use of a whirlpool. In chronically painful sprains, ultrasound provides the best form of therapy. In degenerative disease of the cervical or lumbar region of the spine, heat in the form of ultrasound provides optimal therapy. In patients with slipped disks with secondary muscle spasm, treatment with superficial heat or short-wave diathermy is optimal.

REFERENCES

1. Bingold KC: On splitting plasters. *J Bone Joint Surg* [Br] **61:**3, 1979.
2. Evans RB: An update on wound management. *Hand Clin* **3:**409–432, 1991.
3. Fanciullo JJ, Bell CL: Stress fractures of the sacrum and lower extremity. *Curr Opin Rheumatol* **8:**158–162, 1996.
4. Frost HM: Does the ligament injury require surgery? *Clin Orthop* **49:**72, 1966.
5. Gertzbein SD, Barrington TW: Diagnosis of occult fractures and dislocations. *Clin Orthop* **108:**105, 1975.
6. Gustilo RB, Merkow RL, Templeman D: Current concepts review: The management of open fractures. *J Bone Joint Surg* **2:**299–303, 1990.

7. Heckman JD: fractures: Emergency care and complications. *Clin Symp* **3:**2–32, 1991.

8. Ketchum LD: Primary tendon healing: A review. *J Hand Surg* **2**(6):428, 1977.

9. Krauss MD, Van Meter CD: Longitudinal tibial stress fractures. A case report. *Orthop Rev* **23**(2):163–166, 1994.

10. Lehman JF, et al.: Therapeutic heat and cold. *Clin Orthop* **99:**207, 1974.

11. Matsen KA, Krugmire RB: The effect of externally applied pressure on post-fracture swelling. *J Bone Joint Surg* **56:**8, 1975.

12. Meyer Scott A, et al.: Stress fractures of the foot and leg. *Clin Sports Med* **12**(2):395–413, 1993.

13. Monteleone GP: Stress fractures in the athlete. *Orthop Clin North Am* **26:**3, 1995.

14. Reeder MT, et al.: Stress fractures: Current concepts of diagnosis and treatment. *Sports Med* **22**(3):198–212, 1996.

15. Stanifer E, Wertheimer S: Review of the management of open fractures. *J Foot Surg* **4:**350–354, 1992.

2
CHAPTER

MUSCLE DISORDERS

Muscles are commonly injured by direct and indirect trauma. A forceful blow can cause a localized contusion or disruption of the overlying fascia resulting in herniation. Indirect mechanisms, such as overstretching, will often result in tearing of the muscle fibers with ensuing hemorrhage and a partial loss of function. *Strain* is the term used for muscle injuries whereas *sprain* is used to indicate injury to a ligament.

FIRST-DEGREE STRAIN

A first-degree strain is usually the result of excessive forcible overstretching of the muscle. The patient complains of mild localized pain aggravated by movement or muscle tension. Mild spasm, swelling accompanied by ecchymosis, localized tenderness, and a temporary minor loss of function and strength usually result.

SECOND-DEGREE STRAIN

A second-degree strain involves a disruption of more fibers and results in more significant symptoms and signs than the first-degree injury. It is the result of more forceful contraction or stretch. The differentiation of a first- or second-degree strain is on clinical grounds. There is a low grade, localized inflammatory response with a partial disruption of the musculotendinous junction in the second-degree strain. The complications include recurrence of strain, tendonitis, and periostitis. (The latter two are uncommon.)

THIRD-DEGREE STRAIN

In third-degree strain there is complete disruption of the muscle fibers, and the overlying fascia may be ruptured. The patient experiences severe pain and muscle spasm accompanied by swelling and ecchymosis. There is usually a large hematoma, localized tenderness, and loss of muscle function. One may see an accompanying avulsion fracture on radiographs indicating a disruption at the musculoskeletal junction. Both second- and third-degree injuries are common in the gastrocnemius, biceps, adductors of the thigh, hamstrings, and quadriceps muscle. Acute disruptions involving any of these muscles may present with a bulging or bunching up of the muscle, particularly if the injury involves the musculotendinous junction.

Treatment

The treatment of these injuries depends on the degree of disruption and functional loss. First-degree injuries are accompanied by minor symptoms, and the patient is advised to place ice packs over the injured muscle and to rest for a few days. Mobilization may safely be started as tolerated. In patients with second-degree strains, the injured muscle must be immobilized, the limb elevated, and ice packs applied for the first 24 to 48 hours. After this, the muscle should be "*placed at rest*" by using crutches for ambulation (lower extremity) or a sling (upper extremity) until the swelling and tenderness subside. Passive stretching should be discouraged when there is significant hemorrhage and swelling as this may result in increased fibrosis resulting in a calcium deposition and a delay in healing. Ambulation (for lower extremity strains) or use of the injured muscle (in the upper extremity) should not be initiated until the pain has resolved. Progressive active exercises can be started to the *limit of pain*. This stage of treatment should be accompanied by heat application. One of the more common complications with second-degree strains is recurrence due to early return to normal activity, particularly in the athlete. Calcium deposition in the muscle leading to prolonged disability, another common complication, is also a result of prematurely returning to activity.

Third-degree strains should be immobilized in a splint, ice packs applied, and the limb elevated. The patient should be referred for consultation as surgical repair may be indicated depending on age, the location of the tear, and which muscle is involved.

MUSCLE HERNIATIONS

Muscle herniations through a rent in the overlying fascia can occur. A soft "tumor" may be palpated through the rent, which is not adherent to the overlying skin. The patient may complain of a swelling or bulge of the muscle when contracted and weakness may be noted. An audible snap associated with severe pain during a strong contraction may be noted. The mass is reduced by compression when the muscle is at rest. The muscles most commonly involved with this condition are the biceps, rectus femoris, and gastrocnemius. The treatment is contingent on the symptoms. If there are significant symptoms, the patient should be referred for repair of the defect.

SHIN SPLINTS

Shin splints are seen quite commonly in athletes presenting to the emergency department. The patient complains of pain and tenderness over the anterior tibial muscles, usually occurring at the beginning of athletic training. The muscles may be swollen in the anterior compartment, but there is no functional impairment noted. Active and passive motion aggravates the pain. The treatment includes rest and ice application (early when swelling is a problem) and anti-inflammatory medications. The patient should be returned gradually to activity.

TRAUMATIC MYOSITIS OSSIFICANS

Myositis ossificans is a localized intramuscular ossification after a focal injury to the involved muscle. This formation of bone in the muscle can follow a simple blow or a series of repeated minor traumas to the muscle. A hematoma is a necessary prerequisite for the process to occur. During resorption and organization, the hematoma is invaded by granulation tissue. Collagen proliferates, and osteoblasts, from nearby injured periosteum or from metaplastic connective tissue (referred to as primitive osteogenic tissue), begin to form osteoid trabeculae. It appears that for bone induction to occur in soft tissue three conditions must be present: (1) an inducing agent, (2) osteogenic precursor cells, and (3) an environment that is permissive to osteogenesis.[1]

Clinical Presentation

The condition most commonly occurs in patients between the ages of 15 and 30 years. The site having the highest predilection for this is the elbow at the lower portion of the belly of the brachialis anticus muscle anterior to the elbow joint, usually after a posterior dislocation of the elbow. The elbow is often quite swollen and tender. When a mass of bone forms, active and passive motion are restricted. Later pain and swelling are reduced and a hard, tumorlike mass is palpable over the anterior aspect of the elbow. Active extension of the joint is limited by "inelasticity" of the muscle. Flexion is also prevented by obstruction from the mass. In some cases, there may be a complete ossifying bridge formed at the joint with extraarticular ankylosis. Another common site of myositis ossificans is the quadriceps muscle, which is discussed further in the section on soft tissue disorders of the thigh.

The process usually ceases spontaneously in 3 to 6 months. Radiographs show the calcified mass beginning by the third to fourth week postinjury (Fig. 2–1). The mass of bone may be connected to the shaft of a long bone by a pedicle or may be completely separated. Spontaneous repair may occur with complete disappearance of the osseous mass.

Treatment

The osseous growth should not be disturbed in its early stage. Prolonged rest is indicated with the extremity

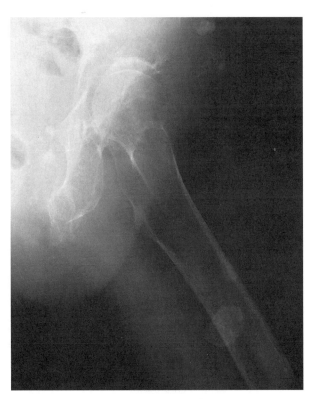

Figure 2–1. Myositis ossificans.

immobilized by a splint or lightweight cast. When the elbow is involved, the proper position of immobilization is with the forearm in a neutral position and the elbow flexed to 90 degrees. No surgery is indicated for 6 to 12 months because spontaneous resorption can occur with complete disappearance of the mass. Early surgical intervention may result in recurrence of the calcification.

MYOSITIS

Two types of myositis have been identified, *polymyositis* and *dermatomyositis*.[2,3] *Myositis* is an inflammation of a muscle that may be due to irritative agents such as bacteria, parasites, or viruses. Also, recent studies have shown that 20 percent of myositis cases are of autoimmune pathogenesis. These individuals test positive for Anti-Jo-1 immunoglobulins, which will reach with a cytoplasmic enzyme (histidyl transfer RNA synthase).[2,3] Patients may present with complaints of difficulty getting off of a chair or toilet seat, getting in or out of a car, climbing stairs, and combing their hair.[2] Another diagnostic feature is an increase in creatinine phosphate levels, which can be noticed in more than 95 percent of the cases.[3] Furthermore, a purplish rash around the eyes or a scaly red, often raised rash on the knuckles are predisposing factors for dermatomyositis.[2] As the inflammation subsides, it is followed by regeneration of the muscle fibers. In patients with systemic infections, myositis with parenchymatous degeneration may develop. Acute sup-

purative myositis with abscess formation in the muscle is an unusual condition. When seen, it is usually secondary to spread of infection from an adjacent focus such as an osteomyelitis or a puncture wound. The most common agents causing this infection are *Staphylococcus* or *Streptococcus* organisms. When swelling occurs early, the muscle fibers are destroyed by compression and toxic degeneration. In severe cases, the muscles may undergo liquefaction necrosis. Clinically, these patients present with fever, chills, localized pain, and edema. The overlying skin may be reddened and the muscle swollen, warm, indurated, and tender to palpation. Loss of muscle power occurs early. The treatment includes an incision and drainage of the abscess and systemic antibiotics. Hot moist compresses with elevation of the limb and splinting of the involved extremity are useful adjuncts. It is imperative that incision and drainage with debridement in the operating room be performed early as the destruction of the fibers ensues very rapidly once the process begins.

REFERENCES

1. Chalmers J, Powers D: Observations on the induction of bone in soft tissues. *J Bone Joint Surg* [Br] **57**:1, 1975.
2. Plotz PH: New understanding of myositis. *Hosp Pract* 33–43, 1992.
3. Targoff IN: Diagnosis and treatment of polymyositis and dermatomyositis. *Compr Ther* **4**:10–24, 1990.

3
CHAPTER

RHEUMATOLOGY

GENERAL PRINCIPLES IN TREATING THE PATIENT WITH ARTHRITIS

In approaching a patient with arthritis, the emergency physician should remember that the pain may be either inflammatory in nature or noninflammatory, with only arthralgia. The physician must first determine when the pain started. Next, the patient should be asked what makes the pain worse or better, and whether there are any constitutional symptoms or a temporal pattern to the pain. Fever and weight loss are important signs because they signify systemic illness. Stiffness is usually an indication of synovitis or gelling.

When a patient indicates that he or she has arthritis and weakness, *four types* of weakness must be considered:

1. Generalized, painless weakness with easy fatigability. This is caused by disuse atrophy; for example, deconditioning after a systemic illness such as mysthenia gravis.
2. Painless loss of power in a specific muscle group. This occurs with complete denervation, such as in polio or localized atrophy.
3. Paresthesias, such as compressive neuropathy or radiculopathy.
4. Weakness associated with pain and cramping, which suggests inflammatory muscle disease or a metabolic disorder.

Rubor and tenderness localized to a joint indicate either crystal-induced or septic arthritis. In cellulitis, one sees diffuse warm, red skin with lymphangitis and adenop-athy.

In *polyarthritis*, *four or more joints* are involved. There are three patterns of polyarthritis:

1. In the additive type of polyarthritis, one sees examples such as rheumatoid arthritis, systemic lupus erythematosus (SLE), and psoriatic arthritis, which all have additive joint involvement that progresses to include additional joints over time.

2. With gonococcal arthritis or acute rheumatic fever and bacterial endocarditis, symptomatic joints subside and then different joints become involved. This is called a *migratory* polyarthritis.
3. In gout, pseudogout, and familial Mediterranean fever, one sees a picture of arthritis with signs and symptoms that come, last a few days, and then go. This is called an *intermittent polyarthritis*.

Whenever one considers the diagnosis of septic arthritis or crystal-induced arthritis, a joint tap is absolutely mandatory. A full discussion of these conditions is presented later in this chapter. Some of the key points in approaching the laboratory test normally performed in patients with arthritis are as follows:

- 20% of patients with acute gout have a normal uric acid level.
- A normal white blood cell count does not exclude infection and, in fact, is quite common.
- In early rheumatoid arthritis, the rheumatoid factor is negative. In addition, other conditions may have positive rheumatoid factors; these are discussed later.
- The erythrocyte sedimentation rate (ESR) responds to inflammatory activity and is quite sensitive. Remember that it is not very sensitive in female patients with rheumatoid arthritis as *half* of these patients have a normal ESR early on.

Skin and Nail Changes Seen with Arthritis

Patients presenting with *Still's disease* have discreet pink-or salmon-colored maculas or slightly elevated papules that are several millimeters in size on the trunk and extremities. Patients with psoriatic arthritis have erythematous scaling plaques over the extensor surfaces and distal interphalangeal joint synovitis.

Erythema multiforme can be associated with fever and polyarthralgias. A high fever and polyarthritis are common with erythema multiforme that is associated with Stevens-Johnson syndrome. The physician who sees a patient with a rash, fever, and intermittent arthritis should think of familial Mediterranean fever, which presents as an erysipelis-like rash in the lower extremity in conjunction with acute monoarthritis and fever.

Papulosquamous lesions are skin lesions that occur in association with arthritic disease in patients with Reiter's syndrome, psoriatic arthritis, and SLE.

Annular lesions are seen in association with rheumatic fever, SLE, and Lyme disease. In rheumatic fever, a migratory polyarthritis is seen in association with an *erhythema marginatum*. This occurs on the trunk and on the proximal extremities. The primary lesion of *erhythema chronicum migrans* is nearly pathopneumonic for acute Lyme disease and occurs at the site of the tick bite, most often in the axilla, groin, thigh, or buttocks. This lesion reaches an average size of 15 cm.

Polyarthritis along with dermatitis involving the face should prompt the physician to consider SLE. *Facial erythematous plaques* and papules that may be confused with discoid-type lesions may be seen. Bacterial infections such as meningococcemia seen in association with arthritis can produce a *petechial* or even a purpuric rash.

Diseases that should be considered when *urticaria* and *arthritis* are present include hepatitis B infection, serum sickness, and primary urticarial vasculitis. Mononucleosis can also present with *urticaria* and *arthritis*. Arthralgias may be seen in patients with chronic urticaria resulting from processes other than leukocytoclastic vasculitis; however, an arthritis generally suggest *vasculitis*.

Erythema nodosum lesions are red- or violet-colored subcutaneous nodules, 1 to 5 cm in diameter, which are usually associated with vasculitis. They typically deve-lop in the pretibial locations and resolve spontaneously after several weeks. When these lesions are seen in association with arthritis, one must consider primary immune processes such as sarcoidosis, inflammatory bowel disease, Behçet's disease, drug-induced causes, pregnancy, and infections such as systemic sepsis.

Oral ulcers are common findings in patients with Crohn's disease, Behçet's syndrome, Reiter's syndrome, and SLE. Ulcers are also seen in the extremities of patients who have vascular spasms secondary to Raynaud's phenomena or other causes. Vascular, infectious, and tumor-associated causes must be considered in patients with cutaneous ulcers and symptoms of arthritis. Lower extremity ulcers in the debilitated rheumatoid patient are common and are a problem in diagnosis. Venous insufficiency ulcers are also common in rheumatoid patients because of reduced skin integrity.

Approach to Acute Monoarthritis

Patients who present to the emergency department with joint pain and swelling require immediate evaluation.

TABLE 3–1. DIFFERENTIAL DIAGNOSIS OF ACUTE MONOARTHRITIS

Finding	Differential Diagnosis
Infections	Bacteria
	Virus (hepatitis B, HIV, rubella, others)
	Lyme disease
	Mycobacteria, fungi
Crystal-induced	Gout
	Pseudogout
Trauma	Fracture involving joint
	Internal derangement (meniscus tear)
	Hemarthrotis
Osteoarthritis or tumor	Metastasis
	Osteoid osteoma
	Villonodular synovitis
Reactive synovitis	Meniscus tear
	Inflammatory bowel disease

The importance of synovial fluid analysis in the diagnosis and management of acute arthritis involving a single joint cannot be overemphasized. If the patient has an undiagnosed or untreated septic arthritis, rapid destruction of articular tissue is inevitable if there is a delay in making the diagnosis. Some infections, if untreated, can destroy cartilage in as little as 2 days.[8] Table 3–1 lists the differential diagnosis for patients who present with acute monoarthritis.

Table 3–2 shows a breakdown of the classification of monoarthritis based on joint fluid analysis. Conditions that present with monoarthritis are listed in the table and highlighted briefly in the pages that follow. They are discussed in more detail later in the chapter.

Infections in the large joints such as the knees and hips occur in nongonococcal bacterial infections. Approximately 80 to 90% of nongonococcal bacterial infections are monoarticular. However, one must remember that 10 to 19% of septic arthritis cases are polyarticular, with the onset in several large joints. When septic arthritis presents in this fashion, it presents as an additive arthritis. Polyarticular involvement is more commonly seen with rheumatoid arthritis. Hematogenous spread is by far the most common route for this infection, making the diagnosis of the primary site an important factor to consider. The most common agents by far are gram-positive aerobes, usually *Staphylococcus aureus*, which accounts for approximately 60% of these infections. Most of these bacteria are resistant to penicillin. *Non−group A, β-hemolytic streptococci* account for approximately 15% of infections, with *Streptococcus pneumoniae* accounting for another 3%. Gram-negative bacteria are found in the remainder of cases. In patients with gram-negative septic arthritis, one must remember to consider immunocompromised hosts, gastrointestinal cancers (which may present with anaerobic infections), and open wounds.

TABLE 3-2. MONOARTHRITIS CLASSIFIED BY JOINT FLUID CHARACTERISTICS

	Group I (Noninflammatory)	Group II (Inflammatory)	Group III (Septic)	Group IV (Hemorrhagic)
Joint Fluid Characteristics				
Viscosity	High	Low	Low	Variable
Appearance	Yellow, transparent	Yellow, transparent	Opaque	Bloody
WBC/mm³	200–2000, mostly lymphocytes	2000–100,000	> 50,000, mostly PMNs	Variable
Differential Diagnosis				
	Traumatic arthritis	Crystal-induced arthritis Gout Pseudogout	Bacterial infection	Trauma
	Osteoarthritis	Rheumatoid arthritis, spondyloarthropathies systemic lupus erythematosus, collagen vascular reactive arthritis Reiter's syndrome, inflammatory bowel disease	Crystalline arthritis	Bleeding, hemophilia, von Willebrand's disease, thrombocytopenia
	Osteochondritis dissecans	Tuberculosis, fungal arthritis		Joint neoplasm
	Early or resolving inflammatory arthritis	Viral arthritis		

PMNs, polymorphonuclear neutrophils; WBC, white blood cell count.

Gonococcal arthritis is more commonly seen than septic arthritis from any other cause, with the frequency being far more common in women than in men. Tuberculous arthritis is uncommon; however, in patients with pulmonary tuberculosis this must be considered. Periarticular bone lesions may accompany bone involvement. *Fungal arthritis* is usually insidious in onset and may be seen in an immunocompromised host. *Viral arthritis* can be monoarticular and is associated with herpes simplex virus, or other viruses. In *Lyme disease*, one usually sees an intermittent arthralgia; however, chronic monoarthritis or even oligoarthritis with erosions may be seen. In patients presenting with this characteristic oligoarthritis, this occurs months after the initial infection in patients who are untreated. Large joints such as the knee are usually infected, and these joints are initially more swollen than painful.

Human immunodeficiency virus (HIV) may be seen in patients presenting with monoarthritis. A syndrome consisting of oligoarticular or monoarticular arthritis involving the lower extremity joints may herald the onset of HIV infection. These patients may have a nonreactive synovial fluid or one that is only minimally reactive. Thus, in patients with an unexplained arthritis who are at high risk for HIV infection, one should consider this diagnosis.

Crystal-induced arthritis is a common cause of monoarthritis. One sees this in gout and pseudogout. Rheumatic arthritis is also commonly seen either with a fracture or delayed from a meniscal tear or ligamentous tear. Osteoarthritis may present in a single joint. Spontaneous osteonecrosis is commonly seen in elderly patients, involving the knee, and can lead to sudden pain with or without any fusion. Penetrating injuries from thorns, wood fragments, or other foreign material can cause a reactive acute synovitis.

Hemarthrosis most commonly is seen after trauma; however, it may be caused by acquired or congenital clotting abnormalities such as hemophilia.

Acute arthritis in patients with *prosthetic* joints is a significant concern as it may indicate infection. The most common source of an infection in a prosthetic joint is hematogenous spread from infective skin lesions. Patients with hip prostheses who present with a monoarthritis may have loosening, which is the most common cause of long-term failure of arthroplasties.

Many *systemic diseases* can present with a monoarthritis initially. This is clearly an uncommon presentation of systemic diseases; however, it should be considered when the other conditions listed earlier and discussed later in the chapter have been ruled out. Systemic diseases that can present with a monoarthritis include SLE, rheumatoid arthritis, arthritis of inflammatory bowel, Behçet's disease, and Reiter's syndrome.

Clinical Presentation

The clinical presentation is extremely useful in deciding how to approach a patient with monoarthritis. A history of previous episodes suggests crystal-induced or other noninfectious causes. If a patient states that he or she has a fever, the physician should think first of septic arthritis. Different types of rashes are suggestive of specific types of arthritis, as previously discussed. Diarrhea, urethritis, or uveitis suggests a reactive type of arthritis. Patients who have a history of trauma should be thought of as possibly having a fracture, which may not be seen on the initial x-ray, particularly in the lower extremity where osteochondral fractures and tibioplateau fractures should be considered.

On examination, one must *distinguish* between arthritis, bursitis, tendinitis, and cellulitis. This is usually not difficult. If one *distracts* the joint, patients with synovitis (arthritis) will have pain. However, those with tendinitis generally will not. Use of the tendon associated with tendinitis causes pain against resistance which will exacerbate the symptoms of tendinitis but not those of arthritis. In patients with cellulitis, the involvement is usually not isolated to the joint alone. If it is, however, then palpating the area where one normally performs an arthrocentesis will reveal this to be the most tender spot in the patient with arthritis, but not in the patient with cellulitis. Even with the most detailed examination, however, cellulitis in the area of the wrist, knee, and sometimes the ankle can mimic arthritis. Painful limitation of motion usually indicates joint involvement. The physician should always observe for mouth ulcers in patients with monoarthritis who are a typical in their presentation. This was discussed earlier, and one must remember that Behçet's syndrome and Reiter's syndrome, as well as SLE, can cause mouth ulcers. As previously discussed, erythema nodosum can be a clue to the diagnosis of SLE.

Synovial Fluid Analysis

Table 3–2 presents some of the common findings in synovial fluid analysis and monoarthritis. Arthrocentesis should be performed on every patient with monoarthritis in whom infection is a possibility. The differential leukocyte count, culture, Gram staining, and examination of the wet preparation for crystals are important laboratory studies to request. If only a few drops of synovial fluid are obtained, then one should send these for a culture, Gram stain, and wet preparation. Differential leukocyte counts can assist in making a diagnosis of infection, as a finding of 90% polymorphonuclear neutrophils (PMNs) should make one think of either infection or crystal-induced disease in early presentations, even if the total leukocyte count is low.

One must remember that the presence of crystals does not exclude infection in patients who have gout, as they are more susceptible to septic arthritis, particularly when the gout is chronic. It is not uncommon for crystal-induced arthritis to produce a high fever and an extremely high leukocyte count suggestive of septic arthritis. Although some authorities suggest that when crystals are found antibiotic therapy can be withheld in patients with recurrent gout involving the same joint, the authors suggest treating with antibiotics until the cultures are negative, in addition to using anti-inflammatory agents.

Approach to Polyarthritis

Polyarthritis generally refers to the involvement of three or more joints. Polyarthritis associated with fever must trigger the clinician to think of infection first and foremost. In patients with bacterial infection and a polyarthritis, the pattern of fever is not a sustained one but rather a quotidian (spiking), intermittent pattern. Usually, there is a daily elevation in the late afternoon or in the evening with a return to normal temperature during the night. The spiking temperature is preceded by shaking chills, which are then followed by profuse sweating. A similar pattern is sometimes seen in Still's disease. In patients with polyarthritis, synovial fluid examination is extraordinarily useful, especially when one is considering bacterial infection as a possibility. Leukocyte counts over $50,000/mm^3$ suggest bacterial infection but can be seen in rheumatoid arthritis, crystal-induced arthritis, and reactive arthritis. When the leukocyte count is relatively low in patients with polyarthritis and the examination is not suggestive of any particular disorder, one must consider three possibilities: viral arthritis, reactive arthritis, or systemic rheumatic illnesses. In addition to ordering tests of antinuclear factor and antistreptococcal antibodies, one should also order antibody tests for *Borrelia burgdorferi*, particularly in patients who live in an area that is suggestive of Lyme disease. Unfortunately, an elevated ESR is of minimal value as this rate is elevated in almost every condition that causes polyarthritis. However, a normal ESR is suggestive of viral infection. One must remember that in infectious arthritis, multiple joint involvement can occur in 10 to 19% of adults. Usually, in infectious arthritis presenting as a polyarticular involvement, there is simultaneous onset in several large joints or additive onset over 1 or 2 days.

Neisserial arthritis is discussed in detail later; however, it is worth noting that it most often is a polyarticular infection presenting as a migratory arthritis with chills, fever, and tenosynovitis involving the wrist or ankle extensor tendon sheaths. The characteristic skin lesion often helps in making the diagnosis. Female patients with neisserial arthritis usually do not report lower abdominal pain or vaginal discharge. Purulent synovial effusions in neisserial arthritis are uncommon, and usually the organism is recovered from blood cultures, particularly in patients who present with fever, chills, and skin lesions. One of the key findings in patients with neisserial arthritis is dramatic improvement in both the fever and arthralgia within 24 hours after treatment is started. Table 3–3 lists the common clinical findings in patients with polyarthritis and fever, and the possible causes to consider.

In *viral arthritis*, one usually sees a migratory arthritis; however, some patients present with symmetric polyarthritis. Patients who present with hepatitis B virus infection may actually have symptoms of arthritis that *precede* the symptoms of hepatitis and resolve once jaundice appears. In these cases, there is moderate fever and sometimes an urticarial or a maculopapular rash. The diagnosis hepatitis can be made because the liver enzyme levels are elevated even though there is no jaundice or liver tenderness. In younger women, rubella and parvovirus B19 can present with a migratory arthritis. In these cases, the patients usually have additive symmetric arthritis, particularly involving the hands. Increasingly, HIV infection as a cause of arthralgia and arthritis is seen. This is usually a symmetric polyarthritis and is discussed in detail later in the chapter.

In patients with *Lyme disease*, one sees a migratory arthralgia with little or no joint swelling accompanied by fever. The large joints are primarily affected, and one of the common features is a large knee effusion with only mild pain, the effusion being disproportionate to the amount of pain. IgM antibodies to *B borgdorferi* may be detected as early as 4 to 6 weeks after the initial infection. One of the characteristic lesions, as discussed earlier under skin manifestation, is erythema migrans.

Bacterial endocarditis can also present with a polyarthritis. In one large series, 44% of patients with bacterial endocarditis had a polyarthritis. Some of the joints have an asymptomatic[8] effusion whereas others are warm, red, and painful.

TABLE 3–3. DIAGNOSTIC FEATURES IN PATIENTS PRESENTING WITH POLYARTHRITIS

Clinical Presentation	Associated Condition	Clinical Presentation	Associated Condition
Skin Lesions		Fever preceding arthritis	Viral arthritis
Papules trunk and extremities	Still's disease		Reactive arthritis
			Lyme disease
Papulosquamous plaques	Psoriatic arthritis		Still's disease
	Reiter's syndrome		Bacterial endocarditis
	SLE	Migratory arthritis	Rheumatic fever
Petechiae	Meningococcemia		Viral arthritis
Erythema multiforme	Stevens-Johnson syndrome		Gonococcemia
Erysipelas-like rash of lower extremity	Familial Mediterranean fever		Meningococcemia
			SLE
Erythema marginatum	Rheumatic fever		Leukemia
Erythema chronicum migrans	Acute lyme disease		Whipple's disease
		Effusion > pain	Inflammatory bowel disease
Facial erythematous papules/plaques	SLE		Lyme disease
			Giant cell arteritis
Annular lesions	SLE		Bacterial endocarditis
	Lyme disease		Tuberculous arthritis
	Rheumatic fever	Pain > effusion	Familial Mediterranean fever
Urticaria	Viral arthritis (hepatitis B)		Rheumatic fever
	Serum sickness		Leukemia
	Vasculitis		AIDS
	Mononucleosis	Morning stiffness	Rheumatoid arthritis
Nodular lesions	Tophi of gout		Still's disease
	Rheumatoid nodules		Viral arthritis
	Rheumatic fever		Reactive arthritis
			Polymyalgia rheumatica
Erythema nodosum	Inflammatory bowel disease	Symmetric small joint involvement	Rheumatic arthritis
	Drugs, Behçet's disease		SLE
			Viral arthritis
Ulcers	Vasculitis	Episodic recurrences	Lyme disease
	Rheumatoid arthritis		Crystal-induced arthritis
			Inflammatory bowel disease
Temperature > 40°C	Bacterial arthritis		Whipple's disease
	Still's disease		Familial Mediterranean fever
	SLE		Still's disease
			SLE

AIDS, acquired immunodeficiency syndrome; SLE, systemic lupus erythematosus.
Modified from Pinals.[66]

Reactive arthritis is discussed in detail later under the specific conditions with which it is commonly associated. Polyarthritis occurs in a number of enteric inflammatory conditions and urogenital infections. One may also see an asymmetric, additive-type of polyarthritis, predominantly involving the large joints of the lower extremity, in these conditions. Again, these specific presentations are discussed in more detail later in the chapter.

Rheumatic fever in children presents with an abrupt onset of polyarthritis and fever. These children have a carditis and may have skin lesions, typically erythema marginatum, which is rarely seen in adults.

Rheumatoid arthritis is discussed in detail later. The systemic form of juvenile rheumatoid arthritis is called *Still's disease*; it is characterized by high fever and polyarthritis. A detailed discussion of this disorder is also presented later.

Systemic vasculitis can present with polyarthritis and fever. In addition, patients usually have concurrent skin lesions, neuropathy, or microscopic hematuria. There may be a small effusion in some of the larger joints. Wegner's granulomatosis may present with fever and polyarthritis before the typical pulmonary or airway findings.

SLE commonly presents with a polyarthritis appearing in the form of a symmetric, peripheral joint involvement that may be intermittent or migratory. These patients are usually afebrile and may have a light sensitivity rash. The antinuclear antibody (ANA) test is very sensitive in SLE.

Patients with *gout* may present with fever and polyarticular involvement. Approximately 10% of these patients have temperatures of 39°C or higher. A detailed discussion of this disorder is presented later in the chapter. *Occult cancer* can present with a polyarthritis and fever. Lymphomas can present in this manner, although this is rare. Oligoarthritis may precede adult carcinomas but is seldom accompanied by fever. Laboratory features in polyarthritis are summarized in Table 3–4.

TABLE 3–4. LABORATORY FEATURES IN POLYARTHRITIS

Leukocytosis > 15,000	Bacterial arthritis
	Still's disease
	Bacterial endocarditis
	Systemic vasculitis
	Leukemia
Leukopoenia	SLE
	Viral arthritis
Positive rheumatoid factor	Rheumatoid arthritis
	SLE
	Viral arthritis
	Bacterial endocarditis
	Tuberculous arthritis
	Systemic vasculitis

SLE, systemic lupus erythematosus.

SEPTIC ARTHRITIS

Inflammation of a joint caused by the presence of a microorganism is uncommon but, perhaps, the most serious arthritic condition presenting to the emergency department. The etiology includes *S aureus, S epidermidis, Streptococcus pneumoniae, Escherichia coli, Pseudomonas aeruginosa,* and *Neisseria gonorrhea.*[34] A prerequisite for the development of septic arthritis is that bacteria must reach the synovial membrane. This may occur in any of the following ways:

1. *Hematogenous spread* occurs as a result of implantation of the organism within the verivascular synovium or rich vascular beds at the articular surfaces. Hematogenous spread often occurs in the sacroiliac joints of drug abusers.[15]
2. A route that is particularly common in small children is dissemination of bacteria from an acute osteomyolitic focus in the metaphysis or epiphysis.
3. An infection in the vicinity of the joint can progress to the joint or spread via the lymphogenic route. This is most often seen in nonpenetrating traumatic and postoperative wound infections and skin and soft tissue infections around the joint, particularly the knee.[44]
4. Another possibility is iatrogenic infections caused by joint puncture for a diagnostic or therapeutic purpose.
5. Penetrating trauma that is caused by dirty objects or by animal or human bites often gives rise to a severe infection because of the high inoculate of bacteria and lacerated tissue.

Clinical Presentation
Although septic arthritis usually presents as a monoarthritis, 10 to 19% of patients have polyarthritis at the onset, involving several large joints. When the condition presents in this fashion, it presents as an *additive-type* of arthritis. Adult and elderly patients with rheumatoid arthritis and inflammation more often have an acute septic arthritis. The lower extremities are most often affected, particularly the hip and knee joints. In the neonatal period up to 1 year of age, the symptoms are usually systemic rather than local. Small children develop high fevers and are usually rather ill. The clinical features are more often characteristic of sepsis than local arthritis. This is a key point to remember if one is considering this diagnosis in children. Older children are also febrile and unwell, but the local signs are more prominent. Distention of the joint capsule and increased intra-articular pressure contribute to pain. Adults often have severe pain and are febrile, but malaise is generally moderate. Patients are reluctant to move and put weight on the joint. The joint capsule is distended and warm, and the skin is often erythematous and edematous.

Fever, decreased range of motion, and joint pain provide initial clues to the emergency physician of an infectious arthritis. Joint effusion is present in 90% of these patients. Tenderness is also invariably present, but erythema and warmth may be imperceptable early on. The pain and physical findings are usually obvious and directly related to the infected joint.

Diagnosis

A tentative diagnosis of deep infection, particularly by hematogenous spread, may sometimes be difficult. In acute septic arthritis, the microbes are generally localized to the synovial fluid, particularly in the initial stage. It is advisable to dilute the aspirative material in a blood culture bottle in a proportion of about 1 to 10 to inhibit the bactericidal components of the joint fluid.[44] Bacteria may be identified in a Gram stain of the synovial fluid in 50 to 75% of cases and on culture in more than 90% of cases.[66] The radiographic finding is symmetric soft tissue swelling around the involved joint; marginal erosion or erosions of the bone occur later. The hallmark of septic arthritis is the loss of the white cortical line over a long contiguous segment.[15] Unfortunately, the radiographs have limited diagnostic value in the early stages of this disease. Radionuclide scanning and magnetic resonance imaging (MRI) may identify juxta-articular osteomyelitis and effusions in deep locations such as the hip and sacroiliac joint.[66] Because delay in treatment is the best predictor of an unfavorable outcome, prompt arthrocentesis is essential.

Treatment

Therapy consists of systemic antibiotics, closed or open drainage of the septic joint, and later, rehabilitation. Currently, the mainstay of treatment is closed drainage, at least once daily. If fluid cannot be obtained from the joint or there is a poor response to antibiotic therapy, then open drainage is performed. Antibiotic treatment is initiated as soon as the specimens have been collected and blood cultures are obtained. Gram staining of the joint fluid should be carried out if possible, prior to initiation of treatment.

Prosthetic Joint Infection

If an infection is present soon after surgery, staphylococci and streptococci are the more common causes and the symptoms are more intensive, with high fever, generalized malaise, and a wound that discharges pus. Later, when the wound has healed or a sinus tract has developed, the patient may still have pain with soft tissue swelling. In late infections, local signs can be rather discreet, with slight tenderness and pain. In some cases of hip joint infection, the joint effusion and pressure can be so high that dislocation occurs. In hematogenous infec-

tion, the onset is usually acute, with high septic fever and increasing pain, even at rest. A prosthetic joint infection is always serious with high morbidity and mortality. Patients with rheumatoid *S aureus* infection around the hip or knee prosthesis have a mortality rate of about 10%.

The diagnosis is made by performing arthroscopy, or when synovectomy is indicated, tissue samples can be used for culture.

Treatment

Prosthetic joint infections can be treated with oral clindamycin or ciprofloxacin, depending on the bacteriologic findings. These cases are often treated operatively, with local infiltration of antibiotics containing bone cement or other vehicles to deliver the antibiotic to the site of infection.

OSTEOMYELITIS

Bone infections are currently classified etiologically by the Wald Vogel system as being either hematogenous osteomyelitis or osteomyelitis, secondary to a contiguous focus of infection.[54]

Hematogenous osteolyelitis develops after bacteremia, most often in prepubertal children and in elderly patients. In children, infection is usually located in the metaphyseal area of the long bones (particularly the tibia and femur). Typical clinical features of this form of osteomyelitis are chills, fever, and malaise with local pain and swelling. Infecting organisms differ according to the age of the patient.[76] *S aureus* and streptococci in neonates are common causes, but *S aureus* is also found in older patients. Gram-negative rods are seen in the elderly as a cause. Fungal osteomyelitis is a complication of catheter-related fungemia and the use of illicit drugs contaminated by *Candida* species; prolonged neutropenia may also be a factor. *P aerugenosa* can be isolated from infection in drug addicts, often from cervical vertebrae, and from patients who have had urinary catheters in place for long periods of time (often affecting the lumbar vertebrae). Children and adults with sickle cell disease most commonly have infection caused by *S aureus* or *Salmonella* species.[9] *Haemophilus influenzae* and *E coli* can also occur in neonatal osteomyelitis.[44] In all forms of osteomyelitis, the typical clinical features are chills, fever, malaise, and local pain and swelling.

The diagnosis is made by needle aspiration of the bone, and this should be performed to establish a bacteriologic diagnosis and determine the presence or absence of abscesses.[76] Any material obtained is prepared for Gram stain and culture. An open biopsy may be required to obtain sufficient material.

Treatment

In treating hematogenous osteomyelitis in children, the parenteral administration of antibiotics may be followed by several weeks of oral therapy, provided the organism has been identified, clinical signs abate rapidly, and patient compliance with therapy is good. β-Lactam antibiotics, clindamycin, ciprofloxacin, and rifampin are known to penetrate bone tissue in sufficient amounts to treat infection. In acute hematogenous osteomyelitis, abscesses should be drained, as decompression prevents further obstruction of blood vessels and the resulting bone necrosis.[44]

Osteomyelitis Caused by a Contiguous Focus of Infection

Osteomyelitis occurring after injury is the most prevalent type. This is usually associated with an open fracture or occurs postoperatively following reconstruction of bone.[76] Infections associated with prostheses are also common. Extension of soft tissue infection into the bone following a dental or sinus infections can also be seen. Sternal infections after median sternotomy and foot infections after puncture wounds are other important causes.[9] Patients may initially present with pain, fever, swelling, and erythema, but as the infection continues or recurs, fever subsides and typical features are pain and drainage from a persistent sinus tract or ulcer.[76] The most common pathogen is S aureus; however, other organisms that can cause contiguous infection include enteric gram-negative bacilli or P aeruginosa.[76] To make the diagnosis, surgical exploration of the infectious focus and tissue biopsies are needed to obtain suitable culture material.

Treatment

Surgical therapy of chronic osteomyelitis requires removal of the dead bone, devitalized tissue, and any foreign material, as well as drainage of the abscess and obliteration of any dead space. This is the treatment recommended in most cases.[9] Antibiotic therapy is reserved for chronic refractory osteomyelitis.

Acute Osteomyelitis

Acute osteomyelitis principally affects children and young adults. In children under 1 year of age, acute osteomyelitis presents with arthritis in about 75% of cases and with septicemia in almost all cases. The epiphysis is sometimes involved. Older children will not move or put weight on the infected limb. The metaphysis may be involved, mostly in the lower extremities around the knee joint, and the trochanteric region also can be involved. In the humerus, one can also see metaphyseal involvement. The area is tender to touch or can be swollen and warm. In the proximal humerus and the femur, the joint may be involved owing to the insertion of the joint capsule below the metaphysis. If the infection is diagnosed and treated within 2 to 3 days of onset, the prognosis is good and chronic complications are rare. Both the diagnosis and the treatment of acute osteomyelitis are similar to those of osteomyelitis caused by hematogenous spread.

Chronic Osteomyelitis

Chronic osteomyelitis can occur from an untreated acute osteomyelitis or, more commonly, as a complication of an infected fracture or a postoperative infection. Often, the vessels are lacerated. The massive bacterial invasion into the area promotes a propagation of the infection, often in the whole diaphysis. Destruction of the bone is prominent and sequestra and circumscribed abscesses arise. Lysis is followed by new bone formation. Sinus tracts originating from the interosseous cavities are common, with subsequent drainage of pus and infected material and small bone pieces to the skin surface. Defective healing and malformation are common features. The treatment is the same as that previously discussed for contiguous focus of infection.

CRYSTAL-INDUCED ARTHROPATHIES*

Gout and pseudogout are inflammatory syndromes caused by crystal deposition in the joints and soft tissues. Features of these two syndromes are compared in Table 3–5.

Gout

Gout is caused by the precipitation of uric acid crystals in the joints and soft tissues. Uric acid precipitates from solution at about 7 mg/dL, so a slight rise in the serum concentration of urate from the normal range of 4 to 5 mg/dL may lead to gouty arthritis. Levels of uric acid are normally higher in men than in premenopausal women, and rise with age in both sexes. Hence, the typical patient afflicted with gout is a middle-aged man. Gout is unusual in men younger than 30 years of age and in premenopausal women.

Although up to 5% of adults have some degree of hyperuricemia, only one fifth of these (1% overall) will ever develop gout. Hyperuircemia may be caused by either overproduction of uric acid, or decreased excretion in the urine. Although a discussion of disorders of urate metabolism is beyond the scope of this text, the emergency physician should be familiar with a few causes of decreased urate excretion as these may precipitate an attack of gouty arthritis: loop diuretics (furosemide, thiazides), salicylates, the antimicrobials pyrazinamide and ethambutol, and ethanol. Because uric acid solubility is temperature-dependent, environmental cold or poor circulation can lead to precipitation as well.

*This section was contributed by Robert Feldman, MD.

TABLE 3–5. CLINICAL FEATURES OF GOUT AND PSEUDOGOUT

	Gout	Pseudogout
Joints affected	First MTP, foot, ankle, knee	Knee
Initial attack	90% monoarticular	90% monoarticular
Distribution	Asymmetric, additional joints added with subsequent attacks	Usually monoarticular, more than three joints unusual
Onset	Hyperacute, within a few hours	Acute, within 6–24 h
Tophi	Present in chronic gout	May develop tophi-like deposits
Provocants	Disorders of urate metabolism Diuretics Ethanol Cold	Joint trauma Systemic illness Endocrine disorders
Crystals	Monosodium urate Needle-shaped Negatively birefringent	Calcium pyrophosphate dehydrogenate Rod-shaped, or rhomboidal Positively birefringent
Cell count	Inflammatory, usually > 50,000, mostly PMNs	Usually inflammatory, may be < 50,000, mostly PMNs
Viscosity	Markedly decreased	Decreased, but variably
Treatment	NSAIDs Analgesics Colchicine	Joint aspiration and injection NSAIDs Early mobilization

MTP, metatarsophalangeal; NSAIDs, nonsteroidal anti-inflammatory drugs; PMNs, polymorphonuclear neutrophils.

Clinical Presentation

The presentation of gout can be divided into four stages, as described next.

Stage 1 (Asymptomatic Hyperuricemia). Symptoms are usually not present, although a small percentage of patients develop urinary calculi.

Stage 2 (Acute Gouty Arthritis). This stage is heralded by the rapid onset of severe pain and swelling of the affected joints. The first metatarsaophalangeal (MTP) joints are affected in over half of initial attacks and eventually in up to 90% of patients with gout.[44] Other sites commonly affected are other joints in the foot, the ankle, and the knee. Almost 90% of initial attacks are monoarticular. The affected joints are markedly erythematous, more so than in other types of noninfectious arthritis. As well as joints, tendons and bursae may be affected.

Although mild attacks may resolve within a few days, more severe attacks may require several weeks to resolve completely. Patients are occasionally systemically ill, and may even appear septic; of course, actual sepsis resulting from joint infection or another source must be ruled out in these cases. Elderly patients may have a more indolent presentation, with multiple joints affected more mildly, leading to confusion with other forms of arthritis.

As an acute attack resolves, the skin overlying affected joints may desquamate. Single attacks do not cause joint damage; however, most patients will have more than one attack. Chronic gout (see later discussion) will lead to joint injury.

Stage 3 (Intercritical Gout). Between attacks of gouty arthritis, the patient is asymptomatic but may still have urate crystals present in both previously affected and unaffected joints.

Stage 4 (Chronic Gout). About half of patients who have had attacks of gout for a period of 10 years or more develop tophi, nodules in the skin and soft tissues containing precipitated uric acid crystals. Tophi and the associated inflammatory reaction to urate crystals can damage cartilage, subchondral bone, tendons, and skin, leading to cosmetic and functional deformities.

Diagnosis

Serum uric acid levels are usually elevated between attacks in patients with gout. However, during an acute attack, uric acid precipitates into the affected tissues and the serum uric acid level may normalize. *Thus, serum uric acid levels are of no use during an acute attack of gout.*

Aspiration of the inflamed joint is the key to the diagnosis of gout. Synovial fluid from a gouty joint reveals:

- *Needle-shaped urate crystals.*[44] If polarized light microscopy is available, they will appear yellow when oriented parallel to the axis of slow vibration marked on the microscope's compensator (i.e., negatively birefringent). The crystals are found intracellularly (within neutrophils) during an acute attack of gout.
- *Low viscosity.*
- *High leukocyte count*, often greater than 50,000/mm^3. Seventy percent or more will be neutrophils.

- An *absence of bacteria* on Gram stain and culture (see later discussion).

Because little fluid is usually obtained from aspiration, especially from the small joints of the foot, a few guidelines for the use of synovial fluid are in order:

- Often, only 2 drops of fluid, one for microscopy and one for culture, are necessary.
- Do not discard the small amount of fluid remaining in the needle or its hub. This may be enough fluid to make the diagnosis!
- Fluid aspirated from around the joint while withdrawing the needle often contains additional crystals, and this may increase the total amount of fluid obtained.
- If only a tiny amount of fluid is available, the preferred order of aπnalysis is culture, then crystal examination, Gram stain, and cell count; any other studies can then be performed if sufficient fluid has been obtained.

Radiographic changes, such as joint erosion, occur long after the diagnosis of gout should be made by other means[44] (Figs. 3–1, 3–2, and 3–3).

Treatment

Strategies for managing gout vary, depending on the acuity of the disease.

Acute Gout. For the patient who has had 3 or fewer attacks, with recovery between attacks, treatment is aimed at decreasing the pain and inflammation during the acute attacks. Plasma urate concentrations are not treated at this point in the disease, as most patients do not go on to develop chronic gout.

Nonsteroidal anti-inflammatory drugs (*NSAIDs*) are the mainstay of treatment. Indomethacin at the dose of 50 mg every 6 to 8 hours is usually effective. This dose is maintained until the pain and swelling decrease, and is then reduced to 25 mg every 6 to 8 hours until the attack resolves completely. Ibuprofen, initially 800 mg every 6 to 8 hours, or naproxen, initially 500 mg twice a day, are alternatives.

Colchicine has been used since the early 1800s to treat gout. Although it is effective, the side effects of vomiting and diarrhea limit its use. Intravenous rather than oral administration decreases the gastrointestinal effects, but may lead to local tissue necrosis if the medication extravasates, as well as the failure of other organs. The use of colchicine in the acute care setting, now that effective NSAID therapy is available, should be reserved for patients who do not respond to or cannot tolerate NSAIDs. Colchicine is given 0.5 mg at a time every hour until inflammation decreases, vomiting or diarrhea develops, or a maximum dose of 6 to 8 mg per day (depending on body mass) is reached. Intravenous colchicine should be given only on the advice of a consultant.

Other analgesics, such as acetaminophen and opiates, may further alleviate pain.

Intra-articular steroid injection may be performed by a consultant. Systemic steroids are not recommended, because of the variable response and frequent recurrence of attacks after the medication is discontinued.

Finally, *eliminate any medications*, such as diuretics, *that precipitated the attack.* The sooner treatment is initiated after an attack begins, the better the response will be.

Chronic Gout. The management of chronic gout is beyond the scope of this text; however, the emergency physician should be familiar with the medications used to treat this condition, and their side effects.

Allopurinol decreases serum urate concentration. About 5 to 10% of patients develop hypersensitivity reactions, usually a pruritic maculopapular rash. A full-blown systemic hypersensitivity syndrome, including fever, eosinophilia, erythema multiforme, and multi-organ–system dysfunction, occurs occasionally and may be fatal. Any patient suspected of having such a reaction should be admitted to the hospital, and the patient's rheumatologist notified.

Probenecid decreases serum urate concentration. It decreases the renal excretion of other drugs, such as penicillins, NSAIDs, and dapsone. Aspirin completely blocks probenecid's therapeutic effect. Gastrointestinal side effects and hypersensitivity reactions may occur in patients receiving probenecid. Probenecid should not be started during an acute attack, as it may increase urate precipitation during the initiation of treatment, worsening the acute gout.

Colchicine may be given prophylactically for up to 9 months following normalization of serum urate levels in a patient with chronic or recurrent gout. Long-term colchicine therapy should only be undertaken by a consultant.

Complications

Patients with long-standing gout have a higher incidence of nephrolithiasis, proteinuria, and hypertension.

Septic arthritis may occur in the same joint as crystal-induced arthritis. In these cases, the inflammatory response caused by the joint infection probably leads to precipitation of urate or calcium pyrophosphate crystals and thus an attack of gout or pseudogout. Because the synovial fluid cell counts of patients with crystal-induced arthritis and infectious arthritis are similar, *synovial fluid obtained from patients with acute arthritis should always be cultured, even if crystals are seen.* Any patient with known gout or pseudogout who is systemically ill in the setting of an acute attack of arthritis, or whose arthritis seems worse or different than usual, should have his or her joint fluid cultured, and empiric antibiotic treatment should be considered.

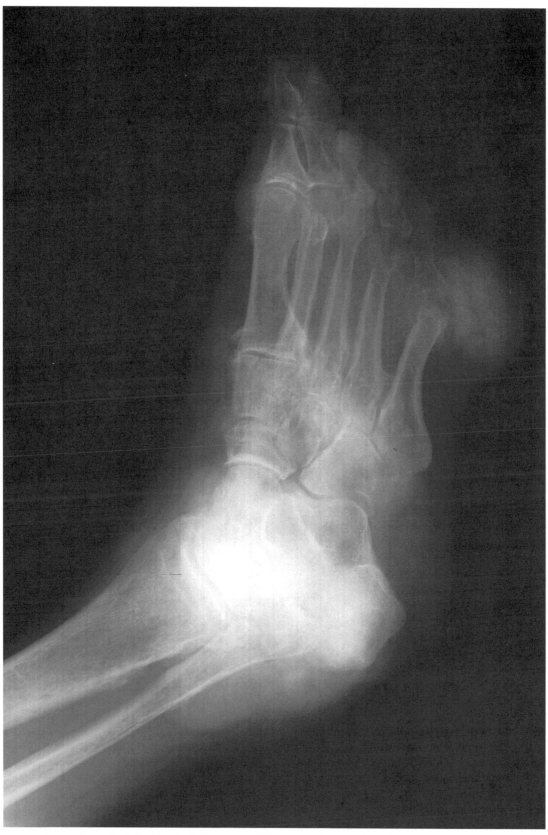

Figure 3–1. Gouty tophi of the foot and knee. *(Courtesy of J. Fitzpatrick, MD, Cook County Hospital.)*

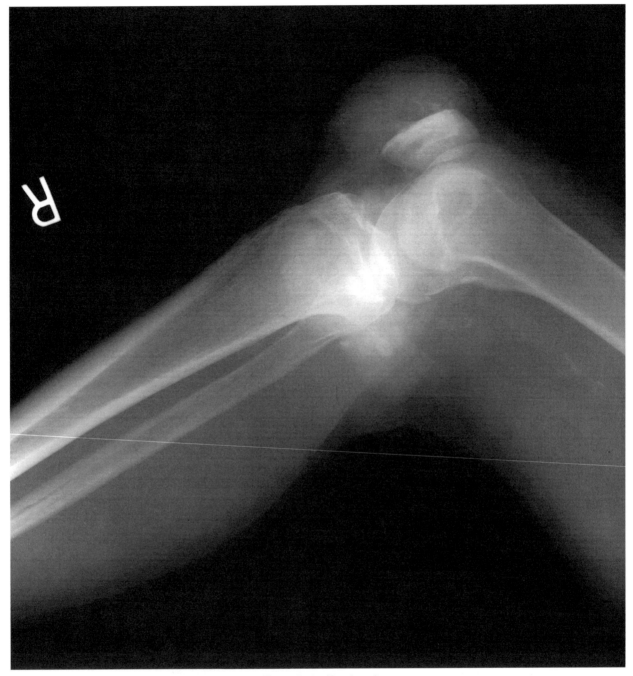

Figure 3–1. *(Continued)*

Finally, *rheumatoid arthritis and gout rarely occur together*, so if a patient with rheumatoid arthritis presents with what appears clinically to be an acute case of gout, an infected joint should be strongly suspected.

Calcium Pyrophosphate Dihydrate Crystal Arthropathy

Calcium pyrophosphate dihydrate (CPPD) crystal deposition in joints occurs primarily in elderly patients. It may present as an acute monoarticular arthritis or as chronic arthritis (usually complicating underlying osteoarthritis). CPPD crystals may be also be found incidentally at arthrocentesis in over 40% of patients with osteoarthritis,[27] and x-rays may show incidental calcification of joint cartilage, synovial tissues, and tendoninsertions (Figs. 3–4 and 3–5). This section deals only with the acute presentation.

Acute Arthritis ("Pseudogout"). Acute CPPD arthritis is *the most common cause of acute monoarticular arthritis* in the elderly. Although any joint may be

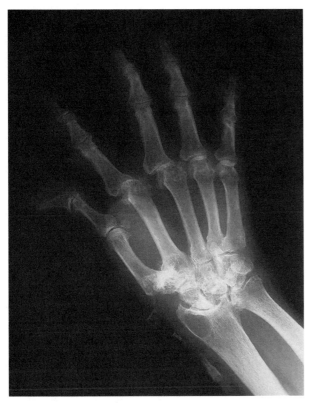

Figure 3–2. Gouty degenerative changes of the hand and wrist.

involved, the *knee is most commonly affected*, followed by the wrist, shoulder, ankle, and elbow joints. Pain and inflammation are severe, and develop rapidly over 6 to 24 hours. As with gout, overlying erythema is common, and the patient may be febrile. Patients with subclinical cognitive impairment may become confused, and sepsis must be ruled out in such cases.

Over 90% of cases affect a single joint, and involvement of more than a few joints is rare and should prompt a search for another etiology for the patient's arthritis. Attacks may be precipitated by joint trauma, concurrent severe illness, surgery, initiation of thyroid replacement therapy, or other systemic diseases such as Wilson's disease, hemochromatosis, and hyperparathyroidism. Most attacks are, however, idiopathic.

Diagnosis is made by joint aspiration, which reveals:

- *Rhomboidal or rod-shaped CPPD crystals*, which are weakly positively birefringent, and appear blue when oriented parallel to the axis of slow vibration marked on a polarizing microscope's compensator.
- Fluid that is usually *blood-stained or cloudy*.
- *Decreased viscosity*.
- *Elevated leukocyte count*, usually greater than 50,000/mm^3, primarily neutrophils.

However, cell counts vary more than in gout and may be much lower.

As with gout, the *presence of crystals does not rule out infection*, and *all synovial fluid specimens must be cultured and Gram-stained*.

Radiologic studies may be normal, may show changes of osteoarthritis, or may show calcification of cartilage, synovial tissues, and tendons.

Treatment

Treatment of acute pseudogout is similar to treatment of acute gout. NSAIDs are effective, but may have gastric and renal toxicities. Dosage is as noted previously for gout. Other analgesics, such as acetaminophen and opiates may be necessary.

Complete joint drainage by aspiration is therapeutic as well as diagnostic, and may resolve the attack of pseudogout. Intra-articular steroid injection may be performed by a consultant after infection is ruled out.

Any underlying illnesses that triggered the attack should be treated. The affected joint should be mobilized as soon as the patient can tolerate. Because patients are usually elderly and have preexisting osteoarthritis, prolonged immobility can rapidly lead to permanent functional disability.

Hydroxyapatite Crystal Arthropathy. Besides urate and calcium pyrophosphate crystals, hydroxyapatite crystals can also provoke an acute arthritis. Apatite crystals can be found in nearly half of osteoarthritic joints, usually in combination with CPPD crystals.[27]

Although hydroxyapatite crystals usually are incidental findings at arthrocentesis, they can occasionally provoke an acute inflammatory reaction resembling gout or pseudogout. The apatite crystals may also lead to rapid erosion of joint cartilage in the setting of osteoarthritis, with pain and loss of joint function.

The crystals may be needle-shaped or may coalesce into larger irregular clumps or rods; they may be difficult to identify on microscopy. Apatite crystals are often found with CPPD and urate crystals in the setting of gout or pseudogout. In these cases, the role of the apatite crystals is unclear.

NSAIDs, analgesics, and referral to an orthopedic or rheumatologic specialist are indicated if apatite arthropathy is suspected. Joint aspiration may be therapeutic as well as diagnostic. Intra-articular steroid injection may be performed by a consultant once infection is ruled out.

OSTEOARTHRITIS

Osteoarthritis is the most common form of arthritis in older patients, causing pain that can significantly reduce function and the quality of life. Osteoarthritis is such a common condition at midlife and in elderly patients that it is almost safe to say that it is ubiquitous.[76]

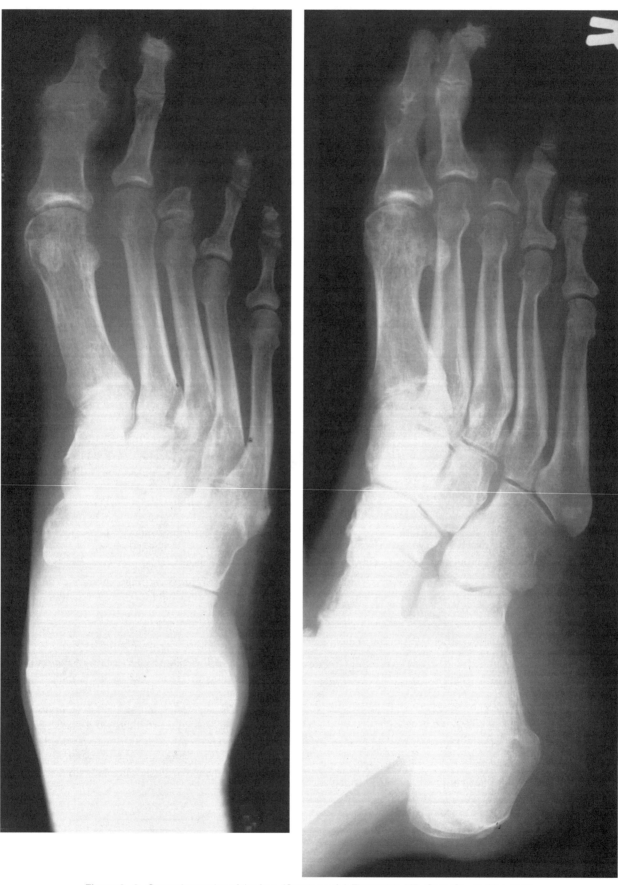

Figure 3–3. Gouty destruction of the foot. *(Courtesy of J. Fitzpatrick, MD, Cook County Hospital.)*

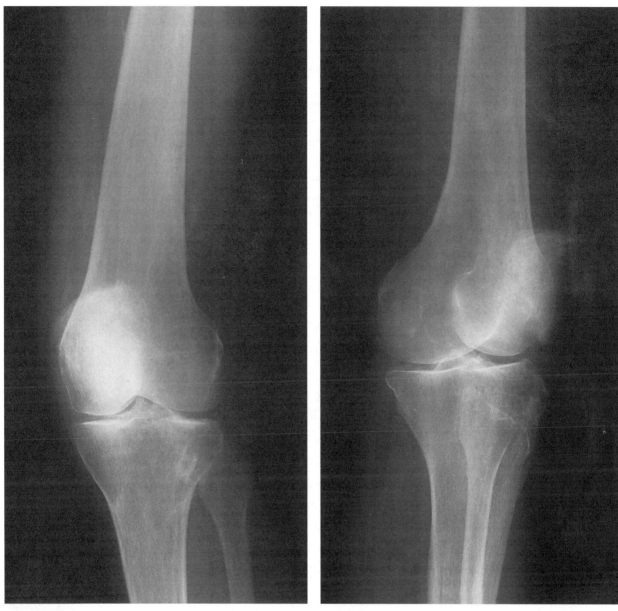

Figure 3–4. Chondrocalcinosis of the knee.

Risk Factors for Osteoarthritis

Obesity is a major risk factor, particularly for osteoarthritis of the knee in women, and to a lesser degree, for hips and hands. Weight loss can prevent the onset of symptomatic osteoarthritis, delay radiographic progression, and lessen symptoms.

Reproductive and hormonal variables also can predispose to generalized osteoarthritis in women. The predilection is for the onset to occur in the perimenopausal years. Genetic factors also raise the risk as there is a strong familial link, particularly in women. Trauma and overuse are other major causes of joint involvement, particularly in the knee and in the hand. Repeated minor trauma may cause increased osteoarthritis with occupational overuse. Recreational overuse or habit-ual physical activity is not associated with symptomatic knee osteoarthritis; however, there is an increased risk of this disorder in elite athletes and an increase in radiologic changes in the knees of women with a history of weight-bearing sports, such as long-distance runners.[55]

Clinical Presentation

Pain is undoubtedly the most prominent and important symptom of osteoarthritis. Pain occurs during active use of an extremity but is also present at rest. Patients experience night pain and tenderness. Stiffness after inactivity, particularly in the early morning hours, is related to gelling, which is usually relieved after 30 minutes of use. Loss of movement, along with the feeling of instability, are problems that occur later in the disease course.

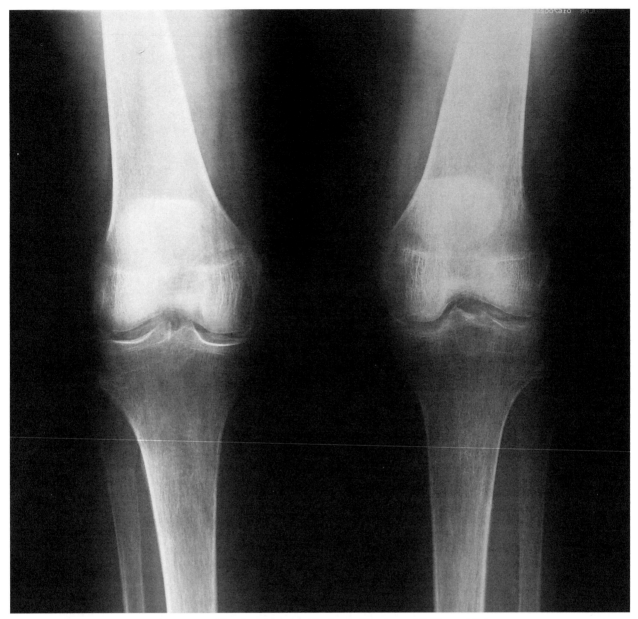

Figure 3–5. Chondrocalcinosis of the knee. *(Courtesy of G. Shove, MD.)*

On examination, the patient has tender spots around the joint margin, and there is firm swelling of the joint margin. The patient has course crepitus signs of mild inflammation. Movements are painful and restricted and there is tightness in the joint. The hip joint is most likely to be painful, and the hand is least likely. The severity of radiographic changes is associated with an increased likelihood of pain, although severe joint damage can be asymptomatic (Fig. 3–6). Pain in osteoarthritis may be the result of raised intraosseous pressure; however, this is unclear. Other features include joint stiffness, loss of function, and, ultimately, joint deformity as the disease progresses. Any joint may be affected, but those of the

hands, feet, knees, and hips, and the apophyseal joints of the spine are most commonly involved. Joints may be affected in isolation or as part of the primary generalized osteoarthritis.[55] Patients with nodal hand osteoarthritis are generally women, and peak onset is in middle age. Patients with a strong family history of osteoarthritis are predisposed to this condition.

Hand Osteoarthritis

The first carpometacarpal joint and the distal and proximal interphalangeal joints are the most commonly affected joints. Patients have pain and bony swelling at the base of the thumb with "heberdons nodes" (distal

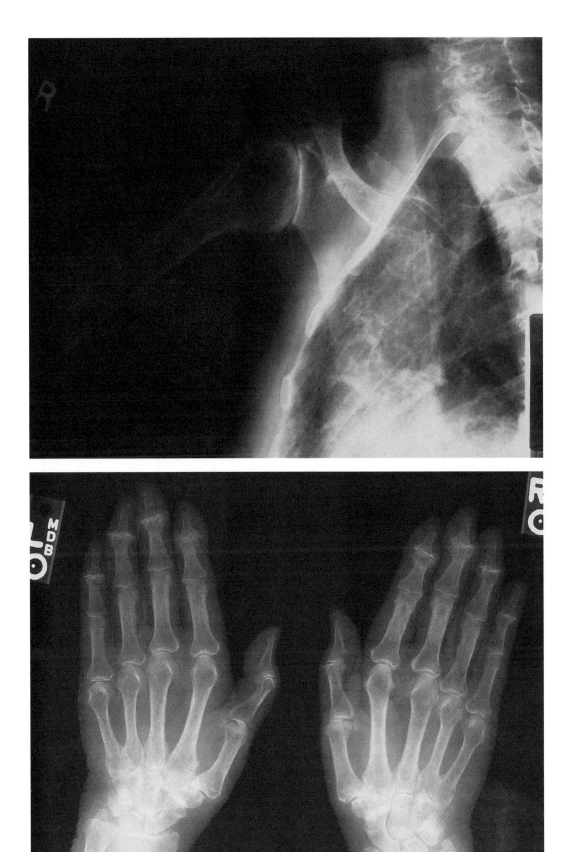

Figure 3–6. Severe osteoarthritis of the hands and shoulder. *(Courtesy of G. Shove, MD.)*

interphalangeal joints). Loss of function in the hands may be quite marked in the beginning as the joints go through phases of inflammation, perhaps lasting for months; however, the long-term outlook for function is generally good despite residual bony deformities.

Knee Osteoarthritis

Symptoms tend to have a gradual onset and deteriorate with time. Mechanical abnormalities, obesity, and poor quadriceps muscle strain can contribute to progression and associated disability. The knee may be affected in any or all of its three compartments, and the medial compartment is more frequently affected than the lateral. Joint line pain and tenderness and bony swelling with loss of articular cartilage leads to joint space narrowing and gradual varus deformity. Osteoarthritis in the patella femoral joint contributes to retropatellar crepitus and pain, particularly going up and down stairs and slopes.[55] In approximately 15 to 20% of patients with knee osteoarthritis, there are effusions which may be of long standing and may result in synovial cyst development, particularly in the popliteal fossa (Baker's cyst), but medial extension along the anserine bursa is also common. Baker's cyst may occasionally rupture and mimic deep vein thrombosis, with pain, swelling, and inflammation in the calf and lower leg.

Hip Osteoarthritis

Hip osteoarthritis often occurs in the elderly population and tends to be more common in men. Pain is characteristically present in the groin (Fig. 3–7). Involvement may be unilateral or bilateral. Symptoms of pain or tenderness around the pelvic girdle region (e.g., in the buttocks or lateral aspect of the thigh) may indicate osteoarthritis of the hip, but other possibly co-existing conditions should be considered, such as referred pain from the spine, or trochanteric bursitis. In the early stages, patients may experience pain with extremes of motion, with internal rotation usually being the earliest movement affected. Patients with advanced disease may experience referred pain in the knee.

Diagnosis

The most useful findings in the diagnosis of osteoarthritis are radiographic x-rays. These are normal early in the disease, but narrowing of the joint space develops as the disease progresses. Other x-ray features are subchondral sclerosis,[76] marginal osteophytes, and subchondral cysts. In osteoarthritis, subchondral cysts are surrounded by a dense rim of bone that differentiates them from the marginal erosions that occur in rheumatoid arthritis. Ninety percent of individuals over the age of 40 years have x-ray changes characteristic of osteoarthritis; however, only 30% have symptoms of osteoarthritis. Labora-

tory features in arthritis are nonspecific and are generally not helpful in making the diagnosis.

Treatment

The aim of treatment in osteoarthritis is to relieve pain and allow the patient to be as active and independent as possible. The drugs used in the management of osteoarthritis are simple analgesics to relieve pain and NSAIDs to reduce the symptoms. Intra-articular corticosteroids provide local relief of symptoms and are used only in advanced disease by rheumatologists. Although not part of the emergency medicine management, one should be aware that intra-articular radiocolloids and sclerosing agents have been used to provide symptomatic relief through obliteration of the synovium and synovitis. Antidepressants and other agents are also used by the primary care physician. Exercise therapy, hydrotherapy, and walking aids and appliances are all adjuncts that are used in this disease process. Ultimately, many patients need joint replacement surgery, particularly in cases of advanced hip and knee osteoarthritis.

RHEUMATOID ARTHRITIS*

Rheumatoid arthritis (RA) is an autoimmune disease that affects about 1% of the world's population. It is characterized by a *symmetric, progressive polyarthritis*. Unlike osteoarthritis, RA often has *systemic manifestations*. Although the cause of RA is unclear, and its course in each patient can be unpredictable, it is generally progressive and leads to tremendous pain, suffering, and disability.

RA has widely varying onset, severity, and progression. RA may actually encompass several diseases with similar manifestations. It is twice as common in women as in men, and has its usual onset in the fourth and fifth decades of life. Prevalence of RA increases with age. (Note: Juvenile rheumatoid arthritis [JRA] is a distinct syndrome and is discussed separately.)

There is thought to be a genetic predisposition to RA, with development of the disease triggered by an inciting environmental factor, such as a viral infection.

RA is characterized by an autoimmune attack on synovial tissue, leading to marked (up to 100-fold) proliferation of synovium. Adjoining tissues are affected by this synovial neoplasia, including *joints*, with their cartilage, bone, and ligaments; *tendons* (as a result of tenosynovial tissue inflammation), and *bursae*. This *inflammation, combined with physical stress*, destroys the joint's structure and function. Additionally, *extrasynovial manifestations may affect nearly any organ*. A diffuse, small vessel vasculitis leads to the formation of

---

*This section was contributed by Robert Feldman, MD.

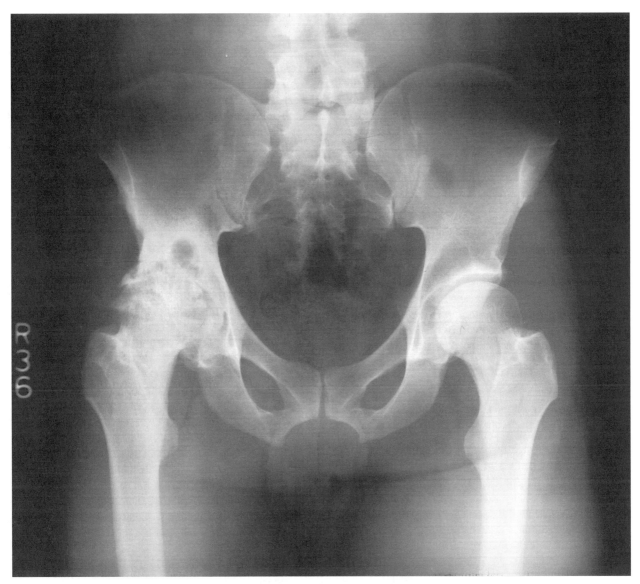

Figure 3–7. Osteoarthritis of the hip. *(Courtesy of J. Fitzpatrick, MD, Cook County Hospital.)*

cutaneous rheumatoid nodules in 20% of patients with seropositive RA.

A basic understanding of the pathophysiology of RA allows the emergency physician to suspect the disease in the undiagnosed patient, and to tailor treatment and detect systemic complications in all patients with RA.

Emergency Department Approach

The emergency physician will encounter two main groups of patients with RA: (1) *those who have not yet been diagnosed as having RA*, who present with polyarticular arthritis; and (2) *those who have been previously diagnosed* and present with an acute flare, systemic manifestations of the disease, or an unrelated medical problem.

Patients with New or Undiagnosed Disease

Onset of RA often follows a prodromal flu-like illness. Onset is usually, but not always, articular, symmetric, and gradual. However, up to 20% of patients may have an acute onset of arthritis over a few weeks, or even a few days. The variability of symptoms and progression in RA often makes initial diagnosis difficult: onset may be over weeks to months, duration of illness may last weeks or decades, and severity may vary from mild arthritis to crippling deformity. Objective clinical findings may not correlate with the patient's symptoms or with the degree of disability.

RA is an autoimmune disease, and many patients have *rheumatoid factor*, an immune complex, circulating in their serum. Seventy to 80% of patients with RA are seropositive during the course of their disease.

Therefore, *about one quarter of patients with RA will be seronegative*. Rheumatoid factor is not specific for RA, and may be found in other diseases as well.

Because there is no specific serologic test for RA, the diagnosis is based on clinical criteria. The classification system requires observation of the patient over time (at least 6 weeks), so the initial diagnosis of RA is unlikely to be made in the acute care setting. The goal in the acute care setting is, therefore, to suspect rheumatologic disease, alleviate any acute symptoms, and refer the patient to the appropriate provider for definitive diagnosis and long-term management. The emergency physician should:

- *Rule out joint infection* with mono- or oligoarticular involvement (see later discussion)
- *Attempt to differentiate RA from other poly-arthropathies*, such as osteoarthritis and gonococcal arthritis
- *Arrange for baseline laboratory studies*, including ESR, complete blood count (CBC), and creatinine level. Rheumatoid factor and ANA tests may also be requested.
- *Rule out serious extra-articular disease* (see later discussion)
- *Treat symptoms* of pain and inflammation (see later discussion)

Any patient suspected of having RA should have a primary care provider, as many of these patients will develop systemic co-morbidities, such as pulmonary or renal disease. Specialty referral may be deferred to the primary care provider if the patient is not severely ill. Studies suggest that RA patients have less morbidity when a rheumatologist is involved in their care.

Pharmacologic Treatment. A variety of agents with varying therapeutic and side effects are used, and must often be combined for optimal results (Table 3–6). A treatment regimen should be tailored for each individual patient. Therapy with agents other than NSAIDs, and perhaps a brief course of steroids, should only be undertaken after consultation with the physician who will be following the patient.

Nonsteroidal Anti-Inflammatory Drugs. NSAIDs are the mainstay of treatment for the pain and inflammation of RA and should be used if they are not contraindicated. They can adversely affect renal function and may exacerbate or cause acid-peptic disease. Cytotec may protect the gastric lining.

Three main types of NSAIDs are available:

- *Salicylates*: Aspirin is the prototype agent. It often causes gastrointestinal (GI) upset and requires frequent dosing, but it is inexpensive and readily available.

- *Salsalate* (and other) *agents*: These drugs require less frequent dosing but are more expensive and still have GI side effects.
- *Other NSAIDs*: Numerous agents are available, with variable dosage and cost. Unfortunately, a given patient's therapeutic response to each drug is not predictable, nor are the exact side effects the patient will experience. New selective cyclo-oxygenase inhibitors may be better tolerated by patients with a history of peptic disease, but they can still cause GI hemorrhage. Often, several agents from different classes are tried to find the best one for patient. If a patient with known RA presents with pain, the physician should ask whether, the patient already knows what is effective for him or her.

Corticosteroids. These drugs may be given systemically or by local injection. Systemic corticosteroids (e.g., methylprednisolone, 100 to 1000 mg/day for 3 days) can improve the symptoms of an acute RA flare. However, systemic corticosteroids do not prevent joint destruction and thus have no sustained benefit for RA patients. They also have serious side effects on many organ systems. Chronic use of systemic corticosteroids should be limited to severe, unremitting disease (e.g., prednisone, 5 to 7.5 mg/day); use for RA-associated systemic disease should be discussed with a consultant prior to initiation.

Local corticosteroid injection decreases symptoms of acute inflammatory synovitis. Joint infection must be ruled out prior to administration, particularly if the flare is mono- or pauciarticular. Generally, this procedure is perfomed by the patient's rheumatologist or primary care physician.

Slow-acting Anti-Rheumatic Drugs (SAARDs). Unlike corticosteroids, SAARDs may alter the destructive course of RA. They are expensive, and require several weeks of use for maximal benefit. SAARDs are usually combined with NSAID therapy, and sometimes with corticosteroids (Table 3–7).

SAARDs have severe side effects, and their use requires close follow-up and careful dose titration. Most patients cannot tolerate these medications for more than 1 or 2 years at a time.

Initiation of SAARD treatment without consultation is beyond the acute care scope of practice. The emergency physician should refill or resume prescriptions for SAARDs on the advice of the patient's primary care provider or rheumatologist; the slow onset of benefits does not justify the acute risk and expense of prescribing these agents from the emergency department. Because patients may present with iatrogenic complications, the emergency physician should have some familiarity with the major agents used and their side effects.

TABLE 3–6. SELECTED NONSTEROIDAL ANTI-INFLAMMATORY DRUGS

Generic Name	Trade Name(s)	Usual Adult Dosage	Comments
Celecoxib	Celebrex	100–200 mg qd–bid	Selective CO inhibitor; *May cause hypersensitivity in patients who are sulfa-allergic.*
Diclofenac	Voltaren	50 mg bid	100 mg qd SR available
Etodolac	Lodine	200–400 mg bid–tid	400 and 600 mg qd SR available
Ibuprofen	Motrin, Advil	600–800 mg tid	Generic available
Indomethacin	Indocin	25–50 mg tid	Generic available
Ketoprofen	Orudis	50–75 mg tid	200 mg qd SR available
Ketorolac	Toradol	10 mg PO q 4–6 h; IM/IV dosing varies	Not to be used more than 5 days due to renal toxicity
Nabumetone	Relafen	1000–2000 mg qd–bid	
Naproxen	Naprosyn, Aleve	250–500 mg bid	Variety of SR and EC preparations available
Piroxicam	Feldene	20 mg PO qd	
Sulindac	Clinoril	150–200 mg bid	

CO, Cyclooxygenase; EC, enteric coated; SR, sustained release.

TABLE 3–7. DRUGS USED IN TREATMENT OF RHEUMATOID ARTHRITIS

Agent	Major Side Effects
Antimalarials (e.g., hydroxychloroquine)	Retinal lesions
Gold: IM more effective and more toxic than PO	Rash, oral ulcers, leukopenia, thrombocytopenia, proteinuria
Penicillamine	Side effects similar to gold
Sulfasalazine	Gastrointestinal (GI) upset, rash
Methotrexate (MTX)	Rash, GI upset, pulmonary toxicity, hepatitis, immunosuppression
Imuran	GI upset, abdominal pain, leukopenia, immunosuppression, hepatitis

Other therapeutic modalities useful for RA include:

- Joint immobilization or bed rest, or both; these may be useful for patients with an acute flare, but joint rest must be weighed against with the effects of deconditioning.
- Physical therapy.
- Reconstructive surgery; this is sometimes necessary to correct deformities, particularly in the hand.
- Specific cytokine antagonists, such as anti–tumor necrosis factor antibodies, which may be of benefit for selected patients. The exact dosage and indications for initiation of such treatments are still under investigation.

Patients with Known Disease

The goals in the acute care setting are to treat the patient's pain and inflammation, limit tissue destruction, and improve daily functioning. *These patients are often on immunosuppressive drugs, which predispose them to infections and may obscure signs of serious infection.*

Both RA and the medications used to treat it may cause systemic complications.

Useful laboratory tests include *ESR* and *CBC*. *Renal function* should be assessed, given the potential nephrotoxicity of many of the medications used to treat RA. Elevation of serum glutamic-oxaloacetic transaminase *(SGOT)* and *alkaline phosphatase* may indicate systemic involvement.

Specific syndromes are discussed in the following sections. Once acute care has been completed, the patient should be referred back to the primary care provider or rheumatologist for further treatment, such as SAARDs.

Specific Syndromes Presenting to the Emergency Department

Table 3–8 summarizes clinical findings and treatment considerations for several specific syndromes of RA.

Articular Disease

Usually *symmetric* and *progressive* joint deterioration is seen, with exacerbations and remissions over the course of the disease (Figs. 3–8 and 3–9). Function is worse after immobility or sleep and *improves with activity during the day.* Patients report morning stiffness, usually lasting more than 30 minutes, with a median duration of 1.5 hours.

Clinical findings include pain in the affected joints, both at rest and with motion, along with, joint swelling, warmth, and tenderness. Erythema may be present with acute onset or flare; if present, the physician should consider infection. Pain, inflammation, and disuse atrophy of muscles lead to progressive functional impairment and loss of range of motion. Radiologic signs of soft tissue swelling, symmetric joint space narrowing, and osteopenia of adjoining bones are present.

TABLE 3–8. SPECIFIC SYNDROMES IN RHEUMATOID ARTHRITIS

Region	Diagnostic Findings (synovial inflammation)	Frequency	Treatment Considerations
Upper Extremities		Usual site of initial inflammation	Immobilization for 2–3 weeks
Hand tendons	*Flexors:* Decreased ROM, tendon rupture, trigger effect, carpal tunnel syndrome *Extensors:* Dorsal hand mass, tendon rupture	Common	Medications, splint, physical therapy, reconstructive surgery
PIP	Fusiform swelling, boutonnière deformity, swan-neck deformity, flail joint	Usual, early	Reconstructive surgery sometimes needed
DIP	Swelling	Rare, never initial or isolated finding	
MCP	Swelling, ulnar drift, volar subluxation (fixed)	Usual, early	
Thumb	Boutonnière deformity, CMC dislocation ("duckbill thumb"), flail IP joint	Common, except duckbill thumb	
Wrist	Carpal subluxation, radiocarpal dislocation, synovial cysts, carpal tunnel syndrome, fracture due to osteoporosis	Almost universal, early CTS may be initial complaint	Same
Elbow	Subcutaneous nodules, synovial cysts, bursitis, limited extension	Common, late	Same as above; nerve compression at elbow may require decompression
Shoulder	Synovitis, bursitis, rotator cuff inflammation, AC joint pain, biceps rupture	Variable, late	Joint injection
Lower Extremities			Immobilize for 6–8 weeks
Foot	Synovitis, bone erosion, valgus deformity, "claw foot," ulcers or MTP–cutaneous fistulae	Common (90%), especially first and fifth MTPs	Local wound care
Ankle	Tendonitis, may lead to Achilles tendon rupture. May compress posterior tibial nerve	Common, but not as sole joint involved	Medications, rest
Knee	Effusion; ligament destruction, which may cause instability; valgus deformity; popliteal (Baker's) cyst formation and rupture (crescent-shaped hemorrhage below malleolus with cyst rupture)	Most common single joint early in disease	Medications, bed rest, injection Be alert for ligamentous instability Ruptured cyst: rule out DVT, occasionally requires decompression
Hip	Synovitis, bursitis	Less common	Medications, bed rest, injection
Spine			
Cervical	C1–C2 subluxation: odontoid–C1 arch space over 3 mm (can cause cord compression and vertebrobasilar insufficiency); discitis; nerve root compression	Spine involvement common in patients with severe disease, although actual subluxation is about 5% overall, and cord or vessel compression is rare	Use caution during airway maneuvers Immobilization and spinal fusion, if needed
Thoracic, lumbar, sacral	Synovitis, spinal stenosis, ostoporotic disease	Rare—consider other diagnoses	
TMJ	Pain with chewing, limited opening, posterior subluxation	Common	
Any of the above	Septic synovitis	Increased over general population	Drainage, antibiotics

AC, acromioclavicular; CMC, carpometacarpal; CTS, carpal tunnel syndrome; DIP, distal interphalangeal; DVT, deep venous thrombosis; IP, interphalangeal; MCP, metacarpophalangeal; MTP, metatarsophalangeal; PIP, proximal interphalangeal; ROM, range of motion.

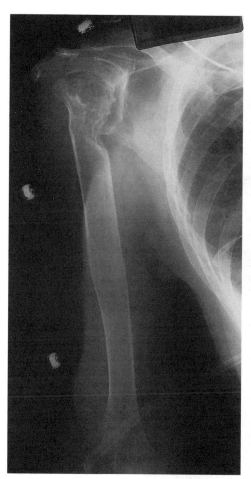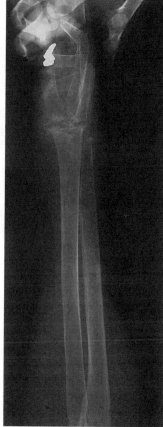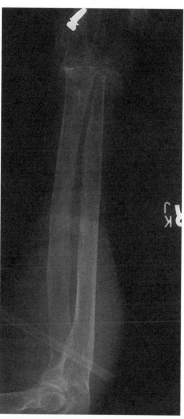

Figure 3–8. Rheumatoid arthritis of the wrist, elbow, and shoulder.

The *"rheumatic hand"* is characteristic (see Fig. 3–9): the proximal interphalangeal (PIP), metacarpophalangeal (MCP), and wrist joints are inflamed, while the distal interphalangeal (DIP) joints are spared.

Treatment. Initial treatment is with NSAIDs and modification of activity. Rest, splinting, and preferential use of large rather than small joints (e.g., carrying a bag on the shoulder rather than in the hand) can delay joint destruction. SAARDs are added, with consultation, for progressive disease.

Acute Rheumatoid Arthritis Flare
In this presentation, the patient has acutely increased synovial inflammation with variable systemic and constitutional symptoms. Joint involvement is usually symmetric, usually with six or more painful, tender, swollen joints. Morning stiffness worsens, typically lasting over 1 hour. Elevated ESR (greater than 30 mm/hour) and C-reactive protein levels are often present.

The immediate goal of treatment is alleviation of the acute pain and inflammation, followed by prompt referral to the patient's primary care provider or rheuma-tologist. Joint infection must always be considered, particularly with mono- or pauciarticular flares (see later discussion).

Treatment. Bed rest may be sufficient in some patients. NSAIDs should be prescribed, unless contraindicated. The patient should be referred promptly to a specialist for SAARDs treatment.

A systemic steroid bolus (e.g., methylprednisolone, 100 to 1000 mg/day for 3 days), given after consultation, can help control a severe, generalized flare. Some patients may require up to 1 month of daily, low-dose, systemic steroid therapy. Local steroid injection into the most acute joints, after infection is ruled out, can decrease local inflammation. Injection is generally performed by the patient's rheumatologist or primary care provider.

Finally, the emergency physician should be alert for signs of new systemic disease, either rheumatic or iatrogenic.

Septic Rheumatic Joint
Patients with RA are at increased risk of joint infection as a result of inflammation and immunosuppression.

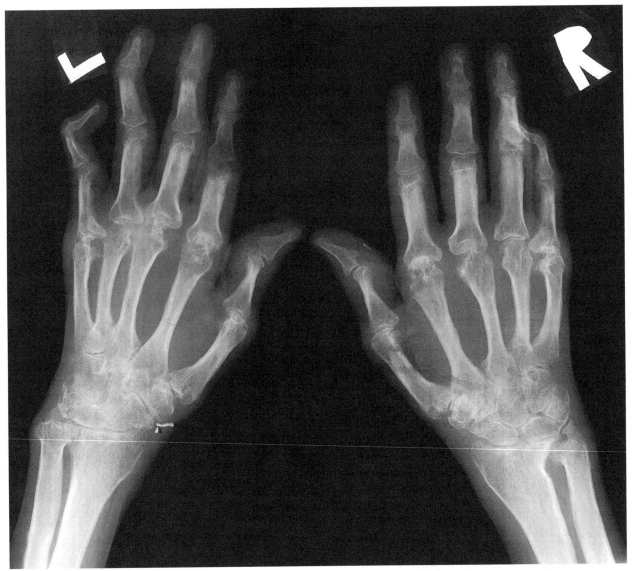

Figure 3–9. Rheumatoid arthritis of the hand. *(Courtesy of J. Fitzpatrick, MD, Cook County Hospital.)*

Furthermore, anti-inflammatory and immunosuppressive medications may suppress clinical signs of infection and delay the diagnosis.

There is no definitive test or finding, other than a positive synovial fluid Gram stain or culture, that can diagnose a septic joint in the setting of rheumatic inflammation. However, a number of findings can guide the clinician's diagnosis and treatment decisions.

Joint infection is usually *monoarticular*. Diagnosis is much more difficult if the infection is polyarticular. Pain greater than the patient's usual flare, fever, and systemic toxicity may indicate infection. Polyarticular infection is usually *asymmetric*, because of hematogenous spread.

Diagnosis

Diagnosis necessitates joint aspiration for culture, Gram stain, and cell count. The physician must ensure that a specimen of synovial fluid is obtained for culture before starting antibiotic therapy.

Empiric antibiotic treatment should be started if clinical suspicion is high, or if the aspirate demonstrates positive Gram stain; leukocyte count greater than 50,000 mm^3 (unusual in RA, but possible); or PMNs greater than 90%. Blood and other specimens, such as urine, should be cultured to increase the yield of any infecting organism, and to search for a site of initial infection.

Treatment

Usually, a parenteral antistaphylococcal antibiotic, such as cefazolin, is administered along with an aminoglycoside, such as gentamycin, unless otherwise indicated by the Gram stain or culture. Serial drainage is performed and early range-of-motion exercises are begun to preserve function.

If the diagnosis is unclear and clinical suspicion is not high, the patient should be referred urgently to a specialist. Empiric treatment without the proper diagnostic workup may commit the patient to an unnecessary course of antibiotics and may delay initiation of appropriate anti-inflammatory therapy.

Popliteal (Baker's) Cyst

Popliteal cysts are common because of the synovial proliferation that characterizes RA. A cyst may rupture spontaneously, or as a result of physical activity, leading to acute calf pain and swelling. The most difficult task facing the emergency physician is ruling out an acute deep venous thrombosis (DVT). Heparinization following a misdiagnosis of DVT can lead to continuing hemorrhage into the calf, with subsequent compartment syndrome.

Diagnosis

Ultrasound is the least invasive test and is widely available. Venography or a contrast arthrogram is occasionally necessary. Note that a crescent-shaped hemorrage below either malleolus is characteristic of a ruptured cyst and not a DVT.

Treatment

Rest, elevation, and analgesia are usually all that is required. Intra-articular corticosteroid injection (after consultation) may help alleviate symptoms before and after rupture. Actual compartment syndrome is rare, but must be treated immediately to prevent permanent disability. Residual calf swelling usually lasts several weeks, and may persist over 3 years.

Atlanto-Axial Subluxation

Although spinal arthritis is common in RA, actual C1–C2 subluxation is uncommon, with an incidence of approximately 5%, overall, in RA. The incidence increases with increasing severity of the patient's overall disease. Actual cord or vascular compromise is rare, but it does occur and can be iatrogenic, resulting from manipulation, such as intubation.

Symptoms and signs of cord compression include severe neck pain, usually radiating to the occiput; extremity weakness, which may be upper or lower, or both (often difficult to assess because of the patient's severe and long-standing arthritis); numbness or tingling in the fingers or feet; loss of vibration sense, with preservation of proprioception; "jumping legs," caused by spinal reflex disinhibition; and bladder dysfunction. Patients may also have vertebral artery insufficiency, including syncope or vertigo.

Diagnosis

An atlanto-dens interval greater than 2.5 mm in adults and 5 mm in children is diagnostic. An emergent computed tomography (CT) or MRI scan should be ordered if cord compression suspected.

Treatment

A hard cervical collar is applied and the patient referred for traction and fusion if there are signs of neurologic or vascular compromise. The physician should avoid aggressive airway maneuvers in patients with signs of RA, or a history of RA, if at all possible.

Systemic Disease

RA may affect nearly any organ. Systemic disease is common, and may be life-threatening. Systemic complications may be caused by the primary rheumatic disease process, or medications, or a combination of both. Signs of serious sytemic disease may be missed, particularly in the patient in whom the diagnosis of RA has not yet been made. The organs that are most often affected include the lungs, heart, liver, and spleen. Blood vessel involvement is also common.

Pulmonary Disease. Mild and asymptomatic pulmonary disease is common in RA. Patients may have pulmonary nodules, pleural effusion, or fibrosis. They occasionally present with restrictive, chronic obstructive pulmonary disease like symptoms. Acute obliterative bronchiolitis is uncommon, but may be fatal; it is unclear if it is caused by the RA itself, or by the medications (SAARDs) used to treat RA.

Cardiac Disease. Pericarditis is the most common cardiac disorder. Usually asymptomatic chronic inflammation is detected only at autopsy, but inflammation may be acute and constrictive. Rheumatic myocarditis and endocarditis occasionally occur. With endocarditis, the physician must rule out bacterial endocarditis; these patients are predisposed to bacteremia as a result of open wounds and immunosuppression.

Hepatic Disease. Hepatitis is often subclinical but may be overt. Liver abnormalities often occur as a result of drug side effects, as well.

Spleen. Felty's disease is defined as RA that occurs in association with an enlarged spleen and leukopenia. It usually occurs in a patient with long-standing RA, including rheumatoid nodules and marked joint deformity. Patients are subject to neutropenia and severe bacterial infections, as well as thrombocytopenia. Any patient suspected of having Felty's disease requires emergent consultation, admission, and aggressive treatment of any suspected bacterial infections. Treatment of RA may improve the manifestations of Felty's disease, but plasmapheresis or splenectomy may be required.

Blood Vessel Disease. Small vessel inflammation is integral to the pathophysiology of RA. Clinically diagnosable vasculitis may be chronic or acute. With chronic vasculitis, leg ulcers and nailfold infarcts are common. Distal sensory neuropathy may also be seen. Acute systemic vasculitis is rare and usually occurs in patients with long-standing disease.

Summary

Rheumatoid arthritis is a common disease with substantial morbidity and occasional mortality. The emergency physician will see numerous patients with RA who desire relief from their symptoms. These patients will be well-served if the physician is able to treat pain and inflammation, preserve limb function, refer promptly for advanced management, diagnose and treat acute infection, and detect acute systemic rheumatic disease.

JUVENILE RHEUMATOID ARTHRITIS (STILL'S DISEASE)

JRA may develop at any age and is characterized as a chronic synovial inflammation without a known cause (Fig. 3–10). No laboratory tests are diagnostic of this condition, although rheumatoid factor and ANAs are commonly seen. About 20% of children with this condition have a systemic onset. The clinical manifestations include *spiking fever*, a salmon-pink rash, generalized lymphadenopathy, and a large spleen. Patients often present with fatigue, weight loss, and anemia. In 50% of patients, the temperature is over 40°C and there is polyarticular involvement. The evanescent pink rash blanches with compression and may be pruritic, and thus confused with a drug sensitivity reaction. The polyarthritis seen initially is a migratory arthritis that eventually becomes a persistent arthritis.

A polyarticular onset of JRA without systemic manifestations occurs in about 40% of patients, and this variety is not referred to as Still's disease. Malaise and weight loss, as well as low-grade fever, are often present. This form may begin at any age during childhood.

In another 40% of children, the onset of this condition is characterized by an asymmetric arthritis affecting predominantly the lower extremity joints. Some patients present with an inflammation of the anterior uveal tract called an iridocyclitis.

Salicylates remain the medication of choice, with the dose starting at approximately 80 to 90 mg per kg per day. Serum salicylate levels must be carefully monitored. Other NSAIDs have also been used successfully. These patients should be referred to a rheumatologist early in the disease course.

SYSTEMIC LUPUS ERYTHEMATOSUS

Although SLE is not usually thought of as a joint disorder, inflammatory arthritis occurs in most patients. SLE is, like RA, an autoimmune disorder that has a variable expression in each individual patient. SLE may also be triggered by medications, such as procainamide.

Clinical Presentation

SLE follows a *relapsing and remitting course.* It typically affects *multiple organ systems*, with different systems affected at different times over the course of the disease (see Table 3–11). Onset early in life is associated with more severe disease than is late onset.

Arthralgias and arthritis are commonly present at the onset of SLE, in about 75% and 50% of patients, respectively. Over the course of their disease, over 90% of patients suffer musculoskeletal involvement. Symmetric synovitis affecting the hands, wrists, and knees, is typical and may be difficult to differentiate clinically from RA. Bone destruction is not usually present in SLE, unlike RA. The combination of synovial inflammation and chronic corticosteroid usage (see the discussion of treatment that follows) causes tendon and ligament damage along with the arthritis. Other musculoskeletal structures are often affected. *Typical musculoskeletal deformities* are summarized in Tables 3–9 and 3–10.

Although musculoskeletal involvement in SLE is generally symmetric, it is not always so. However, if only a single joint is involved, or if one joint is much more acutely inflamed than others, intra-articular infection should be ruled out (see the earlier discussion of RA for details).

Any organ in the body can be affected by SLE. Although a complete discussion is beyond the scope of this text, the provider should *be alert for signs of systemic illness in any patient presenting with inflammatory arthritis* (Table 3–11).

There are a number of interesting laboratory abnormalities in patients with SLE, including a variety of autoantibodies, but most tests are not available emergently and no single antibody is completely sensitive nor specific for SLE. A *CBC and renal function studies* should be checked in a patient who is acutely ill. The ESR is usually elevated, but unfortunately does not correlate with clinical disease activity. Serum IgM rheumatoid factor is present in up to half of patients with SLE.

Treatment

Systemic corticosteroids are the *mainstay of treatment for SLE.* Both low- (less than 0.5 mg/kg/day) and high-dose (1.0 mg/kg/day) regimens of prednisone are used, depending on the lupus manifestation being treated. Unlike RA treatment, chronic corticosteroid usage is

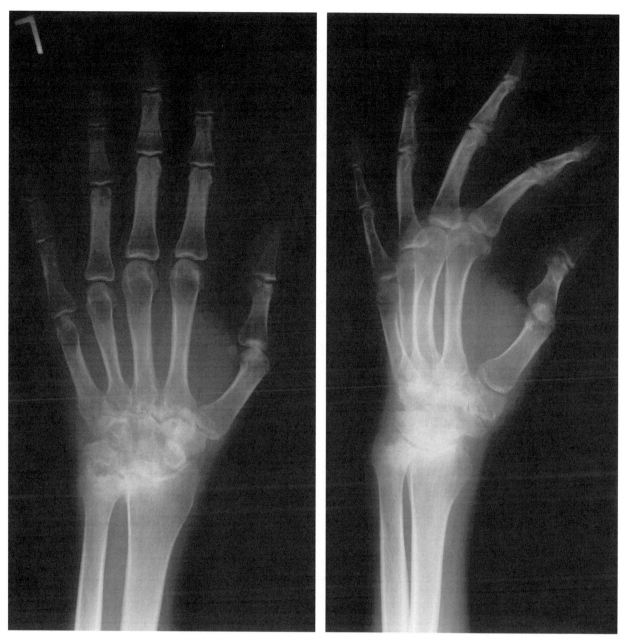

Figure 3–10. Juvenile rheumatoid arthritis of the hand. *(Courtesy of J. Fitzpatrick, MD, Cook County Hospital.)*

often necessary for SLE. As with RA, antimalarials and immunosuppresive drugs are also used; refer to the section on RA for a discussion of toxicities. The physician should remember that all these agents are immunosuppressive, and that patients are therefore more susceptible to serious infections. Furthermore, the immunosuppressive medications may mask signs of infection.

VIRAL ARTHRITIS

Arthritis is a sequel to several common viral infections, but with hepatitis B virus infection the arthritis precedes the symptoms of hepatitis and resolve when jaundice appears. In *hepatitis B virus infection*, during the 1- to 3-week prodromal phase, polyarthritis may be accompanied by moderate fever and, sometimes, by an urticarial or a maculopapular rash. Usually, the small joints are affected symmetrically with arthralgis or arthritis.[44] Aminotransferase levels are usually elevated at this stage, and hepatitis B surface antigen is detectable.

As 10% of the cases of septic arthritis involve more than one joint, the treatment requires that all acutely inflammed joints be tapped to exclude bacterial infection. In some cases of persistent arthritis, it may be helpful to treat hepatitis B virus infection with interferon-α.[44]

TABLE 3–9. JOINT DEFORMITIES ASSOCIATED WITH SLE

Joints Affected*	Deformities	Comments
Fingers	Subluxations, swan-neck deformity, contractures	Subluxation initially reducible, later fixed; usually ulnar deviation
Thumb	Hyperextension of interphalangeal joint (hitchhiker's thumb)	Seen in 30% of patients
Elbow	Flexion contractures	
Hips	Avascular necrosis (osteonecrosis)	May be due to long-term steroid usage; in approximately 10% of patients
Knees	Patellar tendon laxity	
Feet	Gangrene of toes (vasculitis), arthritic deformities	

*Nonerosive arthritis and synovitis.

TABLE 3–10. OTHER MUSCULOSKELETAL FINDINGS ASSOCIATED WITH SLE

Associated Tissues	Deformities	Comments
Muscles	Myositis, myalgias, atrophy (may include diaphragm)	Myositis occurs in about 5–10% of patients with SLE
Tendons	Tenosynovitis, rupture	Often seen early in disease; rupture may be due to SLE or steroid use
Skin	Rheumatoid nodules, other manifestations (see text discussion)	Occurs in about 10% of patients with SLE

TABLE 3–11. COMMON EXTRA-ARTICULAR MANIFESTATIONS OF SLE

System or Organ Affected	Pathology	Incidence at Presentation*	Cumulative Prevalence
Constitutional	*Fever, malaise*	73%	73–90%
Skin, Hair, Mucosa	Rashes: malar, photosensitivity, discoid	57%	66–81%
	Alopecia (diffuse)	—	50–70%
	Mucosal ulcers	7–18%	7–54%
Serosa	Pleurisy	23%	37–64%
	Pericarditis	20%	20–64%
Kidney	Glomerulonephritis	33–44%	33–77%
	Azotemia	3%	8%
Nervous system	CNS (cognitive change, stroke, psychosis, seizures, etc.) *Peripheral neuropathy*	24%	25–66%
Cardiovascular	*Venous thrombosis*	2%	5–26%
	Vasculitis (including digit infarcts)	10%	21–37%
	Myocarditis	1%	4–8%
Pulmonary	Pneumonitis, hemorrhage, "shrinking lung" (diaphragmatic atrophy)	9%	17–65%
Hematologic	*Anemia*	5%	40–58%
	Leukopenia	—	17–49%
	Thrombocytopenia	—	25%

CNS, central nervous system; SLE, systemic lupus erythematosus.

Incidence at presentation refers to the % of patients who manifest the given pathology at time of initial diagnosis.

†*Cumulative prevalence* refers to the % of patients with SLE who will manifest the given pathology at any time during the course of their disease. Based on Klippel and Diepe.[44]

HIV Arthropathy

Several patterns of arthropathy have been described in patients infected with HIV, including brief episodes of severe arthralgia, acute episodic oligoarthritis, and persistent symmetric polyarthritis. Arthritis may be an early feature of acquired immunodeficiency syndrome (AIDS). Arthritis associated with the AIDS is infrequently presents with a fever, but the picture may be confounded by coincidental infection. Arthralgias are common; both a Reiter-like syndrome and a Sjögern-like syndrome occur with increased frequency in this disease.

Treatment

Most patients with HIV who exhibit rheumatic complaints are severely ill as a consequence of other clinical features of HIV. These patients may not tolerate many of the conventional medications used for arthritis. In general, most patients exhibit a mild to severe rheumatic disorder that is self-limiting and experience a good response to a combination of analgesics and NSAIDs.

Rubella Virus Arthritis

Arthralgias and arthritis are reported to occur in up to 50% of infected women as compared with up to 6% of men with this disease. This is an uncommon presentation in children with rubella. Rubella vaccine may cause symptoms in 15% or more of recipients. Joint symptoms usually start within 1 week of the skin rash in natural infection or within 10 to 28 days after immunization. Fingers, wrists, elbow, hip, and knee, as well as toe joints, are most frequently affected, usually asymmetrically. Sudden onset of symptoms is characteristic. Arthralgia and joint stiffness, as well as arthritis, may be accompanied by tenosynovitis and even carpal tunnel syndrome. Usually both the natural and the vaccine-induced arthritis resolve without residua within 30 days; however, some patients experience recurrent arthralgias and episodes of arthritis for up to 2 years and sometimes even longer. There are no abnormal laboratory findings in analysis of synovial fluid.

Parvovirus Arthritis

Most of the interest in arthritis syndrome in this disease has focused on the human B19 parvovirus. In children, complications of parvovirus infection can be severe, including the development of chronic hemolytic anemia with aplastic crises, hydrops vitalis, and erythema infectiosum (Fifth disease). Rheumatoid-like polyarthritis may occur in adults. Arthropathy occurs in up to 5% of children infected with parvovirus B19, often with a characteristic skin rash that may produce a slapped cheek appearance; however, less than 50% of patients have evident joint swelling. Human parvovirus B19 can also cause an acute, and occasionally persistent, arthropathy

in adults. The arthropathy is more common in women (60%) and is characterized by symmetric polyarthropathy with pain, swelling, and morning stiffness in the affected joints. The finger joints, wrists, and knees are occasionally painful. Acute costochondritis has been reported. Although the median duration of joint symptoms is about 10 days, pain and stiffness may persist longer and may even recur. A patient with acute parvovirus arthritis exhibits significant levels of IgM and IgG antibodies to parvovirus B19.

Treatment

Immunoglobulin preparations have been reported to be successful in patients with parvovirus B19–induced red cell aplasia. Acyclovir in postviral fatigue and NSAIDs have been used in cases of myalgia and arthralgia.[44]

LYME DISEASE

Lyme disease is caused by the spirochete *B burgdorferi* and is transmitted by the ixodes tick.[38] Lyme disease is endemic in the northern Atlantic states, the upper Midwest, and the Pacific West.

Clinical Presentation

The clinical progression of Lyme disease is generally described in three stages. Dissemination of *B burgdoferi*, the causative agent, is often accompanied by fever and migratory arthralgia, with little or no joint swelling, but frank arthritis may appear weeks or months later. Arthritis is usually episodic, affecting primarily large but also some small joints.

Stage 1 (Early Infection). The first sign of infection occurs within 3 to 30 days of the tick bite. It is characterized by erythema chronicum migrans. This rash occurs in 60 to 80% of patients and usually fades within 3 to 4 weeks regardless of the treatment, although the lesions may recur.[38] Other signs and symptoms include fatigue, malaise, fever, arthralgia, headache, sore throat, and lymphadenopathy. The spirochete may be isolated from the patient's skin or blood at this stage.

Stage 2 (Disseminated Infection). This stage of infection begins weeks to months later and is associated with cardiac, neurologic, skin, and musculoskeletal abnormalities. Predominant symptoms in stage 2 are debilitating fatigue and malaise. Fluctuating symptoms of meningitis accompanied by facial palsy and peripheral radiculopathy are the usual pattern. At this stage, musculoskeletal pain is common and migratory in joints, bursae, tendons, muscles, and bones. Pain usually occurs without joint swelling and lasts hours or days at a given location. Secondary skin lesions resembling erythema chronicum migrans occur in about 50% of patients.

During stage 2, about 60% of patients develop brief attacks of asymmetric iligoarticular arthritis, primarily in large joints. The knee joint is affected in about 80% of these patients. These attacks occur within 2 weeks to 2 years, begin about 6 months after the onset of the disease, and usually follow intermittent episodes of arthralgia or migratory musculoskeletal pain. Attacks involving the periarticular structures, including the peripheral enthesis (e.g., tendonis insertion into bone) have been reported.

Stage 3 (Late Infection). This stage occurs in approximately 60% of untreated patients and is characterized by chronic or intermittent arthritis as well as by the other chronic abnormalities. In stage 3, the duration of arthritic attacks increases to months, but individual attacks may be separated by remission of months or even years. Synovial lesions may show villous hypertrophy and mononuclear infiltrate. Chronic arthritis may lead to loss of cartilage, subchondral sclerosis, periarticular soft tissue ossification, bony erosion, osteopenia, osteofite formation, and even permanent joint disability. In this stage, spirochetes have been found in joint fluid, synovial tissue, and in blood vessels, mimicking endarteritis obliterans.

Diagnosis

The diagnosis may be difficult in early disseminated stages before zero conversion, unless one identifies the characteristic erythema migrans lesion. The diagnosis is based on the clinical picture, including opportunities for exposure in an area of endemic disease and a prompt response to antibiotic therapy. IgG antibodies are almost always present when synovitis is a prominent feature of late Lyme infection and often persist in cases of successfully treated inactive disease. The Western blot method should be used to confirm the presence of antibodies to *B burgdorferi.*

Treatment

Table 3–12 outlines the various antibiotic therapies available. In stage 1 of the disease, the recommended treatment in adults is tetracycline, 250 mg orally per day for 10 days. Doxycycline, 100 mg twice daily for 10 days is another alternative. Amoxicillin, 500 mg orally per day for 10 days is also used. Erythromycin, 250 mg per day for 10 days is a second-line agent. In children with stage 1 disease, amoxicillin, 50 mg per kg per day orally for 10 days is recommended; children should not be given more than 2 g per day. Erythromycin, 30 mg per kg per day orally for 15 to 20 days is an alternative drug.

In late stage 3 disease, adults should be given penicillin G, 20 million units intravenously per day for 14 days. Ceftriaxone is another alternative; 2 g per day for 14 days intravenously is recommended and will halt the progression of the disease in the majority of cases.[38] In children, amoxicillin 50 mg per kg per day for 10 days can be used in late-stage disease. Tetracycline, 30 mg per kg per day, can also be used orally for 28 days; another alternative is penicillin G 20 million units per day for 10 days.

SERONEGATIVE SPONDYLOARTHROPATHIES*

The seronegative spondyloarthropathies (SNS) are a group of related disorders that may lead to inflammation and fusion of the sacroiliac (SI) joint and, in some cases, of peripheral joints. The term *seronegative* refers to the lack of IgM rheumatoid factor in the patients' serum. Most patients with SNS possess the HLA-B27 antigen, and males are generally affected more often and more severely than females.

This group of disorders is, like RA, characterized by morning sickness, owing to the inflammatory nature of the disease. Unlike RA, these disorders lack serum rheumatoid factor and rheumatoid nodules, and tend to affect predominantly the axial skeleton rather than the small joints of the distal extremities. These diseases are compared in Table 3–13.

Although each disease has its own characteristics, there is significant overlap between them. As in RA, patients present to the emergency department either with an exacerbation of previously diagnosed disease or with new or undiagnosed disease. With the exception of Reiter's syndrome, patients with SNS usually have a subacute presentation. As long as the emergency physician suspects the diagnosis of SNS and refers the patient for timely follow-up, a definite diagnosis of a specific SNS need not be made in the emergency department.

Ankylosing Spondylitis

Ankylosing spondylitis is characterized by inflammation of the SI and intervertebral joints. Inflammation at the sites of ligamentous insertion (enthesopathy) leads to calcification and loss of motion of the joints.

Clinical Presentation

The presence of ankylosing spondylitis is suggested by gradual onset of back discomfort (often dull and difficult to localize), onset before 40 years of age, persistence of discomfort for 3 months or longer, and morning stiffness that improves with exercise. If there is no evidence of Reiter's syndrome, psoriasis, or inflammatory bowel disease (see later discussion), ankylosing spondylitis is the likely disease. Radiographs of the SI joints should

---

*This section was contributed by Robert Feldman, MD.

TABLE 3–12. RECOMMENDED ANTIBIOTIC THERAPIES FOR LYME DISEASE

Early Disease (Stage 1)	
Adults	
Tetracycline	250 mg PO qid × 10 days*
Doxycycline	100 mg PO bid × 10 days*
Amoxicillin	500 mg PO qid × 10 days*
(Second-line agents)	
Phenoxymethylpenicillin	500 mg PO qid × 10 days*
Erythromycin	250 mg PO qid × 10 days*
Children	
Amoxicillin/phenoxymethylpenicillin	50 mg/kg/d PO (not > 2 g/d) × 10 days*
Erythromycin	30 mg/kg/d PO × 15–20 days*
Late Disease (Stage 3)	
Adults	
Penicillin G	20 million units IV qd × 14 days*
Ceftriaxone	2 g/d × 14 days*
Children	
Amoxicillin/phenoxymethylpenicillin	50 mg/kg/d PO (not > 2 g/d) × 10 days*
Tetracycline	30 mg/kg/d PO × 28 days*
Penicillin G	20 million units IV qd × 10 days*

*Up to 30 days if symptoms persist or recur.

TABLE 3–13. COMPARISON OF SERONEGATIVE SPONDYLOARTHROPATHIES

	Ankylosing Spondylitis	Reactive Arthritis (Reiter's Syndrome)	Enteropathic Spondyloarthropathy (IBD)	Psoriatic Arthropathy
Age at onset	20–40 (average: 25)	20s and older	Adult	Any age
Onset	Gradual	Acute	Usually gradual	Variable
Sacroiliitis/Spondylitis	Symmetric (nearly all)	Asymmetric (common)	Symmetric (< 20%)	Asymmetric (20%)
Peripheral joints	Lower limb, hip (~ 25%)	Lower limb (90%)	Lower > upper extremity (< 20%)	Upper > lower extremity (> 90%)
Cardiac aortic insufficiency	< 5%	5–10%	Rare	Rare
Eye (conjunctivitis, uveitis)	Primary uveitis (25%)	Conjunctivitis > uveitis (50%)	Uveitis (< 20%)	Conjunctivitis > (20%)
Skin or nail involvement	None	Common (< 40%)	Uncommon	Nearly all (~ 100%)
HLA-B27 (20%	90%	75–90%	50% with SI/spine	50% with SI/spine
			(5% without)	without)

IBD, inflammatory bowel disease; SI, sacroiliac.

show at least some evidence of sacroiliitis. Spinal films show progressive syndesmophytes and kyphosis.

The symptoms of inflammatory back disease are particularly characteristic of ankylosing spondylitis. Some patients may continue to have only low back pain related to sacroiliitis, whereas others show progressively more widespread back pain and limitation of motion as a result of involvement of the lumbar, dorsal, and cervical spine. Few patients progress to develop the classic rigid bamboo spine. Patients may, however, have involvement to a lesser degree of the dorsal spine and costosternal and costovertebral muscle insertion causing ill-defined dorsal spine pain and pleuritic-type chest pain. Peripheral joint involvement frequently accompanies the back disease, with hips and shoulders being affected most frequently. Other joints affected are the wrist, MCP, and the MTP joints. Most typically, involvement is in an asymmetric pattern, but in some patients, the polyarthritis is symmetric, clinically indistinguishable from RA. Patients may experience a single episode of peripheral arthritis or have recurrent flares. Other manifestations of ankylosing spondylitis include fatigue, weight loss, and *iritis* in up to 25% of patients. *Acute iritis* is more common in HLA-B27–positive than in HLA-B27–negative individuals.

Pulmonary fibrosis, particularly of the upper lobe, is associated with cough, dyspnea, and sputum production. Aortic insufficiency caused by fibrosis involving the aortic ring and valve has been recognized for many years. HLA-B27–positive spondyloarthropathies are associated with severe bradyarrythmias, and these patients may present with symptomatic complete heart block.

Physical examination may initially be unremarkable. With progressive disease, the normal lumbar lordosis is lost, and marked kyphosis of the spine may develop. In advanced disease, the patient develops severe flexion deformities of the lumbar spine, with compensatory (and occasionally primary) flexion of the hips and knees. Laboratory studies are nonspecific. The ESR is elevated in up to 75% of patients with ankylosing spondylitis, but this does not correlate with disease activity. The HLA-B27 marker is usually present, but it is not readily tested in acute care settings.

Systemic involvement is less common and less severe than in RA. Acute anterior uveitis develops in about 25% of patients during the course of their disease and requires ophthalmologic referral for possible corticosteroid treatment. Patients with severe disease may develop restrictive pulmonary disease because of their stooped posture, and occasionally pulmonary fibrosis and cavitation with *Aspergillus* colonization are seen. Less than 10% of patients with severe ankylosing spondylitis will develop cardiac disease, including aortic incompetence and conduction defects.

The diagnosis of ankylosing spondylitis is frequently based primarily on the history, with typical features of inflammatory back disease and other manifestations as previously described. Standard criteria for the diagnosis of ankylosing spondylitis include the presence of sacroiliiatis. Radiographic changes range from vague loss of definition of the edge of the SI joint with some sclerosis to more definite sclerosis, indistinct margins, erosions, and subsequent fusion. Additional techniques such as radionuclid bone scan, CT scan, and MRI are occasionally helpful in clarifying an uncertain picture.

Treatment

The most effective treatment for ankylosing spondylitis is physical therapy, which attempts to prevent the progressive and disabling spinal kyphosis that characterizes the disease. Analgesic and anti-inflammatory medications are used to allow the patient to participate actively in physical therapy. NSAIDs, including indomethacin and naproxen, can be effective in decreasing morning stiffness and increasing physical activity. NSAIDs without physical therapy are of little benefit, and any patient seen in the emergency department who is using NSAIDs alone should be informed of this fact and referred to the appropriate provider.

Patients with ankylosing spondylitis should also be informed of the potential systemic complications so that they can recognize them, especially uveitis, and seek treatment before permanent disability results.

Reactive Arthritis (Reiter's Syndrome)

Inflammatory arthritis may occur in a previously healthy patient following an episode of infectious enteritis, cervicitis, urethritis, or less commonly, pneumonia or bronchitis. The arthritis occurs several weeks after the initial infection, and the infecting organism is not present in the joints at the time arthritis develops. Hence, the arthritis is reactive rather than infectious (e.g., disseminated gonorrhea).

The original description of Reiter's syndrome requires the presence of arthritis, urethritis, and conjunctivitis. The complete triad is not present in most patients with infectious arthritis. Organisms that may cause reactive arthritis include *Chlamydia trachomatis, S pneumoniae, Salmonella, Shigella, Campylobacter,* and *Yersinia enterocolitica.* HIV has also been implicated. The association of gonococcus and other organisms with HLA-B27–associated reactive arthritis is unclear.

Men are affected more often than women. About 75% of patients with reactive arthritis have HLA-B27. Although rheumatic fever is, in a sense, a reactive arthritis, it is not associated with HLA-B27 and is not included in the group of seronegative spond loarthropathies. The incidence of reactive arthritis following infection with a responsible organism varies but is on the order of 1 to 2% or less.

Clinical Presentation

Acute onset of arthritis occurs 2 to 6 weeks after the inciting infection. Distribution of arthritis is asymmetric, primarily affecting the knees and ankles. Inflammation is centered about the sites of ligament and tendon insertion (enthesopathy), including the Achilles tendon and planter fascia insertions.

Entire fingers or toes are often swollen, leading to "sausage digits." As with the other SNS disorders, low back pain associated with sacroiliitis may occur.

Nonmusculoskeletal manifestations include sterile conjunctivitis, which occurs in about 40% of patients. Iritis occurs in up to 5% of patients and may lead to permanent visual impairment and mucous membrane involvement with oral and genital ulcers. These ulcers occur early in the course of the disease and are usually painless; painful ulcers are most often the result of other disorders or superinfection. Cardiac (conduction system and aortic valve) and neurologic (central or peripheral) involvement occur but are uncommon.

Diagnosis

Synovial fluid analysis shows inflammatory cell counts, with leukocytes counts of 500 to 75,000/mm^3 mostly neutrophils. HLA testing is useful in making a definitive diagnosis, but is not available on an emergent basis. X-rays show bony erosion at sites of tendon and fascia insertion. Radiologic sacroiliitis tends to be asymmetric, but may be indistinguishable from the lesions of ankylosing spondylitis.

Treatment

Eradication of the inciting infectious organism may or may not affect the course of the reactive arthritis but seems prudent, particularly in the case of chronic infections such as *Chlamydia*. Some consultants recommend a prolonged (e.g., 3-week) course of antibiotic treatment in the hope that this will decrease relapses. Chronic prophylactic antibiotics are not recommended at this time.

The arthritis is treated with NSAIDs, usually indomethacin (25 to 50 mg every 6 to 8 hours). Sulfasalazine, or other immunosuppressive drugs, may be given by a consultant for refractory cases. Corticosteroid injection of a particularly symptomatic joint may also be performed by a specialist after infection is ruled out.

Patients often relapse; however, relapses are not related to recurrent infection. Treatment of a relapse is, as described earlier, primarily NSAIDs.

Enteropathic Spondyloarthropathy

Up to 20% of patients with inflammatory bowel disease (IBD; ulcerative colitis or Crohn's disease) will develop arthritis. This arthritis may be peripheral, affecting primarily the ankles and knees, or central, affecting the SI joints. Peripheral arthritis symptoms tend to occur late in the course of IBD, and tend to follow the course of the underlying IBD. IBD-associated spondylitis is unrelated to the stage or course of the patient's IBD and may occur before the onset of IBD symptoms. The joints involved are large and small joints, predominantly in the lower limbs. Frequently, there is a tendonitis with inflammation at the insertion of the tendon, which is the hallmark of this disorder. A peripheral arthritis, mainly asymmetric, appears in 17 to 20% of cases of IBD. Although GI inflammation usually occurs first, articular symptoms may precede the intestinal symptoms by months or even years. This is seen especially in Crohn's disease. The type of arthritis seen in IBD is an *asymmetric additive polyarthritis*. Erythema nodosum can be seen in the pretibial area with the lesions varying from 1 to 5 cm in diameter. One of the key findings in all of the inflammatory bowel diseases is that the effusion is disproportionately greater than the pain. Rarely, one sees no bowel signs at all, only fever, arthritis, malaise, and anemia as a presentation.

The prevalence of Crohn's disease has increased during the past three decades to about 75 per 100,000 population. Crohn's disease is characterized by the classic triad of diarrhea, abdominal pain, and weight loss.

Peripheral arthritis, mainly articular and asymmetric, appears in about 17 to 20% of patients with an equal sex ratio, as previously indicated. The peak age of this disease is between 25 and 45 years. Large and small joints are involved, predominantly those of the lower limb (most commonly the knees and the ankles but also the MCP and MTP joints). The arthritis is mainly migratory and transient and subsides within 6 weeks, but it may become chronic and destructive. In most cases, GI symptoms antedate or coincide with the joint manifestations, but the articular symptoms may precede the intestinal symptoms by years. Colonic involvement increases the susceptability of peripheral arthritis in Crohn's disease. Attacks of arthritis may be related temporarily to flares of bowel disease, although this is less pronounced than in ulcerative colitis.

In *ulcerative colitis*, the prevalence is 50 to 100 per 100,000 population. The disease seems to be more frequent in whites and Jews than in nonwhites. Abdominal manifestations of ulcerative colitis are diarrhea and blood loss. A pattern of peripheral arthritis and findings are identical to those seen in Crohn's disease, but their prevalence is much lower (5 to 10%). The disease onset usually precedes the joint symptoms, but a coincidental onset of joint and abdominal symptoms is not uncommon. In the course of the disease, the temporal relationship between attacks of arthritis and the flares of bowel disease is more marked than in Crohn's disease. Joint symptoms are more common in total than in partial colon involvement. Surgical removal of the inflamed colon has a therapeutic affect on joint symptoms.

Treatment of enteropathic spondyloarthropathy should be undertaken after consultation with a rheumatologist or gastroenterologist. Systemic glucocorticoids and sulfasalazine may be indicated, but initiation of treatment of IBD is beyond the scope of acute care practice.

Psoriatic Arthropathy

Fewer than 10% of patients with psoriasis will develop an associated arthritis. About 5% of these patients will have exclusively spinal involvement, and another 40% will have both peripheral and axial arthritis, with about 20% of the remaining patients having sacroiliitis. Some patients have a symmetric polyarthritis resembling RA; if serum rheumatoid factor is present, the patient is considered to have both RA and psoriasis.

Initial treatment of psoriatic arthritis utilizes NSAIDs. After a firm diagnosis is made, methotrexate and antimalarials may be initiated by a consultant.

Juvenile Spondyloarthropathy

Spondyloarthritis in children may be difficult to diagnosis. It often begins with peripheral joints and may simulate JRA. Arthritic symptoms may precede the development of underlying diseases such as psoriasis or IBD by many years.

The emergency physician should have a high index of suspicion for juvenile spondyloarthropathies in children presenting with arthritis. Joint infection must be ruled out by aspiration and culture. A history of preceding dysentary would likely lead to a diagnosis of reactive arthritis. Early referral to the appropriate specialist is essential.

ENTEROGENIC REACTIVE ARTHRITIS

Different enterogenic bacteria are capable of initiating peripheral arthritis: *Shigella flexneri, Salmonella typhimurium, Y enterocolitica* (especially serotype 3), *Y pseudotuberculosis*, and *Campylobacter jejuni* are the most common species. The disease is termed reactive arthritis, because the causative organisms cannot be isolated from the joint.

The peripheral arthritis related to intestinal bacterial infections resembles the clinical picture of spondyloarthropathies: an asymmetric oligoarticular pattern of joint involvement, predominantly of the lower limbs, accompanied by tendonitis (10%). Monoarthritis is a common finding as well as dactylitis (sausage-like toes and fingers). Men are more frequently affected than women (1:5). The arthritis develops generally 6 to 14 days after the diarrhea. The joint symptoms take longer to subside than the abdominal symptoms. Other symptoms are oral ulcers and erythema nodosum. The most common extra-articular lesion are ocular. Acute anterior uveitis and conjunctivitis occur in 5 to 30% of cases and are usually self-remitting. Urogenital symptoms (urethritis, balanitis, vaginitis) occur in about 12 to 20% of cases, although the infectious agent is usually absent from the urogenital tract.

The causative organism can be cultured from stool. The increase in IgM is short-lived, but IgG is persistently elevated. The joint fluid is inflammatory and contains 400 to 120,000 cells/mm^3, mainly PMNs. A characteristic of reactive arthritis is that the causative organism is not detected in the joint fluid of synovium. Endoscopic confirmation can be obtained, and the histology mainly demonstrates an infiltrate with PMNs, mucosal ulceration, and crypt abscesses.

Whipple's Disease
Whipple's disease is probably a form of enterogenic reactive arthritis caused by an infection of the gut, although no classic organism has been described. Characteristic periodic acid Schiff (PAS) staining deposits are found in macrophages of the small intestine and in the mucosa nodes; the cells contain rod-shaped bacilli. These bacilliform bodies are considered to be an etio-

logic agent as they disappear when the patient is successfully treated with antibiotics. Men are affected more often than women by a ratio of 9:1.

Clinical Presentation
Whipple's disease is characterized by weight loss, pyrexia, lymphadenopathy, abdominal pain, and migratory polyarthritis. Diarrhea with steatorrhea is usually the chief complaint and is observed in 75% of the cases.

Peripheral arthritis may be transient or chronic, involves large joints more often than small ones, and is predominantly polyarticular and symmetric. The arthritis may antedate the intestinal complaints.

Diagnosis
Synovial fluid contains a high number of cells (4000 to 100,000/mm^3), predominantly PMNs (up to 100%). Erosive lesions on radiographs are absent, although destructive lesions have been reported. As noted, PAS staining deposits are found in macrophages of the small intestine and in the muscuteric nodes.

Treatment
Treatment consists of tetracycline, 1 g per day for more than 1 year. Additionally, a high fiber diet can help.

Blind Loop (Klippel) Syndrome
Intestinal bypass surgery can cause a syndrome associated with arthritis and dermatitis. The involves bacterial overgrowth and mucosal alteration in the blind loop and is probably immune mediated.

Polyarthritis develops in 20 to 50% of these patients 2 to 3 months after surgery. The arthritis is polyarticular, symmetric, and migratory and may become chronic. The most frequently affected joints are the knee, wrist, MCP, and MTP joints. Radiographic erosions or deformities are not seen. Surgical reanastomosis gives complete resolution.

Coeliac Disease
Coeliac disease is known to be associated with abnormal intestinal permeability. Bowel symptoms are absent in 50% of the cases. Many disorders, such as dermatitis, herpetiforms disease, hyposplenism, and antoimmune disorders, have been associated with coeliac disease. Clinical features of coeliac disease are diarrhea (usually steatorrhea); constitutional disturbances such as fatigue, weight loss, and malaise; neuropathy; and osteomalacia.

The distribution of arthritis varies widely but is mainly polyarticular and symmetric, involving predominantly the large joints, hips, knees, and shoulders. Radiographic changes are rare. There is a striking response of the joint manifestation to gluten-free diet.

REFLEX SYMPATHETIC DYSTROPHY

Reflex sympathetic dystrophy (RSD) is the exaggerated response of an extremity to an injury. Although the precipitant is usually known, the pathogenesis of RSD remains controversial.[36] Most investigators suggest an abnormality of the central or peripheral autonomic nervous system. Some authors suggest a psychiatric etiology or a predisposition in patients who are sympathetic hyperreactors, emotionally labile, have a dependent personality with a low pain threshold. It has been suggested that secondary gain is a factor causing the symptoms.[36] Another widely accepted modern view is that injury causes an initial vasomotor reflex spasm. The resulting persistent vasodilatation with rapid bone resorption causes modeled rarefaction radiographically, progressing to frank osteoporosis. Meanwhile, decreased motor activity results in fibrosis, stiffening, and a "frozen" extremity. Neural disturbances then cause increased sympathetic tone and hyperesthesia, exaggerating the cycle.

Clinical Presentation

Pain in RSD is often but not invariably characterized as burning, although many other descriptions may be used. Pain out of proportion to the nature of the injury or pain persisting beyond the expected healing period (usually 6 weeks and almost always 12 weeks) should always raise the suspicion of RSD. This is actually the hallmark of this disorder. Tenderness is usually present and is diffuse. Allodynia (pain with light touch, a breeze, or cool air) or hyperpathia (pain with normal palpation or pain that lingers after a normal nonnoxious stimulus) are highly suggestive of RSD. Other signs and symptoms include dystonia, tremor, spasm, weakness, and difficulty initiating movement.[46] Classic features of RSD are the pain (often burning), tenderness that is diffuse with periarticular prominence, allodynia (touch sensitivity), hyperpathia (pain following repetitive stimuli), swelling, dystrophic skin changes (usually shiny skin), and vasomotor changes (color and temperature changes). Predisposing factors to RSD include trauma, peripheral nerve injury, myelopathy, brain injury or stroke, cardiac ischemia or infarction, malignancy, and some drugs.

Diagnosis

The diagnosis of RSD is best made by clinical assessment with careful attention to the symptoms and signs previously described. Pain, unfortunately, may be the only manifestation of RSD. Plain radiographs should be checked for osteoporosis. Local or regional sympathetic blockade may be used as a diagnostic tool. A triple phase bone scan will show diffusely increased uptake or delayed images. There are three clinical stages of RSD.

Stage 1. At this stage, early in the disease course, one sees erythema and increased heat in the extremity. There is a soft, puffy swelling of the extremity which is diffuse. The patient experiences hyperesthesia, and there is increased hidrosis. Contractures are not present at this stage; however, the patient has spotty osteoporosis.

Stage 2. This stage usually begins 3 months after the onset of the symptoms. The extremity is cyanotic, there is loss of creases, and skin is tight and shiny. If the hand is involved, which is quite common, then palmar nodules are present and the fingers show tapering. A brawny fusiform swelling is noted. The patient, again, has hyperesthesia as in stage 1, and increased or neutral hidrosis is present. Osteoporosis is more diffuse than in stage 1, and contractures are variable and may be present.

Stage 3. This stage occurs 6 to 9 months after the onset of symptoms. The extremity appears pale, cool, and glossy with tight skin. There is minimal swelling. Sensation may be increased or decreased. The skin is dry. Osteoporosis now is homogenous, and there are thinned cortices at the joint. Contractures are usually present.

Treatment

Treatment in the emergency department is primarily directed at making the diagnosis and referring the patient. Treatment methods include physical therapy, medication, peripheral nerve blockade, or sympathectomy. The goal of physical therapy is to counteract the clinical changes seen. Use of hot and cold treatments, massage, and transcutaneous nerve stimulation is aimed at desensitization. Active motion exercises are used to maintain or improve motion. Soft tissue contractures are treated with dynamic splinting. Medical treatment of RSD is controversial, and most authors agree that vasodilators should be used if vasospasm is present. Use of β-blockers such as propranolol has been advocated by some. Tranquilizers may help to decrease anxiety. Somatic nerve block may be helpful for well-localized lesions. Sympathetic blockade is useful as a diagnostic and therapeutic tool. The middle and the lower stellate ganglia are blocked in RSD that involves the upper extremity. In RSD that involves the lower extremity, the sympathetic chain at the level of L2 and L3 is blocked. If the patient responds initially but relapses, the blockade may be repeated several times. However, if there is still no long-term relief after three or four attempts at sympathetic blockade, then sympathectomy is indicated.[36]

FIBROMYALGIA

Fibromyalgia is an idiopathic disorder that causes chronic pain and manifests few objective clinical features.[89] The basic pathophysiologic abnormalities in fibromyalgia are unknown.[88] Clinical features include abnormal pain threshold, most prominent in the tender points region; paravertebral muscular tightness; limb girdle co-contraction; dermatographia; and allodynia.[44] Other characteristic features include fatigue, sleep disturbance, and morning stiffness. "Pain all over" and parathesis, headache, and anxiety are moderately common symptoms of this disorder.[86]

The diagnosis is based on clinical presentation of fibromyalgia and is 10 times more common in women than in men, with the typical age at onset between 35 and 60 years.[72] When fibromyalgia is primary, results of standard laboratory procedures will be normal or negative. A careful "point count" should be made in the patient suspected of fibromyalgia. This entails manual palpation of several areas of the body. Newly proposed criteria for classification of fibromyalgia are (1) widespread pain in combination with (2) tenderness at 11 or more of the 18 specific tender point sites.

The treatment includes reassurance, NSAIDs, and tricyclic antidepressants (e.g., amitriptyline), especially in patients with sleep disturbances.[72,86]

SARCOID ARTHRITIS

Acute sarcoid arthritis is usually associated with erythema nodosum and hileradenopathy and is frequently accompanied by low-grade or moderate fever.[20] The ankle and knee joints are most frequently involved in acute sarcoidosis. The patient generally has an atraumatic, tender, warm, erythematous swelling that often is clearly periarticular rather than synovial.

Diagnosis
Roentgenograms show only soft tissue swelling. Joint aspiration often yields no synovial fluid. When effusion is aspirated from the joint, it is most often mildly inflammatory; however, with leukocyte counts of less than 1,000/mm^3 predominantly, lymphocytes and large mononuclear cells are seen. Cultures are negative and crystals cannot be identified by compensated, polarized light.

Treatment
Acute sarcoid arthritis may respond dramatically to cholchicine.

GIANT CELL ARTERITIS

Giant cell arteritis is a relatively common disorder of the elderly and has an unknown cause. The onset may be abrupt or insidious. The most common complaint is frequently severe and generally well localized. Patients typ-

ically have proximal muscle stiffness and may also have fever. Malaise and fatigue may also be present. Patients may have pain with swallowing and chewing as well as with talking. Less common symptoms include occular signs and symptoms and jaw and tongue claudication, sore throat, arthritis, neuropathy, and large artery involvement. The most severe consequence of untreated giant cell arteritis is blindness.

Diagnosis
The diagnosis is established by the combination of a typical clinical picture and evidence of vasculitis on temporal artery biopsy. The ESR is elevated, generally to 50 mm/hour and frequently above 100 mm/hour, with a normochromic normocytic anemia noted.

Treatment
Treatment should be instituted immediately if there is imminent risk of visual loss. Confirmation biopsies can then be scheduled within the following week. When the diagnosis of giant cell arteritis is established, patients are started on daily doses of 40 to 60 mg of prednisone.

HEMORRHAGIC ARTHRITIS:

Hemorrhagic joint fluid is most commonly caused by trauma. In the absence of trauma, acute joint hemorrhage suggests the presence of a bleeding diaphysis, the rare entities of joint neoplasm, or pigmented villonodular synovitis.

Hemophilic Arthropathy
Acute hemarthroses are frequently seen in male patients with severe hemophilia of either the classic type (hemophilia A, factor VIII deficiency) or Christmas disease (hemophilia B, factor IX deficiency). The knee is most commonly affected, followed by the elbow and the ankle, but any large joint may be involved. Some degree of joint trauma usually initiates the bleeding, although it may be quite insignificant, particularly in patients with recurrent hemarthrosis.

Three stages of hemophilic arthropathy are recognized. The first is an acute bleeding phase into the joint that occurs in childhood after the child has begun to walk. The joints become warm and often are held at about 30 degrees of flexion. This allows maximal volume of fluid. The second stage is a chronic synovitis that occurs in response to repeated hemorrhages within the joint. The third and final stage is a destructive arthro-pathy.

In hemophilic arthritis, larger joints are affected more commonly than smaller joints. X-ray changes include subchondral bone cysts as well as broad osteophytes, which appear late in the disease and are similar to those seen in severe osteoarthritis. Findings on x-ray

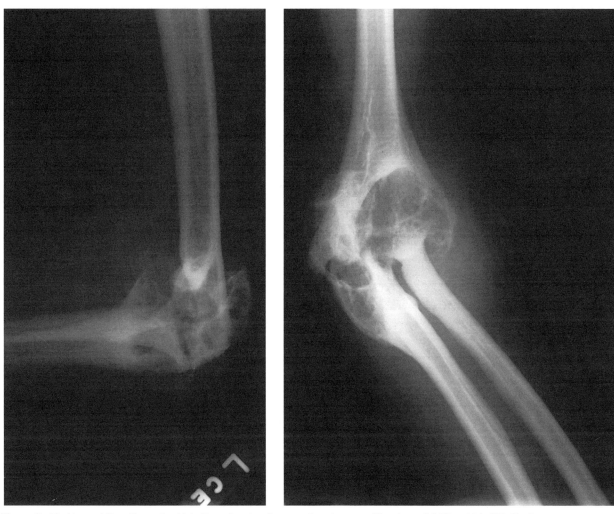

Figure 3–11. Hemophilic arthropathy. Note the extensive degenerative changes. *(Courtesy of J. Fitzpatrick, MD, Cook County Hospital.)*

that are specific to hemophilic arthropathy include widening of the intercondylar notch of the femur, squaring of the distal patella, and enlargement of the proximal radius (Fig. 3–11).

Before the availability of specific therapy with replacement of the deficient clotting factor, the recurrent hemarthroses of hemophilia led inexorably to chronic degenerative arthropathy. The repeated presence of blood in the joint space leads to pigmentation, hypertrophy, and ultimately to fibrosis of the synovium. Cartilage deteriorates and range of motion is decreased. The final result is clinically similar to severe osteoarthritis, with chronic pain, swelling, and loss of mobility. Osteophyte formation, diminished joint space, and periarticular osteopenia may be seen on radiographs in advanced cases.

Treatment

Therapy for acute hemarthrosis in hemophiliacs involved replacement of the deficient clotting factor, aspiration of

the hemarthrosis in selected cases, analgesia, and immobilization. In severe hemorrhage, repeated doses of clotting factor once or even twice daily for 1 to 3 days may be necessary. Patients must be referred for close follow-up and physical therapy to minimize long-term disability.

Replacement of the clotting factor may be accomplished with a number of blood products and concentrates. The patient or family members generally know the type of hemophilia present, which, in turn, dictates the necessary treatment. Hemophilia A may be treated with fresh frozen plama, cryoprecipitate, or factor VIII concentrates. The risk of transmission of hepatitis and the AIDS is increased in concentrates made from multiple-donor blood, but the large volume of fresh frozen plasma needed to adequately restore clotting activity usually precludes its use.

To calculate the amount of concentrate needed, the classic hemophiliac presenting with a bleeding emergency is first assumed to have a native factor VIII activity of 0%. It is recommended that the activity be raised acutely to 20 to 30% of normal in the treatment of hemarthrosis. The number of units of factor VIII clotting activity (the activity contained in 1 mL of normal plasma) required to accomplish this can be calculated as follows:

- It has been found that each unit of factor VIII activity transfused per kilogram of body weight will raise the patient's factor VIII level by approximately 2%. Therefore, to raise the levels to the desired 20 to 30% of normal for treating acute hemarthrosis, 10 to 20 units per kg of factor VIII activity are administered as an initial dose.
- If factor VIII is being used, the number of units of activity can simply be read from the container.
- If cryoprecipitate is used, each bag contains a volume of about 10 mL with 5 to 10 units of factor VIII activity per mL, or about 80 units of activity per bag.
- If, as a last resort, fresh frozen plasma is used, each milliliter contains one unit of activity, so 10 to 20 mL per kg must be given. Simultaneous administration of diuretic may be needed to prevent serious volume overload if fresh frozen plasma is used.

To summarize, a 70-kg patient with classic hemophilia and an acute hemarthrosis should receive about 15 units per kg, or approximately 1000 units, of factor VIII activity to raise the factor level 25 to 30% of normal. This can be accomplished by administering 1000 units of factor VIII concentrate, 120 mL of cryoprecipitate (10 to 14 bags), or 1000 mL of fresh frozen plasma.

Patients with factor IX deficiency (hemophilia B, or Christmas disease) are treated in an analogous fashion, but with different blood products. Concentrated factor IX is available in combination with factor II, VII, or X as prothrombin complex. The dose, in units of factor IX activity, which is indicated on the package, is twice the dose of factor VIII in treatment of hemophilia A because of the rapid diffusion of factor IX out of the vascular space after treatment. Fresh frozen plasma can be used as an alternative.

The duration of treatment of hemophilic hemarthrosis depends on the severity of the bleeding and the persistence or resolution of symptoms. Minor bleeding that is accompanied by little or no swelling may be treated with a single infusion of clotting factors. Because the half-life of exogenous factor VIII is only about 12 hours, however, any significant bleeding requires one or more repeated doses of one half the original amount of factor VIII until symptoms resolve. Consultation with the patient's own physician should be sought in these cases. Factor IX has a half-life of approximately 20 hours.

Large, tense hemarthroses seen in the first few hours after the onset of symptoms must be aspirated to prevent persistent pain and the development of chronic joint dysfunction. This is particularly true if the patient has had few or no previous bleeding episodes in the affected joint. Hemarthroses more than 24 hours old are usually clotted and cannot be aspirated. Aspiration must be performed during the infusion of factor VIII to avoid excessive bleeding or performed immediately after to avoid the early coagulation of the hemarthrosis. After aspiration, plasma factor VIII levels of 25 to 50% should be maintained for several days.

Whether or not a joint is aspirated, immobilization should be instituted and maintained until all symptoms have resolved. The patient must be referred to a consultant who will be able to immediately start a program of physical therapy to limit muscle wasting and restore joint mobility as early as possible. Ice and analgesics are important adjuncts in the treatment of hemarthrosis, but care must be taken to avoid salicylates and nonsteroidal agents that may aggravate the bleeding diathesis by inhibiting platelet function.

A brief mention of factor VIII antibodies is in order. A small percentage of hemophiliacs fail to respond to factor replacement because of high levels of circulating antibodies to factor VIII. A number of treatment modalities have been tried in these case, of which infusion of activated prothrombin complex is currently preferred. The emergency physician must seek consultation if the patient fails to respond to standard therapy or if a history of high antibody levels is obtained. Therapy with activated prothrombin complexes may be complicated by intravascular coagulation of embolus. Joint aspiration should not be attempted in patients with antibodies.

Thrombocytopenia may be present in acute hemarthrosis. Management, which depends on the underlying cause, is described elsewhere.

Joint neoplasms are rare, but they should be suspected in acute hemarthroses without trauma in which no bleeding diaphysis can be demonstrated. Symptomatic treatment and referral for biopsy are indicated.

Pigmented villonodular synovitis is a rare disorder of unknown etiology that may be present with acute hemorrhagic monarthritis.

TRAUMATIC ARTHRITIS

Traumatic arthritis may arise as an early sequela of joint injury or much later as a reaction to mechanical derangement of the joint such as a meniscal injury in the knee. There may or may not be a discreet history of injury to the joint, as occasionally the original insult is trivial enough to pass unnoticed by the patient. Joint effusions after trauma may be small or large. The fluid indices range from normal to frankly hemorrhagic. The rapid development of hemarthrosis after trauma suggests a major ligamentous injury or interarticular fracture. The presence of fat globules in the joint aspirate is diagnostic of a cortical fracture. Symptomatic joint effusion should be aspirated completely to avoid damage to cartilage from elevated pressure in the joint and to allow adequate examination of the joint for ligamentous injuries. In the absence of joint instability requiring early surgical intervention, immobilization and rest are usually adequate therapy. Repeat evaluation for a ligament or a cartilage injury after recovery is necessary.

NEUROPATHIC ARTHROPATHY

Neuropathic arthropathy follows a number of neurologic conditions. Although neurologic conditions are associated with this type of arthritis, controversy exists as to the true mechanism. Neuropathic osteoarthropathy is also referred to as Charcot's joints. A number of conditions have been associated with this form of arthritis, including peripheral nerve injury, spinal cord injury, multiple sclerosis, tuberculosis, uremia, and tabes dorsalis.

These patients present with a swollen, deformed, and unstable joint. Early in the course of this condition, the joint is usually warm and erythematous with hyperemia. Sensory loss and the absence of deep tendon reflexes are common in this condition. Two types of neuropathic joints are noted on x-ray. An atrophic joint occurs rapidly over a period of weeks and typically is seen in a non–weight-bearing area. A hypertrophic joint develops over a longer period of time and appears in weight-bearing joints. In the atropic variety, there is destruction and resorption of the joint. In the hypertrophic variety, there is massive juxta-articular joint inflammation with very large osseous debris accompanied by deformity and subluxation of the joint. The atrophic or acute variety poses a diagnostic problem in that it has been associated with rampant infection or tumor. Also, one sees virtual total destruction and resorption of the joint. The bone around the resorbed area is normally mineralized.

Treatment of this condition basically involves immobilization of the affected joint and restriction of weight bearing. Mechanical devices fitted to prevent accelerated bone destruction have been used. When possible, surgical arthroplasty can be tried, but it often fails. The emergency physician is primarily functioning as a diagnostician in this condition.

ACKNOWLEDGEMENT

The author would like to thank Robert Feldman, Assistant Professor, Department of Emergency Medicine, Cook County Hospital for his valued contributions to this chapter.

REFERENCES

1. Adams EM, Plotz PH: The treatment of myositis: How to approach resistant disease. *Rheum Dis Clin North Am* **21**(1):179–202, 1995.
2. Altman RD: The syndrome of osteoarthritis. *J Rheumatol* **24**:766–767, 1997.
3. Altman R, et al: The American College of Rheumatology Criteria for the classification and reporting of osteoarthritis of the hand. *Arthritis Rheum* **33**:11, 1990.
4. Altman R, et al: Arthritis and rheumatism: The American College of Rheumatology Criteria for the classification and reporting of osteoarthritis of the hip. *Arthritis Rheum* **34**:5, 1991.
5. Altman R, et al: Development of criteria for the classification and reporting of osteoarthritis of the knee. *Arthritis Rheum* **29**:8, 1986.
6. Arnett FC, et al: The American Rheumatism Association 1987 revised criteria for the classification of rheumatoid arthritis. *Am Rheum Assoc* **31**(3):315–324, 1987.
7. Baer PA, et al: Coexistent septic and crystal arthritis. Report of 4 cases and literature review. *J Rheumatol* **13**:3, 1986.
8. Baker DG, Schumacher HR Jr: Current concepts: Acute monoarthritis. *N Engl J Med* **329**(14):1013–1020, 1993.
9. Bamberger DM: Osteomyehtis: A commonsense approach to antibiotic and surgical treatment. *Postgraduate Med* **94**(5):177–82, 1993.
10. Bianchi S, et al: Sonographic examination of muscle herniation. *J Ultrasound Med* **14**:357–360, 1995.
11. Bohlmeyer TJ, et al: Evaluation of laboratory tests as a guide to diagnosis and therapy of myositis. *Rheum Dis Clin North Am* **20**:4, 1994.
12. Boumpas DT, et al: Systemic lupus erythematosus: Emerging concepts. Part 1: Renal, neuropsychiatric, cardiovascular, pulmonary, and hematologic disease. *Ann Intern Med* **122**(12):940–950, 1995.
13. Bradley JD, et al: Comparison of an antiinflammarory dose of ibuprofen, and acetaminophen in the treatment of patients with osteoarthritis of the knee. *N Engl J Med* **325**(2), 1991.
14. Brandt KD: Should osteoarthritis be treated with nonsteroidal anti-inflammatory drugs? *Rheum Dis Clin North Am* **19**:3, 1993.
15. Brower AC: Septic arthritis. *Radiol Clin North Am* **34**:2, 1996.
16. Chapnick EK, Abter EI: Necrotizing soft-tissue infections. *Infect Dis Clin North Am* **10**:4, 1996.
17. Crosby CA, Wehbe MA: Early motion after extensor tendon surgery. *Hand Clin* **12**:1, 1996.
18. Dagan R: Management of acute hematogenous osteomyelitis and septic arthritis in the pediatric patient. *Pediatr Infect Dis J* **12**:88–93, 1993.
19. Dalakas MC: Current treatment of the inflammatory myopathies. *Curr Opinion Rheum* **6**(6):595–601, 1994.
20. Dalakas MC: Polymyositis, dermatomyostis, and inclusion-body myositis. *N Engl J Med* **325**(21):1487–1498, 1991.
21. Dearborn JT, Jergesen HE: The evaluation and initial management of arthritis. *Primary Care* **23**:2, 1996.
22. Dieppe PL: Management of hip osteoarthritis. *BMJ* **311**:853–857, 1995.

23. Dieppe PL: Management of osteoarthritis of the hip and knee joints. *Curr Opinion Rheum* **5**:487–493, 1993.

24. Doherty M, et al: Inorganic pyrophosphate in metabolic diseases predisposing to calcium pyrophosphate dehydrate crystal deposition. *Arthritis Rheum* **34**:10, 1991.

25. Dzwierzynski WW, Sanger JR: Reflex sympathetic dystrophy. *Hand Clin* **10**(1):29–44, 1994.

26. Fox DA: Biological therapies: A novel approach to the treatment of autoimmune disease. *Am J Med* **99**:82–88, 1995.

27. Gibilisco PA, et al: Synovial fluid crystals in osteoarthritis. *Arthritis Rheum* **28**(5):511–515, 1985.

28. Ginzler EM, Schorn K: Outcome and prognosis in systemic lupus erythematosus. *Rheum Dis Clin North Am* **14**:1, 1988.

29. Goldenberg SA: Treatment of fibromyagia syndrome. *Rheum Dis North Am* **15**(1), 1989.

30. Harris C: Osteoarthritis: How to diagnose and treat the painful joint. *Geriatrics* **48**:8, 1993.

31. Harris ED: Rheumtoid arthritis: Pathophysiology and implications for therapy. *N Engl J Med* **322**:18, 1990.

32. Hayashida KI, et al: Bone marrow changes in adjuvant-induced and collagen-induced arthritis. *Arthritis Rheum* **35**:2, 1992.

33. Heffner RR: Inflammatory myopathies. A review. *J Neuropathol Exp Neurol* **52**(4):339–350, 1993.

34. Ho G Jr: Bacterial arthritis. *Curr Opin Rheumatol* **5**:449–453, 1993.

35. Hoffman G, et al: Calcium oxalate microcrystalline-associated arthritis in end-stage renal disease. *Ann Intern Med* **97**:36–42, 1982.

36. Inhofe RD, Garcia-Moral CA: Reflex sympathetic dystrophy. *Orthop Rev* **23**(8):655–661, 1994.

37. Jones A, Doherty M: Osteoarthritis. ABCs of rheumatology. *BMI* **310**:457–460, 1995.

38. Jouben LM, et al: Orthopaedic manifestations of lyme disease *Orthop Rev* **23**(5):395–400, 1994.

39. Kaplan D, et al: Arthritis and hypertension in patients with systemic lupus erythematosus. *Arthritis Rheum* **35**:4, 1992.

40. Khan MA: Spondyloarthropathies. *Curr Opin Rheumatol* **10**:279–281, 1998.

41. Khan MA: Spondyloarthropathies. *Curr Opin Rheumatol* **6**:351–353, 1994.

42. Khan MA, Van Der Linden SM: Ankylosing spondylitis and other spondyloarthropathies. *Rheum Dis Clin North Am* **16**:3, 1990.

43. Klenerman L: The Charcot joint in diabetes. *Diabetics Med* **13**:S52–S54, 1996.

44. Klippel J, Dieppe P: *Practical Rheumatology*. St Louis: Mosby, 1995.

45. Kolstoe J, Messner RP: Lyme disease: Musculoskeletal manifestations. *Rheum Dis North Am* **15**(4), 1989.

46. Kozin F: Reflex sympathetic dystrophy syndrome. *Curr Opin Rheumatol* **6**:210–216, 1994.

47. Krane SM, Simon LS: Rheumatoid arthritis: Clinical features and patogenetic mechanisms. *Med Clin North Am* **70**(2), 1986.

48. Kumar R, Madewell JE: Rheumatoid and seronegative arthropathies of the foot. *Radiol Clin North Am* **25**(6), 1987.

49. Laughlin RT, et al: Osteomyelitis. *Curr Opin Rheumatol* **6**:401–407, 1994.

50. Laughlin RT, et al: Osteomyelitis. *Curr Opin Rheumatol* **7**:315–321, 1995.

51. Lawry G, et al: Polyarticular gout: A prospective, comparative analysis of clinical features. *Rheumatology* **67**(5):335–343, 1988.

52. Lew DP, Waldvogel FA: Osteomyelitis. *N Engl J Med* **336**(14), 1997.

53. Machado EBV, et al: Trends in incidence and clinical presentation of temporal arthritis in Olmsted county, Minnesota, 1950–1985. *Arthritis Rheum* **31**(6), 1988.

54. Mader JT, et al: Update on the diagnosis and management of osteomyelitis. *Clin Podiat Med Surg* **13**(4), 1996.

55. March L: Osteoarthritis. *MJA* **166**(20), 1997.

56. McCarty DJ: Gout without hyperuricemia. *JAMA* **271**(4), 1994.

57. Medical Letter: Drugs for rheumatoid arthritis. *Med Letter* **31**:(795), 1989.

58. Medical Letter: Treatment of Lyme disease. *Med Letter* **31**:(794):57–59, 1989.

59. Mikolich D, et al: Polymicrobial polyarticular arthritis. *J Rheumatol* **21**:5, 1994.

60. Miller FW: Classification and prognosis of inflammatory muscle disease. *Rheum Dis Clin North Am* **20**:4, 1994.

61. Mongey B-A, Hess EV: Advances in rheumatology. *Radiol Clin North Am* **26**:6, 1988.

62. Ochi T, et al: Effect of early synovectomy on the course of rheumatoid arthritis. *J Rheumatol* **18**:12, 1991.

63. Oddis CV: New perspective on osteoarthritis. *Am J Med* **100**(suppl 2A), 1996.

64. Oddis CV: Therapy of inflammatory myopathy. *Rheum Dis Clin North Am* **20**:4, 1994.

65. Osial T, et al: Arthritis-associated syndromes. *Primary Care* **20**:4, 1993.

66. Pinals RS. Polyarthritis and fever. *N Engl J Med* **330**(11):770, 1994.

67. Puett DW, Griffin MR: Published trials and noninvasive therapies for hip and knee osteoarthritis. *Ann Intern Med* **121**:133–140, 1994.

68. Rahn DW: Treatment of Lyme disease. *Postgrad Med* **87**:6, 1990.

69. Ramos-Remus C, Russell AS: Clinical management of ankylosing spondylitis. *Curr Opin Rheumatol* **5**:408–413, 1993.

70. Reinherz RP, et al: Identification and treatment of the diabetic neuropathic foot. *J Foot Ankle Surg* **34**:1, 1995.

71. Rider LG: Assessment of disease activity and its sequalae in children and adults with myositis. *Curr Opin Rheum* **8**:495–506, 1996.

72. Romano TJ: The fibromyalgia syndrome. *Postgrad Med* **83**:5, 1988.

73. Schoen RT: Identification of Lyme disease. *Rheum Dis Clin North Am* **20**:2, 1994.

74. Schumacher RH, et al: Arthritis associated with apatite crystals *Ann Intern Med* **87**:411–416, 1977.

75. Sequeira W: The neuropathic joint. *Clin Experim Rheum* **12**:325–337, 1994.

76. Stanton RP, et al: Chronic recurrent multifocal osteomyelitis. *Orthop Rev* **22**(2):229–233, 1993.

77. Steinberg A, et al: Systemic lupus erythematosus. *Ann Intern Med* **115**:7, 1991.

78. Tan EM, et al: The 1982 revised criteria for the classification of systemic lupus erythematosus. *Arthritis Rheum* **25:**11, 1982.
79. Toivanen A, Toivanen P: Epidemiologic aspects, clinical features, and management of ankylosing spondylitis and reactive arthritis. *Curr Opin Rheumatol* **6:**354–359, 1994.
80. Towheed TE: Acute monoarthritis: A practical approach to assessment and treatment. *Am Fam Phys* **54:**7, 1996.
81. Trentham DE: Rheumatologic therapy for the 1990s. Evolution or revolution? *Rheum Dis Clin North Am* **15:**3, 1989.
82. Vitali C, et al: Disease activity in systemic lupus erythematosus: Report of the consensus study group of the European Workshop for Rheumatology research. *Clin Experim Rheum* **10:**527–539, 1992.
83. Wang A, Gupta A: Early motion after flexor tendon surgery. *Hand Clin* **12:**1, 1996.
84. Williams DN, Schned ES: Lyme disease: Recognizing its many manifestations. *Postgrad Med* **87:**6, 1990.
85. Wolfe F, Cathy MA: The assessment and prediction of functional disability in rheumatoid arthritis. *J Rheumatol* **18:**9, 1991.
86. Wolfe F, et al: The American College of Rheumatology 1990 criteria for classification of fibromyalgia. *Arthritis Rheum* **33:**2, 1990.
87. Wright SW, Trott AT: North American tick-borne diseases. *Ann Emerg Med* **17:**9, 1988.
88. Ytteberg SR: Infectious agents associated with myopathies. *Curr Opin Rheumatol* **8:**507–513, 1996.
89. Yu T-F: Milestones in the treatment of gout. *Am J Med* **56:**676–685, 1974.

COMPLICATIONS

COMPARTMENT SYNDROMES

Various muscle groups in the body are surrounded by fascial sheaths that enclose the contained muscles in a "well-packed" fashion, leaving no space for swelling should an injury occur. Several sites have been implicated where compartment syndromes can occur: interossei of the hand, volar and dorsal compartments of the forearm, gluteus medius, anterior compartment of the leg, peroneal and deep posterior compartments of the leg. An increase in intracompartmental pressure within these sheaths is the principal pathogenic factor in "compartment syndromes."[8] One must suspect a compartment syndrome early to prevent contractive deformities that result from ensuing muscle necrosis. The appearance of inappropriate pain, sensory symptoms, and muscle weakness requires examination to rule out a compartment syndrome.

In performing a neurologic examination, each potentially involved nerve traveling through the compartment is examined thoroughly using two-point discrimination or light touch. Both of these tests are more sensitive than pinprick.[8] The motor examination is performed grading the strength of all potentially involved muscles. Passive stretch of the involved muscles causes pain and palpation discloses tenderness and tenseness over the ischemic segments. The skin may be warm and erythematous even though the peripheral pulses and capillary filling may be entirely normal. Also, if the serum creatine phosphokinase (CPK) levels are 1000 to 5000 units/mL (normal is less than 130 units/mL), then a compartment syndrome could be suspected. Note that further tests must be performed for a definitive diagnosis.[9]

Four signs are reliable in diagnosing a compartment syndrome:

1. Paresthesias or hypesthesias in nerves traversing the compartment
2. Pain with passive stretching of the involved muscles
3. Pain with active flexion of the muscles
4. Tenderness over the compartment

If one "remotely" suspects a compartment syndrome, frequent reexamination in the hospital and measurement of compartment pressures must be carried out. Once the diagnosis of 30 mm Hg or greater within the compartment is made, decompression via a fasciotomy must be performed.[9] Myoglobinuria may complicate the syndrome and adequate hydration to maintain urinary output is essential.

VOLKMANN'S ISCHEMIC CONTRACTURE

Volkmann's contracture is the end result of an ischemic injury to the muscles and nerves of a limb. Volkmann's ischemia is an acute episode of pain aggravated by passive stretching and neurologic deficit resulting from ischemia of the muscles and nerves, which may result from a compartment syndrome. A compartment syndrome is a symptom complex caused by elevated pressure of the tissue fluid in the closed osseofascial compartment of a limb that interferes with the circulation to the nerves and muscles in that compartment. Volkmann's ischemia, if left untreated, will lead to Volkmann's ischemic contracture. Ischemic musculonecrosis and subsequent contracture classically follow a supracondylar fracture of a humerus but may occur with other fractures about the elbow, forearm, wrist, tibia, and femur. It can result from unaccustomed vigorous prolonged exercise in a young adult; in such cases, the anterior tibial compartment is most commonly affected. Here it is referred to as the *anterior tibial syndrome.* Vigorous contraction leads to excess metabolites that cause swelling and increased tissue pressure leading to a rigid fascial compartment resulting in ischemia. The patient is usually male and presents with an aching pain over the anterior aspect of one or both legs. The area is firm, tender, and swollen. If allowed to persist, paralysis of the anterior compartment muscles may ensue and result in a foot drop.

Passive motion of the involved muscles is painful and the skin overlying them is usually erythematous, glossy, and edematous. A sensory loss on the dorsum of the foot between the first and second toes is commonly described. This condition, as with other types of compartment syndromes, requires immediate fasciotomy as soon as the diagnosis is made.

Pathogenesis

There are two distinct types of ischemia that can result from circulatory injury: in type I, a proximal arterial injury gives rise to ischemia distally; in type II, a direct injury gives rise to ischemia at the site of the injury.[5] A severe ischemic insult may have three possible outcomes. Complete recovery may occur if there is good collateral circulation or gangrene may result. A "middle course" may ensue leading to contractures. Gangrene involves all the tissues, especially the most distal (fingers and toes), and typically demarcates to a level determined by the location of the arterial insult. A contracture is a selective ischemia of the muscles and nerves of the distal segment of the limb (the arm below the elbow, or leg below the knee), and the most distal tissues, such as the hand and foot, are not ischemic.[9] They are numb and paralyzed but this is due to ischemia of the muscles and nerves more proximally.

The ischemic process occurs in muscles that are confined within an osteofascial compartment: the anterior tibial, peroneal, and deep posterior compartments of the leg, and the flexor and extensor compartments of the forearm are the most common locations.

Clinical Presentation

Pain is the most important sign and is characterized as deep, unremitting, and poorly localized. It is aggravated by passive stretching of the ischemic muscle. Rarely, pain may be absent altogether. In upper extremity fractures, passive finger extension causes worsening pain, which is an early finding.

Nerve is the tissue most sensitive to ischemia, and the most important physical sign is an increasing neurologic deficit occurring in the nerves that traverse the compartment.[9] The sensory loss in the extremity may begin distally and extend proximally.

The distal pulse is rarely obliterated by the compartment swelling even though there is no circulation to the muscles and nerves within the compartment until late in the course.[5] The diagnosis of ischemia in an injured limb is usually based on clinical examination alone.

Treatment

Because more than a 12-hour delay may lead to necrosis and contracture formation, prompt early action is needed. Nerve injury alone is usually a neuropraxia; when it accompanies a closed fracture it is best treated by observation. Arterial injury warrants immediate operative repair, and the compartment syndrome itself requires immediate decompressive fasciotomy.

One must remove all circular constrictive dressings and relieve flexion if the elbow and forearm are involved. In partially reduced supracondylar fractures, skeletal traction is recommended. In some patients, interruption of the sympathetic reflex arc by stellate ganglion block in the neck may relieve arterial spasms. If relief is not obtained within 30 minutes, then surgery is indicated. When pain, inability to passively extend the fingers or toes, and sensory deficit are present, then fasciotomy is indicated. One must not watch and wait as the goal is to restore circulation before irreparable damage ensues.

OSTEOMYELITIS

Osteomyelitis is a suppurative process occurring in bone, and caused by pyogenic organisms. The bacterium most often isolated, in cases that are secondary to hematogenous spread, is *Staphylococcus aureus*. A mixed flora may be noted when osteomyelitis is secondary to spread directly from an adjacent wound. There are three types of osteomyelitis: hematogenous osteomyelitis; osteomyelitis that is secondary to contiguous focus that becomes infected, such as with an open fracture; and osteomyelitis associated with peripheral vascular disease.

In hematogenous osteomyelitis, the infection is localized to the metaphysis and then dissipates through the subperiosteal space to involve the bone. In osteomyelitis resulting from direct contamination, it is more likely to remain localized at the site of the initial infection. Hematogenous osteomyelitis usually occurs in children and is destructive to the long bones at the metaphysis where active growth is taking place. This type commonly occurs in the upper tibia or lower femur. This type of osteomyelitis may be secondary to a minor skin infection where bacteremia has occurred. The destroyed bone is absorbed by osteoclastic activity. In cases where the circulation is compromised, a sequestrum forms that is separate from surrounding decalcified bone and appears radiographically dense when compared to the surrounding normal bone.

Osteomyelitis secondary to a contiguous focus of infection is most often caused by an open reduction of a fracture. The long bones of the extremities such as the tibia and femur are typically involved. This type of osteomyelitis is polymicrobial in 30 to 50 percent of cases and blood cultures are less likely to be positive. Nevertheless, *S aureus* is still the most common pathogen isolated.[1]

Osteomyelitis associated with peripheral vascular disease is usually seen in elderly patients with diabetes mellitus. Also, the bones of the toes and feet are involved, usually the metatarsals and proximal phalanxes.[1]

Clinical Presentation

The onset is insidious, often preceded by an upper respiratory infection in cases of hematogenous osteomyelitis. There is often a slight fever, and minimal pain. When the process progresses, tenderness over the involved site is noted. In the direct form, pain and edema as well as erythema are noted around the wound and drainage occurs in most cases. The involved extremity is held in semiflexion and passive movement is resisted by muscle spasm secondary to pain that is noted as the process progresses. Initially there is no swelling; however, the soft tissues later become edematous as a subperiosteal abscess develops.

The leukocyte count may not be high although a shift does occur, and the sedimentation rate is almost always elevated. In more advanced cases of hematogenous osteomyelitis, the child is irritable and complains of headache, vomiting, and chills. There is often a high fever and tachycardia with an elevated leukocyte count.

Roentgenograms are of little value early in either form of osteomyelitis. In the direct type, demineralization and periosteal elevation followed by sclerosis can be seen after 10 to 21 days (Fig. 4–1). The most common finding in early infection is rarefaction indicating diffuse demineralization. A culture of a bone biopsy is the only reliable method for isolating the causal bacteria.[1]

Treatment

Antibiotics that penetrate the infected bone as well as joint cavity must be started. Good levels are obtained with the penicillin analogs. Surgical drainage of any abscess and debridement of necrotic bone must be done. Appropriate blood and wound cultures must be obtained to select the appropriate antibiotics. Antibiotics that demonstrate good blood levels as well as tissue levels in bones and joints are chloramphenicol, tetracycline, and cephalosporins. Also, hyperbaric oxygen therapy can facilitate the healing process in those areas with satisfactory cutaneous oxygen tension.[7]

GAS GANGRENE

Traumatic wounds may be contaminated and develop an anaerobic clostridial cellulitis several days after an inadequately debrided wound has been closed. This is the most

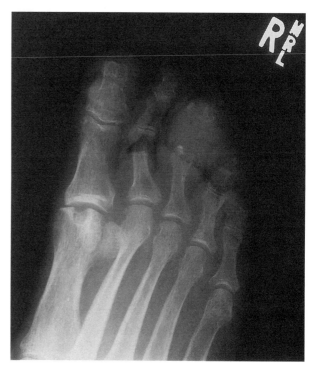

Figure 4–1. Osteomyelitis in the foot.

serious complication of traumatic wounds. In anaerobic cellulitis, the onset is gradual and very little toxemia is noted. The exudate is brown, and the gas that develops in the wound is foul smelling. No muscle invasion is usually present early in the disease. Anaerobic cellulitis can also be caused by streptococcus aerobacter or bacteroides. As the process develops, the original injury penetrates deeply into the muscles, and anaerobic myonecrosis evolves.

The initial symptoms are pain and a "heavy" sensation in the affected area. This is followed by localized edema and exudation of a thin dark fluid from the wound. There is tachycardia early, and the initial temperature is usually minimally elevated.[11] The condition progresses rapidly with increasing toxemia and local spread of infection. A musty odor to the wound is noted. Mental status changes often described as the "terror of death" on the face may be noted.

The treatment is prompt surgical decompression and debridement. Large intravenous doses of penicillin, 3 million units every 3 hours, should be started. When penicillin allergy is present, tetracycline is the recommended alternative at the dosage of 2 to 4 grams intravenously per day.[11] Hyperbaric oxygen chambers are used that presently yield excellent results. Fluid and electrolyte replacement is important in these patients. Studies have recommended the use of sodium salt over potassium salt in order to prevent secondary hemolysis and renal failure.[11] Polyvalent tetanus antitoxin administration with 50,000 units every 4 to 6 hours for the next 24 to 48 hours is indicated.

POSTTRAUMATIC REFLEX DYSTROPHY

Many terms are used that are synonymous with posttraumatic reflex dystrophy, such as Sudeck atrophy, reflex dystrophy, shoulder–hand syndrome, and causalgia. These are painful conditions that may follow trauma or serious infections involving the extremities. There are many theories that exist regarding the etiology, but no known cause has been found.

The syndrome can be divided into three clinical stages: early, dystrophic, and atrophic. In the *early stage*, the patient complains of a constant burning or aching pain in the extremity. This increases with external stimuli or motion out of proportion to the severity of the preceding injury. Following this presentation over the ensuing months, the skin becomes cold and glossy with limited range of motion. The *dystrophic stage* is characterized by the presence of chronic pain with neuropathic descriptors (burning, allodynia, dysthesia, hyperalgesia to cold) in an extremity.[13] The *atrophic stage* is characterized by skin atrophy contractures and severely limited muscle and joint motion. Intractable, osteomyelitis is commonly noted. In the shoulder–hand syndrome, a type of reflex dystrophy, the condition may follow contusion or myocardial infarction. Note that a diagnosis must be made before the early stage progresses to the atrophic stage.

In patients with a mild form, recovery may be spontaneous. The injured extremity should be immobilized, and the patient referred. A temporary block of the sympathetic nervous system has been proposed to treat the dystrophic stage. Several procedures include a local anesthetic, guanethidine or bretylium given intravenously, and chemical or operative sympathectomy.[13] No emergency treatment is needed; however, it is incumbent on the emergency physician to recognize the condition early, before the atrophic stage develops so appropriate follow-up can be obtained.

FAT EMBOLISM SYNDROME

The fat embolism syndrome (intravascular fat droplets) often results after major trauma, particularly long bone fractures. There are many theories and controversies concerning its etiology. An increase of intramedullary pressure transmitted via the draining veins to the pulmonary capillaries is called the *mechanical theory*.[4] The *metabolic theory* suggests that emboli arise in the plasma from conglomeration and fusion of pre-existing physiologic suspensions of tiny chylomicrons. The clinical syndrome is not uncommon and occurs in 19 percent of patients admitted with major trauma.[4] About one third, of cases are mild and require no treatment. Pulmonary involvement is the most common feature of the syndrome with tachypnea, dyspnea, and bilateral diffuse pulmonary edema noted.[6] The syndrome is seen in a number of unrelated conditions including respiratory distress syndromes, diabetes, sepsis after massive blood transfusions, and in patients with collagen vascular disease.

Clinical Manifestations

All cases have a latent period that varies from 4 hours to several days after the injury. The average time of onset is 46 hours. The clinical features of the disorder are divided into major and minor categories.[4,10] The major features are respiratory insufficiency, cerebral involvement, and petechial rash. Minor features include pyrexia, tachycardia, retinal changes, jaundice, and renal problems. The most common etiologic factor is long bone fractures in patients in the second or third decade, usually involving the tibia or femur. In patients in the sixth decade of life, fractures of the hip are a common cause of the syndrome.

About 25 percent of patients will develop symptoms in the first 12 hours and 75 percent will have symptoms by 36 hours. Many mild cases go unrecognized. Studies indicate that 60 to 70 percent of patients with skeletal injuries show some degree of hypoxemia.[12,14] The incidence is greater in fractures involving the femur or tibial shaft, or both, followed by hip fractures. The Po_2 commonly falls to between 60 and 70 mm Hg.

Early recognition is the key to adequate treatment, because fat embolism could lead to the development of a coma, severe acute respiratory distress syndrome (ARDS), pneumonia, or superimposed congestive cardiac failure.[6] Dyspnea and tachypnea are the earliest manifestations. Moist rales are noted over the whole lung field. These symptoms are followed by restlessness and confusion. The temperature may be elevated. Changing neurologic status is a reliable indicator of the syndrome's onset. Typically, petechiae are initially observed over the anterior axillary folds and the root of the neck. They are found in the buccal mucosa and conjunctiva also, and the distribution and intensity of the rash varies at times. It can only be detected in many patients with the aid of a magnifying glass.[4]

Fat in the urine occurs in 50 percent of cases within the first 3 days after injury. It is suggested that the detection of a rise in the serum lipase might be of value in diagnosing the condition early.[3] Chest roentgenograms show a patchy pulmonary infiltrate.

Treatment

The management of respiratory failure secondary to fat embolism is similar to the management of the adult respiratory distress syndrome.[2] Respiratory support with oxygen to keep the PaO_2 above 70 mm Hg is necessary. The injured part should be immobilized, and no excessive motion permitted. Although there is insufficient controlled data to confirm the probable value of parenteral steroids in the treatment of this condition, many recommend their empiric use. Massive doses such as 30 mg/kg of intravenous methylprednisolone are recommended. Controversy remains over the value of heparin, which is recommended by some as a lipolytic agent. Low molecular weight dextran may improve the microcirculation and is also recommended by some authors. It is contraindicated in patients with pulmonary edema, renal failure, congestive heart failure, or dehydration. The mainstay of treatment is respiratory support, which must be started early.

Blood gases should be obtained serially for the first few days in all patients with major lower extremity fractures who are somewhat compromised. When a prolonged stay is necessary in the emergency center, the respiratory rate must be monitored closely, and blood gases analyzed serially as the onset of the syndrome may occur much earlier than previously thought, and has been demonstrated as early as 4 hours after injury.[4]

REFERENCES

1. Bamberger DM: Diagnosis and treatment of osteomyelitis. *Compr Ther* **8**:48–53, 1990.
2. Gossling HR, et al: Fat embolism. *J Bone Joint Surg* **56**:7, 1974.
3. Gurd AR: Fat embolism: An aid to diagnosis. *J Bone Joint Surg* [Br] **52**:4, 1970.
4. Gurd AR, Wilson RI: The fat embolism syndrome. *J Bone Joint Surg* [Br] **56**:38, 1974.
5. Holden CEA: Compartmental syndromes following trauma. *Clin Orthop* **113**:95, 1975.
6. Levy D: The fat embolism syndrome. A review. *Clin Orthop* **261**:281–286, 1990.
7. Mader JT, Calhoun JH: Long bone osteomyelitis. An overview. *J Am Podiatr Med Assoc* **10**:476–481, 1989.
8. Matsen FA: Compartmental syndrome. *Clin Orthop* **113**:8, 1975.
9. Moore RE, Friedman RJ: Current concepts in pathophysiology and diagnosis of compartment syndromes. *J Emerg Med* **6**:657–662, 1989.
10. Murray DG, Racz GB: Fat-embolism syndrome. *J Bone Joint Surg* **56**:7, 1974.
11. Present DA, Meislin R, Shaffer B: Gas gangrene. A review. *Ortho Rev* **4**:333–341, 1990.
12. Tacharkra SS, Sevitt S: Hypoxemia after fractures. *J Bone Joint Surg* [Br] **57**:2, 1975.
13. Wilder RT, Berde CB, Wolohan M, et al: Reflex sympathetic dystrophy in children. *J Bone Joint Surg* **6**:910–919, 1992.
14. Wrobel JJ, et al: Inapparent hypoxemia associated with skeletal injuries. *J Bone Joint Surg* **56**:2, 1974.

BIBLIOGRAPHY

Eaton RG, Littler JW: Joint injuries and their sequelae. *Clin Plas Surg* **3**:1, 1976.

Feil E, et al: Fracture management in patients with hemophilia. *J Bone Joint Surg* [Br] **56**:4, 1974.

Frost HM: Inserting a needle into a dry joint. *Clin Orthop* **103**:37, 1974.

Gutman AB: View on the pathogenesis and management of primary gout. *J Bone Joint Surg* **54**:2, 1972.

Hassmann GC: Acute respiratory failure complicating multiple fractures in the absence of fat embolism. *J Bone Joint Surg* **57**:2, 1975.

Heppenstall BR, et al: Fracture healing in the presence of chronic hypoxia. *J Bone Joint Surg* **58A**:8, 1976.

Kleinert HE, Meares A: In quest of the solution to severed flexor tendons. *Clin Orthop* **104**:23, 1974.

Lancourt E, et al: Management of bleeding and associated complications of hemophilia in the hand and forearm. *J Bone Joint Surg* **59**:4, 1977.

Patzakis MJ, et al: The role of antibiotics in the management of open fractures. *J Bone Joint Surg* **56**:3, 1974.

Shea JD: Pressure sores. *Clin Orthop* **112**:89, 1975.

Tsuge K: Treatment of established Volkmann's contracture. *J Bone Joint Surg* **57**:7, 1975.

Warner T, et al: The cast syndrome. *J Bone Joint Surg* **56**:6, 1974.

White AA, et al: The four biomechanical stages of fracture repair. *J Bone Joint Surg* **59**:2, 1977.

5
CHAPTER

SPECIAL IMAGING TECHNIQUES

Plain radiographs are a sufficient adjunct to the history and physical examination for the evaluation of most acute extremity complaints. Several other imaging techniques, however, have become available that offer additional information. These techniques, which include radionuclide bone scanning, conventional and computerized tomography, and nuclear magnetic resonance imaging, are valuable in the evaluation of certain acute disorders. These techniques and the clinical situations in which they are useful are discussed in this chapter.

RADIONUCLIDE BONE SCANNING

Technique

In radionuclide skeletal imaging, bone-seeking isotopes are administered to the patient intravenously and allowed to localize to the skeleton. The photon energy emitted by the isotopes is then recorded by using a gamma camera. Numerous isotopes have been used for this purpose in the past.[24] Currently clinical bone scanning chiefly employs technetium 99 complexed with organic phosphates.[2] These compounds combine a low absorbed radiation dosage with high resolution images of the skeleton, which are recorded 2 to 3 hours after injection of the isotope.

The bone scan is an extremely sensitive, but fairly nonspecific tool for detecting a broad range of skeletal and soft tissue abnormalities. The pathophysiologic basis of the technique is complex,[6] but depends on localized differences in blood flow, capillary permeability, and metabolic activity that accompany any injury, infection, repair process, or growth of bone tissue. These

processes, as well as similar activity in the soft tissue overlying the skeleton, cause increased uptake of isotope resulting in "hot spots" on the scan. Comparison of the affected and nonaffected sides is generally used to detect differences in uptake.

Applications

Applications of the radionuclide bone scan in the evaluation of acute extremity complaints can be divided into traumatic and nontraumatic categories as follows:[19]

I. Traumatic
  A. Fractures
    1. Anatomically difficult locations
    2. Occult fractures (nondisplaced or stress fractures)
  B. Traumatic osteonecrosis without fracture
II. Nontraumatic
  A. Osteomyelitis
  B. Tumor, primary or metastatic
  C. Occult fractures
  D. Hip pain
    1. *Adults:* Aseptic necrosis, arthritis, transient osteoporosis, occult femoral neck fracture
    2. *Children:* Transient synovitis, arthritis, Legg-Perthes disease

Radionucleid scanning is used to diagnose a number of conditions, as indicated above. Some of the subtle problems that can be identified with this process are occult fractures, facet arthritis, and even difficult to diagnose inflammatory conditions that may not be clearly evident or may be confused with other entities. Tendonitis and tenosynovitis are both inflammatory

TABLE 5–1. SPECIAL IMAGING

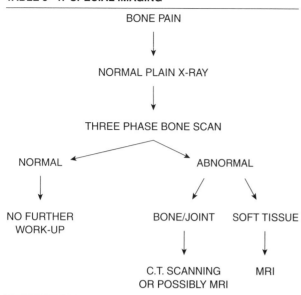

conditions of the tendon that may be diagnosed by bone scanning when it is difficult to separate them from other problems. Achilles tendonitis and patellar tendonitis have both been diagnosed by bone scanning in difficult cases.[10] Epiphyseal injuries, as well as facet syndrome, can be diagnosed by this technique. Table 5–1 indicates a procedure recommended by Holder that may be followed when one encounters difficult cases of potentially osseous pain with a normal plain radiograph.[10]

Traumatic Bone Pain

The radionuclide scan generally reveals the metabolic disturbance at an acute fracture site within 24 hours of the injury. The bone scan can, therefore, be used to diagnose fractures of such structures as the scapula, sternum, sacrum, and portions of the pelvis that are clinically suspected but anatomically difficult to demonstrate with plain radiographs.[23]

More important, the scan is useful in evaluating the possibility of fracture in certain locations that are notorious for having occult, nondisplaced fractures that do not show on initial plain films. The carpal scaphoid,[12] the radial head, and the femoral neck can be evaluated this way. Stress fractures of the metatarsals and other bones are seen on bone scan up to 2 weeks before becoming visible on plain radiographs. Thus, if a fracture is clinically suspected, but not confirmed with plain films, appropriate immobilization and referral for bone scan should be considered.

Rarely, part or all of a bone may infarct after trauma in the absence of fracture. The carpal lunate and metatarsal bones are most often affected[23] The bone scan shows increased uptake at these sites before the appearance of abnormalities on plain films.

Nontraumatic Bone Pain

In addition, the radionuclide bone scan can be used to evaluate any nontraumatic skeletal complaint that appears serious enough to deserve further investigation.

Osteomyelitis[4] causes localized increased uptake of isotope, which is visible on bone scan within 48 hours of the beginning of infection. In the emergency department, the technique is particularly useful because in many patients it is difficult to differentiate between acute osteomyelitis and a localized cellulitis that does not involve bone. However, false-negative scans have been seen after treatment with antibiotics or corticosteroids.

Tumors, both primary and metastatic, are usually detectable by bone scan by the time they cause symptoms. The ability of the scan to cover the whole skeleton is particularly useful for determining the presence and extent of metastatic disease. Care should be taken to obtain plain radiographs of areas suspected of harboring metastases, however, to rule out the possibility of benign lesions such as degenerative joint disease or old fractures.[5]

The bone scan is particularly useful in the evaluation of nontraumatic hip pain, in both adults and children[23] when plain films are normal or nondiagnostic. In adults, degenerative or inflammatory arthritis, avascular necrosis, transient osteoporosis, and occult stress fractures commonly present with hip pain. The bone scan is useful in distinguishing among these. Avascular necrosis appears either as a hot spot overlying the femoral head or as a cold central area surrounded by a ring of increased uptake. Transient osteoporosis, an entity mainly affecting young men, also demonstrates increased uptake of the femoral head when viewed under a bone scan. However, transient osteoporosis displays a decreased bone density when viewed on plain films. If osteonecrosis occurs, the plain films will reveal normal to increased density. Arthritis causes increased uptake of isotope in periarticular bone on both sides of the joint. Finally, occult femoral neck fractures resulting from normal stress placed on bones weakened by osteoporosis are seen on bone scan as bands of increased uptake localized to the neck of the femur.

The three-phase bone scan is very sensitive and is a study of choice in the evaluation of patients with suspected osteomyelitis and a normal radiograph.[21] An indium-111–labeled autologous leukocyte scan is the most cost-effective second study. This study can also be used in the evaluation of shin splints, stress fractures, and occult fractures.[21]

In young children presenting with unexplained hip pain, the differential diagnosis includes transient synovitis, Legg-Perthes disease, infectious arthritis, and osteoid osteoma.[24] The radionuclide scan is also useful in this population, although specialized scanning techniques may be necessary to produce high resolution skeletal images in smaller patients.

The bone scan in Legg-Perthes disease reveals decreased uptake at the femoral head early in the disease. Later, a ring of increased uptake may surround the cold spot. The bone scan is normal in transient synovitis. As mentioned earlier, inflammatory arthritis, including septic arthritis causes increased uptake of isotope by periarticular bone. Finally, osteoid osteoma, a common benign neoplasm that may not be visible on plain films when it arises in the hip joint, causes a very localized point of increased uptake on bone scan, surrounded by a diffuse area of increased uptake caused by abnormal vascularity. Plain films may reveal osteoporosis in periarticular bone.

TOMOGRAPHY

Conventional Tomography
Conventional tomograms are useful to evaluate injured extremities in areas where the three-dimensional configuration of the limb makes the plain radiographs difficult to interpret. The images are produced by rotating the x-ray beam through an arc around the patient's head such that structures of a certain depth will be stationary in the beam and appear with enhanced clarity, whereas tissue superficial and deep to this level will be relatively obscured by motion. The technique can be applied to any area where plain films give inadequate visualization. In emergency practice, tomograms are frequently requested to evaluate injuries of the spine and axial skeleton. Certain extremity injuries, however, may require the use of this technique. These include fractures of the tibial plateau, in which the degree of communication and displacement may be difficult to appreciate on plain films. Nondisplaced femoral neck fractures and pelvic fractures may also be evaluated by this method.

Computed Tomography
In computed tomography (CT), numerous individual radiographic density readings are assembled by the computer in a two-dimensional image of bone and soft tissue structures. The great advantages over plain radiographs are improved soft tissue visualization and the ability to produce images in the axial plane. Although the technique has revolutionized radiography of the cranium and spine, it is also useful in the evaluation of the appendicular skeleton for both traumatic and non-traumatic lesions.

CT has proven useful in the evaluation of pelvic fractures.[8,9] The axial format allows better visualization of anterior and posterior displacement than do plain radiographs. The acetabulum is well visualized by this technique, and the data provided by the CT scan may influence the decision to proceed with open reduction and the type of procedure needed.[14] The cost and radiation exposure of this technique, however, should be borne in mind and it should not be used routinely on all pelvis fractures. Simple fractures not involving the acetabulum, which are stable on clinical examination, are usually adequately evaluated on plain films.

The femoral head and femoral neck can also be evaluated by CT for the possibility of nondisplaced fractures.[20] The axial projection allows good visualization of the head of the femur and its relationship to the acetabulum. Bone fragments or distortions of the joint surface, which are not appreciated on plain films, should be seen routinely on high resolution CT.

There is some evidence that CT may be superior to conventional tomography in the evaluation of tibial plateau injuries. Rafii[17] and co-workers have reported that CT provided more accurate information on the degree of communication and displacement and, in some cases, changed the therapeutic plan in a significant percentage of patients with this injury who were evaluated by both techniques.

The role and technique of CT and magnetic resonance imaging (MRI) in the assessment of the Salter injuries to the physis, epiphysis, and methaphysis, and the analysis of growth disturbances and injuries to these structures has clearly become much easier with the introduction of these two imaging techniques.[18]

Computed Tomography in the Evaluation of Neoplasms of the Extremities
CT has been demonstrated to be an extremely valuable tool in the evaluation of bone and soft tissue neoplasms in the extremities.[1,7,23] Ordinarily, the emergency physician will refer patients with suspected bone tumors, but the increasing availability of CT may make this a routine part of the initial evaluation. Although the CT scan may not be diagnostic,[13,23] it often provides important information about the density of the mass, its relation to normal bone, nerves, and vessels, and the presence or absence of recurrence in patients who have been treated surgically. As mentioned earlier, the radionuclide scan is a more sensitive tool for the initial detection of neoplasms of the extremities. CT is probably more specific in narrowing the diagnostic possibilities and planning biopsy and definitive therapy.

Nuclear Magnetic Resonance Imaging
There is an increasing application of MRI in patients with acute musculoskeletal trauma; causing the identification of more occult traumatic lesions of bone.[16] MRI has been shown to be sensitive in the detection of occult bone lesions, and it can also detect and help assess both occult and traumatic bone lesions. It is indispensable in the diagnosis of a number of soft tissue problems. MRI is sensitive to the detection of occult stress and posttrau-

matic fracture and around various joints. The types of injury detected by MRI include bone bruises, stress or insufficiency fractures, and osteochondral fractures.[3] In addition, ligament injuries are easily detected by this modality.[11] Thus, anytime one has a diagnosis that does not show up on plain films and is unlikely to show up on CT scans, MRI should be ordered.[11,15,16,22]

REFERENCES

1. Caravelli JF, Heelan RT: Computed tomography of bone and soft tissue tumors. In Goldman AB (ed): *Procedures in Skeletal Radiology*. Orlando, FL: Grune & Stratton, 1984.
2. Carty H: *Radionuclide Bone Scanning. Regular Review.* Liverpool, England: Department of Radiology, Royal Children's Hospital.
3. Dalinka MK, Meyer S, Kricon ME, Vanel D: Magnetic resonance imaging of the wrist. *Hand Clin* 1:87–97, 1991.
4. Galasho CSB: Infection. In Galasho CSB, Weber DA (eds): *Radionuclide Scintigraphy in Orthopedics*. Edinburgh: Churchill Livingstone. (1984).
5. Galasho CSB: tumors. In Galasho CSB. Weber DA (eds): *Radionuclide Scintigraphy in Orthopedics*. Edinburgh: Churchill Livingstone. 1984.
6. Galasho CSB: The pathophysiological basis for skeletalscintigraphy. In Galasho CSB, Weber DA (eds): *Radionuclide Scitigraphy in Orthopedics.* Edinburgh: Churchill Livingstone, 1984.
7. Genant HK, et al: Computed tomography of the musculoskeletal system. *J Bone Joint Surg* [Br] 62:1088, 1980.
8. Gill K, Bucholz RW: The role of CT scanning in the evaluation of major pelvic fractures. *J Bone Joint Surg* [Br] 66:34, 1984.
9. Goldman AB (ed): *Procedures in Skeletal Radiology*. Orlando, FL: Grune & Stratton, 1984.
10. Holder LE: Bone scintigraphy in skeletal trauma. *Radiol Clin North Am* 31:4, 1993.
11. Horton MG, Timins ME: MR imaging of injuries to the small joints. *Radiol Clin North Am* 35:3, 1997.
12. King JB, Turnbull TJ: An early method of conforming scaphoid fracture. *J Bone Joint Surg* 63B:287, 1981.
13. Magid D: Computed tomographic imaging of the musculoskeletal system. *Radiol Clin North Am.* 32:2, 1994.
14. Manco LG, Berlow WME: Mensical tears—comparison of arthrography CT, and MRI. *Crit Rev Diagn Imaging* 2:151–179, 1989.
15. Moon KL, Helms C: Nuclear magnetic resonance imaging: Potential musculoskeletal applications. *Clin Rheum Dis* 9:473, 1983.
16. Newberg AH, Wetzner SM: Bone bruises: Their patterns and significance. *Semin Ultrasound CT MRI* 15:5, 1994.
17. Rafii M, et al: Computed tomography of tibial plateau fractures. *AJR* 142:1181, 1984.
18. Rogers LF, Poznanski AK: Imaging of epiphyseal injuries *Radiology* 191:297–308, 1994.
19. Schneider R: Radionuclide bone scanning applications to orthopedics in practice. In Goldman AB (ed): *Procedures in Skeletal Radiology*. Orlando, FL: Grune & Stratton, 1984.
20. Souser DD, et al: Computed tomography in the diagnosis of skeletal and soft tissue trauma. In Goldman AB (ed): *Procedures in Skeletal Radiology*. Orlando, FL: Grune & Stratton, 1984.
21. Sutter CW, Shelton DK: Three-phase bone scan in osteomyelitis and other musculoskeletal disorders. *Am Fam Physician* 54:5, 1996.
22. Walker CW, Moore TE: Imaging of skeletal and soft tissue injuries in and around the knee. *Radiol Clin North Am* 35:3, 1997.
23. Watt I: Radiology in the diagnosis and management of bone tumors. *J Bone Joint Surg* [Br] 67:520, 1985.
24. Weber DA: Radioactive traces used in skeletal procedures. In Galasho CSB, Weber DA (eds): *Radionuclide Scintigraphy in Orthopedics*. Edinburgh: Churchill Livingstone, 1984.

6
CHAPTER

PEDIATRIC ORTHOPEDICS

Children present with a different set of injuries than are commonly seen in adults. Ligamentous injuries are generally less common in children than bone avulsions. In addition, fractures in children are associated more commonly with growth abnormalities.[13]

The following terms used in pediatric orthopedics must be understood.[15]

- *Physis:* The cartilaginous growth plate that appears lucent on x ray

- *Epiphysis:* A secondary ossification center at the ends of long bones that is separated by the physis from the remainder of the bone
- *Apophysis:* A secondary ossification center at the insertion of tendons onto bones
- *Diaphysis:* The shaft of a long cortical bone
- *Metaphysis:* The widened portion of the ends of a bone adjacent to the physis

SALTER-HARRIS CLASSIFICATION

The Salter-Harris classification[9,13,17] refers to physeal fractures (Fig. 6–1). *A Salter I* fracture is a fracture through the physis. This accounts for 6 percent of all physeal fractures. These fractures may be displaced or undisplaced; there is no extension proximally or distally. A *Salter II* fracture is a fracture through the physis which continues on into the metaphysis (Fig. 6–2). This accounts for 75 percent of all physeal fractures. In a *Salter III* fracture, the fracture extends through the physis and continues into the epiphysis. This accounts for approximately 8 percent of all fractures. *Salter IV* fractures go through the physis and into both the epiphysis and the metaphysis (Figs. 6–3 and 6–4). This accounts for 10 percent of physeal fractures. *Salter V* fractures are the most serious accounting for 1 percent of phy-seal fractures. *Salter V* fractures are crush injuries of the physis.

Clinical Relevance
This classification is a radiological classification and is not anatomic nor related to the mechanism or severity of injury. A Salter I fracture if undisplaced may not be obvious on x ray acutely. Here clinical suspicion is the key to making the diagnosis looking for circumferential tenderness along the physeal area. These fractures commonly occur in the distal tibia and fibula and may present with the same mechanism as a sprained ankle without any ligamentous tenderness. In addition, these fractures occur in the hand and fingers of children.

Salter II fractures are those involving the metaphyseal region and the fracture fragment may be displaced or undisplaced. Undisplaced fractures in this area generally do not cause growth disturbances.

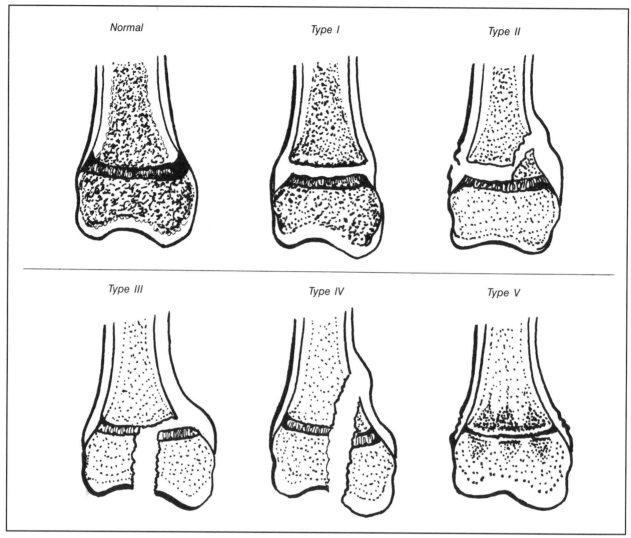

Figure 6–1. The Salter-Harris classification system used in epiphyseal injuries.

Salter III fractures are intra-articular fractures and must be accurately reduced. These usually occur in children who are older with a partially closed physis. These fractures should be referred early in order to have careful and accurate reduction.

Salter IV fractures need accurate reduction to prevent bone bridging between the epiphysis and the metaphysis since these fractures involve fracture through the physis and extend both proximally and distally. This fracture and the subsequent bridging can lead to partial or a complete growth arrest.

Salter V fractures may not be clearly visible at the time of injury and need comparison views and are diagnosed often in retrospect when growth arrest is noted.

A major concern with fractures involving the physis is the potential for growth arrest or growth retardation. One must remember that *any* fracture in children can result in subsequent disturbance of growth and that this is not confined to only those fractures involving the growth plates. Salter I and II fractures generally have the lowest risk of growth disturbance where Salter IV and V fractures have the most significant likelihood of disturbance. The Salter classification does not address mechanism of injury. In general, the greater the mechanism and force generated causing a particular fracture the greater the likelihood of growth disturbance irregardless of the fracture type. In addition, the location of a fracture is of key importance in terms of growth disturbance; a fracture through the physis of the femoral head is of greater significance in terms of growth disturbance as compared to a fracture of higher degree of the digits.

□ EVALUATION OF THE CHILD[16]

In evaluating a child one must remember to carefully palpate the uninjured extremity first in order to obtain the child's confidence. Check into the severity of the

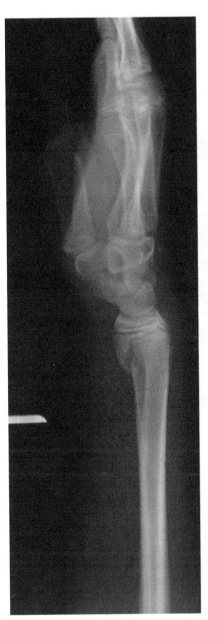
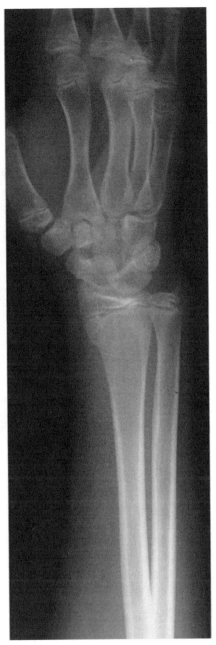
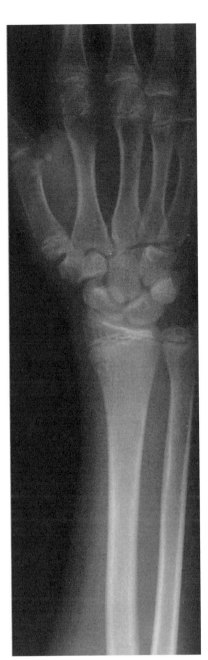

Figure 6-2. A Salter II fracture is demonstrated.

trauma that has caused the injury. Determine whether the history that is given by the parents or guardians is consistent with the observed injuries or whether there is a suggestion of child abuse.

In examining the extremity, neurological evaluation is difficult. Look for a generalized withdrawal response when using pinprick. In examining a child's hand or foot for injury to the nerves one can immerse the extremity for a period of 20 to 30 minutes. One should note wrinkling of skin if the nerve is intact. In assessing the vascular status of the extremity, palpation of pulses may be difficult because of the subcutaneous fat and thus one should assess capillary refill.

It is important to clinically correlate your findings with the history provided. A fracture may be difficult to find in an injured extremity in a child who is crying. On physical examination palpation of areas which are not fractured generally will hurt less than areas which are and the region is usually swollen. Palpation should be gentle but with enough pressure so as to make a comparison between the normal and abnormal region in a child who is irritable.

Radiological Exam

In doing x rays of children always remember that you need at least two views which are perpendicular to one

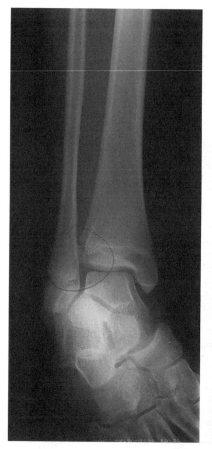
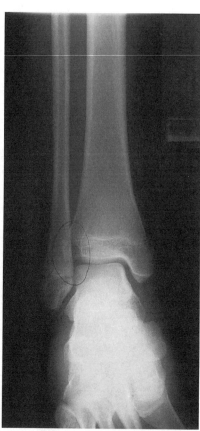

Figure 6–3. A Salter III fracture extending through the distal tibia into the joint is shown.

another. In addition, *comparison views* are invaluable particularly in fractures which are subtle (Fig. 6–5). Look at the growth plates of both sides in comparison views taken in exactly the same position of joints to determine injury there. Order views of an entire extremity and include both joints at either end of long bones. Anterior and posterier fat pad signs will help identify subtle fractures (Fig. 6–6). One should also identify when epiphiseal centers begin to appear (Fig. 6–7).

☐ FRACTURES UNIQUE TO CHILDREN

The bone in children is more porous than that of adults and thus fractures may not appear because the bone may undergo greater plastic deformation causing microfractures not seen in adults. These microfractures are not visualized on routine x rays and the patient may present with tenderness, although with a normal x ray, and the mechanism may suggest significant trauma to the bone or joint.

Torus fractures (buckle) involve a failure of bone with a compressive mechanism. These fractures occur over the metaphyseal region. Traumatic bowing is a deformation that occurs due to the plastic nature of bones in small children without a resulting fracture. Torus or buckle fractures of the distal radius are very common, stable, and heal readily with minimal protection in 2 to 3 weeks.[6] This injury is generally immobilized in a short-arm cast if it involves the forearm; or, a splint can be applied for relief of pain during healing. Complications are quite rare.[6] Greenstick fractures are incomplete fractures that result in a fracture through the tension side of a bone undergoing a deforming stress (Fig. 6–8).

A minimally displaced fracture may result in serious associated soft tissue injury and visceral injuries caused by the displacement of the bone during the fracture mechanism. Thus, a minimally displaced pelvic fracture may be associated with a more significant bladder, sacral plexus, or urethral injury than is seen with a similarly displaced fracture in an adult. Lumbar spine fractures in children who are wearing seatbelts almost invariably are associated with a ruptured viscus due to the elasticity of their bones.[17]

☐ JOINT INJURIES IN CHILDREN

Traumatic joint dislocations are quite unusual in children with the exception of the patellofemoral joint. The ligaments are usually attached to the epiphysis, and the ligaments are virtually the same strength in children as

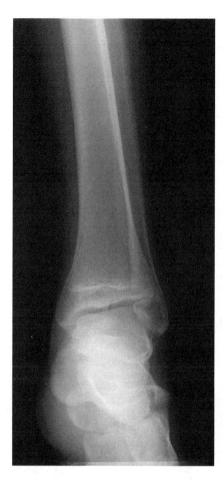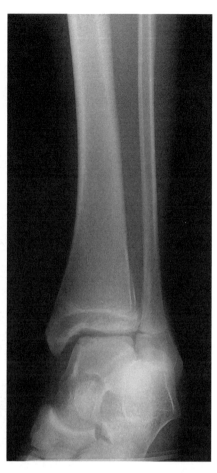

Figure 6–4. A Salter IV fracture of the ankle is shown. (*Courtesy of R. Udesky, MD.*)

they are in adults. Thus, ligamentous injuries are uncommon, however, epiphyseal injuries are more likely to occur. Excessive force on a child's joint usually results in bone failure and not ligamentous injury or dislocation.

☐ Fractures of the Distal Radius and Ulnar

The distal radial physis is the most commonly fractured growth plate. Salter II injuries are the most common, accounting for 58 percent of these fractures.[6] It is sometimes difficult to achieve full reduction of these injuries. The acceptable amount of displacement is not entirely known, although 30 percent physeal displacement seems to heal readily, while 50 percent displacement has remodeled completely with no functional deficit within $1\frac{1}{2}$ years of injury.[6]

Ulnar physeal injuries are less common and occur in only 5 percent of distal forearm fractures. The thick, triangular fibrocartilage complex protects the distal ulnar physis but concentrates force on the attachment to the styloid. Unfortunately, distal ulnar growth arrest occurs in approximately 55 percent of these fractures when they are associated with distal radius fractures.[6] Salter I injuries were the most common pattern occurring in half of the patients. Approximately 70 to 80 percent of the longitudinal growth of the ulnar comes from the distal

physis. Thus, growth arrest can cause significant shortening as well as a milder radial shortening because of a tethering effect.[6] Surgical correction has been advocated mainly for cosmetic improvement when desired by the patient.

Displaced or angulated distal forearm fractures in children, unlike the occurrence in adults, have a great ability to remodel. They rarely lead to dysfunction. Thus, angulation of a distal forearm fracture of at least 20 degrees can be accepted in the younger child, especially under 10 years of age. When a Galeazzi-type fracture occurs in a child, it can usually be treated nonoperatively[6] (discussed in chapter 10). A Galeazzi fracture is defined as a distal radius fracture with disruption of the distal radial ulnar joint.

☐ CHILDREN'S FRACTURES AROUND THE ELBOW

The elbow is a common site for fractures in children. Approximately 9 percent of all fractures in children occur around the elbow joint. The typical history is a fall on the outstretched arm with hyperextension at the elbow. Eighty-five percent of these fractures involve the distal humerus.

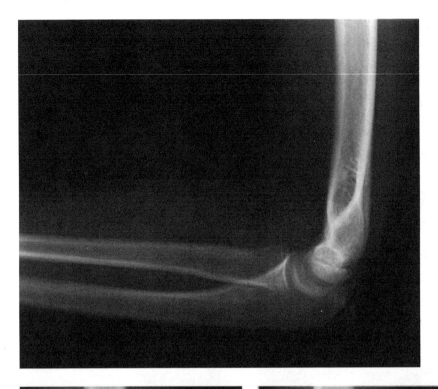

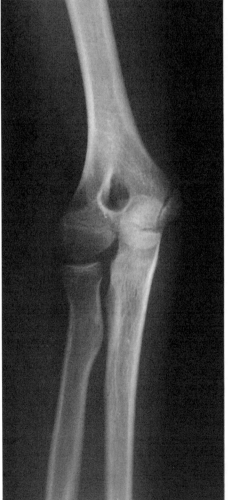

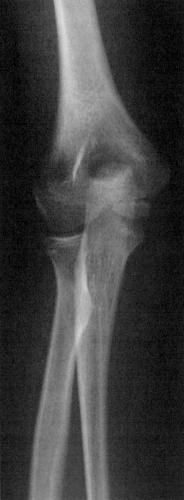

Figure 6–5. Normal growth plates in the elbow of a 13 1/2-year–old girl.

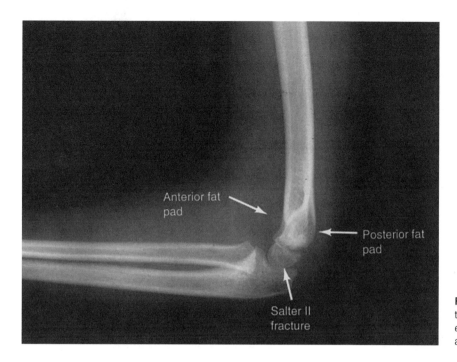

Figure 6-6. A subtle Salter II fracture of the elbow is shown on the lateral view. Notice the anterior fat pad and posterior fat pad.

Radiological evaluation of a child's elbow is made more complicated because of the six ossification centers around the elbow which appear at different ages in both boys and girls. Always remember to get comparison views of the opposite elbow. The age of appearance of common ossification centers in the elbow are as follows:

Appearance of Ossification Center

Radial head	3 to 5 years
Capitellum	1 to 8 months
Trochlea	7 to 9 years
Medial epicondyle	5 to 7 years
Olecranon	8 to 11 years
Lateral epicondyle	11 to 14 years

In assessing the likelihood of a supercondylar fracture in a child look at the *anterior humeral line* (Fig. 6–9). This is a line drawn along the anterior portion of the humeral shaft directed perpendicularly downward on the lateral view (Fig. 6–10). This line should pass through the center of the ossification center of the capitellum in the distal humerus. If the line does not pass through the center it is highly suggestive of a supracondylar fracture at the humerus.

Elevation of the fat pad in the coronoid fossa (anterior fat pad sign) and of the olecranon fossa (posterior fat pad sign) occurring due to an effusion from trauma or an infection is an important feature to investigate.

The elbow is usually swollen with abnormality of the bony landmarks which are often impossible to palpate. Always remember to obtain four views when the elbow is flexed following an injury to accurately assess the elbow in children. These four views obtained in the flexed elbow include the anteroposterior (AP) view of the forearm, the AP view of the humerus, the lateral view of the forearm, and the lateral view of the humerus.

Nerve injury occurs in approximately 7 percent of all supracondylar fractures (Fig. 6–11). The median nerve and radial nerve are injured commonly. When the anterior interosseous nerve is injured there is loss of the thumb interphalangeal (IP) joint in flexion and the index distal interphalangeal (DIP) joint in flexion. Although nerve injury is uncommon with supracondylar fractures; brachial artery compromise which can lead to Volkmann's ischemia (compartment syndrome) is not an uncommon complication with these fractures. The compartment syndrome which may result leads to diminished perfusion and loss of function of the muscles within the forearm. An intact radial pulse at the wrist has no merit in ruling out the evolution of a compartment syndrome or in evaluating the perfusion to the forearm. Review the detailed discussion of compartment syndromes which is presented under complications in Chapter 4.

Fractures that commonly occur around the elbow in children in addition to supracondylar fractures are radial neck fractures, which are usually buckle fractures and are thus easy to overlook. In addition, lateral condyle and medial epicondyle fractures are seen. Medial epicondyle fractures are associated with elbow dislocations. Nursemaid's elbow, which is a subluxation of the radial head, is almost always seen under 5 years of age and is due to a pull on the extended elbow; this is discussed in Chapter 12 on elbow injuries. One must remember that up to 30 percent of nursemaid's elbows tend to recur.

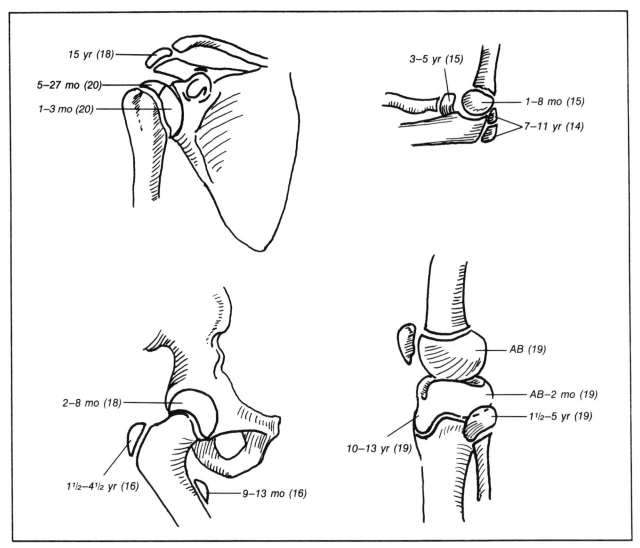

Figure 6–7. The epiphyseal regions at the major joints in the body. The age is shown at which the centers of ossification appear on roentgenograms in months or years. The age at which union occurs is shown in parentheses. AB = at birth. *(Modified from Brashear, Raney).* Shand's Handbook of Orthopaedic Surgery. *St. Louis, Mosby, 1978.)*

□ FRACTURES OF THE RADIUS AND ULNA

The most common childhood fractures are those involving the radius and ulna. When the epiphysis is not yet ossified and one suspects a radial head fracture, look at the *radiocapitellar line* (Fig. 6–12), however, Figure 6–12 demonstrates the fractures to the radial head with displacement which would be difficult to detect otherwise.

In most children who have radius and ulna fractures both bones are usually injured. Monteggia fractures involving the proximal ulna associated with a radial head dislocation are sometimes missed. The radial head should always be in good alignment with the capitellum. Galeazzi fractures involve a distal radius fracture associated with a distal radioulnar dislocation.

□ HIP PROBLEMS IN CHILDREN

A detailed discussion of hip disorders that occur in children is presented under the hip and pelvis in Chapter 26. One must remember that slipped capital femoral epiphysis is a disease that is commonly seen and affects adolescence. Approximately 90 percent of the children are obese and this condition is more common in boys than in girls. In 20 percent of patients the slipped capital femoral epiphysis is bilateral. The classical presentation is that of an externally rotated extremity with a Trendelenburg gait with groin and knee pain.[2] Some of these presentations are painless, however.

Transient synovitis is the most common cause of acute hip pain in children between 3 and 10 years of age. Typically, these children present with hip pain of 1 to 3 days, duration accompanied by a limp or a

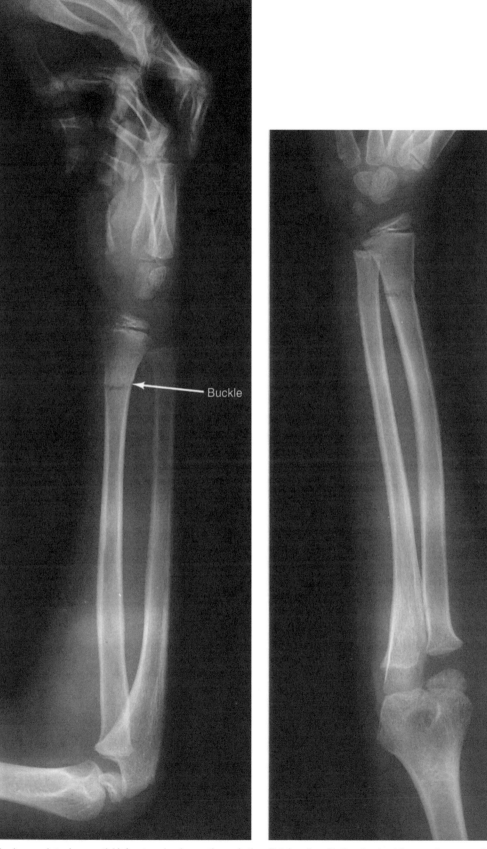

Figure 6–8. An incomplete (greenstick) fracture is shown through the distal radius. Notice the buckling on the opposite side. If a complete fracture was not sustained and only the buckling occurred, this would be called a "torus" fracture.

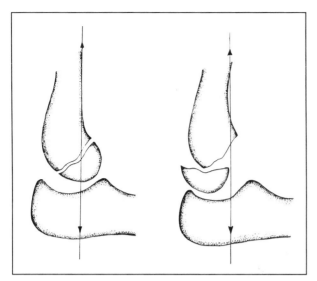

Figure 6–9. The anterior humeral line is a line drawn on the lateral radiograph along the anterior surface of the humerus through the elbow. Normally this line transects through the middle of the capitellum. With an extension fracture of the supracondylar region, this line will either transect the anterior third of the capitellum or pass entirely anterior to it.

refusal to bear weight. This condition has an uncertain etiology and it is diagnosised through a process of exclusion. Septic arthritis must first be ruled out, because femoral head destruction and degenerative arthritis will result if septic arthritis is not treated promptly.[11] In differentiating the two conditions, patients with septic arthritis have a significantly higher temperature, usually greater than 101°F compared with the children with transient synovitis, who have an average temperature of 99°F. One study designed to provide guidance in distinguishing transient synovitis of the hip from septic arthritis found several criteria to be helpful: Severe hip pain and spasm were present in 11 percent of patients with transient synovitis, but in 62 percent of patients with septic arthritis. Tenderness on palpation was present in 17 percent of patients with transient synovitis, but in 86 percent of patients with septic arthritis. A temperature of 38°C or higher was present in 8 percent of patients with transient synovitis, but in 81 percent of patients with septic arthritis. Sedimentation rates greater than or equal to 20 mL per hour were present in 11 percent of patients with transient synovitis versus 91 percent of patients with septic arthritis.[11]

Axiom: *Remember that any child who presents with knee pain who has a normal knee examination must have the hip examined for possible etiology.*

☐ INJURIES OF THE KNEE AND ANKLE IN CHILDREN

Ligamentous injuries involving the knee or ankle are uncommon in children in that the bone is weaker than the ligaments, as indicated earlier. When one has a mechanism of inversion of an ankle, suspect a physeal fracture of the distal tibia rather than a ligamentous injury of the anterior collateral ligament. In the knee, whereas an adult will experience a talofibular ligament rupture, in the child one will see a Salter I or II fracture of the proximal tibia or distal femur. In a rotational injury to the knee or a varus stress of the knee in a child, one will obtain an avulsion of the tibial spine more frequently than an anterior cruciate ligament rupture. By the same token whereas it is more common in the adult to have a rupture of the patellar tendon or quadriceps tendon from an extension block injury to the quadriceps apparatus, in the child an avulsion of the tibial tubercle is far more likely. In children with ankle or knee injuries who present with an effusion, if after obtaining x rays and examining the child one is uncertain whether there is a fracture, one should not aspirate the effusion but rather immobilize the extremity and return the patient to a clinic within approximately 2 weeks.

In dealing with a patellar injury or dislocation, always remember to examine the undersurface of the patellae, as osteochondral chip fractures are more common in children than in adults. The same is true of the ankle, as talar dome fractures are far more common in children than in adults. An osteochondral fracture of the talar dome should be highly suspected whenever one is dealing with a child who presents with an unhealing-ankle sprain or recurrent effusions after an ankle sprain.

Tarsal coalition should be suspected in any child with a history of multiple ankle sprains who demonstrates subtalar stiffness on a physical examination. The typical age is between 8 and 16 years, but may be older. A family history of tarsal coalition may exist. Of all the coalition syndromes, talocalcaneal is the most frequent type. The initial treatment is conservative, consisting of rest and a short-leg cast for 2 to 4 weeks or the use of a well-molded orthotic and physical therapy. Thus, these patients should be referred for appropriate care and follow-up.

Pes planus occurs quite commonly; the incidence of flat feet is approximately 7 to 22 percent.[10] Most patients are asymptomatic. This condition generally does not cause any problems in children. Treatment of symptomatic flat feet with an accessory navicular consists of the use of an orthotic and an exercise program to strengthen the posterior tibial muscles and the peroneal tendons of the foot. Surgery is needed.

Freiberg's disease involves collapse of the articular surface and subchondral bone of the second metatarsal, presumably from a vascular insult.[10] Although this is

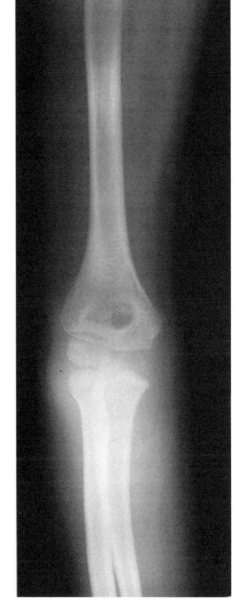

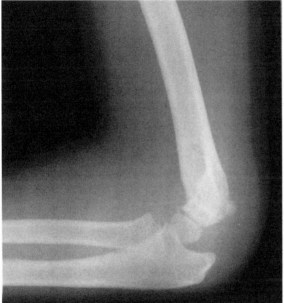

Figure 6–10. Notice on the lateral view, the displacement of the capitellum anteriorly. This would be difficult to see unless drawing the anterior humeral line as shown and discussed earlier.

most commonly seen in the second metatarsal, it can occur in the third metatarsal. Symptoms are pain and tenderness over the metatarsal head with swelling in this area on clinical examination. X rays confirm the diagnosis and treatment consists of decreased weight bearing to the area and a metatarsal pad or orthotic. Surgical excision of loose bodies causing fragmentation of the head is occasionally required.

☐ Osteochondritis Dissecans of the Talus

Most of these lesions are in the middle third of the lateral border of the talus. Lesions are classified into four different stages:

- **Stage 1:** A small area of compression of subchondral bone
- **Stage 2:** A partially detached osteochondral fragment
- **Stage 3:** A completely detached osteochondral fragment remaining in the crater
- **Stage 4:** A displaced osteochondral fragment

Stage 1 and 2 lesions are treated without surgery using a cast, brace, or strap. Stage 3 medial lesions initially should be treated without surgery, but if symptoms persist, surgical excision and curettage is recommended. Stage 3 lateral lesions and all stage 4 lesions are treated surgically with removal of the lesion.

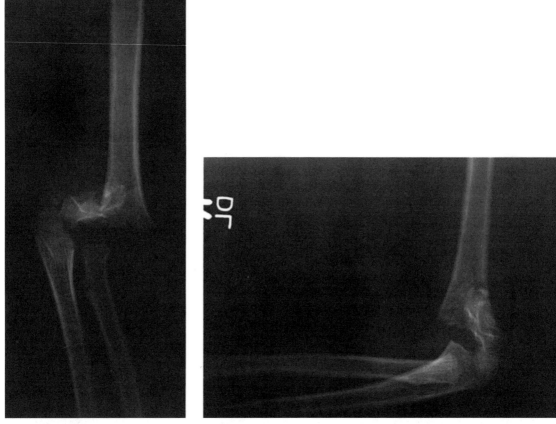

Figure 6–11. A displaced supracondylar fracture with dislocation is shown.

☐ Sever's Disease

Sever's disease, or calcaneal apophysis, is a common entity occurring in patients between 9 and 11 years of age. The child may present with heel pain, particularly with running, and may even be using a tiptoe gait or limping. X rays are often not helpful; however, the patient is tender on palpation of the calcaneal apophysis. Treatment depends on the severity of the symptoms, the primary role being to rest the heel. In very symptomatic patients, a short-leg walking cast for 10 to 14 days may be the treatment of choice.[10]

☐ ORTHOPEDIC INJURIES ASSOCIATED WITH CHILD ABUSE

Whenever there is delay in seeking treatment for an orthopedic injury, one should suspect the possibility of child abuse. If the history is inconsistent with the examination this should also be a sign that increases your suspicion of abuse. Look for skin lesions and evidence of abuse. Fifty percent of fractures in children under the age of 1 are not accidental, and approximately 30 percent of fractures in children under the age of 3 are related to child abuse as well. Anytime a child 1 year of age presents with a fracture, one should suspect child abuse.

Radiographic Evidence of Child Abuse

Fractures of the ribs or sternal area suggest child abuse. Any fractures seen in a child under 3 years of age should be suspect and particularly those seen in a child who is handicapped or premature. Metaphyseal fractures are also suspect. Fractures of the femur and particularly fractures of the distal femur are highly suspicious injuries. Scapular fractures are difficult to obtain and should be suspect.

Several reviews have recently been summarized to demonstrate that all fractures of the humerus in children under the age of 3 years are strongly suggestive of abuse.[3] Supracondylar fractures do occur nonaccidentally once children have begun to walk. They can only happen accidentally with significant trauma.[3] In one study, it was reported that 19 out of 24 children under the age of 2 with femoral shaft fractures had been abused.[3] With this high incidence, clearly when one sees this fracture the first thing one should think of is abuse. Metaphyseal fractures in children secondary to abuse are usually very close to the joint, unlike accidental metaphyseal fractures which are usually at the junction of the

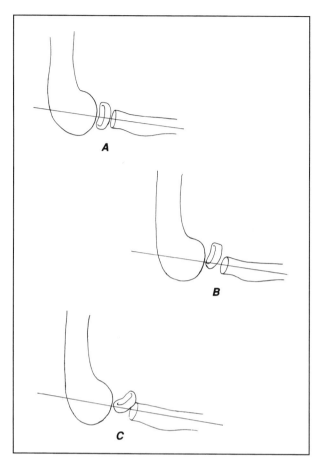

Figure 6–12. A. The radiocapitellar line drawn through the center of the radius should pass through the center of the capitellum of the humerus on the lateral view. **B.** In patients with a fracture of the radial neck in whom the epiphysis has not closed this is useful in making the diagnosis. **C.** This is true particularly when a subtle fracture exists as shown here.

TABLE 6-1. TIMETABLE OF RADIOGRAPHIC CHANGES IN PEDIATRIC FRACTURES

	Early	Peak	Late
1. Periosteal New Bone	4–10 days	10–14 days	14–21 days
2. Soft Callus days	10–14 days	12–21 days	21–28 days
3. Hard Callus	14–21 days	21–40 days	40–90 days
4. Remodeling	3 months	1 year	2 years

Modified from O'Connor J.F., Cohen J. *Dating Fractures*; Kleinman P. (ed): *Diagnostic Imaging & Child Abuse.* Baltimore, Williams & Wilkins, 1987 p 112.

Physicians treating children in the emergency department must have a basic knowledge of the stages of fracture healing that can be detected radiographically. Table 6–1 provides a general timetable of the various phases of fracture healing. One must consider the data in this table as estimates only because very young infants may exhibit an accelerated rate of response.[6]

Risk of Missed Child Abuse

Child abuse must be at the forefront of the emergentologist's mind in examining any child, particularly those under 3 years of age with fractures. There is a 50 percent chance of additional abuse if the child is treated and referred back to the home. In addition, approximately 8 to 10 percent of these children die if this condition is not reported and the child is treated and sent back.

☐ TRANSIENT SYNOVITIS

Transient synovitis or toxic synovitis is presented under hip and pelvis in Chapter 21 however, it is important enough to deserve discussion here. This is the most common cause of painful hips in children. Patients present with pain on passive motion and there is limitation of hip movement. Muscle spasm is present and the child is usually afebrile. The onset is acute but can be insidious. The condition is rarely bilateral with boys being affected more commonly than girls. The average age of this condition is 5 years. In transient synovitis the white blood cell count and the sedimentation rate are both normal.

One must remember to exclude septic arthritis when one suspects this diagnosis. Other conditions that may mimic this include Legg-Calvé-Perthes disease, slipped capital femoral epiphysis, or osteomyelitis. In distinguishing this condition from septic arthritis of the hip, the clinical presentation is usually most helpful. Patients who present with *septic arthritis* of the hip are much *more painful* and *more toxic looking* than those with transient synovitis who will often present with minimal pain and a viral prodrome. In addition, the white

diaphesis and the metaphyseas and are of the torus variety.[3] Metaphyseal fractures are usually caused by a shaking injury.[5] A variant of metaphyseal injury that is not as well known is shown by radiographic translucency in the immediate subphyseal region, similar to that sometimes seen in chronic illnesses such as leukemia.

The three most critical features to look for when examining an x ray of a child and suspecting abuse are the following:

- Bilateral fractures
- Multiple fractures
  - Metaphyseal fractures
  - Rib fractures
  - Scapular fractures
  - Fractures of the outer end of the clavicle
  - Finger injuries in nonambulant children
- Fractures of different ages
- Skull fractures

cell count is much higher with septic arthritis and the sedimentation rate is much higher. If one does a tap, few white blood cells (WBCs) are seen in transient synovitis and greater than 80,000 WBCs in septic arthritis. A tap should be done under fluoroscopic control.

☐ BONE INFECTIONS IN CHILDREN

Septic arthritis and osteomyelitis are not uncommon in children. Each year in the United States, 1 in 5000 children under the age of 13 is diagnosed with osteomyelitis.[18] The pathologic origin is hematogenous seating, local invasion from contiguous infection, or direct inoculation of the bone, either surgically or after trauma. Chapter 21 provides a more detailed discussion of the most common type of septic arthritis that occurs in the hip.

The presentation is usually that of a fever, which may be low grade, and what is called *pseudo-paralysis*, which essentially is a refusal of the child to use that limb.[8] Children with osteomyelitis have tenderness to palpation particularly over the metaphysis, which is commonly affected. Gentle passive motion, however, is usually allowed. Presenting symptoms in neonates may be as vague as increased irritability or poor feeding.[18] When the hip and shoulder are involved in osteomyelitis, the pus can track under the periosteum of the metaphysis into the adjacent joint and thus the patient may have findings of both osteomyelitis and a septic arthritis.

Septic arthritis children will have pain on any motion of the joint whatsoever, which is a distinguishing feature with osteomyelitis in that these children generally will allow passive motion if it is done gently.[8] The diagnosis of osteomyelitis can be made by satisfying any two of the following diagnostic criteria:

• Purulence of the bone
• A positive bone or blood culture
• Localized erythema, edema, or both
• A positive imaging study, either on radiography, scintosgraphy, or magnetic resonance imaging (MRI)

Cultures taken from bone result in a culture yield of 80 percent. Blood cultures should be drawn on all patients suspected of having osteomyelitis; the yield is usually 60 percent.[18] *Staphyloccus aureus* is a pathogen in most cases of hematogenous osteomyelitis with group A β-hemolytic streptococci a distant second. The femur and tibia are by far the most common bones affected. *Haemophilus influenzae* type B occurs more often in infants.[18]

The diagnosis of septic arthritis can be made when a child presents with a fever, an elevation of the white count, and an elevated sedimentation rate. X rays of bone are generally normal and it takes 7 to 10 days for x ray changes to appear in either osteomyelitis or septic

arthritis. Soft tissue, however, may show some changes earlier. Aspiration can be attempted in superficial joints; however, aspiration of the hip joint which is commonly affected should only be done under fluoroscopic control and only after an injection of air or dye to confirm the entry into the joint. Because plain x rays are usually not productive early in the course of this disease, these films should be followed by skeletal scintigraphy. Scinigraphically guided aspiration of the hip evacuates pus, decreases damage to particular surfaces, differentiates joint sepsis from other effusions, and helps direct antibiotic therapy.[12] Hip scintigraphy has been found to be 91 percent accurate in detecting osteomyelitis.[7] Computed tomography (CT) scans are not useful in establishing a diagnosis of acute muscular skeletal sepsis.[7]

A septic hip in a child is a surgical emergency because the intracapsular blood supply is compromised due to the increased joint pressure from the infection. These patients should be referred immediately for drainage. In treating children with osteomyelitis, one should use a β-lactamase–resistant penicillin such as oxacillin, naficillin, or a combination of ampicillin and sulbactam, or a first-generation cephalosporin. The length of antibiotic therapy is at a minimum 4 weeks for acute osteomyelitis.[18]

Initial antibiotic therapy in children with osteomyelitis should be oxacillin, as previously indicated. However, for patients who are allergic to penicillin, cefazolin 100 mg/kg in divided doses over 24 hours is indicated. If patients are allergic to both penicillin and cefazolin, clindamycin 24 mg/kg in divided doses over 24 hours or vancomycin are indicated.[7] In children who have sickle cell disease, the infection is usually located in the diaphysis rather than the metaphyses and the offending organism is frequently *Salmonella*.

In infections of the foot after puncture wounds in children, the causative organism is usually *Pseudomonas aeruginosa*, which causes approximately 95 percent of cases, particularly those in which the sole of a tennis shoe has been punctured. In these cases, after debridement, an aminoglycoside antibiotic such as gentamycin or tobramycin should be administered.[7]

☐ TUMORS IN CHILDREN

The most common site for childhood malignant tumors is around the knee. One must be suspicious whenever there is unilateral knee pain without any associated trauma. Pathological fractures are also suspect, particularly when they occur through weakened bone, which may be a bone cyst. A number of benign tumors occur in children as incidental findings; these include osteochondromas and fibrous cortical defects.

REFERENCES

1. Anderson SJ: Evaluation and treatment of the ankle sprains. *Compr Ther* **22**(1):30–38, 1996.
2. Callanan DL: Causes of refusal to walk in childhood. *South Med J* **75**:20, 1982.
3. Carty HM: Fractures caused by child abuse. *J Bone Joint Surg* **75-B**:6, 1993.
4. Chorley JN, Hergenroeder AC: Management of ankle sprains. *Pediatr Ann* **26**:1, 1997.
5. Cramer KE: Orthopedic aspects of child abuse. *Pediatr Clin North Am* **43**:5, 1996.
6. Dicke TE, Nunley JA: Distal forearm fractures in children. *Orthop Clin North Am* **24**:2, 1993.
7. Dirschl DR: Acute pyogenic osteomyelitis in children. *Orthop Rev* 305–312, 1994.
8. Erasmie U, Hirsch G: Acute haematogenous osteomyelitis in children. The reliability of skeletal scintigraphy. *Z Kinderchir* **32**:360, 1981.
9. Frankel VH, Nordin M: *Basic Biomechanics of the Skeletal System*. Philadelphia: Lea and Febiger, 1980.
10. Griffin TY: Common sports injuries of the foot and ankle seen in children and adolescents. *Foot Ankle Inj Sports* **25**:1, 1994.
11. Hart JJ: Transient synovitis of the hip in children. *Am Fam Phys* **54**:5, 1996.
12. Jaramillo D, et al: Osteomyelitis and septic arthritis in children: Appropriate use of imaging to guide treatment. *AJR* **165**(2):399–403, 1995.
13. Lovell WW, Winter RB: *Pediatric Orthopedics*, 3rd ed. Philadelphia: Lippincott, 1990.
14. Mandell GA: Imaging in the diagnosis of musculoskeletal infections in children. *Curr Probl Pediatr* **26**:218–237, 1996.
15. Marcus RE (ed): *Trauma in Children*. Rockville, MD: Aspen, 1986.
16. Ogden JA: Skeletal injury in the child. *Pediatric Orthopedics*, 3rd ed. Philadelphia: Lea and Febiger, 1990.
17. Rang M: *Children's Fractures*, 2nd ed. Philadelphia: Lippincott, 1983.
18. Sonnen GM, Henry NK: Pediatric bone and joint infections. Diagnosis and antimicrobial management. *Pediatr Clin North Am* **43**:4, 1996.

BIBLIOGRAPHY

Gertzbein SD, Barrington TW: Diagnosis of occult fractures and dislocations. *Clin Orthop* **108**:105, 1975.
Rockwood CA, Wilkins KE, King RE: *Fractures in Children*. Philadelphia: Lippincott, 1984.

PART II

FRACTURES AND RHEUMATOLOGY

UPPER EXTREMITIES

7
CHAPTER
FRACTURES OF THE HAND

DISTAL PHALANGEAL FRACTURES

CLASS A: EXTRA-ARTICULAR FRACTURES
(p. 105)

Type I: Longitudinal   Type II: Transverse   Type III: Comminuted   **Type IV: Transverse with displacement**

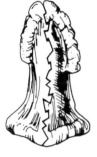
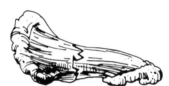
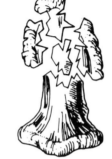
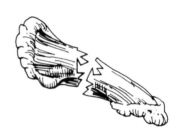

CLASS B: INTRA-ARTICULAR AVULSION FRACTURES
(pp. 106)

Type I: Dorsal avulsion fracture

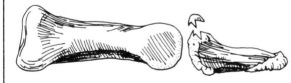
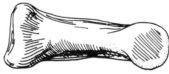

A: "Mallet" fracture (<25% of articular surface)   B: "Mallet" fracture (>25% of articular surface)

Type II: Volar avulsion fracture

(pp. 108)

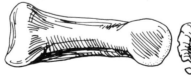

CLASS A: EXTRA-ARTICULAR SHAFT FRACTURES
(pp. 114)

Type I

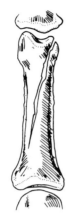

A: Greenstick
   fracture

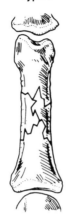

B: Nondisplaced nonangulated
   comminuted midshaft

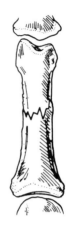

C: Nondisplaced nonangulated
   transverse midshaft

Type II

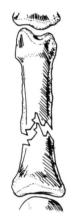

A: Displaced transverse
   midshaft

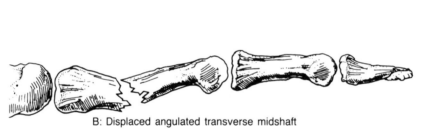

B: Displaced angulated transverse midshaft

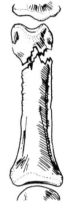

C: Displaced angulated
   transverse neck

Type III: Spiral

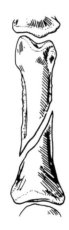

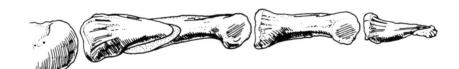

MIDDLE PHALANGEAL FRACTURES

CLASS B: EXTRA-ARTICULAR SHAFT FRACTURES
(p. 118)

Type I: Nondisplaced transverse

Type II: Displaced or angulated

Type III: Spiral

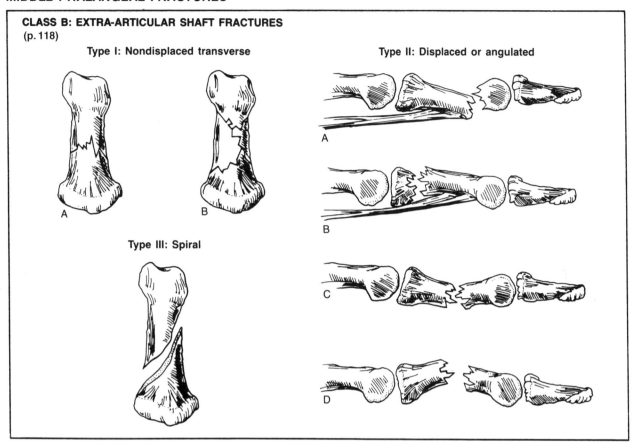

PROXIMAL PHALANGEAL FRACTURES

CLASS A: INTRA-ARTICULAR FRACTURES
(p. 119)

Type I

Type II

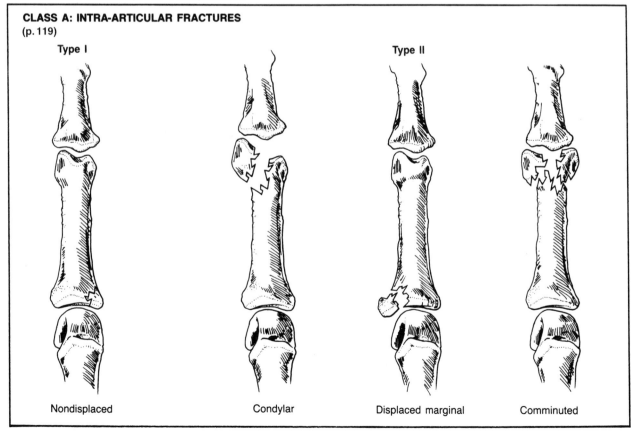

Nondisplaced   Condylar   Displaced marginal   Comminuted

MIDDLE PHALANGEAL FRACTURES

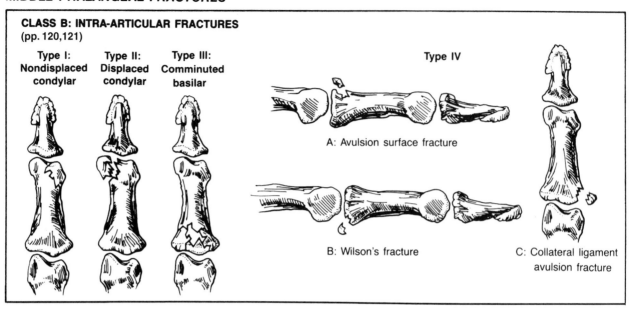

CLASS B: INTRA-ARTICULAR FRACTURES
(pp. 120,121)

Type I:
Nondisplaced
condylar

Type II:
Displaced
condylar

Type III:
Comminuted
basilar

Type IV

A: Avulsion surface fracture

B: Wilson's fracture

C: Collateral ligament
avulsion fracture

METACARPAL FRACTURES 2 THROUGH 5

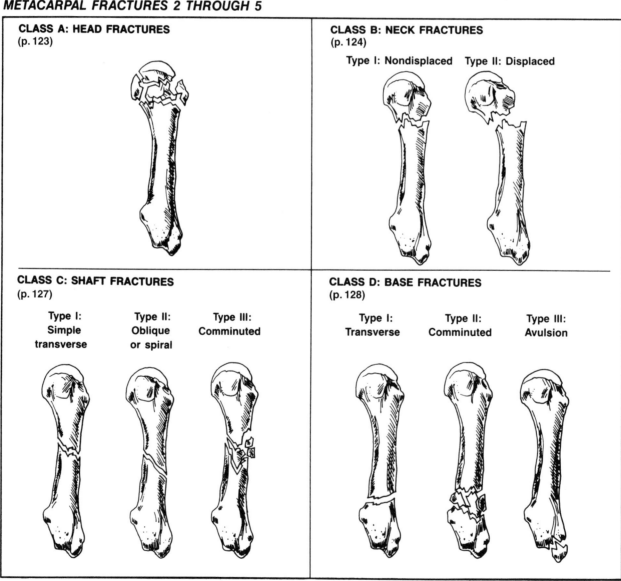

CLASS A: HEAD FRACTURES
(p. 123)

CLASS B: NECK FRACTURES
(p. 124)

Type I: Nondisplaced   Type II: Displaced

CLASS C: SHAFT FRACTURES
(p. 127)

Type I:
Simple
transverse

Type II:
Oblique
or spiral

Type III:
Comminuted

CLASS D: BASE FRACTURES
(p. 128)

Type I:
Transverse

Type II:
Comminuted

Type III:
Avulsion

CLASS A: EXTRA-ARTICULAR BASE AND SHAFT FRACTURES
(p.130)

Type I: Transverse base fracture

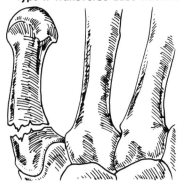

Type II: Transverse shaft fracture

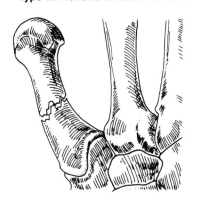

Type III: Epiphyseal plate fracture (in children)

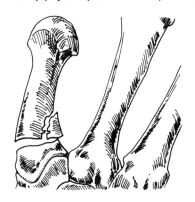

CLASS B: INTRA-ARTICULAR BASE FRACTURES
(p.131)

Type I: Bennett fractures–dislocation

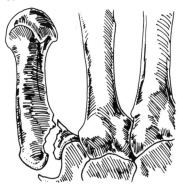

Type II: Rolando fracture

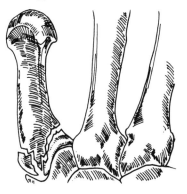

The emergency center management of hand fractures is complex, requiring an exhaustive physical examination and the implementation of therapy based on sound medical judgment. Frequently, these fractures are seen and treated as minor injuries without realizing that improper management can result in lifelong crippling disabilities. For example, a small degree of rotational malalignment with a metacarpal or proximal phalanx fracture will, if uncorrected, result in a poorly functioning partially disabled hand. Only with a thorough understanding of the essential anatomy can one hope to diagnose hand injuries and to initiate appropriate therapy.

Essential Anatomy

The design and versatility of the human hand has impressed anatomists and authors for centuries. Anatomically, the hand is a group of highly mobile gliding bones connected by tendons and ligaments to a "fixed center."[6] This fixed center consists of the second and third metacarpal bones. The remainder of the hand is suspended from these two relatively immobile bones. All of the intrinsic movements of the hand are relative to and dependent on the stability and immobility of these two bones. Mobility is a critical consideration in the management of fractures. Those bones with a high degree of mobility can withstand a greater degree of angulation with the retention of normal function. Those bones with less mobility require a much more precise reduction in angulation to ensure a return to full function.

Another important consideration in diagnosing and treating hand injuries is the concept of rotation. For the hand to function smoothly all of its parts must work together as a team. An example of this is shown in Figure 7–1, which demonstrates that normally all of the fingers of a fist point to the tubercle of the scaphoid. Rotational deformities interrupt this teamwork resulting in malpositioning or overlap as shown in Figure 7–2. It is imperative that the emergency physician understand the importance of angulation and rotation in the management of hand fractures.[7,10]

Axiom: *Rotational malalignment is never acceptable in fractures of the metacarpals or phalanges. Acceptance of angulation deformities in meta-carpal or phalangeal fractures is dependent on the degree of angulation and bony mobility. Angulation is acceptable in more mobile bones but is unacceptable in stationary bones (ie, second and third metacarpals).*

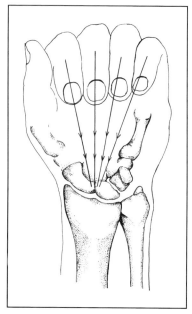

Figure 7–1. Note that lines drawn through the fingernails will meet at the scaphoid in the normal hand.

Examination

It is of critical importance when treating patients with hand injuries to initially examine and document neural, vascular, and tendon injury before manipulation or therapy. In addition, rotary malalignment must be recognized clinically and corrected.

X Ray

All significant hand injuries, including those with any degree of swelling, should be evaluated radiographically

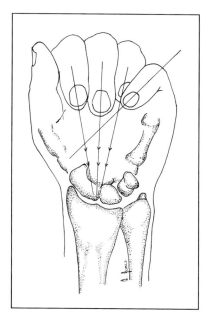

Figure 7–2. In the patient with rotational malalignment of a fracture, the fingernail of the involved digit does not point to the scaphoid.

even if the likelihood of a fracture seems remote. Chip or avulsion fractures may not be suspected on the basis of clinical examination and yet if undetected and untreated may result in a significant disability. A minimum of three views should be obtained when a hand fracture is suspected (anteroposterior [AP], lateral, and oblique). Metacarpal injuries may require special views for adequate radiographic visualization. For example, fractures of the fourth and fifth metacarpals are frequently undetected until a lateral view with 10 degrees of supination is obtained. Second and third metacarpal injuries are often detected on a lateral view with 10 degrees of pronation. Finger injuries require a true lateral view without superimposition of the other digits. One should not accept and subsequently base a diagnosis on inadequate radiographs of the hand.

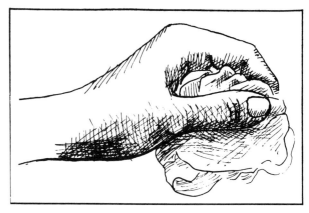

Figure 7–3. The thumb should be immobilized in the fist position as shown and a splint applied dorsally (exclude fluffs in hand).

Treatment

Hand injuries are best anesthetized by nerve blocks, usually at the wrist. Metacarpal blocks are frequently successfully employed in managing phalangeal fractures. Intravenous lidocaine or a *Bier block* results in very effective anesthesia but should be used only by the experienced practitioner. Patients with suspected open fractures should receive perioperative antibiotics. It is the authors' recommendation that clean distal phalangeal fractures without significant tissue disruption or crush injury can be closed in the emergency room (see Fig. 7–9). All other open-hand fractures require consultation, perioperative antibiotics, and operating room management.

Simple traction is rarely used in managing hand fractures owing to the instability of the reduction. Countertraction (splint) or percutaneous Kirschner wires are frequently employed in unstable hand fractures. After reduction, the hand should be immobilized with the wrist in 20 degrees of extension, the metacarpophalangeal (MCP) joints in 50 to 90 degrees of flexion, and the interphalangeal (IP) joints in 15 degrees of flexion. The thumb is typically immobilized in the fist position (Fig. 7–3).

A significant problem in the management of hand fractures is the tendency to develop early lymphatic stasis and edema.[8,10] The exudate consists of a protein-rich fluid that has a tendency to stimulate the development of adhesions among the tendons, synovial sheaths, and joints. This complication often leads to fibrosis and stiffness. Early elevation with gentle compression is often helpful in reducing edema. In addition, early motion of the hand is essential in reducing edema.

The most frequent complications after hand fractures include *deformities* and *chronic joint stiffness*.

Classification

The classification of hand fractures is difficult and at times confusing. The authors have elected to classify hand fractures on the basis of anatomic location and mechanical function. For example, metacarpal fractures are considered as an anatomic group and classified together except for the first metacarpal, which is classified separately because of its distinct mechanical function. Fractures of the hand are classified as shown in the following table.

DISTAL PHALANGEAL FRACTURES
☐ Class A: Extra-articular fractures (Fig. 7–6)
☐ Class B: Intra-articular avulsion fractures—dorsal (Fig. 7–10)
☐ Class B: Intra-articular avulsion fractures—volar surface (Fig. 7–14)

MIDDLE AND PROXIMAL PHALANGEAL FRACTURES
☐ Class A: Extra-articular proximal shaft fractures (Fig. 7–24)
☐ Class B: Extra-articular middle shaft fractures (Fig. 7–27)
☐ Class A: Intra-articular proximal fractures (Fig. 7–28)
☐ Class B: Intra-articular middle fractures, types I, II, and III (Fig. 7–29)

☐ Class B: Intra-articular middle fractures, type IV (Fig. 7–30)

METACARPAL FRACTURES 2 THROUGH 5
☐ Class A: Head fractures (Fig. 7–33)
☐ Class B: Neck fractures (Fig. 7–34)
☐ Class C: Shaft fractures (Fig. 7–37)
☐ Class D: Base fractures (Fig. 7–38)

FIRST METACARPAL FRACTURES
☐ Class A: Extra-articular base and shaft fractures (Fig. 7–40)
☐ Class B: Intra-articular base fractures (Fig. 7–41)

DISTAL PHALANGEAL FRACTURES

Distal phalangeal fractures are classified into extra-articular fractures (longitudinal, transverse, and comminuted) and intra-articular fractures. It is important to understand the anatomy of the distal phalanx when diagnosing and treating these injuries. As shown in Figure 7–4, fibrous septa extend from the bone to the skin and serve to stabilize fractures of the distal phalanx. Traumatic hematomas can form between these septa and may result in severe pain secondary to elevated pressure occurring within this closed space. Two tendons attach to the distal phalanx of digits 2 through 5. As shown in Figure 7–5, the *flexor profundus* attaches to the volar aspect, whereas the *terminal slip of the extensor tendon* attaches on the dorsal surface. In distal phalanx of the thumb, the flexor pollicis longus inserts on the volar base and the extensor pollicis longus on the dorsal base. These tendons can avulse when subjected to excessive stress. Clinically, there will be a loss of function while radiographically small avulsion fractures along the base of the phalanx are often seen. These fractures are considered intra-articular.

□ CLASS A: EXTRA-ARTICULAR FRACTURES (FIG. 7–6)

Mechanism of Injury
The mechanism of injury is always a direct blow to the distal phalanx. The force of the blow will determine the

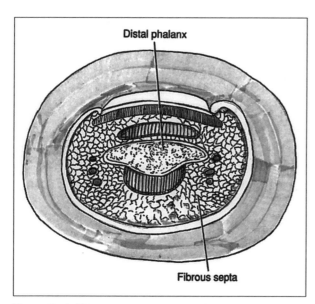

Figure 7–4. Fibrous septa extend from the bone to the skin and serve to stabilize fractures of the distal phalanx.

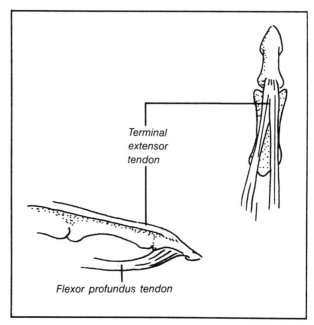

Figure 7–5. The flexor profundus tendon attaches to the volar aspect of the distal phalanx whereas the terminal slip of the extensor tendon attaches to the dorsal surface.

severity of the fracture. The most common fracture is a comminuted fracture.

Examination
Examination typically reveals tenderness and swelling over the distal phalanx including the pulp. Subungual hematomas are also noted frequently and indicate a nail bed laceration.

X Ray
AP and lateral views are generally adequate in demonstrating the fracture and any displacement, if present.

Associated Injuries
As mentioned earlier, subungual hematomas along with nail bed lacerations are frequently seen. Incomplete avulsion of the nail is noted frequently in association with transverse distal phalanx fractures.

Treatment
□ Class A: Type I   (Longitudinal)
             Type II   (Transverse)
             Type III   (Comminuted)

These fractures are treated with a protective splint, elevation to reduce swelling, and analgesics. Either the simple volar splint or the hairpin splint as shown in

DISTAL PHALANGEAL FRACTURES

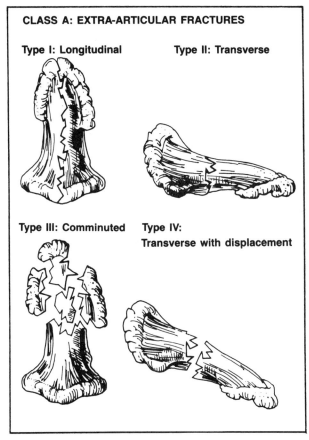

CLASS A: EXTRA-ARTICULAR FRACTURES

Type I: Longitudinal

Type II: Transverse

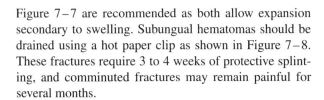

Type III: Comminuted

Type IV:
Transverse with displacement

Figure 7–6.

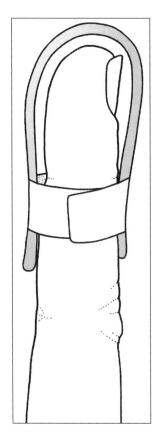

Figure 7–7. Hairpin splint.

Figure 7–7 are recommended as both allow expansion secondary to swelling. Subungual hematomas should be drained using a hot paper clip as shown in Figure 7–8. These fractures require 3 to 4 weeks of protective splinting, and comminuted fractures may remain painful for several months.

□ Class A: Type IV (Displaced)
Transverse fractures with angulation or displacement may be difficult to reduce as soft tissues may be interposed between the fragments. If uncorrected, this may lead to nonunion of the fragments. This fracture can be reduced frequently with dorsal traction on the distal fragment followed by immobilization with a volar splint and repeat radiographs for documentation of position. If this is unsuccessful orthopedic referral is indicated for pinning.

Class A (Open Fractures with Nail Lacerations)
Distal phalangeal fractures associated with nail plate lacerations should be considered as open fractures and treated in a "clean room." The technique for managing these fractures is shown in Figure 7–9, and proceeds as follows:

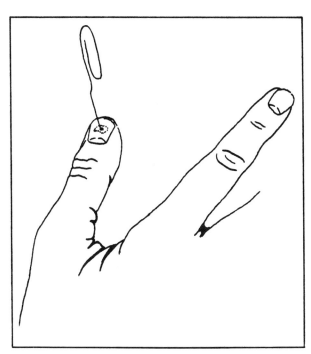

Figure 7–8. The drainage of a subungual hematoma with a paper clip.

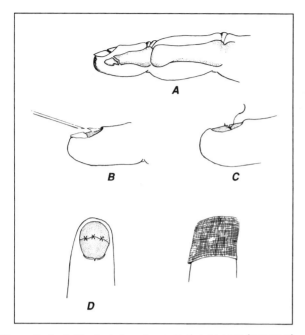

Figure 7–9. *A.* The technique for managing an open fracture of the distal phalanx. *B.* The nail is removed and the nail bed repaired with absorbable suture. *C.* Simple approximation of the nail bed results in good apposition of the fractured phalanx. *D.* A small strip of xeroform gauze should be placed over the nail bed and underneath the eponychial fold.

1. Regional anesthesia using either a metacarpal or wrist block should be used. The hand is then prepared and draped in a sterile manner.
2. The nail plate should be dissected bluntly (using a spoon or probe) from the nail bed and root matrix.
3. With the plate removed, the nail bed laceration can be explored and thoroughly irrigated with normal saline. The nail bed can then be elevated and the fracture reduced. The nail bed is then sutured using a minimum number of 5-0 absorbable interrupted sutures.
4. Adaptic or xeroform gauze should be placed under the roof matrix separating it from the root. This prevents the development of synechia that can result in a deformed nail plate.
5. The entire digit should be dressed with gauze and splinted for protection. The outer dressing can be changed as needed, but the adaptic separating the root from the roof matrix should remain in place for 10 days.
6. A broad spectrum cephalosporin antibiotic should be initiated and continued for 7 to 10 days.
7. Repeat radiographs for documentation of reduction are indicated. If the fracture remains unstable a pin may be inserted.

Complications

Distal phalangeal fractures may be associated with several serious complications.

1. Osteomyelitis is often associated with open fractures. Open fractures include those associated with nail plate lacerations and those associated with a subungual hematoma that has been drained.
2. Nonunion is usually secondary to interposition of the nail bed between the fracture fragments.
3. Delayed union is commonly seen in comminuted fractures.

□ CLASS B: INTRA-ARTICULAR AVULSION FRACTURES—DORSAL SURFACE (FIG. 7–10)[22]

Mechanism of Injury

This injury is typically referred to as a mallet finger and results from forced flexion of the distal phalanx with the finger in taut extension. The fracture is commonly seen in baseball players when the ball accidently hits the tip of the finger causing forced flexion. Three injuries are possible to the extensor tendon with this mechanism and they are diagrammed in Figure 7–11.

1. The tendon may stretch resulting in a 15- to 20-degree loss of extension.
2. The tendon may rupture resulting in up to a 45-degree loss of extension.
3. The tendon may avulse a fragment from its attachment to the distal phalanx.

Examination

On examination, there will be a 40- to 45-degree loss of extension at the distal interphalangeal (DIP) joint with an avulsion injury. The patient will be unable to extend the distal phalanx, and there will be swelling and tenderness over the dorsal aspect of the joint.

DISTAL PHALANGEAL FRACTURES

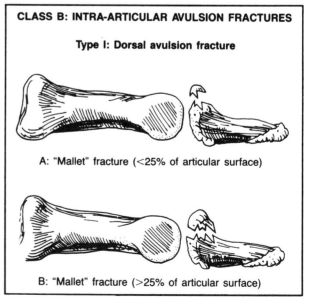

CLASS B: INTRA-ARTICULAR AVULSION FRACTURES

Type I: Dorsal avulsion fracture

A: "Mallet" fracture (<25% of articular surface)

B: "Mallet" fracture (>25% of articular surface)

Figure 7–10.

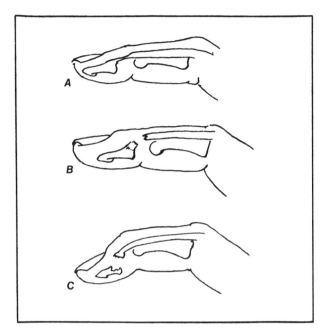

Figure 7–11. Three ways the extensor tendon can be disrupted. **A.** A stretch of the tendon without division of the tendon. **B.** When the tendon is ruptured from its insertion on the distal phalanx there is a 40-degree flexion deformity present, and the patient cannot actively extend the tendon at the distal interphalangeal joint. **C.** A fragment of the distal phalanx can be avulsed with the tendon.

X Ray
A true lateral view is essential in selecting a management program for avulsion fractures. It is essential to distinguish if the fragment is less than or greater than 25 percent of the articular surface.

Associated Injuries
The tendon may stretch or elongate without any associated fracture.

Treatment
The therapeutic program selected is dependent on two variables: patient reliability and the size of the avulsion fragment.

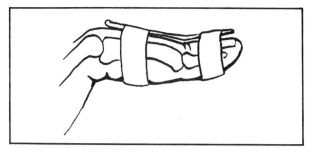

Figure 7–12. A dorsal splint on the distal interphalangeal joint.

□ Class B: Type IA (Less than 25 Percent of Articular Surface)
In the reliable patient, this fracture can be treated with immobilization in a splint. The DIP joint should be extended with flexion at the proximal interphalangeal (PIP) joint. Either a volar or dorsal splint should be applied, although in the authors' experience dorsal splints provide better fixation because there are fewer soft tissues interposed between the splint and the fracture (Fig. 7–12). The finger must be maintained in this position for 6 to 8 weeks. After this, the splint can be removed during the daytime with the patient cautioned against finger flexion for an additional 4 weeks.

If the patient is unreliable, the hand and finger can be casted in the position described in the Appendix. The cast should remain in place for 6 weeks followed by 2 to 3 weeks of splinting of the digit.

□ Class B: Type IB (Greater than 25 Percent of Articular Surface)
This fracture is frequently associated with some degree of subluxation of the DIP joint. The emergency department management is immobilization with orthopedic referral. Controversy exists regarding the benefits of continued immobilization compared with surgical intervention.[2,11,20,21,25]

If the fracture is improperly treated, a hyperextension PIP deformity may result. This is secondary to the imbalance between the ruptured extensor tendon and the unopposed distal flexor tendon as shown in Figure 7–13.

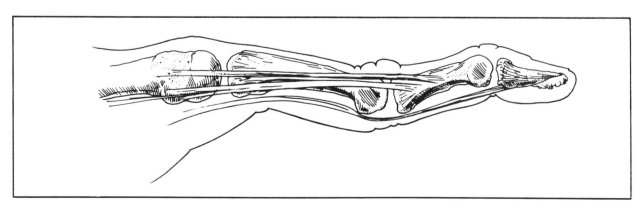

Figure 7–13. If the fracture is treated improperly, a hyperextension deformity will occur at the proximal interphalangeal joint. This is secondary to an imbalance between the ruptured extensor tendon and the unapposed distal flexor tendon.

□ CLASS B: INTRA-ARTICULAR AVULSION FRACTURES—VOLAR SURFACE (FIG. 7–14)

The flexor profundus tendon inserts on the base of the distal phalanx. Avulsion injuries are classified as intra-articular fractures.

Mechanism of Injury
This is an uncommon injury resulting from forceful hyperextension while the flexor profundus tendon is tightly contracted.

Examination
The patient will be unable to flex the distal phalanx. There will be tenderness over the volar aspect of the distal phalanx or palm. This is secondary to tendon retraction after rupture.

Axiom: *Patients with traumatic swelling and tenderness over the volar aspect of the distal phalanx with additional palmar pain have a rupture of the flexor profundus tendon until proven otherwise.*

X Ray
The lateral view is best for demonstrating this fracture.

Associated Injuries
Associated injuries are rarely seen with this fracture.

Treatment
The emergency center management consists of a volar splint and referral. Early surgical fixation is the treatment of choice.

Complications
Intra-articular flexor surface distal phalanx avulsion fractures are often complicated by malunion.

Fractures of the middle and proximal phalanx have

DISTAL PHALANGEAL FRACTURES

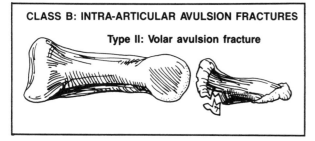

CLASS B: INTRA-ARTICULAR AVULSION FRACTURES

Type II: Volar avulsion fracture

Figure 7–14.

MIDDLE AND PROXIMAL PHALANGEAL FRACTURES

many similarities in their anatomy, mechanisms of injury, and treatment; therefore, they will be discussed together with their differences highlighted.

Essential Anatomy
There are no tendons that attach to the proximal phalanx. There are, however, tendons that lie in close proximity to the proximal phalanx that can at times complicate fracture management. Proximal phalanx fractures tend to have volar angulation secondary to the traction exerted by the interosseous muscles in conjunction with the action of the extensor tendons (Fig. 7–15).

Fractures of the middle phalanx are less common than those of the proximal phalanx because the majority of the axial force applied to a digit is absorbed by the proximal phalanx. This results in a higher incidence of proximal phalangeal fractures or PIP dislocations than middle phalangeal fractures. The middle phalanx has a narrow shaft, and this is where most fractures occur. It is also important to recognize that the flexor superficialis attaches over nearly the entire volar surface of the phalanx whereas the attachment of the extensor tendon is limited to the proximal dorsal portion. The flexor superficialis tendon is divided and inserts along the lateral margins of the bone (Fig. 7–16).

The flexor superficialis, with its broad insertion, exerts the predominant deforming force in middle phalangeal (MP) fractures. For example, a fracture at the base of the middle phalanx will typically result in volar displacement of the distal segment whereas a distal shaft fracture will usually present with volar displacement of

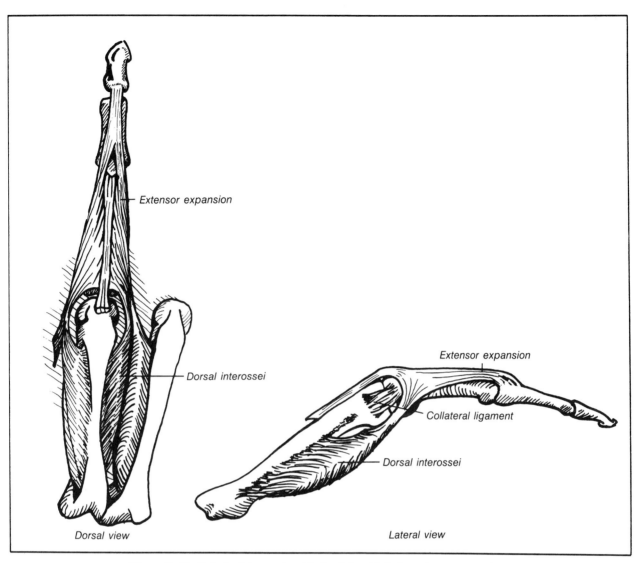

Figure 7–15. Note the interossei and their relationship to the extensor expansion.

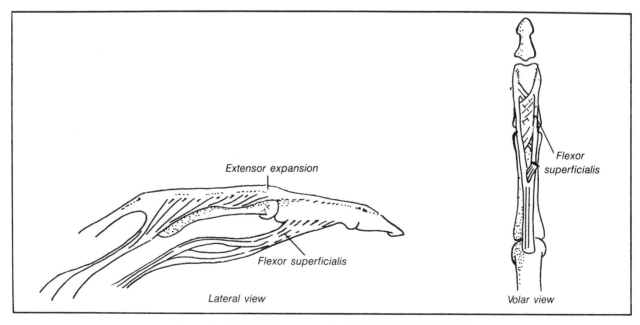

Figure 7–16. Note the tendons attaching to the middle phalanx.

the proximal segment and dorsal displacement of the distal fragment.

A final anatomic point to consider is the cartilaginous volar plate at the base of the middle phalanx (Fig. 7–17). Intra-articular fractures may be complicated by displacement of this cartilaginous plate.

Examination

All patients require a thorough examination with documentation of nerve function distal to the fracture site. Rotational malalignment must be discovered and corrected early in the management of these fractures. As mentioned earlier, rotational deformities can be suspected when all of the fingers of the closed fist do not point to the tubercle of the scaphoid.[3] Another method of diagnosing this disorder is to compare the plane of the fingernails on each hand. In a normal person, the plane of the nail plate for the extended right long finger will be similar to that on the left. With rotation, there will be a discrepancy between these planes as shown in Figure 7–18.

X Ray

Rotational deformities can be detected radiographically by comparing the diameter of the phalangeal fragments. If there is asymmetry, a rotational deformity should be suspected (Figs. 7–19 and 7–20).

Treatment

Patients with suspected open fractures should receive perioperative antibiotics. Prophylactic coverage with a

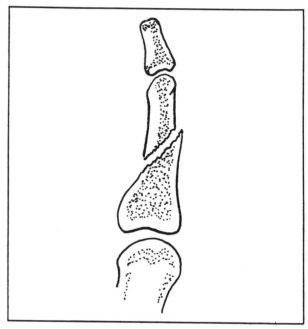

Figure 7–19. With rotational malalignment, there is asymmetry of the diameters of shaft at the fracture site.

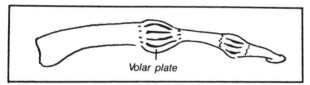

Figure 7–17. The volar plate at the base of the middle phalanx.

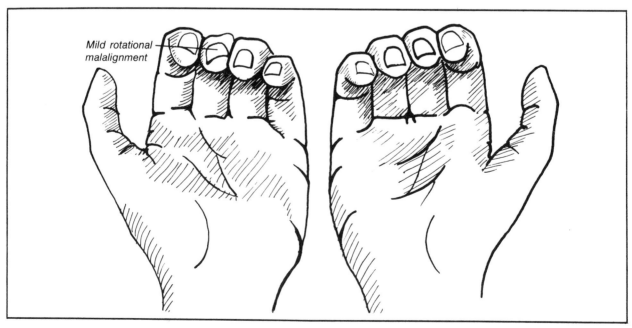

Figure 7–18. With rotational malalignment, the planes of the fingernails are not parallel when one compares the plane of the injured nail to the normal fingernail of the opposite hand.

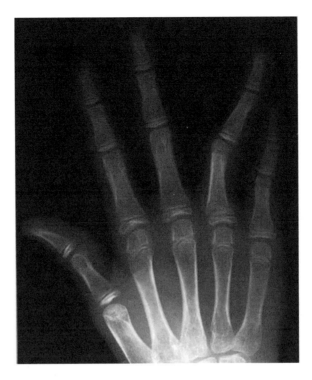
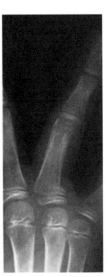

Figure 7–20. Angulated and rotated proximal phalanx fracture.

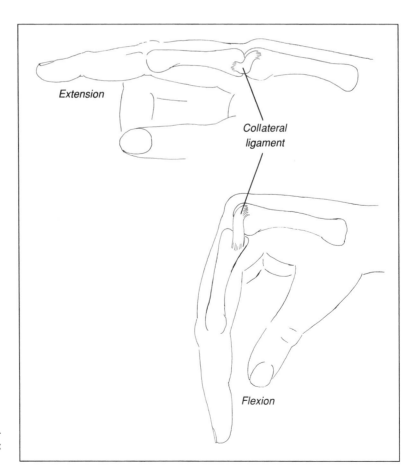

Figure 7–21. Note that the collateral ligament is taut in flexion and lax in extension.

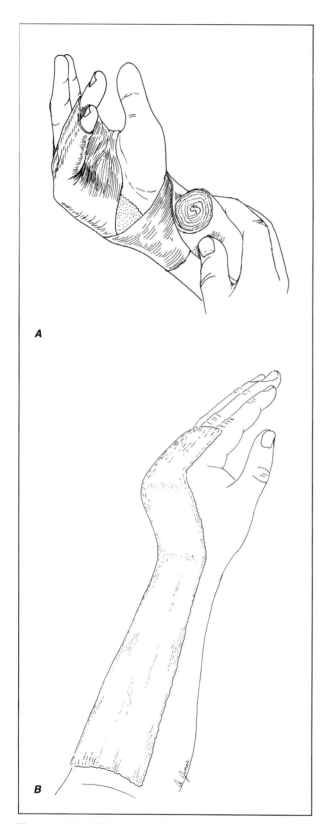

A

B

Figure 7–22. *A.* The gutter splint. Once applied, the MCP joint should be 50 to 90 degrees of flexion. ***B.*** An alternative to the gutter splint would be a volar splint or a dorsal splint with an extension hood extending to the PIP joints can be used.

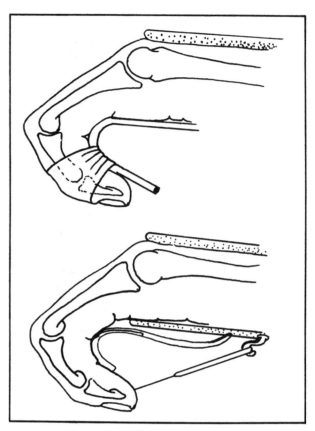

Figure 7–23. Böhler traction splints.

cephalosporin is recommended although patients with contaminated wounds should also receive penicillin and an aminoglycoside. The value of a routine single swab culturing of the wound preoperatively is questionable. Consultation for operating room exploration, irrigation, and stabilization is recommended.[23] There are two general principles that need to be emphasized when treating closed middle and proximal phalangeal fractures.

1. Never immobilize a finger in full extension. Fingers should be immobilized in the position of function with about 50 degrees of flexion at the MCP joint and 15 to 20 degrees of flexion at the IP joints to prevent stiffness and contracture. If a stable reduction is only possible in full extension, the patient requires internal fixation before immobilization in flexion. In flexion, the collateral ligaments are taut and will aid in maintaining a reduction (Fig. 7–21).
2. Never cast beyond the distal palmar crease. If distal plaster immobilization is required a gutter splint (Fig. 7–22) immobilizing the involved digit along with the adjacent normal digit or a cast with a traction device should be used (see Appendix).

Conceptually speaking there are three methods of treating middle and proximal phalangeal fractures. The method selected is dependent on the type of fracture, its stability, and experience of the physician.

Dynamic Splinting. This form of therapy simply involves taping the injured digit to the adjacent uninjured one. This allows maximal use of the hand with early mobilization and prevents stiffness. It is indicated only for stable nondisplaced, impacted, or transverse fractures (stable) (see Appendix). Recently, dynamic splinting was effectively utilized in uncomplicated proximal phalangeal fractures and those that were stable after reduction.[4] Articular, oblique rotated, or unstable fractures are typically not candidates for dynamic splinting.[4]

Casting, Splinting, and Traction Devices. These methods are applied generally only by orthopedic or hand surgeons with the exception of the gutter splint (see Fig. 7–22 and Appendix). The gutter splint is used in fractures that are stable, in no need of traction, and not complicated with rotation or angulation. The gutter splint offers more immobilization than is possible with dynamic splinting. Traction splints as shown in Figure 7–23 are used in complicated fractures and are generally applied only by the consulting orthopedic surgeon.

Internal Fixation. Internal fixation usually with Kirschner wires is used for unstable fractures or intra-articular avulsion fractures where precise reduction is necessary.

Classification

Proximal and middle phalangeal fractures are divided into three types. Type I fractures are nondisplaced stable fractures that can be treated by the emergency physician. Type II fractures are displaced and may be stable or unstable after reduction. Type II fractures should be referred for orthopedic follow-up. Type III fractures are unstable and often complicated by rotational deformities and require referral for reduction and immobilization.

☐ CLASS A: EXTRA-ARTICULAR PROXIMAL SHAFT FRACTURES (FIG. 7–24)

Mechanism of Injury
There are two mechanisms of injury commonly associated with extra-articular proximal phalanx fractures.[8] A direct blow to the proximal phalanx can result in a type I or type II fracture. An indirect blow that results in twisting or torque applied along the longitudinal axis of the digit frequently causes a type III spiral fracture.

Examination
Pain and swelling will be localized over the site of the fracture. Longitudinal compression of the digit results in pain referred to the fracture area. Rotational deformities are commonly associated with proximal phalangeal fractures. Clinical recognition of rotation, as shown in Figures 7–1, 7–2, and 7–18, is essential as any rotational deformity is unacceptable.

X Ray
An AP view of the hand as well as an oblique and true lateral view of the digits are essential. As mentioned earlier, rotational deformities should be suspected when there is a discrepancy in the diameter of the phalangeal fragments as shown in Figures 7–19 and 7–25.

Associated Injuries
Digital nerve injuries including contusion and transection may be associated with proximal phalangeal fractures. Arterial injuries may be associated with open or closed fractures and usually require no treatment. Tendon injuries are infrequently associated with proximal phalangeal fractures. These may present acutely as a tendon rupture or the symptoms may be delayed as with a partial rupture with limited motion due to adhesions.

Treatment
There is a tendency to underestimate the potential disability encountered with proximal phalangeal fractures. A thorough physical examination followed by the correction of angulation and rotation with immobilization will in most cases result in a full restoration of function.[19,23] Rotational deformities may be clinically inapparent unless enhanced by one of the three following tests:

1. Convergence test toward the scaphoid tubercle
2. Comparison of the finger and nail planes
3. Radiographic diameter of the fracture fragments

☐ Class A: Type IA   (Greenstick Fracture)
This is a stable fracture with no tendency for displacement or angulation because the periosteum is intact. The fracture should be treated with dynamic splinting followed by early motion exercises (see Appendix). A radiographic examination should be repeated in 7 to 10 days to exclude delayed displacement or rotation.

☐ Class A: Type IB   (Nondisplaced Nonangulated Comminuted Midshaft) (Fig. 7–26)
            Type IC   (Nondisplaced Nonangulated Transverse Midshaft)
These nondisplaced transverse or comminuted fractures may not have an intact periosteum and are therefore potentially unstable. These fractures can be treated by one of two methods depending on stability:[19,22,23]

PROXIMAL PHALANGEAL FRACTURES

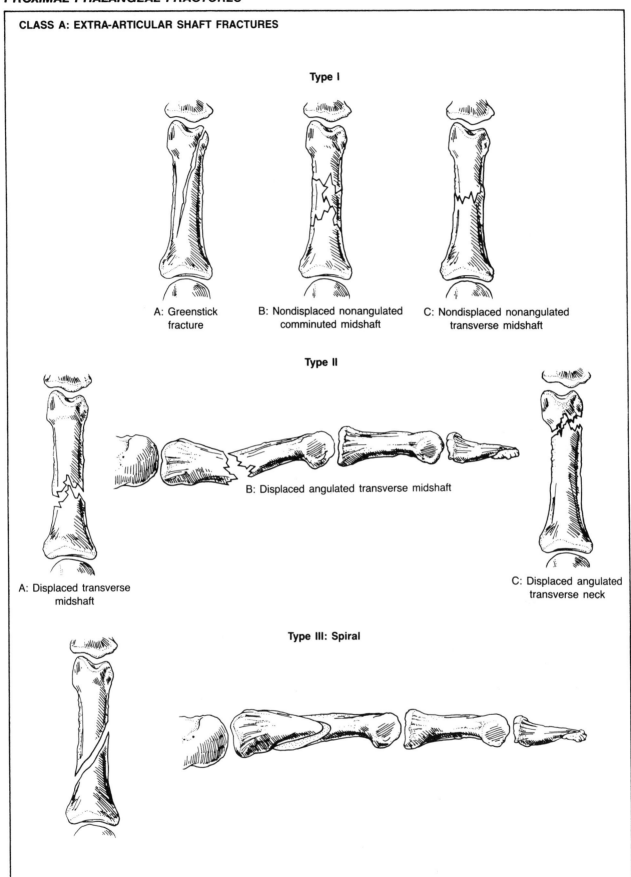

CLASS A: EXTRA-ARTICULAR SHAFT FRACTURES

Type I

A: Greenstick fracture

B: Nondisplaced nonangulated comminuted midshaft

C: Nondisplaced nonangulated transverse midshaft

Type II

A: Displaced transverse midshaft

B: Displaced angulated transverse midshaft

C: Displaced angulated transverse neck

Type III: Spiral

Figure 7–24.

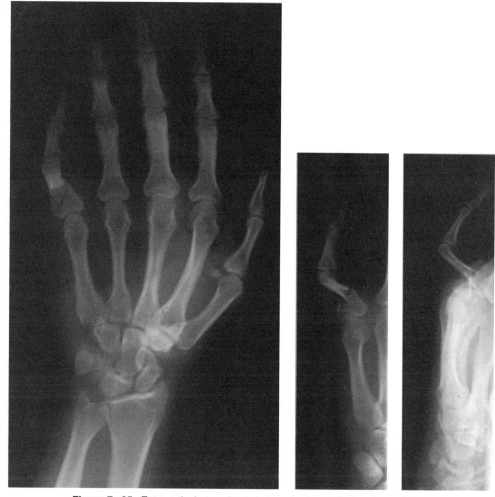

Figure 7–25. Extra-articular proximal phalanx fracture with dorsal angulation.

1. Dynamic splinting (see Appendix) with early motion exercises followed by a repeated radiographic examination in 5 to 7 days to ensure proper placement is the most simple method of treatment.
2. It is the authors' recommendation that these fractures be treated with a gutter splint for 10 to 14 days (see Appendix). This should be followed by a repeat x ray examination, and if the fragments are properly positioned a dynamic splint can be used (see Appendix).

☐ Class A: Type IIA   (Displaced Transverse Midshaft)
            Type IIB   (Displaced Angulated Transverse Midshaft)
            Type IIC   (Displaced Angulated Neck)

These fractures are unstable and may or may not be stable following reduction.[12] The emergency center management of these fractures includes immobilization, ice, elevation, and orthopedic referral. If this is not available

these fractures may be reduced by the emergency physician. The method of reducing type IIB fractures is as follows:

1. Anesthesia using either a wrist or metacarpal block is recommended.
2. While flexing the MCP joint longitudinal traction should be applied to gain length. The MCP joint should be flexed to 90 degrees to tighten the collateral ligaments and reduce the displacing force of the intrinsic muscles.
3. At this point, traction should be continued while the PIP is flexed to 90 degrees. The fracture should be reduced in this position. If, with slight extension of the PIP, there is loss of reduction, the fracture is unstable and will require internal fixation. If the fracture cannot be reduced using this method, interposition of tissue should be suspected.
4. If the reduction is stable, a short arm cast to the palmar crease with a dorsal extension to the PIP should be applied with the MCP in some flexion.

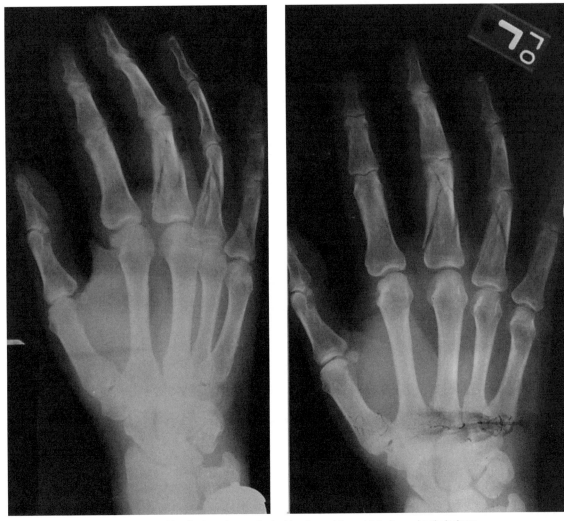

Figure 7–26. Nondisplaced comminuted fracture of the midshaft proximal phalanx.

More MCP flexion may be necessary in order to achieve near anatomic alignment.[5] Postreduction radiographs for documentation of position are recommended.

5. Referral for close orthopedic follow-up is strongly urged.

☐ Class A: Type III (Spiral)

The emergency center management of these fractures consists of immobilization, ice, elevation, and orthopedic referral. In many instances, internal fixation may be necessary.

Complications

The complications of proximal phalangeal fractures may result in permanent disability[10] and are as follows:

1. Rotational malalignment is a disabling complication that must be ruled out initially and on all subsequent examinations.
2. The extensor mechanism is in close proximity with the periosteum and adhesions may form after injury. This complication is commonly seen following type II or III fractures and results in a loss of motion that may require surgical intervention.
3. Adhesions may form between the flexor profundus and the superficialis tendons following immobilization. These debilitating injuries require surgical intervention for restoration of function.
4. Nonunion is rarely encountered except with inadequately immobilized fractures or open fractures.

☐ CLASS B: EXTRA-ARTICULAR MIDDLE SHAFT FRACTURES (FIG. 7–27)

Mechanism of Injury

A direct blow to the middle phalanx is the most commonly encountered mechanism for fractures. Indirect trauma, such as twisting along the longitudinal axis, frequently results in PIP dislocations rather than spiral fractures of the middle phalanx.

Angulation deformities resulting from the pull of the flexor and extensor tendons are commonly associated with these fractures. The flexor mechanism exerts

MIDDLE PHALANGEAL FRACTURES

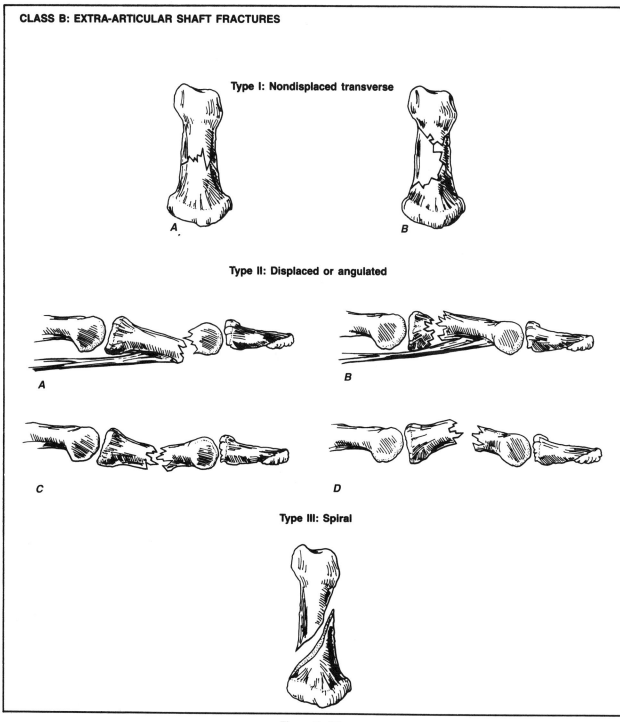

CLASS B: EXTRA-ARTICULAR SHAFT FRACTURES

Type I: Nondisplaced transverse

A.   B

Type II: Displaced or angulated

A   B

C   D

Type III: Spiral

Figure 7–27.

the predominant force and tends to displace the larger of the fracture fragments in a volar direction.

Examination
Pain and swelling will be localized over the fracture area. Clinical and radiographic recognition of rotational deformities, as shown in Figures 7–1, 7–2, and 7–18, are essential.

X Ray
AP, lateral, and oblique views are essential to identify fracture lines as well as angulation and rotational deformities.

Associated Injuries
Digital neurovascular structures may be damaged with middle phalanx fractures. In addition, tendon rupture (acute or delayed) along with the formation of adhesions may be associated with these fractures.

Treatment

□ Class B: Type I (Nondisplaced Transverse)
These fractures may be treated with dynamic immobilization or a gutter splint (see Appendix) for 10 to 14 days followed by a repeat radiographic examination to ensure proper reduction.[12,13]

□ Class B: Type II (Displaced or Angulated Transverse)
These fractures are unstable and may remain unstable after reduction. The emergency department management of these fractures includes immobilization, ice, elevation, and orthopedic referral. If emergent consultation is not available these fractures may be reduced by the emergency physician. The method of reducing a type IIB fracture is as follows:

1. Anesthesia using either a wrist or metacarpal block is recommended.
2. Gentle longitudinal traction in conjunction with flexion and manipulation of the distal fragment generally results in reduction.
3. If the fracture is unstable with slight extension, internal fixation is indicated.
4. If the reduced fracture is stable, immobilize the digit in a gutter splint in the position of function for 4 to 6 weeks (see Appendix). Postreduction radiographs for documentation of position are recommended.
5. Referral for orthopedic follow-up is strongly urged.

□ Class B: Type III (Spiral)
The emergency center management of these fractures consists of immobilization, ice, elevation, and emergent orthopedic referral. Many consultants will use a *Böhler traction device* (see Fig. 7–23) in managing these fractures.

Complications
The complications are similar to those of proximal phalanx injuries.

1. Rotational malalignment must be diagnosed and corrected early in the management of these fractures.
2. Scarring of the extensor mechanism with subsequent reduced motion may complicate these fractures.
3. The development of flexor tendon adhesions is a disabling complication of these fractures.
4. Nonunion secondary to inadequate immobilization or incomplete reduction may complicate the management of these fractures.

□ CLASS A: INTRA-ARTICULAR PROXIMAL FRACTURES (FIG. 7–28)

These fractures can be divided on the basis of therapy into two types. Type I fractures are uncommon and are treated as closed injuries whereas type II fractures are more common and require surgical reduction.

Mechanism of Injury
The most frequent mechanism is avulsion secondary to collateral ligament traction. The indirect transmission of a longitudinal force, however, may result in a condylar fracture.

Examination
There will be a fusiform swelling with tenderness over the involved joint.

X Ray
AP, lateral, and oblique views are usually adequate in demonstrating these fractures.

Associated Injuries
Avulsion fractures may result in detachment of the collateral ligament with subsequent joint instability.

PROXIMAL PHALANGEAL FRACTURES

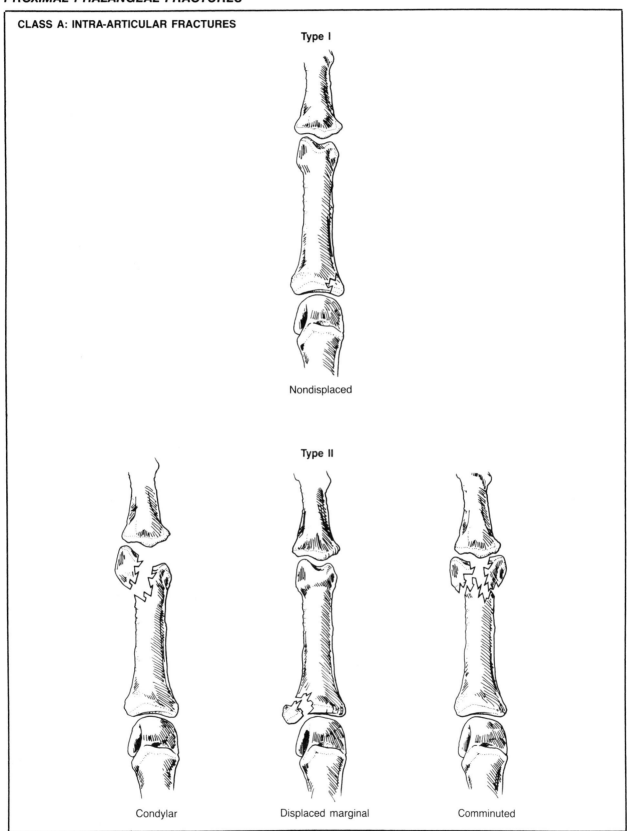

CLASS A: INTRA-ARTICULAR FRACTURES

Type I

Nondisplaced

Type II

Condylar   Displaced marginal   Comminuted

Figure 7–28.

Treatment

□ Class A: Type I   (Nondisplaced)

Intra-articular avulsion fractures of the base of the proximal phalanx of the index through the fifth finger may be treated conservatively if the fragment is stable and involves less than 20 percent of the articular surface. Buddy taping with active motion exercises along with early referral for close monitoring are recommended.[11-20]

□ Class A: Type II   (Displaced or
                        Comminuted)

Emergency management includes immobilization, ice, elevation, and referral for open reduction and internal fixation.

Complications

The most common complications include chronic joint stiffness or arthritis.

□ CLASS B: INTRA-ARTICULAR MIDDLE FRACTURES, TYPES I, II, AND III (FIG. 7-29)

These fractures can be divided into four types on the basis of anatomy and therapy. Type I fractures are nondisplaced condylar fractures whereas type II includes displaced condylar fractures. Type III includes comminuted basilar fractures of the middle phalanx. Type IV fractures are avulsion injuries and are distinct. They share no common therapeutic principles with the preceding three types. Type IV fractures will be discussed separately.

Mechanism of Injury

There are two mechanisms that commonly result in intra-articular middle phalangeal fractures. Direct trauma only infrequently results in these fractures, but the most common mechanism of fracture is secondary to a longitudinal force transmitted from the distal phalanx.

Examination

There will be a fusiform swelling with tenderness over the involved joint.

X Ray

AP, lateral, and oblique views are usually adequate in demonstrating these fractures.

Associated Injuries

None are commonly encountered.

MIDDLE PHALANGEAL FRACTURES

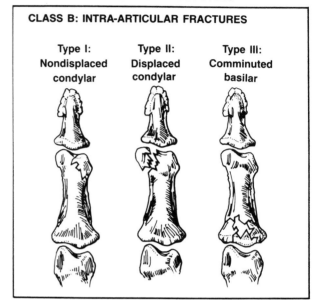

CLASS B: INTRA-ARTICULAR FRACTURES

Type I: Type II: Type III:
Nondisplaced   Displaced   Comminuted
condylar   condylar   basilar

Figure 7-29.

Treatment

□ Class B: Type I   (Nondisplaced Condylar)

Dynamic splinting (see Appendix) with early motion exercises is the recommended mode of therapy.

□ Class B: Type II   (Displaced Condylar)

Emergency management includes immobilization, ice, elevation, and referral.

□ Class B: Type III   (Comminuted Basilar)

Emergency management includes immobilization, ice, elevation, and referral for traction splinting.

Complications

The most frequent complications include joint stiffness or arthritic degeneration, which may occur despite optimum therapy.[17]

□ CLASS B: INTRA-ARTICULAR MIDDLE FRACTURES, TYPE IV (FIG. 7-30)

Avulsion fractures of the middle phalanx are generally referred to as *boutonnière injuries*. These fractures have been divided into three groups on an anatomic and therapeutic basis. Group A injuries are secondary to an avulsion of the central slip of the extensor tendon and if untreated will result in a boutonniere deformity. Group B injuries are due to an avulsion of the volar plate. Group C injuries represent an avulsion of the collateral ligament.

MIDDLE PHALANGEAL FRACTURES

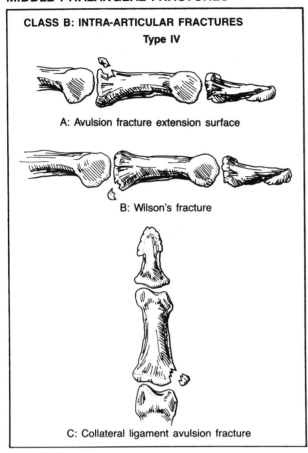

CLASS B: INTRA-ARTICULAR FRACTURES
Type IV

A: Avulsion fracture extension surface

B: Wilson's fracture

C: Collateral ligament avulsion fracture

Figure 7–30.

Mechanism of Injury

Each group of type IV fractures is associated with a different mechanism of injury. In type IVA injuries, forced flexion with the finger in rigid extension may result in a tendon tear or an avulsion injury. In type IVB, extreme hyperextension at the PIP joint will result in avulsion of the volar plate that is frequently accompanied by dorsal subluxation or dislocation of the middle phalanx. In type IVC, extreme medial or lateral traction of the digit will result in an avulsion of the collateral ligaments.

Examination

This is a difficult fracture to diagnose early. Initially, there will be a point of tenderness without swelling or deformity at the PIP joint. Later, there will be fusiform swelling and tenderness of the PIP joint. Early diagnosis can be made by anesthetizing the digit and examining for range of motion and for joint stability. Dorsal avulsion fractures will prevent full extension whereas PIP laxity will accompany collateral ligament injuries.

X Ray

AP and lateral views are usually adequate (Fig. 7–31).

Associated Injuries

Injuries commonly associated with these fractures include type IVA where there may be a complete tear of the central slip of the extensor tendon without avulsion of bone. Type IVB fractures are associated with a subluxation or dislocation of the PIP joint. This may be difficult to diagnose on clinical grounds secondary to pain and swelling. The type IVC fracture is commonly associated with lateral joint instability.

Treatment

Type IV fractures should be immobilized for only a minimum period of time to reduce the incidence of joint stiffness. In addition to early referral, periodic radiographic examinations to ensure proper positioning during healing are indicated.

☐ Class B: Type IVA (Avulsion Extensor Surface)

Avulsion surface fractures require internal fixation, therefore, urgent referral is indicated. Tendon avulsions without fractures can be treated by splinting the PIP joint in full extension for 5 to 6 weeks. The DIP joint should not be splinted and should receive active and passive range of motion exercises throughout the splinting period.

☐ Class B: Type IVB (Wilson's Fracture)

If the fragment is less than 30 percent of the joint surface, closed treatment can be recommended. The PIP joint should be splinted in 45 to 50 degrees of flexion for 4 weeks after any dislocation or subluxation has been reduced. This therapeutic program is controversial as some hand surgeons will elect internal fixation for all of these fractures to repair the volar plate. In the other camp, recent literature supports a conservative treatment approach for fractures where there is no subluxation of the joint.[2] Early consultation is therefore advised so that the appropriate therapeutic program can be selected.

☐ Class B: Type IVC (Collateral Ligament Avulsion)

Surgical fixation is recommended by most surgeons. Early consultation is recommended strongly so that the appropriate therapeutic program can be selected.

Complications

Class B, type IV fractures may be associated with several disabling complications.

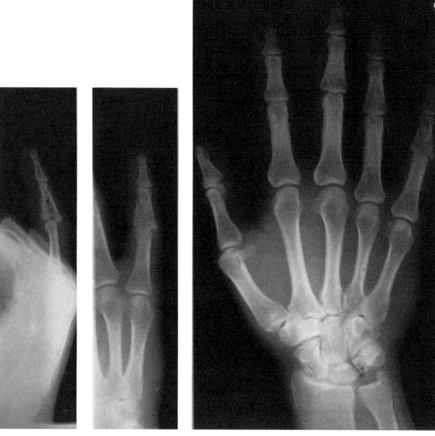

Figure 7–31. Comminuted intra-articular fracture of the middle phalanx.

1. Joint instability secondary to ligamentous damage may be noted.
2. Chronic degenerative arthritis may complicate the management of these fractures.
3. Loss of extensor tendon function as a result of nonunion may occur.
4. A boutonnière deformity, as shown in Figure 7–32, may result if this fracture is not diagnosed or is improperly treated.

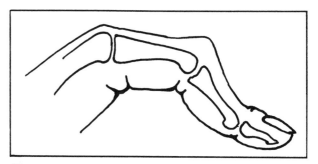

Figure 7–32. A boutonniere deformity resulting from disruption of the extensor tendon.

METACARPAL FRACTURES 2 THROUGH 5

Metacarpal fractures are divided into two groups: those involving the first metacarpal and those involving metacarpals 2 through 5. This distinction is based on the fact that the mechanical function of the first metacarpal is distinct from the remaining metacarpals. First metacarpal fractures will be discussed separately at the end of this chapter.

Essential Anatomy

The heads of the metacarpals are connected by the inter-metacarpal ligaments. At the bases of the metacarpals there is a great amount of variation in mobility. Metacarpals 4 and 5 have from 15 to 25 degrees of AP motion whereas 2 and 3 have virtually no motion at their base. Metacarpals 2 and 3 represent the *fixed center* of the hand from which the remaining bones are suspended. The normal "degree of mobility" is of critical concern when reducing metacarpal fractures. Angulated fractures of metacarpals 4 and 5 do not require a precise reduction because their normal mobility allows for compensation. Angulated fractures of the second and third metacarpals, however, require a precise reduction because angulation will inhibit the normal function.

As shown in Figure 7–21 (p.112), the collateral ligaments are taut in flexion and lax when the digit is extended. Fracture reduction may be facilitated with digit extension and subsequent laxity in the collateral ligaments.

Classification

Metacarpal fractures 2 through 5 are divided into four classes.

- **Class A:** Metacarpal head fractures
- **Class B:** Metacarpal neck fractures
- **Class C:** Metacarpal shaft fractures
- **Class D:** Metacarpal base fractures

☐ CLASS A: HEAD FRACTURES (FIG. 7–33)

These are uncommon fractures with many disabling complications even with optimum therapy. These frac-

METACARPAL FRACTURES 2 THROUGH 5

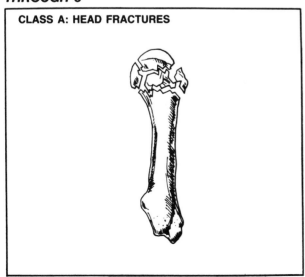

CLASS A: HEAD FRACTURES

Figure 7–33.

tures occur distal to the attachment of the collateral ligaments.

Mechanism of Injury

The most common mechanism is a direct blow or a crushing injury resulting typically in a comminuted fracture.[17]

Examination

There will be tenderness and swelling over the involved MCP joint. Pain will be increased and localized over the MCP joint with axial compression of the extended digit.

X Ray

AP and lateral views are usually adequate for demonstrating this fracture. At times, oblique views may be necessary to adequately visualize the fracture fragments. A 10-degree pronated lateral view may be helpful in assessing index- and middle-finger metacarpal fractures. A 10-degree supinated lateral view may be helpful in assessing ring- and small-finger metacarpal fractures. Collateral ligament avulsions can often be optimally visualized with the Brewerton view taken with the MCP joints flexed 65 degrees with the dorsal surface on the plate and the beam angled 15 degrees radially.[1]

Associated Injuries

Injuries associated with metacarpal head fractures include (1) extensor tendon damage, (2) a crush injury to the interosseous muscle resulting in fibrosis, and (3) collateral ligament avulsion.[1]

Treatment

All metacarpal head fractures require referral for management and follow-up. Fractures associated with adjacent lacerations should be considered open and emergent orthopedic consultation with operative exploration irrigation and repair is recommended. Patients with suspected open fractures should receive perioperative parenteral antibiotics. Prophylactic coverage with a cephalosporin is recommended although patients with contaminated wounds should also receive penicillin and an aminoglycoside. The value of routine single swab culturing of the wound perioperatively is questionable.[23] Emergency management should include elevation, ice, analgesics, and immobilization of the hand in a soft bulky dressing in the position of function. Metacarpal head fractures with large intra-articular defects generally require intraoperative fixation to establish a near normal joint relationship.[14-20] For small intra-articular fragments, most consultants will immobilize the hand only for a short time and then begin motion exercises. Many of these fractures may require arthroplasty later.

Complications

Metacarpal head fractures may be associated with debilitating hand complications.[10]

1. Rotational malalignment must be diagnosed and corrected early in the management of these fractures.
2. Interosseous muscle fibrosis resulting from crush damage is a late complication of this fracture.
3. Extensor tendon injury or fibrosis may be associated with this fracture. Symptoms and signs may present acutely or be delayed in their presentation.
4. Chronic stiffness of the MP joint may complicate these fractures.

□ CLASS B: NECK FRACTURES (FIG. 7–34)

Nearly all metacarpal neck fractures are unstable and have some degree of volar angulation. After reduction there is a tendency for the distal fragment to be displaced in a volar direction.

The accuracy of reduction when treating these fractures is dependent on the mobility of the involved metacarpal. In the fifth metacarpal, where the normal excursion is 15 to 25 degrees, up to 40 degrees of angulation is acceptable without limitation of normal function. In the fourth metacarpal, up to 15 degrees of angulation is acceptable without inhibiting normal motion.[11] This is in contradistinction to fractures of the second and third metacarpals where accurate anatomic reductions are essential for the restoration of normal function.

Mechanism of Injury

Direct impaction forces, such as a punch with a clenched fist, often result in neck fractures. Neck fractures of the fifth metacarpal are called "boxer's fractures," and are very common injuries.

Examination

There will be tenderness and swelling over the involved MP joints. Rotational deformities may accompany these fractures and must be diagnosed and corrected early. Figures 7–1, 7–2, and 7–18 summarize the clinical findings that signify rotational malalignment.

X Ray

AP, lateral, and oblique views are usually adequate in defining the fracture and in determining the amount of angulation and displacement (Fig. 7–35). A 10-degree pronated lateral view may be helpful in assessing index- and middle-finger metacarpal fractures. A 10-degree supinated lateral view may be helpful in assessing ring- and small-finger metacarpal fractures.

Associated Injury

Associated injuries are not commonly seen with these fractures. Occasionally, this fracture will be accompanied by injuries to the digital nerves.

Treatment

Three important points must be stressed in the treatment of metacarpal neck fractures.

1. Rotational deformities must be diagnosed and treated early.
2. The acceptance of volar angulation is dependent on the normal mobility of the involved metacarpal.
3. Fractures associated with adjacent lacerations should be considered open, and emergent orthopedic consultation with operative exploration irrigation and repair is recommended.[1]

Metacarpal neck fractures are divided into two groups: those involving the fourth and fifth and those involving the second and third metacarpals.

□ Class B: Type I (Nondisplaced Nonangulated Metacarpals 4 or 5)

The management of this fracture[16] includes ice, elevation, and immobilization with a palmar plaster splint to the palmar crease and a dorsal splint extending to, but not including the PIP. This should be accomplished with the wrist extended 30 degrees and the MCP joints flexed to 90 degrees.[1,16] Generally, it is recommended to begin PIP and DIP motion without delay. Protected MCP motion can begin in 3 to 4 weeks.[1] There is some evidence to support immediate immobilization of single metacarpal 2 to 5 subcapital fractures after adequate reduction with functional casting applied immediately

METACARPAL FRACTURES 2 THROUGH 5

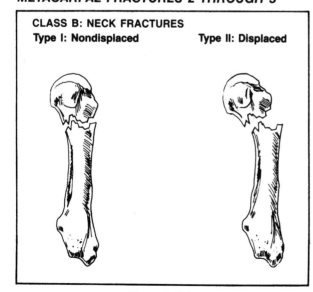

CLASS B: NECK FRACTURES
Type I: Nondisplaced   **Type II: Displaced**

Figure 7–34.

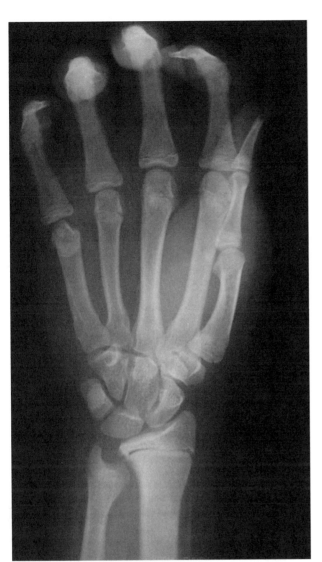 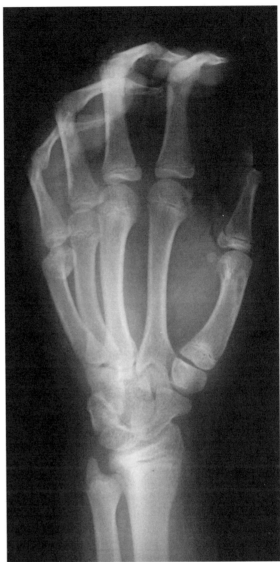

Figure 7–35. Fracture of the metacarpal neck with volar angulation.

prior to reduction.[18] This approach may be considered after orthopedic consultation.

☐ **Class B: Type I   (Angulation of Less than 4 Degrees, Metacarpals 4 or 5)**

Reduction of this fracture is optional when the fifth metacarpal is involved but should be attempted on fourth metacarpal fractures. These fractures can be reduced in most cases by adhering to the following steps:

1. An ulnar nerve wrist block should be used to achieve adequate anesthesia.
2. Finger traps should be placed on the involved digits for 10 to 15 minutes to disimpact the fracture.
3. After disimpaction, the MCP joint should be flexed to 90 degrees as well as the PIP and DIP joints (Fig. 7–36).

4. The physician should now apply a volar directed force over the metacarpal shaft while at the same time applying dorsally directed pressure over the flexed PIP joint. Reduction should be completed with this maneuver.
5. Immobilization with a palmar plastic splint to the palmar crease and a dorsal splint extending to, but not including the PIP, should be accomplished with the wrist extended 30 degrees and the MCP joints flexed to 90 degrees.[1,5]
6. A radiographic examination postreduction and at 1 week is recommended to ensure maintenance of proper position.
7. Generally it is recommended to begin PIP and DIP motion without delay. Protected MCP motion can begin in 3 to 4 weeks.[1] There is some evidence to support immediate immobilization of single metacarpal 2

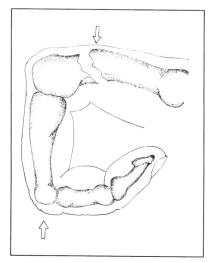

Figure 7–36. The 90–90 method of reduction of a fracture of the metacarpal. the proximal phalanx is used to push the metacarpal fracture into a good position.

to 5 subcapital fractures after adequate reduction with functional casting applied immediately prior to reduction.[18] This approach may be considered after orthopedic consultation.

☐ Class B: Type II   (Angulation of More than 40 Degrees, Metacarpals 4 or 5)

Reduction is mandatory for these fractures and should be accomplished by the 90-to-90 method listed previously and shown in Figure 7–36. After reduction, immobilization with a palmar plastic splint to the palmar crease and a dorsal splint extending to, but not including the PIP, should be accomplished with the wrist extended 30 degrees and the MCP joints flexed to 90 degrees.[1,18] These fractures require close follow-up because they have a tendency to develop volar angulation despite immobilization in a gutter splint. Repeated, frequent radiographic examinations including postreduction views are strongly urged. If the reduction is unstable, pin fixation will be necessary, and early referral is indicated. Generally, it is recommended to begin PIP and DIP motion without delay. Protected MCP motion can begin in 3 to 4 weeks.[1] There is some evidence to support immediate immobilization of single metacarpal 2 to 5 subcapital fractures after adequate reduction with functional casting applied immediately prior to reduction. This approach may be considered after orthopedic consultation.

☐ Class B: Type I   (Nondisplaced Nonangulated Metacarpals 2 or 3)

The recommended therapy includes ice, elevation, and immobilization in a gutter splint (see Appendix) extend-

ing from the distal elbow to the PIP joint. The wrist should be in 20 degrees of extension and the MP joint should be in 50 to 60 degrees of flexion with the PIP free. Close follow-up for angulation or rotational malalignment is strongly urged. *Caution*: These fractures require follow-up radiographic examinations at 4 to 5 days postinjury to exclude delayed displacement. Displacement is difficult to correct if detected beyond this time. Generally, it is recommended to begin PIP and DIP motion without delay. Protected MP motion can begin in 3 to 4 weeks.[1]

☐ Class B: Type II   (Displacement or Angulation More than 15 Degrees, Metacarpals 2 or 3)

The emergency management of these fractures includes ice, elevation, and immobilization in a volar splint with referral. Accurate reduction of these fractures is imperative and frequently can only be maintained with pinning.

Complications

Metacarpal neck fractures are associated with several disabling complications.[13]

1. Collateral ligament damage and asymmetry may be secondary to malposition of the fracture fragment.
2. Extensor tendon injuries may accompany these fractures.
3. Rotational malalignment may accompany these fractures and must be diagnosed and corrected early.
4. Dorsal bony prominence with compromise of the extensor mechanism may complicate these fractures. This complication can be avoided by:
   a. adequate immobilization,
   b. acceptable reduction with close follow-up to ensure proper positioning,
   c. elevation of the extremity to reduce edema.
5. Malposition or clawing of the finger when extension is attempted may complicate these fractures if the reduction is incomplete or unstable.
6. Pain with grasp.

☐ CLASS C: SHAFT FRACTURES (FIG. 7–37)

There are three types of metacarpal shaft fractures: transverse, oblique, and comminuted. Each of these fractures will be discussed separately in the treatment section.

Mechanism of Injury

There are two mechanisms that result in metacarpal shaft fractures. A direct blow to the hand may result in a transverse or short oblique fracture with dorsal angulation secondary to the pull of the interosseous muscles.

METACARPAL FRACTURES 2 THROUGH 5

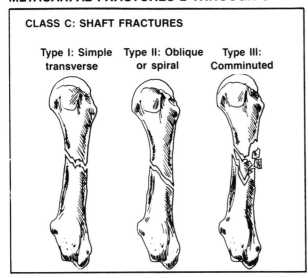

CLASS C: SHAFT FRACTURES

Type I: Simple transverse   Type II: Oblique or spiral   Type III: Comminuted

Figure 7–37.

Comminuted fractures are also seen with this mechanism and are associated with a significant amount of soft tissue damage.

An indirect blow resulting in a rotational torque force applied to the digit is transmitted to the metacarpal shaft and frequently causes a spiral shaft fracture. Angulation is uncommon with these fractures as the tendency of the deep transverse metacarpal ligament is to shorten and rotate these fractures.

Examination

There will be tenderness and swelling over the dorsal aspect of the hand. The pain will be increased with motion and in most cases the patient will be unable to make a fist. Rotational deformities must be excluded early in the management of these fractures (see Figs. 7–1, 7–2, and 7–18).

X Ray

AP, lateral, and oblique views are often necessary for accurate visualization of the fracture. A 10-degree pronated lateral view may be helpful in assessing index- and middle-finger metacarpal fractures. A 10-degree supinated lateral view may be helpful in assessing ring- and small-finger metacarpal fractures. As the metacarpal shaft fracture is more proximal, the tendency for dorsal angulation becomes greater. Rotational malalignment should be suspected if there is a discrepancy in the shaft diameter (see Fig. 7–19) or if there is metacarpal shortening.

Associated Injury

Injury to the neural structures is only infrequently associated with these fractures.

Treatment

Metacarpal shaft fractures are often associated with rotational malalignment. Rotational deformities can be detected clinically on the basis of three tests:

1. Convergence test (see Figs. 7–1 and 7–2)
2. Plane of the nail plate (see Fig. 7–18)
3. Radiographic diameter of the fracture fragments (see Fig. 7–19)

Angulation deformities of less than 10 degrees in the index and middle metacarpals and less than 20 degrees in the ring and fifth metacarpals are acceptable.[1]

☐ Class C: Type I (Nondisplaced Transverse)

These fractures can be treated with a gutter splint extending from the distal elbow to the fingertip. The wrist should be extended 30 degrees with the MCP joint in 90 degrees of flexion and the PIP and DIP in extension. Early referral and repeated radiographic examinations are recommended.

☐ Class C: Type I (Displaced or Angulated Transverse)

All of these fractures require elevation, ice, immobilization, and consultation for reduction and follow-up. Emergency reduction when consultation is unavailable may be accomplished by the following method:

1. A wrist block should be used to achieve adequate anesthesia.
2. The fracture fragments should be manipulated into position using a volar directed force over the dorsally angulated fragment while traction is maintained. Rotational deformities must also be corrected at this time.
3. A well-molded dorsal and volar splint with the wrist extended 30 degrees and including the entire metacarpal shaft but not the MCP joints should be applied.
4. The patient should be referred for follow-up and for frequent radiographic examinations including postreduction views to ensure proper positioning.

☐ Class C: Type II (Oblique or Spiral)

These fractures require ice, elevation, immobilization in a bulky compressive dressing, and referral for reduction and pinning.

☐ Class C: Type III (Comminuted)

The emergency management of these fractures includes ice, elevation, and immobilization in a bulky compressive dressing with early referral. Some orthopedic surgeons prefer a volar splint or even a Böhler traction splint in managing these fractures.

Complications

Complications frequently associated with these fractures may be disabling.

1. Malrotation must be diagnosed and corrected early in the management of these fractures.
2. Dorsal bony prominence with compromise of the extensor mechanism may be associated with these fractures.
3. Interosseous muscle damage with subsequent fibrosis has been associated with these fractures.
4. Nonunion may be secondary to insufficient immobilization, inadequate reduction, or may be associated with osteomyelitis at the fracture site.
5. A chronic painful grip may result from palmar angulation of the distal bone fragment.

☐ CLASS D: BASE FRACTURES (FIG. 7–38)

Metacarpal head fractures are usually stable injuries. Rotational malalignment of the head will be magnified in its presentation at the tip of the digit.

Mechanism of Injury
There are two mechanisms that result in metacarpal head fractures. A direct blow over the head of the metacarpal may result in a fracture. Indirectly, digital torsion exerting a longitudinal torque is an uncommon fracture mechanism.

Examination
There will be tenderness and swelling at the base of the metacarpals. Pain will be exacerbated with flexion or extension of the wrist or with longitudinal compression.

X Ray
AP and lateral views are generally adequate in defining these fractures (Fig. 7–39). Intra-articular base fractures often require tomograms or CT scans to evaluate fully the carpometacarpal relationship.[1] Always exclude a carpal bone fracture when a metacarpal base fracture is detected.

Associated Injury
Fractures at the base of the fourth and fifth metacarpals may cause injury to the motor branch of the ulnar nerve resulting in paralysis of the intrinsic hand muscles with the exception of the hypothenar muscles. This neural

METACARPAL FRACTURES 2 THROUGH 5

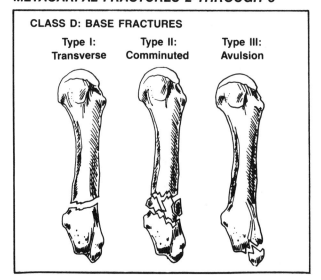

CLASS D: BASE FRACTURES

Type I: Transverse   Type II: Comminuted   Type III: Avulsion

Figure 7–38.

injury is associated frequently with crush injuries. The neural damage may not be apparent initially secondary to swelling and pain. Referral with close follow-up of these injuries is strongly urged.

Treatment
The emergency management of these fractures includes ice, elevation, and immobilization in a bulky compressive dressing with referral. Many orthopedic surgeons prefer a volar splint or even a Böhler traction splint in managing these fractures. Arthroplasty may be necessary if an intra-articular fracture is noted.

Complications
Metacarpal base fractures are associated with several serious complications.

1. Damage to the extensor or the flexor tendons may be associated with these fractures.
2. Rotational malalignment must be detected and corrected early in the management of these fractures.
3. Chronic carpal metacarpal joint stiffness is often noted after these fractures.

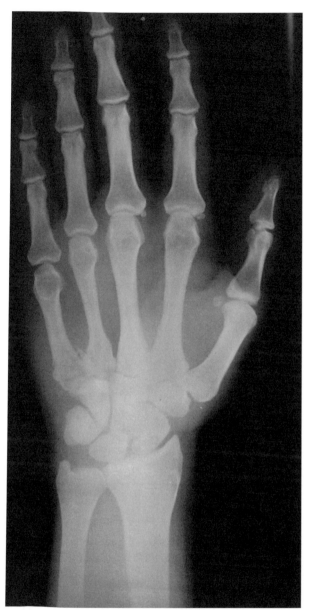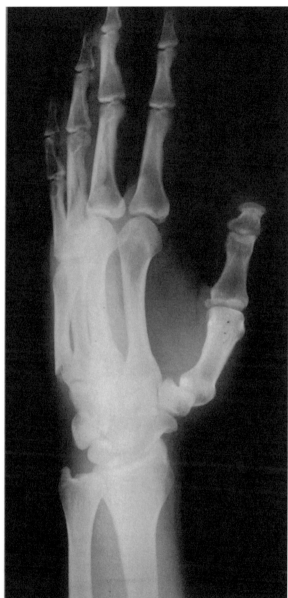

Figure 7–39. Fracture of the base of the fifth metacarpal.

FIRST METACARPAL FRACTURES

The first metacarpal is biomechanically distinct from the remaining metacarpals because of its high degree of mobility. For this reason, fractures of the first metacarpal are uncommon, and angulation deformities can be accepted without functional impairment.

Fractures of the first metacarpal are classified into three types. Class A fractures are extra-articular, Class B fractures involve the metacarpal joint, and Class C fractures involve sesamoid bones of the thumb.

FIRST METACARPAL FRACTURES

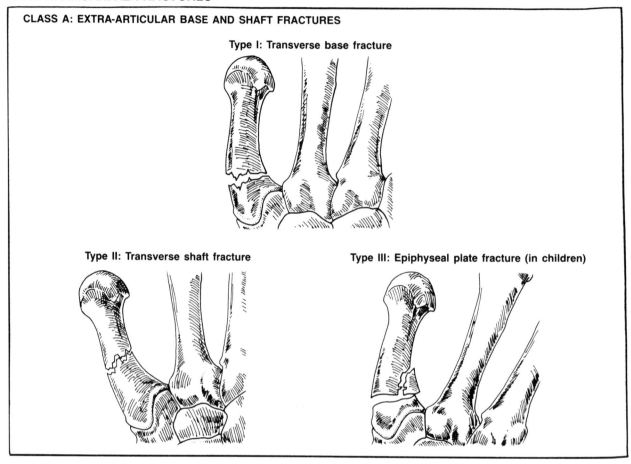

CLASS A: EXTRA-ARTICULAR BASE AND SHAFT FRACTURES

Type I: Transverse base fracture

Type II: Transverse shaft fracture

Type III: Epiphyseal plate fracture (in children)

Figure 7–40.

☐ CLASS A: EXTRA-ARTICULAR BASE AND SHAFT FRACTURES (FIG. 7–40)

Extra-articular fractures are more commonly seen than are intra-articular fractures of the first metacarpal. There are three types of extra-articular fractures: transverse, oblique, and, in children, epiphyseal plate fractures.

Mechanism of Injury
First metacarpal fractures are usually the result of a direct blow, a blow over the distal thumb, or impaction. Longitudinal torque or angular forces distally typically result in a metacarpal dislocation rather than a fracture. Longitudinal torque associated with a direct blow often results in an oblique fracture.[15]

Examination
There will be pain and tenderness over the fracture site, which is increased with motion.

X Ray
AP and lateral views are generally adequate for defining shaft fractures. Intra-articular fractures or epiphyseal plate fractures often require oblique views to accurately define the fracture lines and displacement.

Associated Injuries
Associated injuries are uncommonly encountered with these fractures.

Treatment
Because of the normal mobility of the first metacarpal, 20 to 30 degrees of angular deformity can be accepted without subsequent functional impairment. Fractures with over 20 to 30 degrees of angulation should undergo a closed manipulative reduction under regional anesthesia followed by postreduction radiographs.[15] The thumb should then be immobilized in a short arm thumb spica (see Appendix) for 4 weeks with the metacarpal joint flexed and the thumb in the fist position.

Oblique fractures may be unstable and complicated with rotational deformities. Percutaneous pinning is often required in the management of these fractures. Type III epiphyseal plate injuries require referral for definitive management and follow-up.[15]

FIRST METACARPAL FRACTURES

CLASS B: INTRA-ARTICULAR BASE FRACTURES

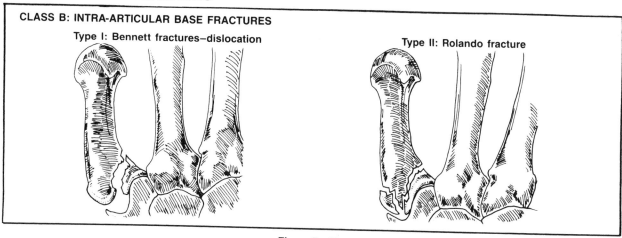

Type I: Bennett fractures–dislocation

Type II: Rolando fracture

Figure 7–41.

Complications

Extra-articular first metacarpal fractures may be complicated by rotational deformities with subsequent impairment of normal hand function.

☐ CLASS B: INTRA-ARTICULAR BASE FRACTURES (FIG. 7–41)

There are two types of intra-articular first metacarpal fractures. The first type is a Bennett fracture, which is a fracture combined with a subluxation or dislocation of the metacarpal joint. The second type of intra-articular first metacarpal fracture is a Rolando fracture, which can be a T or Y fracture involving the joint surface.

Mechanism of Injury

The most common mechanism is an axial force directed against a partially flexed metacarpal such as striking a rigid object with a clenched fist. The major deforming forces are supplied by the abductor pollicis longus which, in conjunction with the extrinsic extensors, result in lateral and proximal subluxation of the metacarpal shaft. The anterior oblique ligament (trapezium to

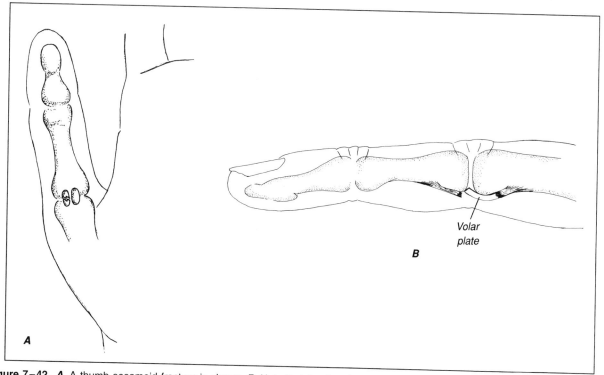

Volar plate

B

A

Figure 7–42. *A.* A thumb sesamoid fracture is shown. ***B.*** Note that the thumb may be hyperextended at the MCP joint and the volar plate of the thumb may become locked at the MCP joint during hyperextension.

metacarpal) and the deep ulnar liga-ment insert on the base of the first metacarpal and have a tendency to hold the proximal fragment in place.

X Ray
Routine views of the thumb are generally adequate in defining the fracture fragments. Intra-articular base fractures often require tomograms or CT scans to evaluate fully the carpometacarpal relationship.[1]

Treatment

☐ Class B: Type I   (Bennett Fracture–Dislocation)

The emergency management of these fractures includes ice, elevation, immobilization, and emergent orthopedic consultation. In some instances, a very carefully molded plaster cast followed by x ray confirmation of anatomic positioning will be elected. The thumb should be abducted and the MCP joint should not be hyperextended. If a satisfactory reduction cannot be maintained or achieved, percutaneous wiring is recommended.[2]

☐ Class B: Type II   (Rolando Fracture)

The emergency management of this fracture includes ice, elevation, immobilization, and referral. This fracture has a poor prognosis and is primarily dependent on the degree of comminution.

Complications
The most common complication is the development of osteoarthritis. In the Bennett fracture this may be secondary to an inadequate reduction whereas in the Rolando fracture it may occur despite optimum management.

☐ CLASS C: SESAMOID FRACTURES OF THE THUMB (FIG. 7–42)

Commonly, the hand has five sesamoids. Two of these sesamoids are present at the MCP joint of the thumb nearly 100 percent of the time. The ulnar sesamoid sits over the ulnar condyle of the distal first metacarpal. The radial sesamoid sits over the narrow radial condyle of the first metacarpal head.

The sesamoids of the thumb are embedded in the fibrous plate of the MCP joint. The accessory collateral ligaments insert into the lateral margins of the sesamoids while the tendon of the adductor pollicus inserts on the ulnar sesamoid and the flexor pollicus brevis on the radial sesamoid.

Mechanism of Injury
Typically, the patient will present with an MCP hyperextension injury. On examination there will be tenderness and swelling on the volar surface of the MCP joint.[2] The collateral ligaments should be stressed to assess their integrity. Palmar plate injuries determined by hyperextension instability or hyperextended locked MCP joint should be assessed and documented.[2]

X Ray
Routine views of the hand may demonstrate the fracture. If in doubt radial and ulnar oblique views of the thumb along with comparison views may be helpful.

Treatment
Closed fractures of the sesamoids without hyperextension instability can be treated with a splint with the MP joint in 30 degrees of flexion for 2 to 3 weeks.[15] In open fractures, those locked in hyperextension or those with clinical MCP instability, consultation for operative repair is recommended.[2]

Complications
Hyperextension deformity of the MCP joint of the thumb can complicate unstable palmar plate injuries.

REFERENCES

1. Ashkenaze DM, Ruby LK: Metacarpal fractures and dislocations. *Orthop Clin North Am* **23**(1):19, 1992.
2. Barton N: Conservative treatment of articular fractures in the hand. *J Hand Surg* **14A**(2):386–389, 1989.
3. Bowman SH, Simon RR: Metacarpal and phalangeal fractures. *Emerg Med Clin North Am* **11**(3):671–702, 1993.
4. Burdett-Smith MA: Displaced phalangeal fractures and associated injuries. *J Hand Surg* **17**(3):332–336, 1992.
5. Burkhalter WE: Closed treatment of hand fractures. *J Hand Surg* **14A**(2):390–393, 1989.
6. Burnham PJ: Physiological treatment for fractures of the metacarpals. *JAMA* **169**:815, 1962.
7. Burton RI, Eaton RG: Common hand injuries in the athlete. *Orthop Clin North Am* **4**(3):809, 1973.
8. Butt WE: Fractures of the hand. *Can Med Assoc J* **86**:731, 1962.
9. Butt WE: Fractures of the hand: Treatment results. *Can Med Assoc J* **86**:815, 1962.
10. Clinkscales GS: Complications in the management of fractures in hand injuries. *South Med J* **63**:704, 1970.
11. Corley Jr FG, Schenck Jr RC: Fractures of the hand. *Clin Plast Surg* **23**(3):447–462, 1996.
12. Curry GJ: Treatment of finger fractures, simple and compound. *Am J Surg* **71**(1):80, 1946.
13. Golden GT, et al: Fractures of the phalanges and metacarpals: An analysis of 555 fractures. *JACEP* **6**(3):79, 1977.
14. Green DP, et al: Fractures of the hand with associated injuries. *J Hand Surg* **8**:383, 1983.
15. Green DP, et al: Fractures of the thumb metacarpal. *South Med J* **65**(7):807, 1972.
16. Jahss SA: Fractures of the metacarpals. *J Bone Joint Surg* **26**(1):178, 1938.

17. Kaplan L: The treatment of fractures and dislocations of the hand and fingers. *Surg Clin North Am* **20:**1695, 1940.
18. Konradsen L, Nielsen P, Albrecht-bests E: Functional treatment of metacarpal fractures. *Acta Orthop Scand* **61**(6):531–534, 1990.
19. Lamphier TA: Improper reduction of fractures of the proximal phalanges of the fingers. *Am J Surg* **94:**926, 1957.
20. Light TR, Bednar MS: Management of intra-articular fractures of the metacarpophalangeal joint. *Hand Clin* **10**(2):303–314, 1994.
21. Lubahn JD: Mallet finger fractures: A comparison of open and closed technique. *J Hand Surg* **14A**(2):394–396, 1989.
22. Mansoor IA: Fractures of the proximal phalanx of fingers. *J Bone Joint Surg* **51**(1):196, 1969.
23. McLain RF, Steyers C, Stoddard M: Infections in open fractures of the hand. *J Hand Surg* **16A**(1):108–112, 1991.

BIBLIOGRAPHY

Brasher HR, Rainey RB: *Shand's Handbook of Orthopedic Surgery.* St. Louis: Mosby, 1978.
Kilgore EG, Graham W: *The Hand.* Philadelphia: Lea & Febiger, 1977.
Lipscomb PR: Management of fracltures of the hand. *Am Surg.* **29**(4):277, 1963.
Posner MA: Injuries to the hand and wrist of athletes. *Orthop Clin North Am* **8**(3):593, 1977.

8
CHAPTER
FRACTURES OF THE CARPALS

SCAPHOID FRACTURES

CLASS A: FRACTURE THROUGH THE WAIST
(p. 143)   **(MIDDLE THIRD)**

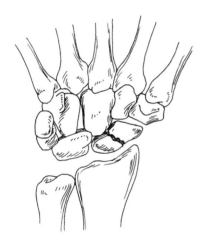

CLASS B: FRACTURE THROUGH THE PROXIMAL THIRD

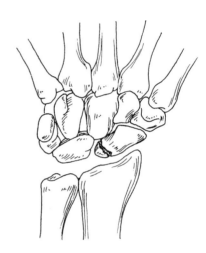

CLASS C: FRACTURE THROUGH THE DISTAL THIRD

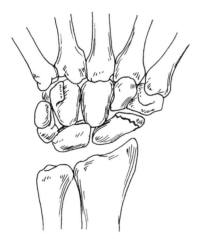

CLASS D: FRACTURE THROUGH THE TUBERCLE

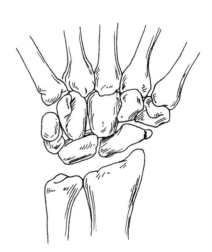

TRIQUETRUM FRACTURES

CLASS A: DORSAL CHIP FRACTURE
(p. 147)

CLASS B: TRANSVERSE FRACTURE

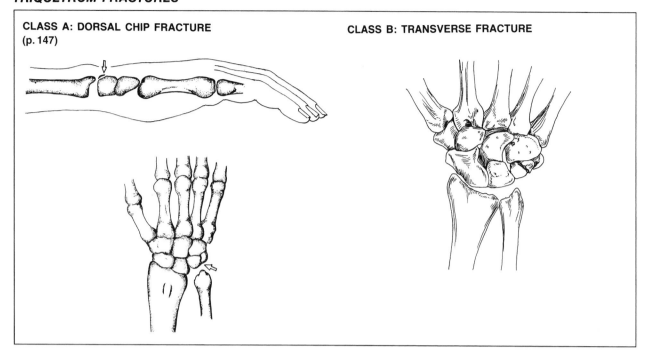

CAPITATE FRACTURE
(p. 150)

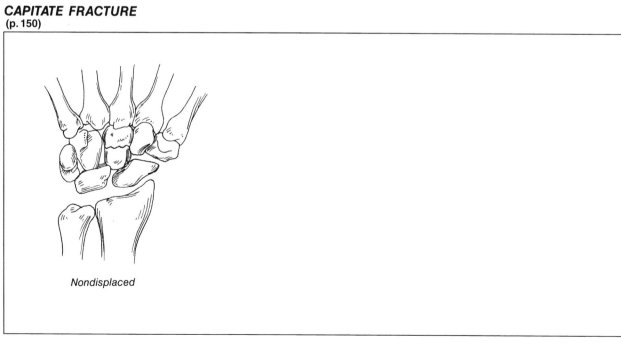

Nondisplaced

HAMATE FRACTURES

CLASS A: DISTAL ARTICULAR SURFACE FRACTURE
(p. 151)

CLASS B: HOOK OF HAMATE FRACTURE

CLASS C: COMMINUTED BODY FRACTURE

CLASS D: PROXIMAL POLE ARTICULAR SURFACE FRACTURE

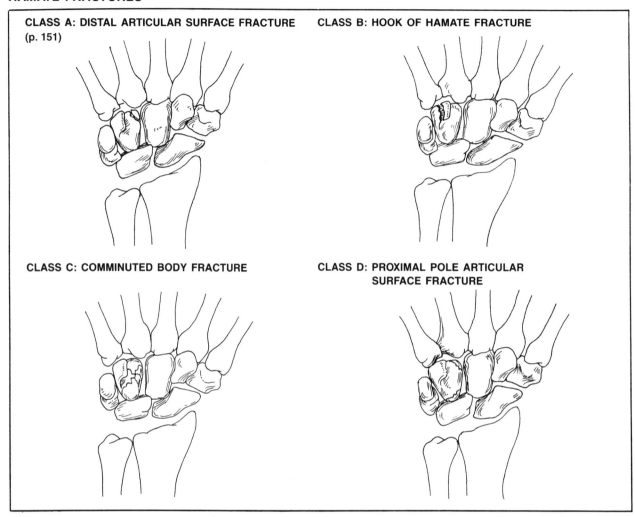

TRAPEZIUM FRACTURES

CLASS A: VERTICAL FRACTURE
(p. 153)

CLASS B: COMMINUTED FRACTURE

CLASS C: AVULSION FRACTURE

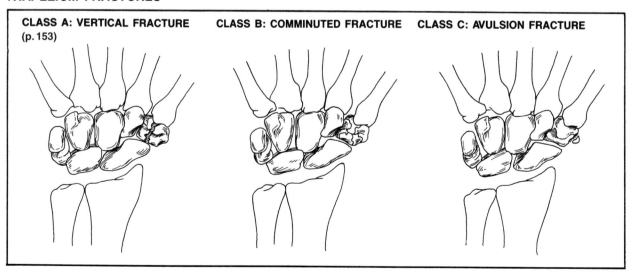

PISIFORM FRACTURES

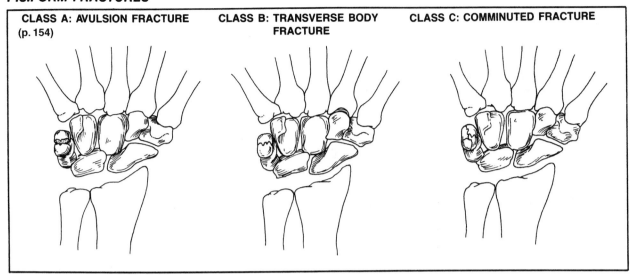

| CLASS A: AVULSION FRACTURE (p. 154) | CLASS B: TRANSVERSE BODY FRACTURE | CLASS C: COMMINUTED FRACTURE |

The carpals are a complex set of bones joined by ligaments forming multiple articulations. Because radiographs often reveal a significant overlap of shadows, a careful history as well as a meticulous clinical examination are often necessary to accurately diagnose these fractures. The scaphoid is not only the most frequently fractured carpal bone, but it is also one of the most fre-

quently missed carpal bone fractures. The triquetrum is the second most commonly fractured carpal bone whereas the lunate is the third most frequently fractured.

Essential Anatomy (Fig. 8–1)

The carpals are divided into a proximal row of four bones and a distal row of four bones. The proximal row

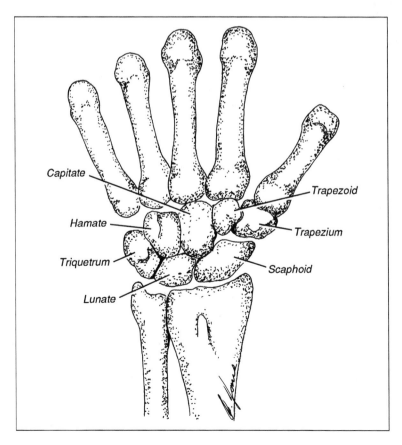

Figure 8–1. The radius articulates with the carpal bones. The ulna has a nonosseous fibrocartilaginous union with the triquetrum.

from the radial to the ulnar surface includes scaphoid (navicular), lunate, triquetrum (triangular), and pisiform. The distal row from the radial to the ulnar surface includes trapezium (greater multangular), trapezoid (lesser multangular), capitate, and hamate. The pisiform lies adjacent to the volar surface of the triquetrum and does not articulate with the shaft of the forearm bones or with any of the remaining carpal bones. Fractures of the pisiform will be considered separately at the end of this chapter.

Of the forearm bones only the radius articulates with the carpal bones. As shown in Figure 8–1, the ulna has a nonosseous fibrocartilaginous union with the triquetrum. As shown in Figure 8–2, the deep branch of the ulnar nerve and artery pass through the palmar canal formed by the pisiform and the hook of the hamate. This deep neurovascular bundle supplies the three hypothenar muscles, the interossei, the two ulnar lumbricals, and the adductor

pollicis. Injury to either the hamate or the capitate may result in neurovascular bundle damage and subsequent impairment of normal function. The median nerve as shown in Figure 8–2 also lies in close proximity to the volar surfaces of the lunate and the capitate.

It is essential to understand the relationship between the tendons and the carpal bones. As shown in Figure 8–2, the tendon of flexor carpi ulnaris virtually engulfs the pisiform in its attachment. The close proximity of the flexor carpi radialis to the tubercle of the trapezium is also noteworthy. Trapezium injuries may result in tendon damage with subsequent pain with normal motion. Figure 8–3 demonstrates the borders of the *anatomic snuff box*. As shown, the ulnar aspect is made up by the extensor pollicis longus whereas the tendons of the extensor pollicis brevis and the abductor pollicis longus form the radial border of the box. At the proximal floor of the box lies the scaphoid and distally the base is formed by the trapezium.

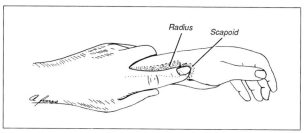

Figure 8–3. Note the borders of the anatomic snuff box.

Examination

A meticulous examination combined with an in-depth knowledge of the anatomy is essential for accurately diagnosing carpal bone fractures. With the hand deviated in a radial direction and the thumb extended, the anatomic snuff box becomes prominent. As mentioned previously, the scaphoid lies at the proximal base of the anatomic snuff box. Tenderness in this area may indicate the presence of a fracture, which in many instances cannot be radiographically visualized. If the thumb is now flexed, the first carpal metacarpal joint can be visualized and palpated as shown in Figure 8–4. Lister's tubercle, as shown in Figure 8–5, can be easily palpated over the dorsal distal radius. This tubercle serves as a landmark in locating the lunate and the capitate. With the hand in a neutral position, there is a small indentation in the skin corresponding to the capitate (Fig. 8–6). With the hand in flexion, the lunate becomes easily palpable just distal to Lister's tubercle (Fig. 8–7). It is important to note that Lister's tubercle, the lunate, and the capitate form a straight line that transects the third metacarpal (Fig. 8–8). It is important to note this imaginary line when reviewing traumatic wrist radiographs. The triquetrum can also be palpated just distal to the ulnar styloid.

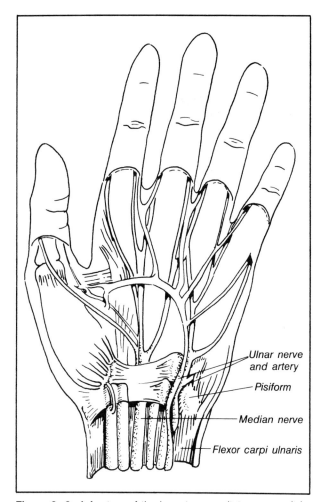

Figure 8–2. A fracture of the hamate or capitate can result in damage to the nerves and vessels, which course in close proximity to them. The median nerve lies close to the volar surface of the lunate and the capitate. The tendon of the flexor carpi ulnaris covers the pisiform at its attachment.

Ulnar nerve and artery

Pisiform

Median nerve

Flexor carpi ulnaris

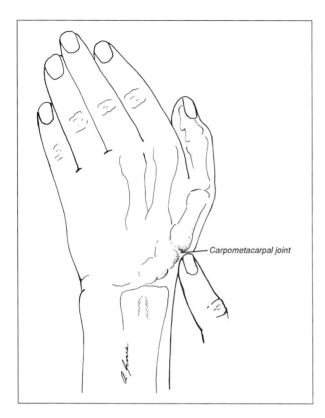

Figure 8-4. With the thumb flexed, the first carpal metacarpal joint can be visualized and palpated.

As shown in Figure 8-9, the pisiform is easily palpated at the base of the hypothenar eminence on the volar aspect of the hand. The hook of the hamate can be palpated by placing the interphalangeal (IP) joint of one's thumb over the pisiform with the distal phalanx directed toward the web space between the thumb and index fingers. With deep palpation, the hook of the hamate can be palpated under the tip of the examiner's thumb (Fig. 8-10).

After the examiner has located the point of maximum tenderness, all patients with suspected carpal injuries must have the function of the ulnar and median nerves documented. The ulnar nerve may be injured directly by trauma or secondarily due to compression resulting from hemorrhage or edema. Ulnar nerve injuries may be present as a delayed complication secondary to intraneural fibrosis or delayed compression. The median nerve may be damaged along with the carpal bone injury resulting in a carpal tunnel syndrome.

X Ray

The minimum number of radiographic views include an anteroposterior (AP), lateral, and oblique with the wrist in a neutral position. The following additional views may be obtained to better visualize suspected fractures:

1. AP with maximum radial deviation
2. AP with maximum ulnar deviation
3. Lateral with maximum flexion
4. Lateral with maximum extension

Ninety percent of all carpal fractures will be visualized with these views. Other imaging techniques including computed tomography (CT), bone scans, or tomograms may be necessary, but are typically not utilized on the initial visit.[4]

The normal angle between the scaphoid and the lunate is 30 to 60 degrees and between the capitate and the lunate is less than 20 degrees. Angles greater than normal reflect ligament instability.

The spacing between the carpal bones is normally a *constant*, independent of wrist positioning. A variation in spacing is abnormal and may reflect subluxation, arthritis, or an old fracture. The normal width between the scaphoid and the lunate is 1 to 2 mm in the AP projection. Spaces greater than 3 mm are *abnormal*.

Associated Injuries

Carpal fractures are often associated with other fractures or dislocations of the ipsilateral extremity. In addition, neurovascular injuries often accompany these fractures.

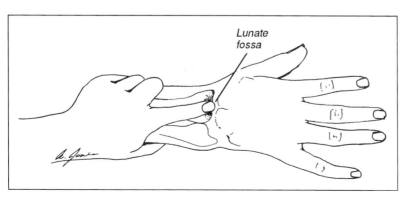

Figure 8-5. Lister's tubercle can be palpated over the dorsal aspect of the radius.

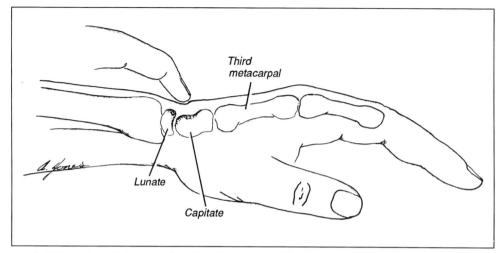

Figure 8–6. With the hand in the neutral position, there is a small indentation noted that corresponds to the capitate.

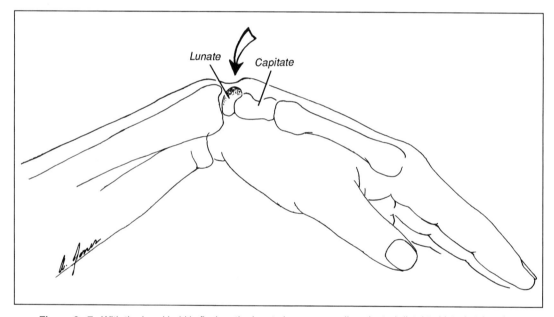

Figure 8–7. With the hand held in flexion, the lunate becomes easily palpated distal to Lister's tubercle.

Complications

Carpal fractures are associated with several common complications.

1. Patients often suffer refractures secondary to minimal trauma.
2. Most carpal fractures are associated with at least a transient median nerve neuropathy. Hook of hamate or pisiform fractures may be complicated by ulnar nerve compromise.
3. Carpal fractures and especially scaphoid fractures often suffer the sequelae of nonunion. In many patients, this is secondary to inadequate immobilization for an insufficient length of time. Malunion and delayed union are also commonly seen.

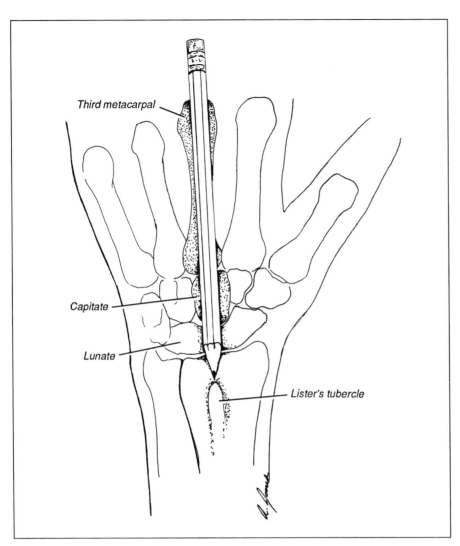

Figure 8–8. Lister's tubercle, the lunate, and the capitate form a straight line that transects the third metacarpal.

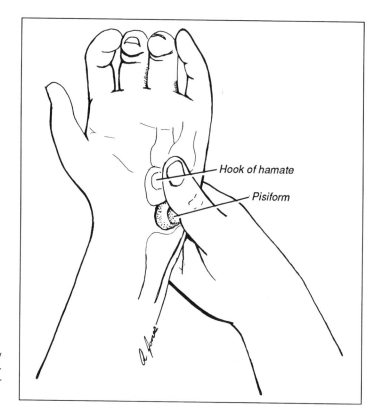

Figure 8–9. The pisiform is easily palpated at the base of the hypothenar eminence on the volar aspect of the hand.

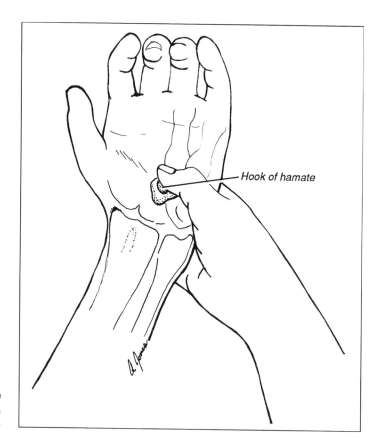

Figure 8–10. The hook of hamate can be palpated with deep palpation, under the tip of the examiner's finger.

SCAPHOID FRACTURES

☐ Class A: Fracture through the
                     waist (middle third)   (Fig. 8–11)
☐ Class B: Fracture through the
                     proximal third   (Fig. 8–11)
☐ Class C: Fracture through the
                     distal third   (Fig. 8–11)
☐ Class D: Fracture through the
                     tubercle   (Fig. 8–11)

TRIQUETRUM FRACTURES

☐ Class A: Dorsal chip fracture   (Fig. 8–13)
☐ Class B: Transverse fracture   (Fig. 8–13)

LUNATE FRACTURES

CAPITATE FRACTURES (Fig. 8–17)

HAMATE FRACTURES

☐ Class A: Distal articular
                     surface fracture   (Fig. 8–18)
☐ Class B: Hook of hamate fracture (Fig. 8–18)
☐ Class C: Comminuted body fracture (Fig. 8–18)
☐ Class D: Proximal pole articular
                     surface fracture   (Fig. 8–18)

TRAPEZIUM FRACTURES

☐ Class A: Vertical fracture   (Fig. 8–21)
☐ Class B: Comminuted fracture   (Fig. 8–21)
☐ Class C: Avulsion fracture   (Fig. 8–21)

PISIFORM FRACTURES

☐ Class A: Avulsion fracture   (Fig. 8–23)
☐ Class B: Transverse body fracture (Fig. 8–23)
☐ Class C: Comminuted fracture   (Fig. 8–23)

SCAPHOID FRACTURES

The scaphoid is the most commonly fractured carpal bone (Fig. 8–11). The high incidence of fractures relates to the size and the position of the normal scaphoid. The scaphoid is classified as a proximal carpal. Anatomically, however, it extends well into the area of the distal carpal bones. Radial deviation or dorsiflexion of the hand is normally limited by impingement of the radius on the scaphoid. With stress, fractures frequently result.

The blood supply to the scaphoid normally penetrates the cortex on the dorsal surface near the tubercle and near the waist area. Therefore, there is no direct blood supply to the proximal portion of the bone. Because of this tenuous blood supply, scaphoid fractures have a tendency to develop delayed union or avascular necrosis.

Axiom: *The more proximal the fracture line in scaphoid injuries, the greater is the likelihood of developing avascular necrosis.*

It is imperative for the clinician to realize that a patient presenting with a "sprained wrist" may have an occult scaphoid fracture. This injury can often be excluded acutely on the basis of physical examination. As will be discussed later, normal radiographs do not exclude this fracture.

Axiom: *Patients presenting with symptoms of a sprained wrist must have the diagnosis of an acute scaphoid fracture ruled out.*

Scaphoid fractures can be divided into four types as shown in Figure 8–11. The four types of scaphoid fractures are as follows:

- **Class A:** Waist or middle third fractures
- **Class B:** Proximal third fractures
- **Class C:** Distal third fractures
- **Class D:** Tubercle fractures

This classification lists scaphoid fractures in order of decreasing frequency. (Class A fractures represent 80 percent of scaphoid fractures.) Using this classification system the complications after scaphoid fracture in order of increasing incidence would be D, C, A, and B.

**CLASS A: FRACTURE THROUGH THE WAIST
(MIDDLE THIRD)**

CLASS B: FRACTURE THROUGH THE PROXIMAL THIRD

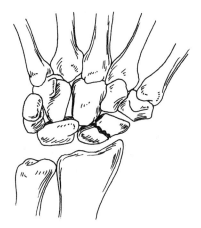

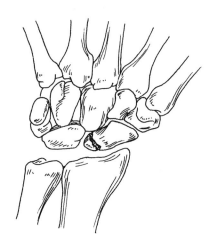

CLASS C: FRACTURE THROUGH THE DISTAL THIRD

CLASS D: FRACTURE THROUGH THE TUBERCLE

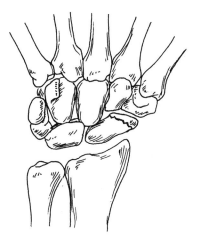

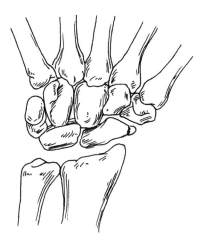

Figure 8–11.

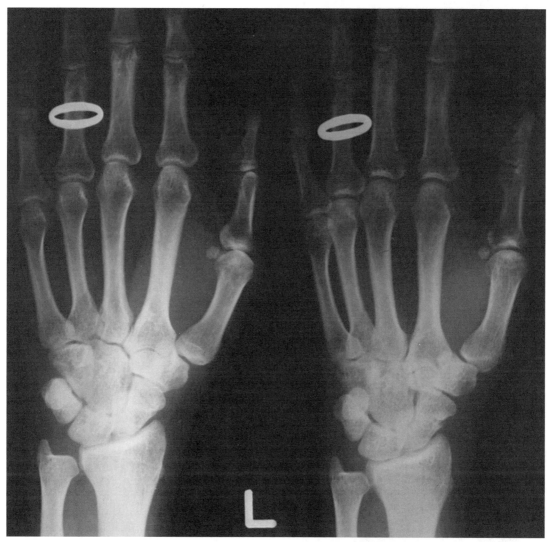

Figure 8–12. Fracture of the waist of the scaphoid. (*Cont.*)

Mechanism of Injury

Scaphoid fractures commonly result from forceful hyperextension of the wrist. The particular type of fracture is dependent on the position of the forearm at the time of injury. Class A fractures are thought to occur secondary to radial deviation with hyperextension resulting in impingement on the navicular waist by the radial styloid process. Scaphoid stress fractures have been reported.[3,7]

Examination

On examination there is generally maximum tenderness over the floor of the anatomic snuff box. In addition, radial deviation of the wrist or axial compression of the thumb also will elicit pain.

X Ray (Fig. 8–12)

Routine radiographs including AP, lateral, and oblique views may not demonstrate the fracture. If a fracture is suspected clinically, right and left oblique views as well as a scaphoid view or tomograms may be necessary to demonstrate the fracture. Despite this, a fracture may not be demonstrated radiographically for up to 6 weeks post-injury.[9] An indirect sign of an acute scaphoid fracture is displacement of the scaphoid fat stripe.[6] In many instances, a comparison view of the uninjured wrist may be helpful.

In addition to the detection of direct or indirect radiographic signs of fracture, a number of important concepts must be recalled before the interpretation of scaphoid radiographs.

Displaced or Unstable Fractures. Displacement between the fracture fragments or an unexplained variation in position between the fragments on different views indicate an unstable fracture. Fracture dislocations usually imply dorsal displacement of the distal fragment and carpal bones. The proximal fragment and lunate generally maintain their normal relationship with the radius.

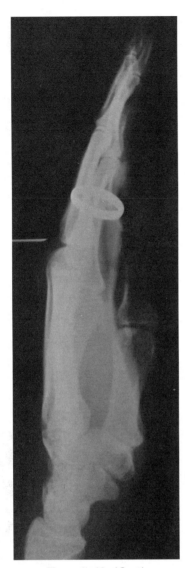

Figure 8-12. (*Cont.*)

Rotary Subluxation of the Scaphoid. This commonly missed injury can be suspected when the distance between the scaphoid and the lunate is greater than 3 mm. This injury is frequently associated with lunate fractures and complicated by posttraumatic joint disease.

Old Scaphoid Fractures. Radiographically, these injuries often will be associated with sclerotic fragment margins. In addition, the radiolucent distance separating the fragments will be similar to the distance between other carpal bones.

Bipartate Scaphoid. This is a normal variant that may be mistaken for a class A fracture. The presence of a normal smooth bony margin is indicative of this normal finding.

Associated Injuries

The majority (90 percent) of scaphoid fractures have no associated injuries. Injuries associated with scaphoid fractures include the following:

1. Radiocarpal joint dislocation
2. Proximal and distal carpal row dislocation
3. Distal radial fracture
4. Bennett's fracture of the thumb
5. Lunate fracture or dislocation
6. Scapholunate disassociation

Treatment

The treatment of navicular fractures is controversial and unfortunately fraught with complications. In general, distal fractures as well as transverse fractures heal with fewer complications when compared with proximal or oblique fractures. Cast immobilization is recommended; however, the position of the thumb and forearm as well as the extent of the forearm and thumb casted is controversial.[11] It is the authors' recommendation that proximal third fractures be immobilized for 12 weeks whereas middle or distal third fractures be immobilized for a minimum of 8 weeks. As with other fractures immobilization, ice, and elevation are important adjuncts in the initial management of navicular fractures.

Clinically Suspected Scaphoid Fractures without Radiographic Evidence. The patient should be treated as having an undisplaced scaphoid fracture, and the forearm placed in a long arm thumb spica cast (see Appendix). The thumb should be in a wine glass position (see Appendix). The wrist should be casted in slight flexion and neither ulnar nor radial deviation.[4] The cast should extend from the IP joint of the thumb to an area proximal to the elbow with the elbow in 90 degrees of flexion.[2] Some orthopedic surgeons do treat suspected, distal pole and tubercle scaphoid fractures with short arm thumb spica casts.[1] After 7 to 10 days, a repeat physical and radiographic examination should be completed. If a fracture is identified, the cast should be reapplied for an additional 4 to 5 weeks (total of 6 weeks). This should be followed by a short arm thumb spica cast (see Appendix) until clinical and radiographic signs of union are clearly seen.[4] If a fracture is not identified, but the examination remains clinically suspicious, the cast should be reapplied and the patient reexamined at 7- to 10-day intervals.[4] If a clinical suspicion of a fracture continues, despite negative radiographs, a bone scan, CT scan, or magnetic resonance imaging (MRI) evaluation may be helpful in confirming the diagnosis. MRI evaluation of the scaphoid may demonstrate viability of the fragments.[4,10]

Nondisplaced Scaphoid Fractures. A long arm thumb spica cast (see Appendix) extending to the IP joint of the thumb should be applied. The forearm and the thumb should be positioned as mentioned in the previous section. After 6 weeks, a short arm thumb spica may be applied for the remaining duration of immobilization totaling 8 to 12 weeks. Typically at this point, clinical and radiographic signs of union are present and casting can be discontinued.

Displaced Scaphoid Fractures. The patient should be placed in a volar splint and referred to an experienced surgeon for an attempt at closed reduction. If this attempt is unsuccessful open reduction is indicated.

Alternate modes of therapy are recommended by some authors, including a long arm thumb spica cast with the wrist slightly dorsiflexed and the forearm neutral for nondisplaced fractures. In addition, some authors

recommend the incorporation of the entire thumb into the spica cast.

Complications

The following complications of scaphoid fractures may occur despite optimum treatment.

1. Avascular necrosis is often associated with proximal third fractures, displaced fractures that are inadequately reduced, and comminuted fractures or fractures that are inadequately immobilized.
2. Delayed union, malunion, or nonunion may be encountered despite optimum management. Significantly, the most important determinate in cases of nonunion is early discontinuation of immobilization.[6]
3. Radiocarpal arthritis with subsequent wrist pain and/or stiffness.[6]

TRIQUETRUM FRACTURES

Triquetrum fractures (Fig. 8–13) can be divided into two types. Class A fractures are usually secondary to hyperextension with ulnar deviation. In this position the hamate forces the triquetrum against the dorsal lip of the radius, resulting in fragment shearing.

Class B fractures are secondary to a direct blow to the dorsum of the hand and are frequently associated with perilunate dislocations.

Examination

There will be dorsal swelling and tenderness localized over the area of the triquetrum.

X Ray

Class A fractures are best visualized on the lateral radiograph with the hand in flexion. Class B fractures are best visualized on AP and oblique radiographs. It is important to exclude other carpal injuries that frequently accompany triquetrum fractures (Fig. 8–14).

Associated Injuries

Triquetrum injuries are associated frequently with scaphoid fractures, distal radial fractures, and ulnar nerve injuries. The deep branch (motor) of the ulnar nerve lies in close proximity to the triquetrum and may be compromised with injuries in this area.

Treatment
☐ CLASS A: DORSAL CHIP FRACTURE

The authors recommend a compressive dressing with splinting, ice, and elevation until the swelling is reduced. This should be followed by a short arm cast or wrist splint for 3 weeks. This in turn can be followed by a short arm removable wrist splint for an additional 3 weeks.

☐ CLASS B: TRANSVERSE FRACTURE

Other carpal injuries must be excluded by clinical and radiographic means before treatment. The recommended treatment is a short arm cast with the wrist neutral and the thumb in the position of grasp or opposition. The cast should include the thumb only to a point just proximal to the MP joint. Orthopedic referral for follow-up is recommended.

Complications

As mentioned earlier, damage to the deep branch of the ulnar nerve with subsequent motor impairment may accompany this fracture.

TRIQUETRUM FRACTURES

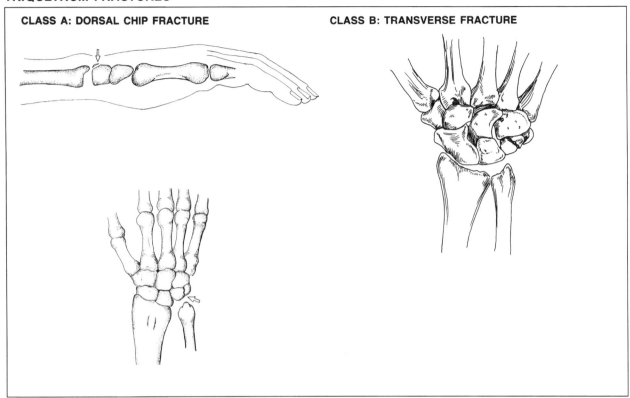

CLASS A: DORSAL CHIP FRACTURE   **CLASS B: TRANSVERSE FRACTURE**

Figure 8–13.

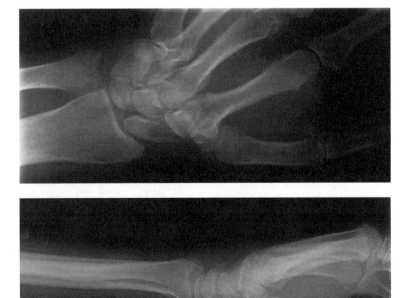

Figure 8–14. Triquetrum fracture.

LUNATE FRACTURES

The third most common carpal fracture is a lunate body fracture (Fig. 8–15). Lunate body fractures may occur in any plane with varying degrees of comminution. As with scaphoid fractures, the clinical suspicion of a fracture mandates treatment to prevent the development of Kienböck's disease (osteonecrosis of the proximal fragment with collapse).

Mechanism of Injury
Lunate fractures generally result from an indirect mechanism such as hyperextension or indirect trauma as with pushing a heavy object.

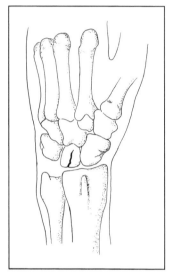

Figure 8–15. A lunate fracture is shown.

Examination
There will be pain and tenderness dorsally over the area of the lunate. In addition, axial compression of the third metacarpal will exacerbate the pain.

X Ray
Coned views in multiple projections are sometimes necessary to demonstrate the fracture line. It is important to exclude other carpal injuries that frequently accompany lunate fractures.

Associated Injuries
Other carpal injuries frequently accompany lunate fractures.

Treatment
As with scaphoid fractures treatment should be initiated on the basis of clinical or radiographic evidence of a fracture. It is the authors' recommendation that the patient be casted in a long arm thumb spica (see Appendix) for a total of 6 to 8 weeks. This should be followed by the application of a short arm cast until union is complete. Orthopedic referral after initial immobilization is strongly recommended.

Complications
Patients under 16 years of age generally have an uncomplicated resolution of their injury. Inadequately treated lunate fractures have a tendency to develop osteonecrosis of the proximal fragment. With time, there will be compression and collapse of this fragment resulting in the development of *Kienböck's disease* (Fig. 8–16).

Lunate fractures also have a tendency to develop lunatomalacia despite adequate treatment.

CAPITATE FRACTURES

The capitate, the largest of the carpal bones, articulates with the scaphoid and the lunate proximally, the trapezoid and the hamate along its lateral surfaces, and the second, third, and fourth metacarpals distally. Capitate fractures compromise 5 to 15 percent of all carpal fractures (Fig. 8–17). Capitate fractures are usually transverse and may be difficult to detect on plain radiographs at times requiring tomograms for diagnosis.

Mechanism of Injury
There are two mechanisms of injury that result in fractures of the capitate. A direct blow or crushing force over the dorsal aspect of the wrist may result in a fracture. Indirectly, a fall on the outstretched hand may result in a fracture.

Examination
Tenderness and swelling over the dorsal aspect of the hand in the area of the capitate will be present. Axial compression or movement of the third metacarpal will exacerbate the pain.

X Ray
Routine views are often adequate for diagnosing this fracture. Some patients however, may require tomo-

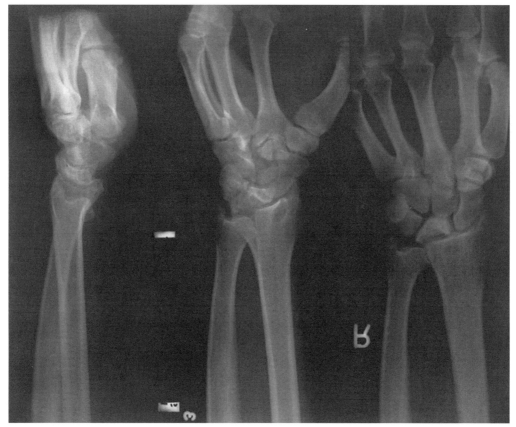

Figure 8–16. Aseptic necrosis of the lunate called Kienböck's disease is shown.

grams for diagnosis. Clinically suspected fractures with normal radiographs may be better evaluated using CT.[5]

Associated Injuries

Capitate fractures may be associated with scaphoid fracture, distal radial fracture, or lunate dislocation or subluxation.

CAPITATE FRACTURES

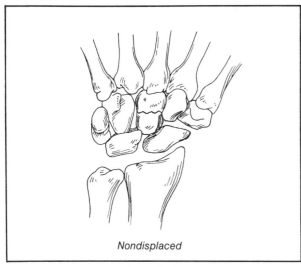

Nondisplaced

Figure 8–17.

Treatment

Nondisplaced Capitate Fracture.[8] The extremity should be immobilized in a short arm thumb spica (see Appendix) with the wrist in slight dorsiflexion and the thumb immobilized to the IP joint in the wine glass position for 8 weeks.

Displaced Capitate Fracture. The patient should be referred for an attempted manipulative reduction followed by immobilization. If unsuccessful, surgical reduction is indicated.

Complications

Capitate fractures may be associated with several complications.

1. Malunion or avascular necrosis may complicate the healing of capitate fractures.
2. Posttraumatic arthritis is noted frequently after comminuted capitate fractures.
3. Fibrosis after the injury may result in a median nerve neuropathy or a carpal tunnel syndrome.

HAMATE FRACTURES

Hamate fractures (Fig. 8–18) can be divided into four types on the basis of the area of the bone involved.

- **Class A:** Hamate fracture involving the distal articular surface
- **Class B:** Hamate fracture involving the hook
- **Class C:** Hamate fracture involving the comminuted body
- **Class D:** Hamate fracture involving the proximal pole articular surface

Mechanism of Injury

Each type of hamate fracture is generally secondary to a particular mechanism of injury.

- **Class A:** These fractures typically result from a fall or blow to the flexed and ulnar deviated fifth metacarpal shaft.
- **Class B:** A fall on the outstretched taut dorsiflexed hand generally results in these fractures.
- **Class C:** Direct crushing forces often result in comminuted body fractures.

HAMATE FRACTURES

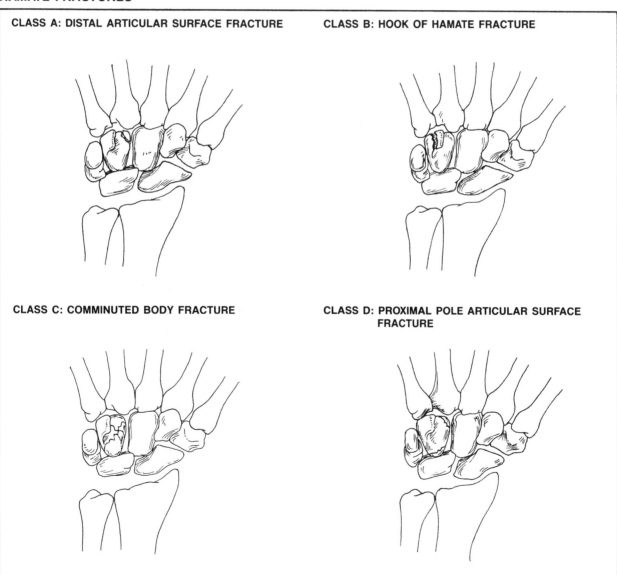

CLASS A: DISTAL ARTICULAR SURFACE FRACTURE

CLASS B: HOOK OF HAMATE FRACTURE

CLASS C: COMMINUTED BODY FRACTURE

CLASS D: PROXIMAL POLE ARTICULAR SURFACE FRACTURE

Figure 8–18.

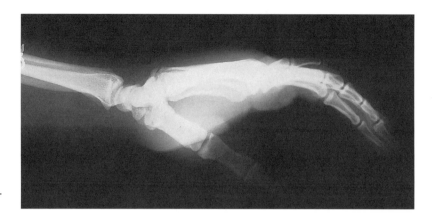

Figure 8–19. Hamate fracture. Lateral view (Note arrow).

- **Class D:** These proximal pole or osteochondral fractures are impaction injuries that generally occur with the hand dorsiflexed and in ulnar deviation.

Examination

With all hamate fractures, there will be tenderness and swelling over the involved area. Class A fractures will exhibit increased pain with axial compression of the fifth metacarpal. Class B fractures will exhibit tenderness over the palm of the hand in the area of the hamate hook. Class C and D fractures will demonstrate increased pain with wrist motion.

X Ray

Routine radiographs including oblique views are generally adequate in demonstrating these fractures (Figs. 8–19 and 8–20). Hamate hook fractures are best demonstrated on a carpal tunnel view.

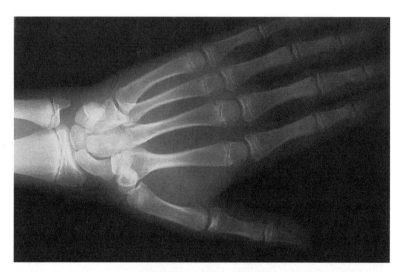

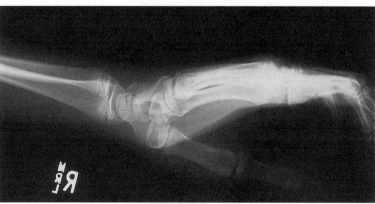

Figure 8–20. Hamate fracture. AP view shows how difficult it is to visualize.

Associated Injuries

Ulnar nerve or arterial injuries frequently accompany these fractures.

Treatment

Nondisplaced hamate fractures are treated with a short arm cast for a period of 6 weeks. Displaced fractures should be referred for reduction after the extremity has been splinted, elevated, and iced.

Complications

Ulnar nerve injuries may accompany these fractures and result in interosseous atrophy. In addition, hamate fractures may be followed by the development of arthritis at the fifth carpometacarpal joint.

TRAPEZIUM FRACTURES

Trapezium fractures (Fig. 8–21) are uncommon and may be classified into types:

- **Class A:** Vertical fractures
- **Class B:** Comminuted fractures
- **Class C:** Avulsion fractures

Mechanism of Injury

Trapezium fractures are generally the result of one of two mechanisms. Class A and B fractures occur when the adducted thumb is driven forcefully into the articular surface of the trapezium.[8] The bone is crushed between the radial styloid process and the first metacarpal. Class C avulsion fractures are secondary to a forceful deviation of the thumb with capsular strain and eventually bony avulsion.

Examination

The patient will note tenderness and swelling over the area of the trapezium. In addition, the pain will be increased with thumb motion or axial compression of the thumb.

X Ray

Routine radiographic views are generally adequate in demonstrating this fracture (Fig. 8–22).

Associated Injuries

Trapezium fractures may be associated with first metacarpal fractures, distal radial fractures, and first metacarpal dislocations seen especially with class A injuries.

TRAPEZIUM FRACTURES

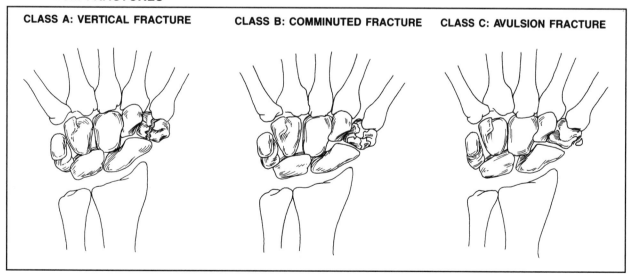

CLASS A: VERTICAL FRACTURE   CLASS B: COMMINUTED FRACTURE   CLASS C: AVULSION FRACTURE

Figure 8–21.

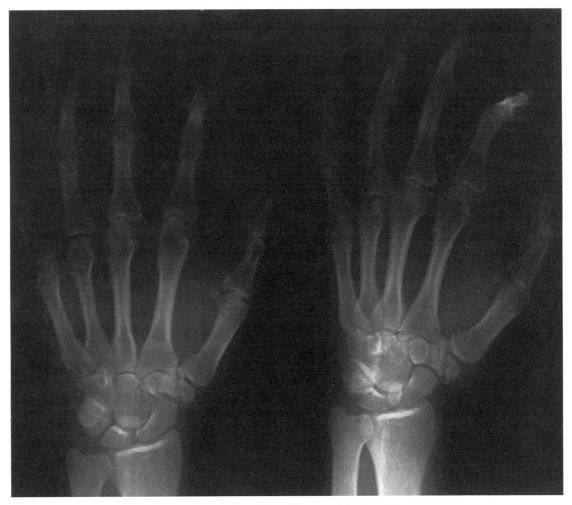

Figure 8–22. Comminuted fracture of the trapezium.

Treatment

The emergency management of these fractures includes elevation, ice, immobilization, and referral as reduction with the restoration of normal anatomy is critical.

Complications

Trapezium fractures may be complicated by the development of arthritis involving the first metacarpal joint or delayed pain with use of the flexor carpi radialis.

PISIFORM FRACTURES

The pisiform is unique in that it articulates only with one bone, the triquetrum. Anatomically it is important to recall that the deep branch of the ulnar nerve and artery pass in close proximity to the radial surface of the bone. In addition, the tendon of the flexor carpi ulnaris attaches to the volar surface of the pisiform.

Pisiform fractures (Fig. 8–23), are classified as follows:

• **Class A:** Avulsion fractures

• **Class B:** Transverse body fractures
• **Class C:** Comminuted fractures

Mechanism of Injury

There are two common mechanisms resulting in pisiform fractures. A direct blow or fall on the outstretched hand will usually result in a transverse or comminuted body fracture. Indirectly, a fall on the outstretched hand with tension on the flexor carpi ulnaris may result in an avulsion fracture.

PISIFORM FRACTURES

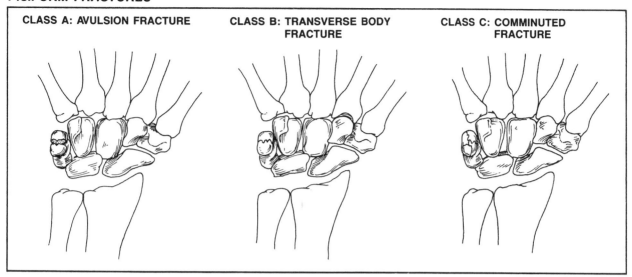

| CLASS A: AVULSION FRACTURE | CLASS B: TRANSVERSE BODY FRACTURE | CLASS C: COMMINUTED FRACTURE |

Figure 8–23.

Examination
There will be tenderness over the area of the pisiform. Always examine and record the function of the motor branch of the ulnar nerve when pisiform fractures are suspected.

X Ray
An oblique palmar view with the hand at an angle of 35 degrees from the casette is usually best for demonstrating this fracture.

Associated Injuries
Pisiform fractures may be associated with:

1. Damage to the motor branch of the ulnar nerve
2. Triquetrum fractures
3. Hamate fractures
4. Distal radial fractures

Treatment
The recommended therapy includes immobilization in a short arm cast for 6 weeks followed by active exercises.

Complications
Complications related to a missed pisiform fracture include pisotriquitral chondromalacia or subluxation, loose fragments in the joint space, and degenera-tive arthritis. Pisiform fractures may be complicated by an impairment of the deep branch of the ulnar nerve.

REFERENCES

1. Amadio PC: Scaphoid fractures. *Orthop Clin North Am* **23**(1):7–17, 1992.
2. Barton NJ: Twenty questions about csaphoid fractures. *J Hand Surg* [Br]:289–310, 1992.
3. Engel A, Feldner-Busztin H: Bilateral stress fracture of the scapoid: A case report *Orthop Trauma Surg* **110**:314–315, 1991.
4. Gelberman RH, Wolock BS, Siegel DB: Fractures and nonunions of the carpal scaphoid. *J Bone Joint Surg* **12**:1560–1566, 1989.
5. Green DP: Fracture of the hand with associated injuries. *J Hand Surg* **8**:393, 1983.
6. Gumucio CA, Young FB, Gilula VL, Kreamer BA: Management of the scaphoid fractures: A review and update. *J Hand Surg* **11**:1377–1388, 1989.
7. Hanks GA, Kalenak A, Bowman LS, Sebastianelli WJ: Stress fractures of the capal scaphoid: A report of four cases. *J Bone Joint Surg* **71A**:938–941, 1989.
8. Rockwood CA, Green DP: *Fractures.* Philadelphia: Lippincott, 1975.
9. Stordahl A, Schjoth A, Woxholt G, et al: Bone scanning of fractures of the scapoid. *J Hand Surg* **9B**:189–190, 1994.
10. Trumble TE: Avascular necrosis after scapoid fracture. A correlation of magnetic resonance imaging and histology. *J Hand Surg* **15A**:557–554, 1990.
11. Verdam C: Fractures of the scaphoid. *Surg Clin North Am* **40**:461, 1960.

BIBLIOGRAPHY

Fleege MA, Jebson PJ, Renfrew DL, Steyers CM Jr, El-Khoury Y: Pisiform fractures. *Int Skeletal Radiol* **20**:169–172, 1991.

Yanni D, Lieppins P, Laurence M: Fractures of the carpal scaphoid. *J Bone Joint Surg* (7):600–602, 1991.

SOFT TISSUE INJURIES, DISLOCATIONS, AND DISORDERS OF THE HAND AND WRIST

In many community emergency departments 25 to 30 percent of all emergency visits involve the hand.[44] The anatomy of the hand must be well understood before contemplating the care of injuries occurring to this "vital organ." The reader is referred to any of the standard anatomic texts for a detailed discussion of the anatomy as we will consider only the essential anatomic points as they relate to the specific sections discussed in this chapter.

When a patient presents to the emergency department with a hand disorder, the physician should first ascertain if there is any history of trauma, which, in most instances, will be obvious. The approach to the traumatized hand and the differential diagnosis to be considered is quite different when compared with the nontraumatized hand. Important historical points to be elicited in evaluating hand injuries include three factors: the time elapsed since the injury, the environment in which the injury occurred (dirty), and the mechanism of injury (crush, laceration, etc.). In the nontraumatized hand, the three historical points of importance to ascertain are:

When did the symptoms begin? What functional impairment has been experienced? What activities worsen the symptoms?

The following discussion is divided into traumatic and nontraumatic conditions of the hand. These are the two regions under which the various conditions presenting to the emergency department will be discussed:

Traumatic Disorders

- Wounds and injuries
- Tendon injuriesa
- Nerve injuries
- Vascular injuries
- Injuries to the ligaments and the joints

Nontraumatic Disorders

- Noninfectious inflammatory conditions
- Constrictive and compressive conditions
- Infections
- Space infections

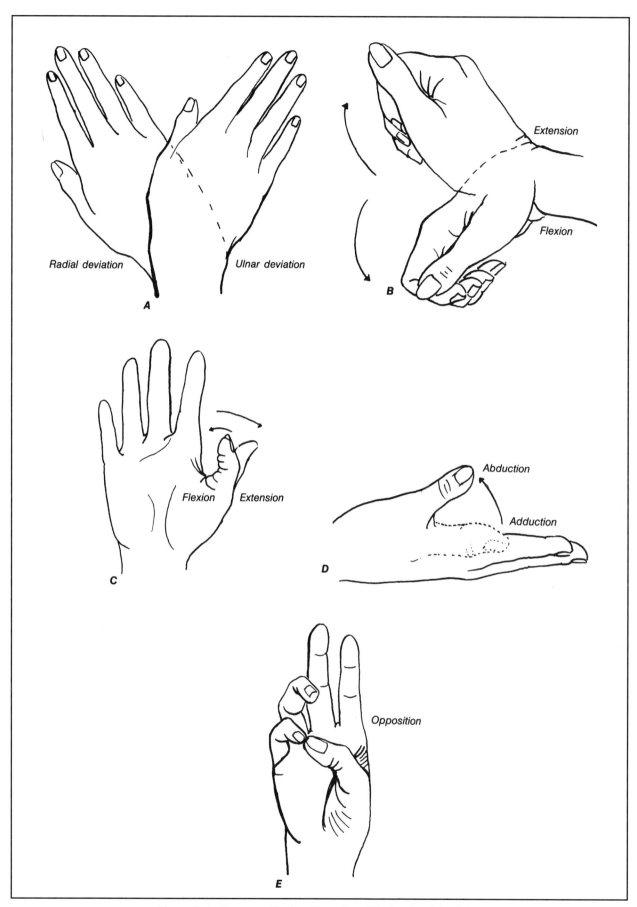

Figure 9–1. Terms used to describe motion of the hand and the digits.

Terminology

Standard terminology must be used to avoid confusion when discussing the disorders of the hand. The terminology used in this chapter is taken from the *Handbook of the American Society for Surgery of the Hand*.

The hand has a *dorsal* surface and a *volar* surface and the same terms are used when discussing the digits. In addition, each digit has a *radial* and an *ulnar* border. The muscle mass at the base of the thumb is called the *thenar* eminence and the muscle mass along the ulnar border of the hand is the *hypothenar* eminence.

The motions of the hand and the wrist are shown in Figure 9–1 and include radial and ulnar deviation (A), and extension and flexion at the wrist (B). Motions at the thumb are complex and the terms used to describe the motions are flexion and extension as shown in Figure 9–1C; abduction and adduction are the motions shown in Figure 9–1D; and opposition is shown in Figure 9–1E. The digits are named the thumb, index, long, ring, and little fingers, respectively to avoid confusion as to which digit (thumb or index finger) should be numbered the first.

TRAUMATIC DISORDERS

☐ WOUNDS AND INJURIES

Wounds of the hand are divided into tidy and untidy injuries. A tidy wound can be converted to an untidy one by poor care within the emergency department and an untidy wound can be converted to a tidy one by debridement and irrigation. The nature of the offending agent must also be considered; wounds from a knife or glass are generally clean whereas wounds in industries or secondary to bites from animals or fish are not. These should be cleansed thoroughly, and delayed closure should be contemplated if there is any question about contamination. Crush injuries always have macerated tissue and are considered untidy wounds. The interval between the insult and the time treatment is rendered should be ascertained because this dictates the need for systemic antibiotics.

Tidy wounds have little contamination and can be closed after irrigation with physiologic saline solutions. Closure may be delayed by 24 to 48 hours after cleansing and the patient placed on systemic antibiotics. Untidy wounds, however, should be debrided and thoroughly cleansed by irrigation under pressure, and closure should be delayed unless the wound can be converted to a clean one.

Control of Bleeding

To assess a wound, one must have control of bleeding. This is usually possible with the application of a sterile pressure dressing. When this is not feasible, however, proximal control is best achieved by the use of a sphygmomanometer placed in the normal position over the arm. Cast padding should be placed under the cuff and the arm should be elevated to permit good venous drainage of the limb after which the cuff is rapidly inflated to 250 to 300 mm Hg or 100 mm Hg above systolic pressure. This provides good control of bleeding for 20 to 30 minutes and permits enough time to clean the wound and ligate bleeding vessels. Examination may be facilitated by the use of a magnifying loop. This should not be done until a precursory evaluation of nerve and tendon function has been performed and only in those cases where bleeding is of such a magnitude that it must be controlled to assess and cleanse the wound.

Types of Wounds

Incised wounds are those caused by a sharp object such as a knife or glass. Although these are usually tidy wounds that can be closed primarily, they can be contaminated in certain occupations such as the fish-handling industry.

The *avulsed wound* may need grafting as contamination may be significant. If clean, these wounds may be closed primarily with a full or a split thickness graft. Full thickness grafts are best obtained from the inguinal region. Other good sites are the wrist crease or hypothenar eminence. The anticubital region should not be used as a donor site because the scar is unpredictable.

Blast wounds are very serious injuries owing to the forceful penetration of foreign objects and early closure may seal in necrotic tissue as well as foreign material. The initial care should be evaluation of nerve and tendon function with careful documentation and local debridement. The nerves may be contused and not disrupted in these injuries. The hand should be rechecked 36 to 72 hours after injury for final debridement and wound closure in the operating room. There is a latent period before the impact of the concussive force on the circulation is clinically apparent.

Initial Treatment of Wounds

The initial care of the wound should include careful assessment and evaluation of the extent of injury followed by cleansing with physiologic saline solution under pressure irrigation. The surrounding skin should be cleansed with an antibacterial solution such as povidone-iodine (Betadine). Judicious debridement and removal of foreign material and nonviable tissue should follow when indicated. Whether or not to close must then be decided and the repair can be done as a primary repair or delayed due to contamination. Several authors have investigated the use of prophylactic antibiotics in uncomplicated soft tissue wounds. It appears that the infection rate in matched groups is no different with or without the use of prophylactic antibiotics.[28,36] Thus, it is recommended that prophylactic antibiotics not be used in simple soft tissue wounds of the hands.

☐ Special Injuries

Injection injuries may involve extensive loss of tissue and are associated with a high infection rate. Depending on the agent, one must decide whether to treat the patient conservatively or open the involved digit or hand for debridement.[25] Most of these injuries involve grease, paint, or other industrial toxins, require surgical debridement, and should be immediately referred. Injections with *water* under pressure may be observed in the hospital.

Gas injected under pressure may dissect widely and penetrate the systemic circulation causing increased tissue tension locally and circulatory embarrassment centrally. This should be treated with elevation of the hand, immobilization, and broad-spectrum antibiotics.

Liquid injection may spread widely and may act to block nerve conduction delaying the onset of pain and thereby deluding the examiner into thinking he or she is dealing with a minor injury. The patient may then complain of a sudden hot feeling in the hand.

When dealing with a high-pressure injection injury, the amount of tissue damage is dependent on the type of material injected, the amount injected, and the velocity of the injected material. Paint and paint thinner generate a large, early inflammatory response resulting in a high percentage of amputations. On the other hand, grease gun injuries do not cause large, inflammatory responses. The local interference to vascular supply may be due to thrombosis of the blood vessels or to digital vasospasm. Within several hours after the digit has been injected, the extremity becomes painful and swollen. Initially, there may be anesthesia and even vascular insufficiency in the extremity. In the late stages, marked breakdown of the skin occurs resulting in ulcers and draining sinuses. Radiographs of the extremity sometimes help determine the spread of the material and the extent of surgical exploration and the debridement necessary. Lead-based paint appear as densities within soft tissues. Nonlead-based paint presents with subcutaneous emphysema on x ray. Grease will appear as a lucency.[63]

When dealing with a chemical irritant, the patient must be hospitalized and observed hourly while antibiotics, steroids, and low molecular weight dextran are given. When known to be a toxin, *fasciotomy* is advocated early. Lead-based paint can be seen on x ray. Grease gun injuries can enter under very high pressures (15,000 pounds per inch^2) and need immediate decompressive surgery and debridement.[25]

☐ Crush Injuries

Crush injuries to the hand are common in industry. The tissue is congested and ischemic whereas the surface wounds are often quite simple and misleading as to the full extent of the injury. Usually these open wounds should be closed later.

☐ Foreign Bodies in the Hand

Glass, metal, and wood are the most common foreign materials seen in hand wounds. Although some particles are inert and cause little reaction, others can cause significant problems. Glass may be radiopaque or radiolucent depending on the presence of lead within the glass fragments. Glass can usually be detected on plain films; however, it is more easily detected using computed tomography (CT) scans.[6] Small pieces may not require removal whereas larger ones tend to migrate and become symptomatic as fibrous reaction envelops them. One may see only a small laceration or puncture wound with local hemorrhage and be unable to find the particle, in which case splinting of the injured hand should be done. In this case, waiting several days to explore may prove beneficial. Small fragments may encapsulate and gradually migrate to the surface. Metallic particles may remain inert and asymptomatic requiring no removal. Particles of metal that are symptomatic may be allowed to remain until a capsule forms around them and facilitates their removal. Wood is usually radiolucent and cannot be seen on x ray. Wood may sometimes be inert with the exception of those that are stained with toxic dyes such as aniline or contain oils or resins that induce an inflammatory response and a chemical cellulitis if not removed and the wound drained. Plastic is perhaps the most difficult substance to detect and one must often use magnetic resonance imaging (MRI).[66]

Mangled Hand Injuries

Treatment of these injuries is difficult in the emergency department. Only a precursory assessment of the circulation and gross neurologic assessment should be done as well as preliminary x rays. Open wounds should not be probed because that increases the chance of infection. The hand should be covered with sterile dressings and immobilized as soon as possible. Immediate surgery is needed when external hemorrhage cannot be controlled (except with an inflated blood pressure cuff) and when rapid, progressive swelling results from internal hemorrhage. Blind clamping of vascular structures should never be performed. If direct pressure does not work, the hand should be elevated and a sphygmomanometer applied proximal to the zone of injury and inflated while maintaining the pressure at 100 mm Hg above systolic pressure. This can be tolerated with no anesthesia for 20 to 30 minutes. Pain control with parenteral narcotics or regional anesthesia is usually warranted. Prophylactic broad-spectrum parenteral antibiotics are also indicated. These antibiotics should cover both gram-positive and gram-negative organisms. Primary closure is usually not indicated. Revascularization attempts and salvage of the digits usually fail. These mangled hand injuries generally occur secondary to use of farming equipment.[63] Tetanus prophylaxis as well as broad-spectrum antibiotics should be administered.

Injuries secondary to snowblowers are common in the Midwest and East. These are usually secondary to a hand being placed in the machine to dislodge impacted snow. Injuries occur to the dominant hand in almost all cases. Usually, the two digits that are injured are the long and ring fingers. These injuries are usually to the dorsal side of the fingers and hand and are characterized by extensive lacerations and contusions. Following digital block and radiographs, debridement and repair should take place in the operating room.[63]

□ Digital Degloving Injuries

This is often called a *ring injury*[5,15] because the ring finger is the most commonly involved digit. When the ring is hooked in a fall, the skin may be *elevated* in which case treatment is with repositioning of the skin and the administration of low molecular weight dextran or heparin as well as elevation and immobilization of the hand. *Complete avulsion* of the skin with intact tendons and ligaments requires either a pedicle flap or amputation of the digit and should be referred.

□ Punctures

Punctures must be carefully assessed and treated depending on the etiology. Animal-induced punctures should be elevated and immobilized and antibiotics given. If the puncture is from a pencil containing aniline dye (from an indelible point), then local excision to avoid cellulitis or other problems is recommended.

□ TENDON INJURIES

The muscles and tendons of the hand are divided into the extrinsic flexors and extensors of which there are 14 of each contained in the forearm and the *intrinsics*, which lie in the body of the hand composed of 20

individual muscles. The tendons of the extrinsics are responsible for most of the "gross" motions that the hand and the digits perform. These tendons are commonly involved in hand injuries whereas fine detailed movement requires the added function of the intrinsics. The tendons are quite mobile and are held in place by pulleys that prevent the tendon from dislodging from its normal position. The tendons are ensheathed by a synovial membrane that acts as a living lubricant membrane to permit normal gliding of the tendon. Although the flexors are capable of a wide range of motion, when compared with the extensors an extensor injury causes a greater impairment of motion than does a similar flexor injury. The tendons become almost avascular in the adult and get their blood supply from the muscles proximally and the site of insertion distally.

Tendons function best when they are at an optimal position of stretch.[32] The *extensor carpi radialis brevis*, which inserts centrally on the transverse arch, is the most important of the wrist extensors acting to stretch the long flexors (extrinsics) to obtain a powerful grasp. The physician should compare the power of his or her own grasp with the wrist in flexion and in about 15 degrees of extension.

The most common site of tendon injury is the extensors over the dorsum of the hand where the tendons are more superficial and exposed to injury. Tendon injuries may be closed or open, partial or complete. One can have 90 percent of a tendon cut with motion still remaining. To detect this, one must test motion *against resistance*.

The position of the hand when injury occurred is important to determine. If the hand was in flexion with a laceration to the volar aspect of the fingers, then the flexor tendons may be transected and the distal stump would lie distally to the wound. However, if the hand was in the extended position, the tendon stumps would lie at the wound edges. When the tendons are injured by a direct blow to the hand or the fingers, the closed injury will hide significant tissue damage. The patient will initially develop edema of the hand and an inflammatory response followed by fibroblastic proliferation, which leads to adhesions of the tendons to surrounding tissues. This is particularly true with blows to the dorsum of the hand where the extensor tendons lie in close proximity to the surface and are subject to peritendinous fibrosis called *Secrétan's disease*.

Great forces are required for a closed injury to cause a rupture of a tendon. With forces acting against the tendon while it is contracting one may avulse the bone at the insertion of the tendon on one of the phalanges or rupture the tendon. In lacerations to the hand where tendons are transected, the prognosis as to function of the tendon without significant adhesions is determined to a large extent by how clean or dirty the wound is. Adhesions are accentuated by touching the tendons and even blood extravasation around the tendon, therefore every attempt should be made to avoid unnecessary manipulation of the injured tendon.

Examination

One can have 90 percent of a tendon cut and still have normal motion. To adequately assess the tendons, one must test motion *against resistance*. A negative examination means nothing with regard to small partial tendon lacerations. With a partially cut tendon, examination at 10 days will disclose decreased strength as compared with the initial examination and later as the tendon heals, strength is regained. Generally, in performing any of the tests for tendon function listed below, one will note that the tendon is placed in as much stretch as is optimal before testing to provide for the greatest strength during contraction.

☐ Extrinsic Flexors
☐ *Flexor Digitorum Profundus and Flexor Pollicis Longus (Fig. 9–2)*
These flexors insert on the distal phalanx of the respective digits and are tested by asking the patient to flex the distal interphalangeal joint while the proximal joints are held in an extended position.

☐ *Flexor Digitorum Superficialis (Fig. 9–3)*
The flexor digitorum superficialis is tested by holding all the other fingers in the hand fully extended and asking the patient to flex the finger to be tested. If the distal interphalangeal joint is permitted to relax, then flexion at the proximal interphalangeal joint is independent of the flexor digitorum profundus.

☐ *Flexor Carpi Radialis*
The flexor carpi radialis inserts on the volar aspect of the index metacarpal and one can palpate this tendon just radial to the midline with the wrist flexed against resistance.

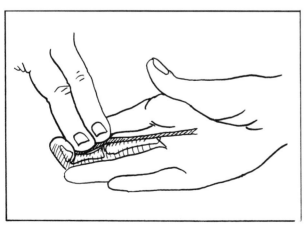

Figure 9–2. Testing the flexor digitorum profundus function.

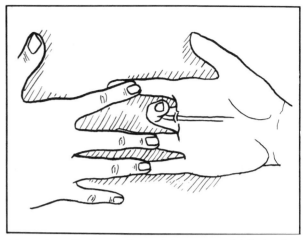

Figure 9–3. Testing the flexor digitorum superficialis function.

☐ *Flexor Carpi Ulnaris*
The flexor carpi ulnaris is palpated under tension when the wrist is flexed against resistance and the thumb and little finger are opposed. It inserts on the pisiform and is easily palpated at this point.

☐ *Palmaris Longus*
The palmaris longus is palpated by flexing the wrist against resistance and opposing the thumb and the little fingers. The tendon lies in the midline where it attaches to the palmar fascia. However, the tendon is congenitally absent in one fifth of the population.

☐ *Flexor Tendons*
The extensor tendons are arranged in six compartments over the dorsal aspect of the wrist (Fig. 9–4).

☐ *Abductor Pollicis Longus and Extensor Pollicis Brevis*
The abductor pollicis longus inserts at the dorsal base of the thumb metacarpal and the extensor pollicis brevis inserts at the base of the proximal phalanx of the thumb. These can be tested by asking the patient to forcefully spread the hand. The abductor pollicis longus can be palpated just distal to the radial styloid. The extensor pollicis brevis can be palpated under tension over the dorsum of the thumb metacarpal.

☐ *Extensor Carpi Radialis Longus and Extensor Carpi Radialis Brevis*
These tendons insert at the base of the index and the middle fingers, respectively. They are evaluated by asking the patient to make a fist and extend the wrist forcibly (Fig. 9–5).

☐ *Extensor Pollicis Longus*
The extensor pollicis longus passes around Lister's tubercle on the dorsal aspect of the radius and inserts on

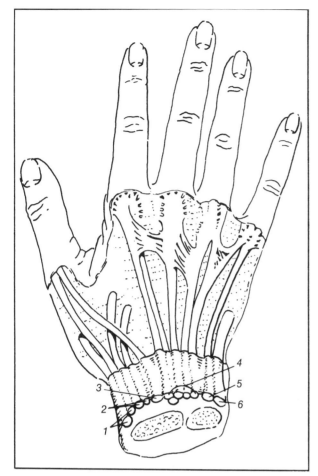

Figure 9-4. The extensor tendons of the wrist. Note that there are six compartments that enclose the extensor tendons. The first contains the abductor pollicis longus and the extensor pollicis brevis. The second compartment encloses the extensor carpi radialis longus and the extensor carpi radialis brevis. Adjacent to these is the extensor pollicis longus tendon in the third compartment. The extensor digitorum communis and the extensor indicis are contained in the fourth compartment. The extensor digiti minimi is enclosed by the fifth compartment and the extensor carpi ulnaris in the sixth.

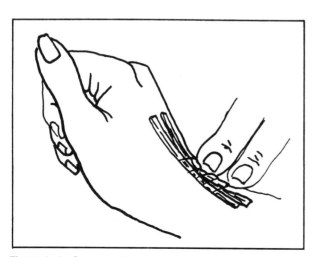

Figure 9-5. One can palpate the extensor carpi radialis longus and brevis tendons as shown. Function can then be tested.

the distal phalanx of the thumb. It forms the ulnar border of the anatomic snuff box and can be easily seen by extending the thumb (Fig. 9-6). Only this tendon can extend the thumb and forcibly hyperextend it at the interphalangeal (IP) joint. It can be tested by asking the patient to hyperextend the distal phalanx of the thumb against resistance.

□ *Extensor Digitorum Communis (Fig. 9-7)*

These tendons are tested by asking the patient to flex the IP joints into a tight claw and actively extend the metacarpophalangeal (MCP) joint. This permits the examiner to visualize the extensor digitorum communis. Although the extensor digitorum minimi is in the next compartment, we will consider it here rather than separately because it is easily tested at this point in the examination.[9] The extensor indicis and extensor digitorum minimi can be tested by asking the patient to first make a fist, then extend the index and the little fingers while the long and ring fingers remain flexed. (Fig. 9-8).

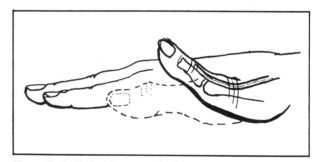

Figure 9-6. To test the strength of the extensor pollicis longus, extend the thumb with the hand positioned flat on a table.

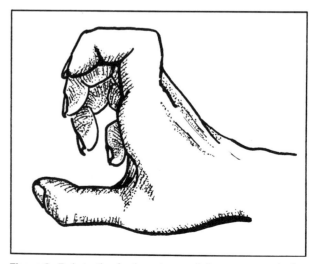

Figure 9-7. In testing for the extensor digitorum communis, the MP joints should be held in extension and the IP joints flexed. Compare the strength of extension at the MP joint to the opposite hand.

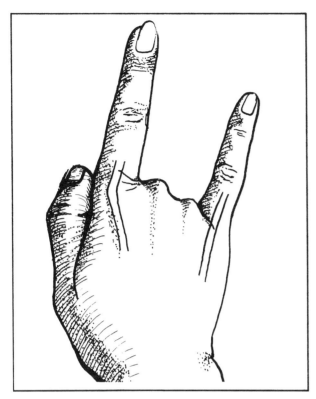

Figure 9–8. The extensor indicis and extensor digiti minimi are tested as shown either individually or together. It is important to hold the adjacent fingers in a flexed position to test for isolated tendons without interference from the communis tendon.

□ *Extensor Carpi Ulnaris*

This tendon inserts at the dorsal base of the fifth metacarpal and is evaluated by asking the patient to ulnar deviate the hand while the examiner palpates the taut tendon over the ulnar side of the wrist just distal to the ulnar head (Fig. 9–9).

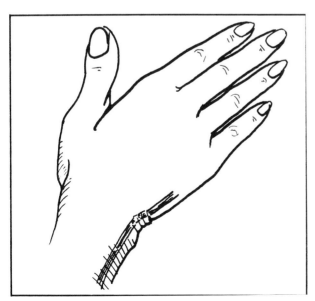

Figure 9–9. The method for testing the extensor carpi ulnaris.

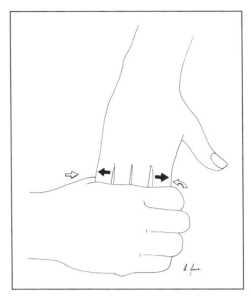

Figure 9–10. To test the dorsal interossei, spread the fingers forcibly against resistance.

□ *Intrinsics*

The *dorsal interossei* can be tested by spreading the hand forcibly against resistance (Fig. 9–10). The *volar interossei* are tested by placing a piece of paper between the extended fingers and asking the patient to resist with drawal of the paper from between the fingers (Fig. 9–11). The *thenar* and *hypothenar* muscles can be tested by asking the patient to cup the palm and pinch the thumb and little fingertips together forcibly. One can feel the tone of these muscles and compare them with the normal side. The intrinsic tendons (lumbricals) can be tested by asking the patient to extend the wrist and the fingers while the examiner presses down on the fingertips.

The Bunnel-Littler test is used to check the intrinsics of the hand. In performing this test, the MCP joint is held in slight extension and the proximal interphalangeal (PIP) joint is flexed. This test evaluates the lumbricals and interossei (Fig. 9–12). A great force should be required to flex the IP joints if the lumbricals are normal.

Thumb adduction is tested by having the patient hold a piece of paper between the thumb and the side of the phalangeal region of the index finger (Fig. 9–13). When the *adductor pollicis* is weak, the IP joint of the thumb flexes with this maneuver and is called a positive *Froment's* sign.

Common Reasons for Misdiagnosis

The physician should be aware of the reasons why an emergency evaluation can lead to an erroneous diagnosis:

1. Patient cooperation is essential and this is often lacking, particularly in the intoxicated patient.

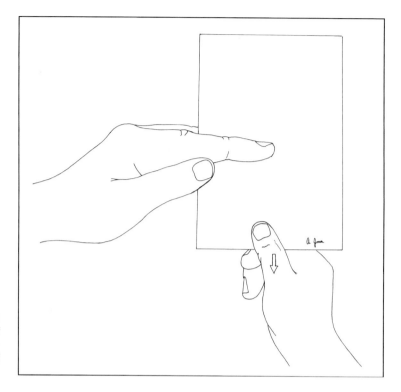

Figure 9–11. The volar interossei are tested by placing a piece of paper between the fingers and asking the patient to resist withdrawal of the paper.

2. In open wounds, an incomplete injury to the tendon is common and may be difficult to assess.
3. Blunt injury to the dorsum of the digit or hand can result in compromise of the extensors, which is not noted initially.
4. Lacerations over the PIP joints and the MCP joints may transect the middle extensor tendon and the diagnosis is not made until the hood mechanism decompensates and leads to deformity.

Treatment

Definitive repair of a tendon injury can be deferred for up to 72 hours and still be considered a primary repair provided the initial emergency wound care has been adequate. This should include: surgical skin preparation of the hand, temporary wound approximation with sutures or an appropriate dressing, immobilization in a splint, elevation, and administration of appropriate antibiotics.

A *primary repair* is defined as a repair done in the first 72 hours postinjury. A *delayed repair* is performed in the first week after injury, and a *secondary repair* is done after all edema has subsided and the scar has softened, usually 4 to 10 weeks after injury.

Axiom: *A negative examination of a patient with a suspected tendon injury should always be reevaluated to be certain of the diagnosis, particularly in the uncooperative patient*

It should be emphatically stated that a primary repair is the treatment of choice whenever possible. Delayed re-

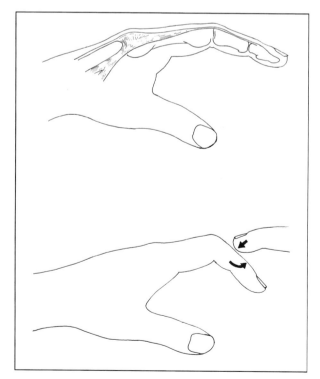

Figure 9–12. The intrinsics are tested with the Bunnel-Littler test. In this test the MCP joints are held in extension and the PIP joint is extended against resistance.

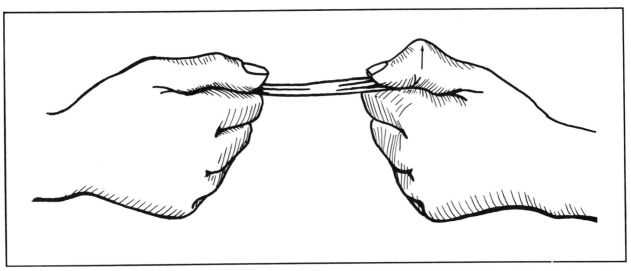

Figure 9–13. A positive Froment's sign. Note the flexed IP joint (*arrow*).

pairs are done when other trauma exists and repair of the hand must be deferred or the wound is not optimal for repair because of infection or swelling. Secondary repair should be performed when associated injuries compromise the patient or wound complications are likely. Partial tendon injuries can be splinted without surgical repair. For flexor tendon repairs 4-0 nylon is used and 6-0 nylon is used at the peritendinous structures along with extensor block splint. Repairs of the complete flexor tendon ruptures are best done by hand surgeons in the operating room.[71] An avulsion injury of the flexor tendon (jersey injury) is best treated surgically rather than with a splint.[10, 41]

Flexor tendon injuries have been categorized into zones in order to assist in planning treatment (Fig. 9–14). Zone 1 extends from the distal insertion of the profundus tendon to the site of the superficialis insertion (see Fig. 9–14). Injuries here generally result in the proximal tendon retracting. Zone 2 injuries are in the area often called "no man's land." The profundus and superficialis tendons interweave closely and injuries here may injure the viniculae providing the blood supply to the tendons. Repairs in this area are quite complex and should only be attempted by a qualified hand surgeon. Zone 2 flexor tendon lacerations are, unfortunately, the most commonly seen flexor tendon lacerations in emergency medicine and technically the most difficult to repair.[33] Zone 3 injuries extend from the distal edge of the carpal tunnel to the proximal edge of the flexor sheath. These injuries generally have a good result with primary repair. Zone 4 injuries include the carpal tunnel and its related structures. Injuries here require careful exploration for associated injuries. In zone 5 injuries, it is essential that the surgeon have adequate exposure and conduct an exhaustive search for major structures that are injured.[33]

Extensor tendon injuries are usually closed. When the injury is a disruption of the tendon to the distal

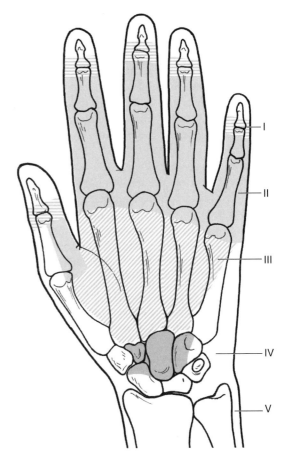

Figure 9–14. Zone classifications for flexor tendon injuries of the hand.

interphalangeal (DIP) joint the treatment should be splinting the joint in extension. Hypertension, as has been previously suggested, should be avoided. In addition, there should be no block to motion at the PIP joint (see Fig. 9–17). The splint should remain in place for 6 weeks. In

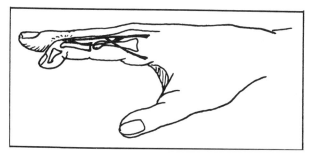

Figure 9–15. A mallet finger deformity without associated fracture.

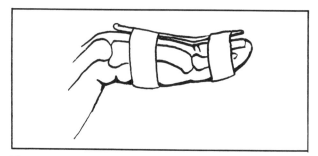

Figure 9–17. The extension splint used for disruption of the extensor tendon slip at the DIP joint.

patients who use the hand a great deal and depend on finger motion at their fingertips, plaster immobilization may be recommended. If nothing is done with these injuries a flexion deformity of the DIP joint with extension at the PIP results and is called a *mallet finger* (Fig. 9–15). A mallet finger is a flexion deformity at the DIP joint area in which there is complete passive but incomplete active extension of the DIP joint. This injury is usually sustained from a sudden blow to the tip of the extended finger. The insertion of the extensor tendon may be avulsed or there may be an avulsion fracture of the distal phalanx with the tendon still attached. Disruptions of the tendon at the PIP joint can cause a *boutonnière deformity* (Fig. 9–16) as a sequel and these should all be referred for repair. A boutonnière deformity of the finger involves flexion of the PIP joint and hypertension of the DIP joint. It usually results from an injury that disrupts the extensor tendon insertion into the dorsal base of the middle phalanx. The lateral bands progressively stretch and slip volar to the axis of the PIP joint, and become flexors of the PIP joint. Boutonnière injuries can be caused by three closed mechanisms: deep contusion of the PIP joint; acute forceful flexion of the PIP joint against resistance; and palmer dislocation of the PIP joint. These findings may not show up for 7 to 14 days. Thus, one should suspect a possible boutonnière injury whenever one encounters a painful swollen PIP joint with any of the above mechanisms. Extension at the PIP joint is

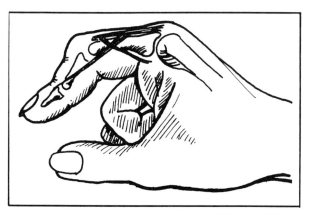

Figure 9–16. The boutonnière deformity.

tested. A 15- to 25-degree extension lag with decreased strength against resistance should make one suspect this injury. The treatment is to keep the PIP joint in constant and complete extension.[5] This deformity is usually not present immediately after injury, but develops as the lateral bands progressively drift in a volarward direction. Ruptures over the proximal phalangeal region should be treated in a similar manner to middle phalanx disruptions for 3 to 4 weeks' duration. Rupture of the extensor tendon at its attachment to the distal phalynx is terated as a mallet finger with a dorsal splint (Fig. 9–17).

A classification system used to divide extensor tendon injuries into zones and aid in treatment decisions has been devised.[33] Zone 1 injuries are over the distal phalynx (Fig. 9–18). Treatment of these injuries is generally nonoperative. A dorsal splint is applied, maintaining the DIP joint and slight hyperextension for 6 weeks. During this time, the PIP joint and MCP joint are allowed to move freely. Zone 2 injuries are over the middle phalanx. The treatment here is identical to that for zone 1 injuries. Zone 3 is over the PIP joint. These injuries can be either open or closed, with the central tendon the most commonly injured structure.[33] This is the injury that leads to a boutonnière deformity. Closed injuries here are treated with a PIP joint splint and extension for 5 to 6 weeks. Some hand surgeons recommend early controlled mobilization. Open injuries are treated with primary repair. Zone 4 injuries include the area over the proximal phalanyx. These injuries are similar to zone 3 injuries and are treated with primary or delayed repair with an appropriate splint for 3 to 6 weeks. Zone 5 injuries are over the MCP joint. When these are secondary to a human bite, the wound must be explored and thoroughly lavaged and left open. This often results in only a partial injury to the tendon. If the joint capsule is injured and it is not secondary to a human bite, this can be repaired with 4-0 or 5-0 absorbable suture. Zone 6 injuries involve the extensor tendons over the dorsum of the hand, which are the superficial locations. Even apparently minor wounds may involve the extensor tendons because they are so close to the skin. Four-0 nonabsorbable material using a figure-of-eight stitch is indicated here. The wrist should then be immobilized at 30 degrees of extension with the

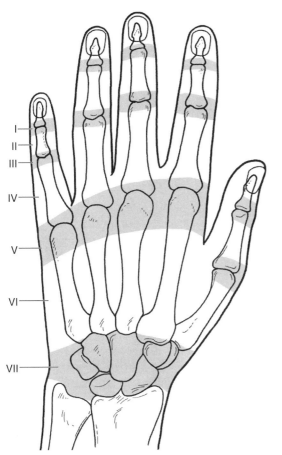

Figure 9-18. Zone classifications for extensor tendon injuries of the hand.

MCP joint fully extended for 4 weeks. This is the optimal treatment for these injuries. Tendons at this site tend not to retract because they are connected to adjacent structures and tendons. Zone 7 injuries are uncommon and involve the extensor retinaculae. These injuries require repair by a hand surgeon.[33]

Extensor tendon injuries at the level of the distal forearm and wrist are usually a result of deep lacerations.[5] The tendon may retract due to the elasticity of the musculotendinous junction. Treatment is surgical with longitudinal exposure to grasp the retracted ends. Nonabsorbable 4-0 nylon is used and the wrist is splinted in 20 degrees of extension and the MCP joint is placed in neutral position for 10 days.

On the dorsal hand lacerations causing extensor tendon rupture will often lead to adhesions.[5]

□ NERVE INJURIES

Three nerves supply the hand with sensory and muscular branches: radial, ulnar, and median. There are three types of injuries to these nerves or their branches. In a *neurotmesis* the nerve is completely disrupted. In an *axonotmesis* there is variable motor and sensory dysfunction. In these patients, the proximal and distal ends of the nerves are separated; however, the Schwann cells are maintained. In a *neuropraxia* there is no loss of continuity.

The sensation of the hand is provided by branches of these nerves as shown in Figure 9-19. The sensory

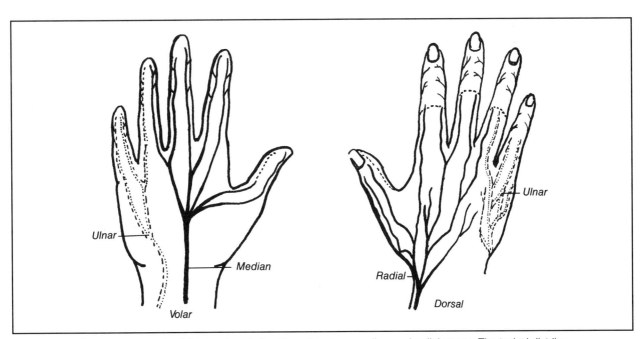

Figure 9-19. The sensory supply of the hand as derived from the ulnar, median, and radial nerves. The typical distribution is shown but variability does occur. The tip of the index finger is the most constant region for examining the median nerve sensory distribution in the hand, and the tip of the little finger for the ulnar.

innervation of the ulnar nerve is very constant whereas others can vary. Of all the sensory nerves, the significance of the median nerve is the most important to normal hand function, whereas the radial nerve is the least significant with regard to sensory distribution and the ulnar nerve being second to the median in its importance as a sensory supplier of the hand.

There are four pure motor nerves of the hand: the posterior interosseous nerve of the radial, the volar interosseous nerve of the median, the deep motor branch of the ulnar, and the recurrent motor branch of the median nerve.

Examination

Two-point discrimination is the most sensitive test for the sensory supply over the distribution of the nerve being tested in the hand. This can best be performed with a paper clip with its two ends separated approximately 5 mm (Fig. 9–20). Two-point discrimination is a static test. An injured hand is able to distinguish two blunt points that are 2 to 5 mm apart at the fingertips and 7 to 10 mm apart at the base of the palm. The dorsum of the hand is the least sensitive, with a normal threshold of 7 to 12 mm for two-point discrimination.[30] The sensory branches are examined in order and compared with the uninjured extremity.

The test of radial nerve sensation is done with pinprick and two-point discrimination over the dorsum of the thumb web space. The motor branches of the radial nerve are tested by the extensors of the wrist and extension at the MCP joint. Ulnar nerve sensation is best tested over the little finger, and motor branches are examined by asking the patient to forcibly spread the fingers and comparing the strength to the normal side. Flexion of the distal joint of the ring and little fingers against resistance is an additional test of ulnar nerve function. Adduction of the thumb is also a function of the ulnar nerve and this

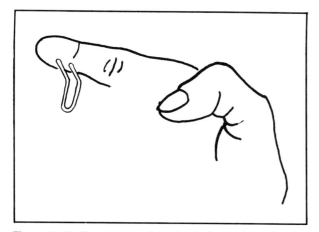

Figure 9–20. Two-point discrimination is the most sensitive indicator of a neurologic deficit involving the sensory branches of the nerves supplying the hand.

should be tested. The median nerve is tested by checking pinprick and two-point discrimination over the eponychium of the index and long fingers. Motor supply is tested by asking the patient to flex the wrist and PIP joints of the thumb and index fingers against resistance. Coin discrimination of different coins in the hand is a good test for sensation of the median nerve.

Nerve injuries can result from contusions, lacerations, and puncture wounds of the hand. One must check for nerve function in every hand injury to avoid delay in diagnosis. Contusions usually result in a neuropraxia with no loss of continuity of the nerve in which case function is usually regained and treatment is simply observation. Lacerations or puncture wounds can result in an axonotmesis or a neurotmesis. To differentiate between these, one must examine the patient meticulously for both sensory and motor function of the tested nerve.

☐ Ulnar Nerve Injuries

Lacerations of the ulnar nerve at the distal forearm and wrist result in hypothenar muscle weakness, loss of finger abduction, adduction (interosseus muscles), and flexion, as well as adduction of the thumb. Hand sensory loss of the ulnar nerve distribution will also occur. Laceration of the ulnar nerve in the proximity of MCP joints of the thumb, ring finger, and middle finger can result in loss of abduction and adduction, weakness of the thumb flexion, and adduction while hypothenar muscles and ulnar sensation remains intact. Deep volar hand lacerations of the MCP joints can cause isolated injury to the digital nerves and distal sensor loss with normal motor function.[30]

The specific signs of ulnar nerve injury are as follows:

- Loss of sensation in the distribution of the ulnar nerve
- Deformity of the hand such as Duchenne's sign (clawing of the ring and the little fingers)
- Inability to actively adduct the little finger
- Hyperflexion of the interphalangeal joint of the thumb on a powerful pinch (Froment's sign).

Intrinsic and hypothenar muscle paralysis with muscle wasting and loss of digital abduction and adduction may also occur. Bouvier's sign, the inability to actively extend the interphalangeal joint on passive flexion of the MCP joint, is also present.[29]

Ulnar neuropathy in bicyclists is not an uncommon overusage injury. Patients experience insidious onset of numbness, weakness, and loss of coordination in one or both hands, usually after several days of cycling.[10] The most common sites are the ring and little fingers on the ulnar side. To prevent this problem cyclists should wear padded gloves and a pad on the handlebars of the cycle. In addition, one should recommend that the top bar of the handlebar be level with the top of the saddle. If symptoms continue, they must cease bicycle riding for a short time.[10]

□ Neuroma

Neuromas are composed of disorganized axons interwoven with scar tissue. These may be quite painful, particularly when they occur over pressure points. They usually occur after injury to the nerve when the nerve remains intact, or in cases where the nerve is divided at the proximal stump of the nerve. Neuromas may follow years after an injury. When the sensory branches of a nerve are involved, neuromas can be very painful and often enlarge insidiously.[40]

The most common sites of neuromas are the sensory branches of the radial nerve at the distal third of the forearm and the wrist. A neuroma in this area may follow trivial trauma which the patient may not recall. Other common sites are the main median nerve, the palmar cutaneous branches at the wrist, and the main ulnar nerve with its dorsal sensory branches to the wrist. The treatment usually depends on how symptomatic the patient is and may include surgical intervention.[40]

□ VASCULAR INJURIES

The vascular supply to the hand is provided by the radial and ulnar arteries, which combine within the hand to form the superficial and deep palmar arches. The integrity of these vessels can best be tested by the *Allen test*. This is performed by compressing the radial and ulnar arteries at the wrist after having the patient make a fist and opening and closing it several times to exsanguinate the hand of its blood (Fig. 9–21A) and finally opening the hand. Next, the radial artery only is released; if blood flows to all the digits then the radial artery is patent and good collateral flow exists into the radial artery system (Fig. 9–21B). The same is done in testing the ulnar artery. If both vessels are injured, then at least one, usually the ulnar, must be repaired.

Vascular injury in the upper extremity is most often caused by repetitive trauma. The ulnar artery is susceptible to injury at the segment between the distal margin of the tunnel of Guyon and the palmar aponeurosis where the superficial palmar arch begins. Repetitive impact can occur among baseball catchers, touring cyclists, and handball players, causing an aneurysm with either thrombosis or vascular spasm. Symptoms of vascular injury include one or more cold digits, pain, intermittent mottling, and stiffness. An aneurysm may present with a probable mass.[57]

□ INJURIES TO THE LIGAMENTS AND THE JOINTS

Ligamentous injuries to the hand are very common and often missed. The consequence of these injuries is stiffness and painful swelling that is chronic in the joint. One

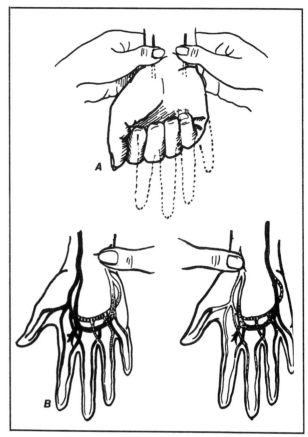

Figure 9–21. Allen test. An Allen test is performed to ascertain the patency of the radial and ulnar arteries supplying the hand. **A.** The patient is asked to make several fists while the examiner compresses the radial and ulnar arteries as shown. The patient then opens the hand and the examiner releases pressure from one of the arteries. In the patient with a patent vessel, an erythematous flush should be noted in the hand when pressure is released. **B.** The same is done with the vessel on the opposite side.

must rule out ligamentous injuries in joints having a history of significant trauma. On examination, one will note hemarthrosis or localized tenderness to one or both sides of the IP joint. A vital part of the assessment is to check stability by *lateral stress tests* (Fig. 9–22) and *active motion* at the IP joints and the MP joints of the hand. Stable joints that are painful on lateral stress testing indicate a partial tear or sprain of the collateral ligaments supporting the joint.

In performing a stress test of the collateral ligaments of the digits, one must always compare the same joint on the opposite hand. Minimal opening of the few millimeters with a good end point indicates that the collateral ligament is ruptured but that the volar plate is intact. If one notices wide opening on stress testing, the volar plate must be ruptured because of the boxlike nature that the collateral ligaments and volar plate form around the joint (Fig. 9–23). Thus, wide opening indicates that both the collateral ligament and volar plate

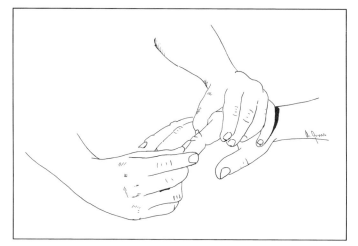

Figure 9–22. The lateral stress test is performed by holding the phalanx on either side of the joint and attempting to open the joint's base. Comparison to the opposite digit should be done. Minimal opening indicates that the collateral ligament is ruptured on that side. Wide opening indicates that the collateral ligament and the volar plate are both ruptured.

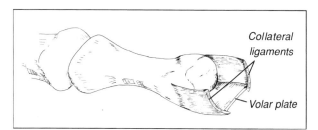

Figure 9–23. The collateral ligaments on either side of the joint and the volar plate form a boxlike support around the joint.

are ruptured. Wide opening of the joint should be treated in a gutter splint and referred for assessment by a hand surgeon to determine whether surgical repair is necessary. Functional stability is evaluated by active motion. If the patient cannot perform motion due to pain, or stress testing is limited by pain, then a digital or wrist block is indicated. In performing stress tests, one should keep the joint in extension and always compare opening with the uninvolved digit. Supplemental stress roentgenograms may be helpful in evaluating difficult cases.

□ Sprains of the IP and MCP Collateral Ligaments

The collateral ligaments provide the support against lateral displacement of these joints. If a partial tear is indicated by appropriate stress testing as described above, the treatment should be rest with complete immobilization for 10 to 14 days. The joints with demonstrable instability to stress must be immobilized for 21 days. Immobilization should be with the IP joint splinted at 30 degrees of flexion and the MCP splinted at 45 to 50 degrees of flexion. When the thumb MCP is involved, it should be splinted in 30 degrees of flexion. One can splint the involved digit with a lightly padded plaster cast or metallic splints that are commercially available. After immobilization of the involved digit,

active motion is encouraged for the remainder of the hand. Capsular thickening noted by palpation and chronic swelling of the involved joint at the end of the period of immobilization suggests the initial damage was greater than at first thought and that more protection is needed. This should be provided by buddy splinting the digit to the adjacent normal one for 5 to 7 days. The problem at this point is no longer instability, but stiffness and decrease in motion with pain at the involved joint later. Swelling may persist for several weeks after a sprain to the joints.

□ DIP Joint Injuries and Dislocations (Fig. 9–24)

The DIP joint is stable in all positions as capsular support consists of tough collateral accessory ligaments laterally and the fibrous plate volarly.[67] Dorsal support is minimal and includes the extensor mechanism that blends with the dorsal capsule. The collateral ligaments are thick, rectangular bands that arise laterally from the condyle and pass distally and volarly to insert into the volar lateral articular margin and the volar plate. The volar plate provides support to the distal joint and is square shaped and 2- to 3-mm thick.

Disruption is only important in terms of joint stability, which can be assessed by the two methods described above: active motion and lateral stress testing. These tests are most valid under digital anesthesia after reduction of the dislocation. If reduction is maintained through full range of motion, then adequate ligamentous support can be assumed and only 10 to 14 days of immobilization is needed. If, however, displacement occurs in the last 15 degrees of joint extension, then major disruption must be assumed and immobilization in 30 degrees of flexion for a full 3 weeks is indicated.

Reduction is by simple longitudinal traction and manipulation into its normal position.

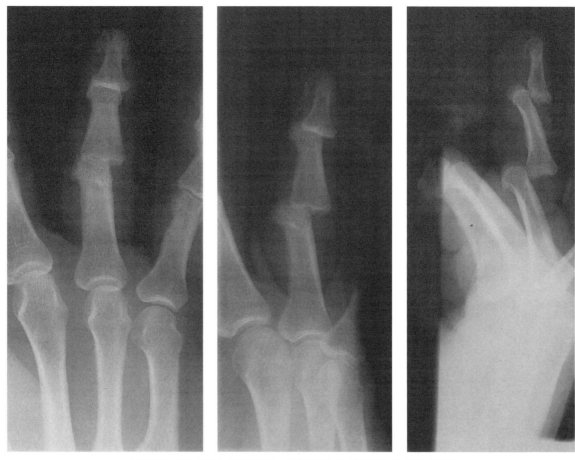

Figure 9–24. Hand dislocation—PIP and DIP. *(Courtesy L. Miller, RN.)*

□ PIP Joint Injuries and Dislocations (Fig. 9–25)

The integrity of the PIP joint is maintained by the two collateral ligaments on either side of this joint and the volar plate on the volar aspect, which together form a boxlike support around the joint (see Fig. 9–23). For instability to occur at the joint there must be disruption of two of these three supporting structures. The PIP joint is prone to develop stiffness after injury even with good immobilization, and this complication must be mentioned to the patient.

Classification. There are three types of injuries that occur at this joint:

1. Dislocations: posterior (common); anterior (rare); lateral (common)
2. Volar plate injuries
3. Fracture–dislocations

Each of these will be discussed separately. Lateral dislocations are often classified as collateral ligament injuries (rupture) because spontaneous reduction is the rule here.

Lateral and posterior dislocations of the PIP joint are quite common, whereas anterior dislocations are rare. Anterior dislocations are invariably associated with disruption of the central slip of the extensor tendon from its insertion at the base of the middle phalanx.[72]

Fracture–dislocations are relatively uncommon injuries.

Mechanism of Injury. Posterior dislocations are caused by hyperextension of the PIP joint such as occurs when the outstretched finger is struck by a ball. For this injury to occur, there must be rupture of the volar plate or collateral ligaments, at least in part.

Lateral dislocations are caused by abduction or adduction stresses to the finger usually while it is in the extended position. The radial collateral ligament is far more commonly injured than the ulnar collateral.

Anterior dislocations are caused by a combination of varus or vulgus forces causing a rupture of the collateral ligament and the volar plate and an anteriorly directed force displacing the base of the middle phalanx forward rupturing the central slip of the extensor mechanism.[72]

Fracture–dislocations occur when the extended finger is struck in such a way that longitudinal compression occurs along with hyperextension causing a fracture through the volar lip of the middle phalanx and dorsal

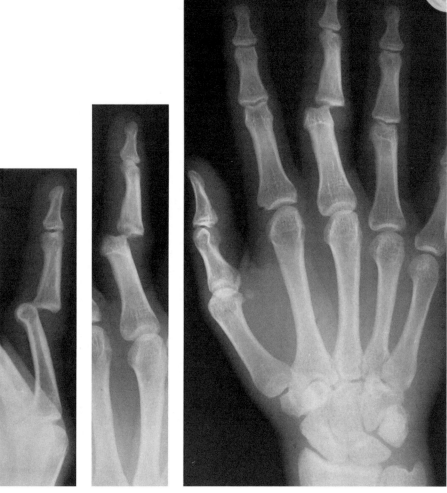

Figure 9–25. A posterior (dorsal) dislocation of the PIP joint of the long finger is shown.

displacement of the middle phalanx and distal portion of the finger. This commonly occurs when the extended finger is struck by a ball.

The volar plate may be ruptured when a blow occurs on the end of the finger causing a hyperextension force. The volar plate may be torn from its distal attachment at the base of the middle phalanx, and a small piece of bone may be avulsed with it.

Examinations. Acute swelling and pain may camouflage an existing deformity or a dislocation; however, this is not often the case and the deformity is usually obvious. One must x ray the digit before reduction is performed, and *after reduction* one must *examine the collateral ligaments* by stress testing and the volar plate.

In patients with lateral dislocations (these usually reduce spontaneously) on examination in the emergency department, the physician will note pain on lateral stress testing and tenderness over the lateral joint. Lateral in-

stability indicating a complete rupture must be assessed while the digit is extended.

Injuries to the volar plate will cause a hyperextension deformity at the PIP joint on extension of the finger, whereas pain and catching or locking are noted with flexion of the digit.

If the hyperextension deformity is severe, the patient may have a compensatory flexion deformity of the DIP joint secondary to the tenodesing effect of the flexor digitorum profundus tendon. There is maximal tenderness over the volar aspect of the finger joint, and pain is increased on passive hyperextension and relieved by passive flexion. In addition, there is loss of normal "check" on extension of the finger provided by an intact volar plate. To do an adequate examination to check for these findings, a digital or metacarpal block is usually indicated.

Patients with fracture–dislocations are unable to flex the PIP joint and in addition have swelling, pain, and deformity. (See Fig. 9–26.)

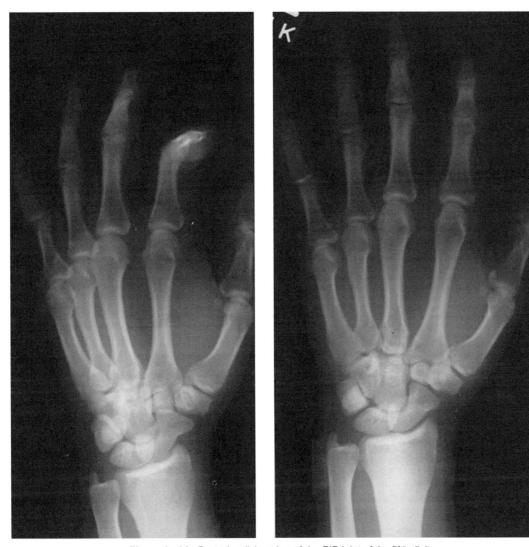

Figure 9-26. Posterior dislocation of the PIP joint of the fifth digit.

X Ray. Routine views of the digit should be taken and with the suspicion of rupture of the collateral ligament or with marked swelling, or a questionable examination stress views may be taken and compared with the normal side.

In injuries to the volar plate with avulsion of the plate, one may see a small bone fragment avulsed from the base of the middle phalanx, but usually the x ray is normal. X rays taken with the finger in extension may show abnormal hyperextension when compared with the normal side.

With fracture–dislocations, there is dorsal subluxation of the middle phalanx with a fracture of the volar lip of the middle phalanx that may involve up to one third of the articular surface.

Treatment

Collateral Ligament Injury. Dynamic splinting for 2 to 5 weeks is indicated in *acute partial rupture*. Major tears require splinting for 3 to 5 weeks with the joint flexed 35 degrees followed by guarded active motion with buddy splinting for protection for an additional 3 weeks.[1] *Acute complete ruptures* with instability on stress testing can be splinted for 6 weeks although some authors prefer surgical repair of unstable injuries. Consultation with the orthopedic service is indicated. *Volar plate injuries* should be treated with splinting the PIP joint in 30 degrees of flexion for 3 to 5 weeks. An alternative is to splint the joint for 3 weeks and follow this with active flexion in an extension block splint set at 15 degrees of flexion for 2 more weeks.

Dislocations. Posterior dislocations are usually easily reduced under metacarpal block anesthesia by longitudinal traction and manipulation back to its normal position (Fig. 9–27). This may require some hyperextension. If the volar plate is trapped in the joint space, open reduction is indicated. After reduction, the joint is splinted in 15 degrees of flexion for 3 weeks to allow healing of the

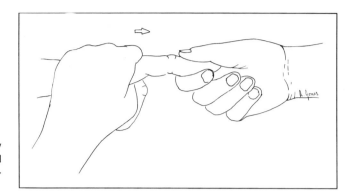

Figure 9–27. The joint is easily reduced by longitudinal traction and manipulation back to its normal position.

volar plate. If the joint is stable, after reduction, then early motion is indicated after initial immobilization with protection by taping to the adjacent finger for an additional 3 weeks. If unstable, then it is splinted for 3 weeks with the PIP joint in 15 degrees of flexion, after which an extension block splint should be used for an additional 3 weeks.

Anterior dislocations are usually easily reduced, but are commonly associated with a boutonnière deformity, which results if the central slip is detached. Because surgical intervention may be needed, referral is indicated.[52,72]

Fracture–dislocations may be reduced as per the routine method and if the fragment is large or unstable then open reduction and fixation are indicated. The authors believe all these should be referred.[52]

With any of the above dislocations, soft tissue may be interposed in the joint space and block reduction of the dislocation. This should be suspected in any case in which one or two attempts at reduction prove unsuccessful. These cases may require open reduction to extract and repair the interposed ligament, tendon, or volar plate and should be referred.[54]

Complications. The complications of PIP joint injuries and dislocations are restricted joint motion, which is a common sequel. The most common complication of which patients complain is *persistent thickening* of the PIP joint. Volar plate and collateral ligament instability are further problems. The patient should be warned that thickening of the joint may persist indefinitely but function should be normal.

☐ MCP Joint Injuries

The MCP joints are condyloid joints that have, in addition to flexion and extension, as much as 30 degrees of lateral motion while the joint is extended. Because of the shape of this articulation, the joint is more stable in flexion when the collateral ligaments are stretched than in extension, which permits lateral motion in the joint. The collaterals have a loose attachment to the proximal neck portion of the metacarpal.[8]

☐ *Injuries to the Collateral Ligament and Volar Plate of the MCP Joint*

These injuries usually occur with hyperextension stresses applied to the MCP joint with the finger extended. The patient presents with massive ecchymosis and swelling of the joint, and the x ray is usually negative for fractures. The treatment of this injury is a gentle compressive dressing with light plaster reinforcement. These patients may require prolonged immobilization depending on the degree of injury and should be referred for follow-up care.

☐ *Dislocations of the MCP Joint*

Dislocations at the MCP joint are usually dorsal (see Fig. 9–28). These are complex irreducible dislocations and are not nearly as common as IP dislocations. The finger on examination appears shortened and is usually ulnar deviated and in extension. The index finger is most commonly involved and the metacarpal head is prominent in the palm. Closed reduction usually fails because the metacarpal head is buttonholed between the flexor tendons and the lumbrical muscles. The volar plate is still attached to the dorsally displaced proximal phalanx, which becomes interposed between the joint surfaces and locks thus necessitating surgical reduction.

In subluxation, the proximal phalanx is locked in 60 to 90 degrees of hyperextension and the articular surfaces are in partial contact. Reduction is performed by flexion of the digit after longitudinal traction is applied to disengage the proximal phalanx.

☐ Injuries to the Joints of the Thumb
☐ *IP Joint Dislocations*

This injury is handled similarly to distal IP joint injuries of the fingers. The most common injury is a dorsal dislocation with lateral dislocations being less frequent. Dorsal dislocations are often associated with open injuries, and reduction is usually simple after a median nerve block. The joint usually remains stable because the volar plate remains attached to the distal phalanx and immobilization of the joint should be done for 3 weeks in slight flexion.

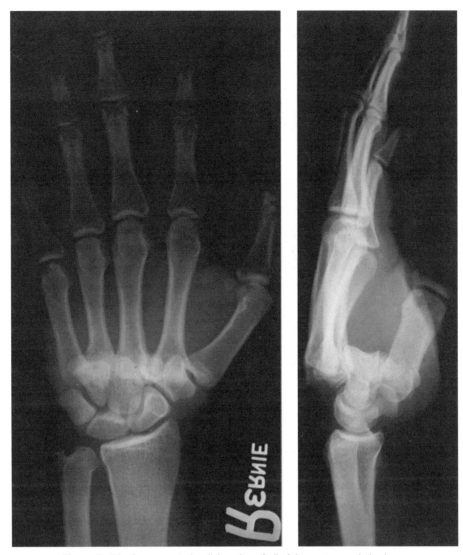

Figure 9–28. A rare posterior dislocation of all of the metacarpals is shown.

☐ *MCP Joint Injuries and Dislocations of the Thumb (Fig. 9–29)*

This joint is very mobile, and dislocations here are quite common. The collateral ligaments are thick and provide good support for the joint. The volar plate contains within its substance two sesamoid bones that serve as the insertions for the flexor pollicis brevis (radial sesamoid) and the adductor pollicis (ulnar sesamoid). Because of the mobility of this joint, dislocations here are far more common than at the digits and are of two types, dorsal and lateral, each with an equal frequency.[70]

Dorsal dislocations occur with extreme hyperextension or shearing forces, and disruption of the volar supporting structures almost always occurs. Displacement varies from a subluxation of the phalanx to the complete dislocation with the proximal phalanx resting over the metacarpal head. For the latter to occur, the volar plate and the collaterals must completely tear. On the x ray, the sesamoids are found to be lying 1 to 2 mm proximal to the base of the proximal phalanx. When dislocation is not associated with this degree of disruption of the supporting structures, reduction is usually easy. Flexion of the metacarpal to relax the muscles and extension of the IP joint which tightens the flexor tendon should be applied. Longitudinal traction is then applied until distraction occurs, and the MCP joint is flexed. After reduction, the digit is splinted for 3 weeks in flexion unless there is more than 40 degrees of lateral instability in which case surgical repair may be indicated. The amount of instability must always be assessed after reduction.

Lateral dislocations present with only local pain and swelling. To diagnose this injury, one must do stress examinations of the ulnar and radial collateral ligaments of the thumb.[70] These are best done under local anesthe-

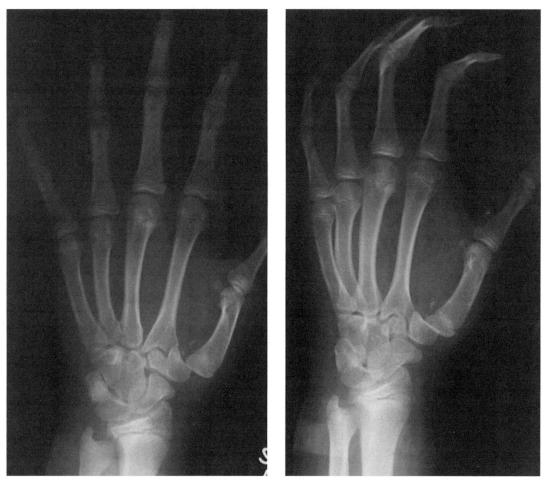

Figure 9–29. A carpal–metacarpal dislocation of the thumb is shown with avulsion fragments.

sia with a block. *Ulnar collateral ligament rupture* is 10 times more common than radial ligament injury and can be very disabling, whereby the patient has a weak pinch and cannot resist an adduction stress.[70] This injury is commonly called *gamekeeper's thumb*.[7] To diagnose this, the examiner checks the thumb in extension and determines if there is greater than 20 degrees of ulnar ligament instability when compared with the normal side (Fig. 9–30). If the joint opens less than 20 degrees, than no surgically correctable instability exists.[7] One can splint the thumb for 3 weeks. If there is greater than 20 degrees of instability, the patient must be referred for repair of this ligament, because the aponeurosis of the adductor pollicis may become interposed between the ends of the disrupted ligament and the ligament ends cannot come together by simple splinting in two thirds of the cases (Fig. 9–31). The same is not true with radial disruption because no tissue is interposed here. Although some surgeons believe that 40 degrees of opening can be treated without surgery,[44] the authors recommend that all those with more than 20 degrees of opening at the joint should be referred. Patients with gamekeeper's thumb

have been treated with a special thumb splint designed to reduce motion simulating the injury and yet provide for mobilization three times a day rather than surgical intervention with good results.[62] This remains controversial. This injury is commonly missed in the emergency department, resulting in disability.[70] It is seen commonly in skiers who have fallen where the ski pole abducts the thumb at the MCP joint, rupturing the ulnar collateral ligament.

☐ *Lunate and Perilunate Dislocations*

Carpal and carpometacarpal dislocations are complex and often difficult dislocations to adequately assess without multiple roentgenograms taken in several projections. The consequences of inadequate evaluation during the initial examination or misdiagnosis may be quite devastating to the patient who depends on a normal functioning wrist for his or her livelihood. It is the authors' belief that the complexity of these injuries requires consultation in all suspected cases and therefore they will discuss only the basics of the more common dislocations.

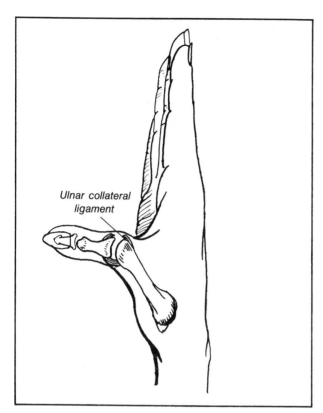

Figure 9–30. Examining for disruption of the ulnar collateral ligament of the thumb at the MCP joint.

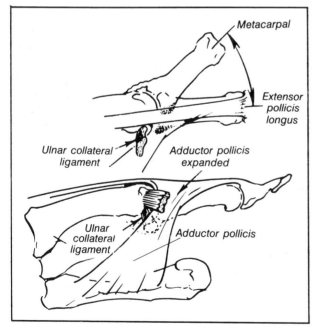

Figure 9–31. Note that the adductor pollicis of the thumb is interspersed between the two ruptured ends of the ulnar collateral ligament and ruptures of that ligament. (*From Kilgore ES Jr, Graham WP III, The Hand. Philadelphia: Lea & Febiger, 1977, p 154, with permission.*)

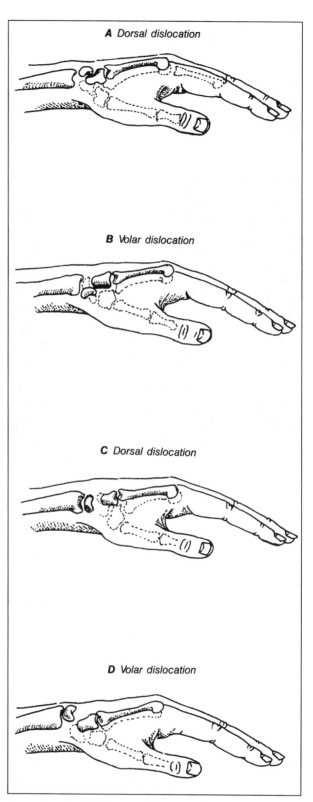

Figure 9–32. *A, B.* Lunate dislocations. *C, D.* Perilunate dislocations.

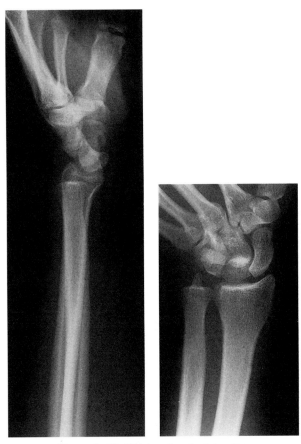

Figure 9–33. Wrist perilunate dislocation.

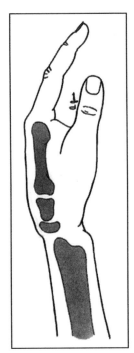

Figure 9–34. A dorsal lunate dislocation.

The lunate may dislocate or the bones around it may be displaced (perilunate dislocations) usually caused by a hyperextension injury (Figs. 9–32 and 9–33). In lunate dislocations, the lunate is displaced volarly or dorsally (Fig. 9–34).

On examination, there is limitation of normal motion of the wrist with a palpable fullness on the volar aspect with tenderness. The median nerve may be compressed in the carpal canal by the lunate, and the patient may display signs of a median nerve injury.

Roentgenograms show the lunate to have a *triangular appearance* on routine anteroposterior (AP) views, and the volar displacement is easily seen on the lateral view (Fig. 9–35). In situations where the remainder of the carpus is displaced, one sees the lunate in its normal position but there appears to be overlap of the remaining carpals in relation to it. One should always, in looking at the lateral view of the wrist, draw an imaginary line between the centers of the radius, lunate, and capitate. This line should always go through the lunate at its midportion (Fig. 9–36). If, however, the lunate is displaced or subluxed, the line connecting the capitate with the midpoint of the radius will either go through only an edge of the lunate or not go through it at all. The lateral radiograph is the single most important view from which to determine correct alignment

of the carpals.[14] When this is properly positioned, the hand is in neutral position and the posterior cortices of the radius and ulna are superimposed on one another. The key elements of the lateral radiographs are linear arrangement of the radius, lunate, and capitate, as discussed above.[16] In addition, on the lateral view, the angle formed between the scaphoid and the lunate by lines drawn through their longitudinal axis is normally 47 degrees and ranges between 30 and 60 degrees in the normal wrist. An angle greater than 70 degrees indicates that carpal instability exists. Occasionally, scapholunate joint laxity may be seen only on the AP view with a tightly clinched fist. This "fist compression" tends to force the capitate head into and widen the scapholunate joint.[55] The scaphoid may lose its normal elongated shape and appear shortened with a dense ring shape around its distal end. This "cortico ring" sign represents a scaphoid seen in an axial projection after volar rotation.[55] Both perilunate and lunate dislocations usually involve either rotary subluxation of the scaphoid or commonly a scaphoid fracture.[55]

All lunate and perilunate dislocations should be immobilized with the wrist in neutral position in a volar splint and referred immediately for reduction and definitive care.

☐ Scapholunate Dissociation
This commonly missed injury is characterized by displacement of the scaphoid to a more vertical position

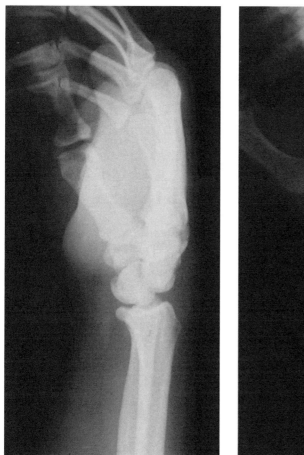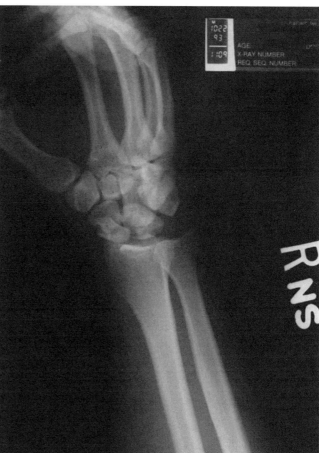

Figure 9–35. *A, B.* A volar lunate dislocation associated with a scaphoid fracture is shown. Notice the triangular appearance of the lunate in (***B***). (*Courtesy of D. J. Manning, MD, Racine, WI.*)

in the proximal row of carpal bones in relation to the lunate. This produces a gap between the lunate and the proximal pole of the scaphoid.[13]

Routine views show the *scapholunate joint space* to be greater than 3 mm. This joint space should always be looked at in any patient with trauma to the wrist in whom one suspects the often diagnosed "sprain." The joint space should never be greater than 3 mm wide on the AP view.

Patients with scapholunate dissociation who are diagnosed within 6 weeks of injury are called *acute scapholunate dissociation.* Those injuries which are diagnosed after 6 weeks are termed *subacute.* There are multiple surgical procedures which have been described for dealing with these cases.[46] Patients with this injury should be placed in a thumb spica splint or cast and referred to a hand surgeon[46] (Fig. 9–37).

A scaphoid shift maneuver provides a qualitative assessment of the stability of the scaphoid and for periscaphoid synovitis. This always has to be compared to the contralateral side. With the patient's forearm slightly pronated, the examiner grasps the patient's wrist from the radial side with the same hand (the examiner's right hand when examining the patient's right hand), placing the thumb palmar prominence of the scaphoid while wrapping the fingers around the patient's distal radius. This enables the thumb to push the scaphoid with counterpressure provided by the fingers (see Fig. 9–37). The examiner's other hand grasps the patient's hand at the metacarpal level to control wrist position. Starting in the ulnar deviation and slight extension, the patient's wrist is moved rapidly and slightly flexed with constant thumb pressure on the scaphoid. The examiner's thumb pressure opposes the normal rotation and creates a subluxation stress, causing the scaphoid to shift dorsally in relation to the other bones in the carpus. This (scaphoid shift) may be subtle or dramatic. As thumb pressure is withdrawn, the scaphoid returns abruptly to its normal position, sometimes with a resounding "thunk."[83]

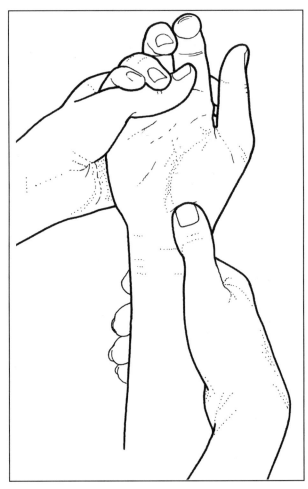

Figure 9-37. The scaphoid shift maneuver to assess for scaphoid stability and periscaphoid synovitis. The patient's forearm is slightly pronated. The examiner grasps the patient's wrist from the radial side, placing the thumb on the prominence of the scaphoid and wrapping the fingers around the distal forearm. The thumb should put pressure on the scaphoid while the examiner's fingers provide counterpressure. The examiner's other hand grasps the patient's hand at the level of the metacarpal heads. The examiner ulnar deviates and slightly extends the patient's hand, then moves the patient's wrist radially and into slight flexion while maintaining thumb pressure on the scaphoid. This maneuver is positive if the scaphoid shifts dorsally.

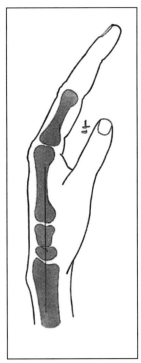

Figure 9-36. Note that a line drawn through the midpoint of the radius and the capitate on the lateral view of the wrist traverses the midpoint of the lunate. If the lunate is dislocated or subluxated, the line will traverse only a fragment of the bone or miss it entirely.

Nontraumatic Disorders

☐ NONINFECTIOUS INFLAMMATORY CONDITIONS

☐ Venous and Lymphatic Congestive States

The drainage of the hand takes place via the lymphatic system and the veins that course on the dorsal aspect.

Any condition that leads to swelling in the hand, whether it be a fracture, strain, or contusion, can lead to lymphatic congestion and a nonpitting edema over the dorsum of the hand. This limits motion and may lead to fibrosis with an impediment to normal tendon function. A principle to follow in all conditions leading to swelling of the hand is to begin motion of the noninjured part early. One should avoid a constrictive dressing and elevate the hand to guard against edema formation.

☐ Myositis

Muscle soreness can occur with activity in an unconditioned patient. One form of this is myositis crepitans that occurs over the abductor pollicis longus and the extensor pollicis brevis. A second common site is the muscles of the wrist and the digital extensors. In this condition, the examiner will note crepitation that is palpable and audible with a stethoscope. The muscle is edematous and tender with increasing pain on stress. The treatment in the acute stage is splinting and injection of triamcinolone, which usually affords good relief.

☐ Desmitis

Desmitis is an inflammatory condition of the ligaments of the hand and usually involves the wrist and IP joint ligaments on the radial or ulnar side of the digit. The condition usually follows trauma or any repetitive stress to the joint.

On examination, pain is usually well localized with minimal tenderness to palpation. Stress of the involved ligament accentuates the pain. Swelling and erythema are infrequent findings with this condition, and x rays are negative.

The treatment is local steroid injections. Recurrences are common, and, therefore, the involved joints should be splinted to avoid any stresses.

☐ Tendonitis

There are three types of noninfectious tendonitis: simple tendonitis, tendonitis with synovitis, and villonodular synovitis. All forms most commonly involve the wrist flexors and extensors.

In *simple tendonitis*, active and passive tension of the tendons accentuates the pain. The tenderness is usually well localized over the involved tendon. The condition may occur de novo, however, usually after repetitive stress of the involved tendon. Swelling and erythema are infrequently seen with simple tendonitis. When the flexors of the digits are involved, the tenderness is most often over the MCP joint area.

The treatment is local injection with a steroid, which usually affords excellent relief.

In *tendonitis with synovitis*, there generally is no recognized precipitating cause; however, a history of excessive stress on the tendon is often obtained. In uncomplicated synovitis, usually no gross synovial thickening is noted. The mechanism of the synovitis is one of friction between the tendon and the sheath leading to an effusion that may even become hemorrhagic if the stress continues and later villonodular as thickening results, leading to ischemic rupture of the tendon. The most common site for this form of tendonitis is the extensor tendon sheaths.

On examination the patient has a soft, nontender, diffuse subcutaneous swelling noted over the base of the hand confined to the area proximal to the extensor retinaculum. In some cases, one may get a dumbbell deformity with swelling seen on either side of the extensor retinaculum. The same condition may be seen with the flexors but not recognized due to the fat padding of the palm and the thickened skin of the palm. Commonly, the flexor tendons distal to the MCP joint are affected and this is easily recognized.

The treatment for this form is rest; injection with steroids usually affords prompt relief and a change in any precipitating activity is advisable.

As the condition continues or becomes more chronic, the synovium thickens and is actually palpable over the dorsal or volar aspects of the hand. Less tenderness along with decreasing excursion of the involved tendon may be noted. This condition is known as *tendonitis with villonodular synovitis*. There is no fluid contained in the synovial sheath; therefore, patients do not respond to an injection with steroids. The thickened synovium obstructs the excursion of the joint and the fingers that become thickened, and the recommended treatment is synovectomy.

Tendonitis involving the extensor pollicis longus is rare, but when it does occur, usually occurs at Lister's tubercle. This may occur after a Colles' fracture.[76] Patients who have tendonitis of the extensor digiti minimi or indicis present with pain at the wrist which can be reproduced by full passive flexion of the wrist.[76] Flexor carpi ulnaris tendonitis may be bilateral and may require surgical excision of the pisiform.[76] Patients who have flexor tendonitis of the digits may present with a stabbing or burning pain proximal to the carpal tunnel. Patients who present with stenosing tenosynovitis of the extensor carpi ulnaris tendon often require surgical release.[76]

☐ CONSTRICTIVE AND COMPRESSIVE CONDITIONS

The constrictive conditions include the various forms of stenosing tenosynovitis and neural entrapment syndromes. In this discussion the compressive conditions such as Volkmann's contractures will be included.

☐ Stenosing Tenosynovitis

There are three types of stenosing tenosynovitidies involving the hand: trigger finger, De Quervain's, and that of the extensor pollicis longus. The condition most commonly involves the flexor tendons at the level of the MCP joint where the tendon passes through the pulley system. The abductor pollicis longus and the extensor pollicis brevis over the radial styloid and the extensor pollicis longus at Lister's tubercle appear to be the most commonly involved extensor tendons. This is most common in women between the ages of 40 and 50 years.

The patient complains of discomfort after excess activity involving the tendon or on first arising, both

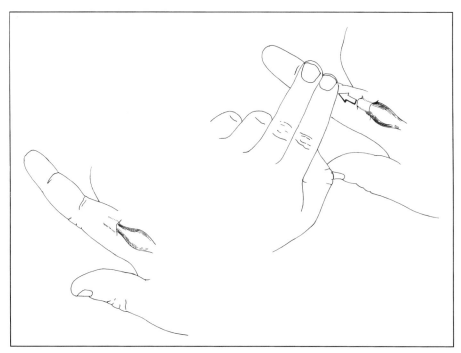

Figure 9–38. Note the fibrous thickening causing the condition known as trigger finger.

corresponding to moments when there is maximal tissue edema. The symptoms may be bilateral. Both the tendon and the pulley hypertrophy are a consequence of excessive repetitive strain. Tenderness is often localized over the proximal flexor pulley.

When there is painful blocking of flexion and extension at the involved joint, the syndrome called *trigger finger* is present. Two types of trigger fingers occur: diffuse and nodular.[24] The nodular type is far more common, representing 93 percent of cases, and responds well to injection with triamcinolone. There is only a 48 percent success rate with the diffuse type.[24] At times, the patient complains only about the PIP joint, which is the site of referred pain from the proximal flexor pulley. The ring and long fingers are the most commonly involved digits. Active closing of the fist reproduces the locking (Fig. 9–38). The site of maximal swelling in relation to the pulley governs the attitude of the digit. If the swelling is proximal to the pulley, then the digit can flex but not extend easily; however, if the swelling is distal to the pulley, then the digit can passively, but not actively, flex. The following treatment is recommended in patients with trigger finger: 2 mL lidocaine and 0.5 mL of steroid suspension mixed together. An injection is given through the web space and over the nodule.[20] After the injection, extension of the finger is usually possible. The finger should be splinted in extension. This will allow the nodule to lie underneath the flexor tendon pulley so the pressure can be applied. A removable splint is fabricated and should be worn for 7 to 10 days. Injection therapy usually works well in most patients.[60] Sometimes one needs to do three injections which

are spaced 2 to 3 weeks apart using Celestone™, which is a water-soluble steroid that does not leave a residue (Schering Corporation, Kenilworth, NJ).[60] When this does not work and surgical intervention is necessary, a longitudinal incision to release the finger is desirable.[73]

De Quervain's stenosing tenosynovitis involves the abductor pollicis longus and extensor pollicis brevis in the first dorsal wrist compartment (Fig. 9–39). Patients complain of pain over the radial aspect of the wrist with radiation proximally and distally. There is localized tenderness over the radial styloid where the pulley may look and feel thickened. A pathognomonic test, which reproduces the pain, is tensing the tendons by holding the thumb in the palm making a fist, and ulnar deviating the wrist, called *Finkelstein's test* (Fig. 9–40). One must differentiate this condition from carpometacarpal arthritis of the thumb, which causes localized tenderness at that joint. Women are more commonly affected than men with a ratio of 10 to 1. Usually, this condition is due to overuse or associated with rheumatoid arthritis.[20] Treatment involves injection of the tendon sheath with a local anesthetic and a steroid (Fig. 9–41).[35,76,86] During the injection one should see a visible swelling proximal to the extensor retinaculum; this is a guide that the needle is in the right spot. The steroid should be injected after the anesthetic and not mixed in the same syringe. Occasionally, one must inject a second time to achieve good results. If there is no good result after two injections, surgical intervention should be recommended. In the majority of cases, injection therapy is all that is needed followed by splinting of the thumb for a short period of time and rotational exercises afterward.[35]

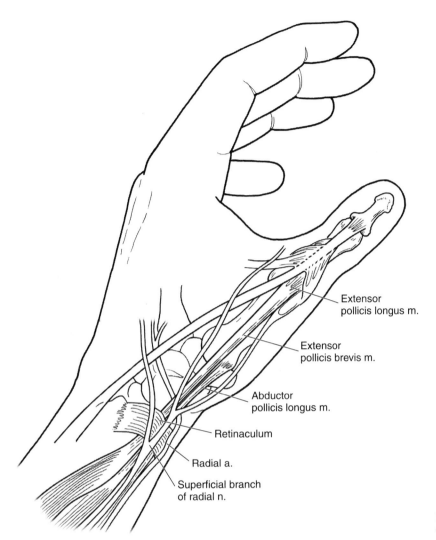

Extensor
pollicis longus m.

Extensor
pollicis brevis m.

Abductor
pollicis longus m.

Retinaculum

Radial a.

Superficial branch
of radial n.

Figure 9–39. Anatomy of the first dorsal wrist compartment.

Stenosing tenosynovitis of the extensor pollicis longus is an infrequent problem. The patient presents with tenderness along Lister's tubercle, which is the most common site of stenosis and rupture.

☐ Carpal Tunnel Syndrome

This syndrome involves compression of the median nerve in the carpal canal as the nerve is brought against the *transverse carpal ligament*. This occurs with the simultaneous flexion of the digits and the wrist (Fig. 9–42). The condition is most common in postmenopausal women and is usually idiopathic, but may follow fractures at the wrist, crush injuries, rheumatoid arthritis, pregnancy, diabetes, or thyroid disease. Any condition causing chronic swelling of the hand and wrist may lead to this syndrome.

Patients often complain of "their hand going to sleep," paresthesias over the distribution of the median nerve, and numbness. The pain may radiate to the shoulder but spares the little finger. The patient may be awakened from sleep with pain in the hand due to fluid reten-

tion. When this occurs, the patient should be instructed to elevate the hand and milk the fluid out. Symptoms develop after repetitive gripping or after acute wrist flexion such as occurs with driving a car or operating a tool that must be held in the hand for prolonged periods of time.

The earliest objective sensory finding in carpal tunnel syndrome is diminished vibratory sensation, tested with a 256-cycle tuning fork. More severe median nerve involvement results in abnormal two-point sensory discrimination.[81]

Tinel's sign will be positive and involves tapping the volar wrist. The patient will note paresthesias in the distribution of the median nerve (Fig. 9–43). This occurs only later in the course of the disorder, however. *Phalen's test* is performed by asking the patient to let the wrist fall into volar flexion for 1 minute and if positive, the physician will note paresthesias in the hand over the nerve distribution (Fig. 9–44). A *tourniquet* applied at the arm inflated to 200 mm Hg pressure for 2 minutes may also produce paresthesias in the hand and

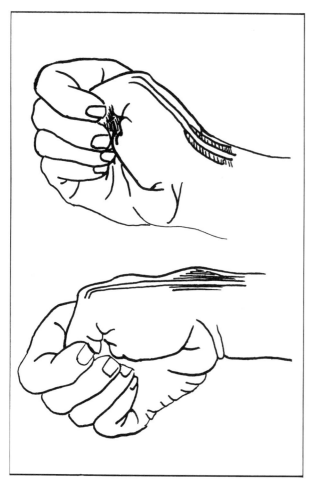

Figure 9–40. Finkelstein's test for examining a patient with suspected De Quervain's tenosynovitis. The patient will complain of pain over the tendon when the thumb is grasped in the hand as shown and the patient's ulnar deviates the wrist.

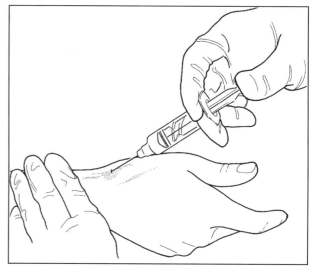

Figure 9–41. Injection for DeQuervain's stenosing tenosynovitis. The needle is inserted between the tendon and the sheath. If the needle is inserted properly, a sausagelike swelling will be noted in the first compartment as the fluid is injected. Lidocaine should be injected after the corticosteroid is injected and before removal of the needle, which helps prevent steroid discoloration or atrophy of the skin.

is another test that may be done when this condition is suspected.

In treating those patients with night pain, the involved wrist should be splinted in neutral or slight extension. Conservative therapy involves the injection of steroids proximal to the transverse carpal ligament. The needle should be placed in the skin just ulnarward to the palmaris longus tendon. Dexamethasone can be injected at this point after inserting the needle beneath the transverse carpal ligament and aim directing the needle at a 30-degree angle to the skin. If a response is not noted, surgical release is needed.

☐ Ulnar Nerve Compression Syndromes

There are three sites where the ulnar nerve may be compressed: the ulnar groove behind the medial epicondyle, the cubital tunnel near the aponeurosis of the flexor carpi ulnaris, and the wrist at the heel of the hand near the pisiform.[79] These conditions are usually the result of trauma such as a direct blow, but may, in the case of compression at the ulnar groove, occur after leaning on the elbow.

Ulnar groove compression leads to paralysis of the flexor carpi ulnaris and profundus to the ring and the little finger and the intrinsics. Compression at the cubital tunnel has no effect on the flexor carpi ulnaris although there is distal paralysis of the interossei and adductor pollicis as well as the two ulnar lumbricals. There is no sensory loss, however, over the distribution of the ulnar nerve.[79] The treatment is operative at the wrist and conservative, with expectant waiting at the elbow for 3 to 4 months after which one explores the area, if no improvement has occurred. Compression of the ulnar nerve in the tight triangular fibrosseous tunnel at the wrist can also cause this syndrome.[20] One must remember that if the intrinsics are involved then the compression is distal to this tunnel. This should be treated surgically.

☐ Radial Nerve Compression

Compression of the superficial radial nerve occurs with contrusive injuries or constrictive dressings. A removable splint is recommended for 7 to 10 days. Compression of the digital nerves occurs with repetitive external compression. The typical example is bowler's thumb. Pain and numbness occur localized to the ulnar aspect of the thumb.

The most common site for compression of the radial nerve is in the axilla called *Saturday night paralysis*. This is typically seen in alcoholic patients who sleep with their arms resting over the back of a chair. The radial nerve is compressed against the humerus in the spiral groove. Most of these compressions clear spontaneously and the treatment is a cock up splint worn to prevent wrist drop.

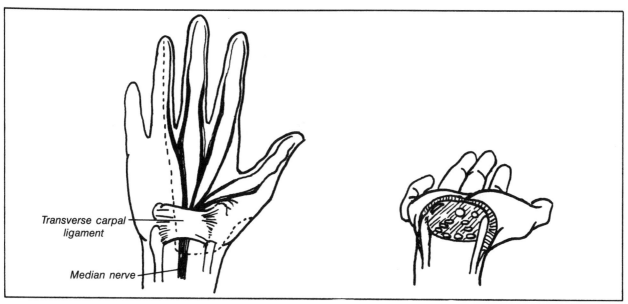

Figure 9–42. The carpel tunnel with the median nerve under the transverse carpal ligament.

☐ Bowler's Thumb

This is a perineural fibrosis which is caused by repeat compression of the ulnar digital nerve of the thumb while grasping a bowling ball. Patients complain of tingling and hyperesthesia at the pulp of the thumb. Usually, a palpable lump which is very tender is present on the ulnar side of the thumb.

☐ Volkmann's Contracture

The key element of importance to the emergency physician in considering this syndrome is its *early recognition and prevention*. The syndrome involves ischemic contracture of the muscles of the forearm and nerves to the hand and follows many compressive states such as com-

pression from a supracondylar fracture of the humerus in which swelling at the fracture site has compromised flow in the forearm and the nerves traversing the area. Once muscle necrosis has occurred, treatment is too late. The presence of peripheral pulses is deceptive. The key is to anticipate this implication by the appearance of *pain*. If one sees a patient with a cast or compressive dressing in the arm, elbow, or forearm who complains of pain and has digital swelling and paresthesias, the physician must remove the dressing or cast immediately. If this does not relieve the pain and paresthesias, the fascial compartment must be opened.

Axiom: *Any patient with a cast or compressive dressing of the upper extremity who complains of increasing pain, swelling, and paresthesias of the digits must have the dressing or cast removed immediately. If this offers no relief, a fasciotomy is indicated.*

If this complaint is not relieved, the full blown picture of Volkmann's ischemic contracture will develop. This syndrome involves three elements: forearm pronation and flexion of the wrist and digits, paralysis of the intrinsics, and diminution of the median and usually the ulnar nerve sensation. Surgery is needed to free the nerves and decompress the flexor compartment.

☐ Compartment Syndrome of the Hand

Isolated acute compartment syndrome of the hand is a relatively rare phenomenon. Acute compartment syndrome occurs when the tissue pressure within an

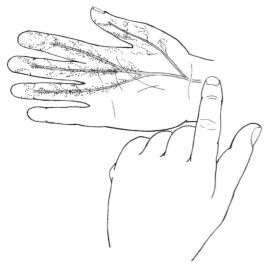

Figure 9–43. The Tinel test is performed by tapping the volar surface of the wrist over the median nerve.

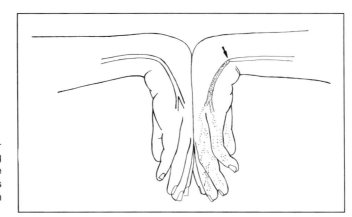

Figure 9-44. Phalen's test is performed by compressing the opposing dorsal surfaces of the hand with the wrist flexed together as shown. This causes tingling over the median nerve distribution.

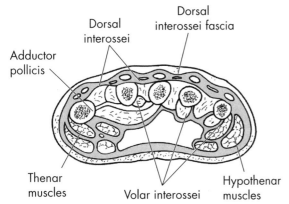

Figure 9-45. Cross section of the palm, through the metatarsal shafts, showing the compartment of the hand.

enclosed space is elevated to the extent that there is decreased blood flow within the space, decreasing tissue oxygenation. There are many compartments within the hand.[3,4] The volar and dorsal interossei are enclosed in fascia between the metacarpals. The thenar and hypothenar muscles are contained in separate compartments, as is the adductor pollicis muscle (Fig. 9-45). The blood supply of the interosseous muscles is variable. The blood supply originates in the superficial ulnar arch and the deep radial arch.

The clinical findings necessary to make this diagnosis are similar to those of other compartment syndromes in the body: pain which is increased upon passive or active stretch, and which increases beyond what is expected for the injury. The hallmark of muscle and nerve ischemia is persistent pain that is progressive and unrelieved by immobilization. Worsening of the pain by passive muscle stretching is the most reliable clinical test in making the diagnosis of compartment syndrome. The intrinsic compartments of the hand are tested by possibly abducting and adducting of the fingers while keeping the MCP joint in full extension and the PIP joint in flexion. The third most important finding is weakness. Nerve abnormalities are late occurrences.

The causes of compartment syndrome in the hand are numerous. They include major vascular injury, postoperative bleeding, embolectomy, cardiac catheterization, lying on a limb, fractures, contusions, exercise with overuse, and thermal injuries, among others. Compartment pressure measurements can be taken using a Stryker device or the technique described under compartment syndromes in the lower limb[22] (see Chapter 28).

☐ Ganglion

A ganglion is the most common tumor of the hand and consists of a synovial cyst from either a joint or the synovial lining of a tendon that has herniated (Fig. 9-46). It contains a jellylike fluid that may become completely sealed off within the cyst or be connected to the synovial cavity and fill or empty into it. The wrist is the region where most ganglia occur, the dorsal and radial aspects being the more common sites. They arise here from the radiocarpal joint or the extensor synovial bursae. The cyst is almost always distal to the extensor retinaculum. The flexor tendon sheaths of the fingers are often sites where ganglia may occur. The dorsal lateral surface of the digits is an alternate site where these tumors are seen.

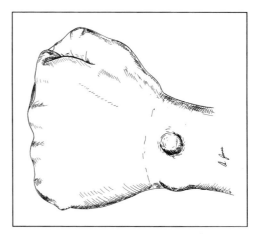

Figure 9-46. A dorsal ganglion is shown.

A specific traumatic event will be elicited from 15 percent of patients.[77] Often, only a history of chronic stress is solicited.[77] Patients complain of a dull ache or mild pain that is noted over the ganglion. Larger ganglia are less painful than smaller ones and the pain decreases after rupture.[77] Dorsal ganglia are more common than volar ganglia. Dorsal wrist ganglia make up about 60 to 70 percent of all soft tissue tumors of the wrists.[31] The occult dorsal ganglion, also arising from the dorsal scapholunate ligament, is less easily detected on clinical examination and may only be palpable with the wrist in extreme flexion. A history of trauma is often missing in patients with occult ganglia. These may form in response to chronic stress.[31] Occult dorsal wrist ganglia produce chronic wrist pain in some patients.

The onset is almost always insidious although some patients give a history of noting the "bump" over a period of a few days. A history of changing size is often obtained because of the filling and emptying into the parent synovial space. On examination one notes a firm, usually nontender, cystic lesion that feels like a bead underneath the skin. Diagnosis is usually easy due to the frequency with which these are seen. Aspiration will disclose a jelly-like material that confirms the diagnosis when doubt exists. One must be aware of a ganglionlike lesion called a *carpal boss* that is seen over the base of the metacarpals of the index and long fingers, as these osseous lesions can look like a ganglion and be confused with it. In fact, some carpal bosses are covered by a fluid-filled sac.

Treatment in the emergency center consists of aspiration with a large bore needle when the patient complains of symptoms. Initial treatment should include steroid injection of the dorsal capsule followed by immobilization.[31] The recurrence rate is very high with this method of treatment, and the patient must be informed of this. Reassurance is important in treating and informing the patient that this lesion is not malignant.

When conservative therapy fails, operative treatment is instituted.[31] For those patients who are symptomatic, surgical excision is also the treatment of choice. Excision of the dorsal ganglion with a portion of the capsule at the joint is the recommended treatment of choice.[77] In 94 percent of cases, a cure was achieved after operation.[20] In approximately 65 percent of cases, cure was achieved after injection with a corticosteroid and or rupture.[20] Patients can be advised of this alternative and referred.

□ INFECTIONS

Many things favor the development of infections, including retained foreign bodies, tight dressings around wounds, or congestive states following fractures. *Staphylococcus aureus* is isolated from 50 percent of all hand infections followed by beta-hemolytic streptococcus, which accounts for 15 percent. Other common organisms are *Aerobacter aerogenes*, *Enterococcus*, and *Escherichia coli*. *Eikenella corrodens* is an organism that is isolated from approximately one third of human bite wounds.[37] *Pasteurella multocida*, a facultative anaerobe, is present in the oral flora of approximately two thirds of domestic cat bites and one half of dog bites.[37] Infection with these organisms is usually rapid and associated with significant cellulitis and lymphangitis. Multiple organisms, however, are isolated from 70 percent of all hand infections. Rapid inflammation occurring within hours usually indicates that *Streptococcus* is the infecting organism in contrast with *Staphylococcus* which usually takes several days to develop an infection. The hallmarks of infection in the hand are heat, erythema, pain, and throbbing. Swelling and tenderness are other signs with fluctuation occurring late. Infections involving the tendons cause a limitation of motion and tenderness over the involved tendon.[2,48]

The mainstay of treatment of any hand infection includes splinting and elevation as well as appropriate antibiotics. Elevation of the hand can be easily accomplished by using stockinette. The stockinette is cut at both ends as shown in Figure 9–47. By making a cut at both ends, the hand can be elevated while the patient is walking, sitting, and so on. This is a cheap dressing and works far better than a sling for elevating the hand. Tetanus prophylaxis must be administered when any wound is noted in patients not already immunized. Splinting should be in a position permitting maximal drainage for all hand infections as shown in Figure 9–48. Because *S aureus* and *beta-hemolytic streptococcus* are isolated from up to 75 percent of hand infections (Table 9–1),[23] the antibiotic chosen must be effective against these organisms. Methicillin, erythromycin, and the cephalosporins are good choices in most hand infections.

□ Furuncle or Carbuncle

Furuncles or carbuncles of the hand are common and occur over the hair-bearing regions of the hand and arm. These infections are usually caused by *S aureus* and when seen early may be treated with rest, immobilization, elevation, and systemic antibiotics. Once the abscess is well localized, drainage occurs either spontaneously or through a small incision made over the point of maximal fluctuance with an 11 blade. Drainage is facilitated by applying warm compresses. If these infections are not treated adequately, they may lead to cellulitis of the hand.

□ Pyoderma

This is a benign type of hemangioma that may occur around a suture site or where there is a retained foreign body of the hand, usually under a moist dressing. The granuloma that forms may be up to 20 mm in diameter, but is usually about 3 to 5 mm. These are painful

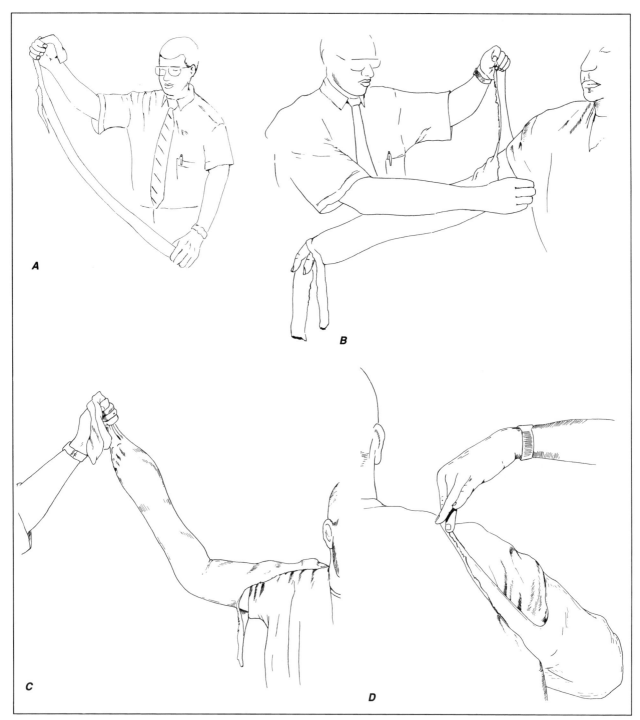

Figure 9–47. A dressing used for elevation of the hand is shown (**A**). The stockinette is applied along the entire upper extremity (**B**). The stockinette is cut at both ends to form a "Y" (**C** and **D**). The stockinette is fitted onto the upper extremity and the ends are then tied together as shown (**E**). The ends can be tied together to maintain elevation of hand or distal end can be tied to "lamp post" when patient is seated to maintain elevation at home. (*Cont.*)

tumors, and should be treated by exposure to air and keeping the area dry in cases of small lesions (3 mm). With larger pyodermas, the tumor should be excised flush with the surface of the skin and treated expectantly.

☐ Cellulitis

Cellulitis can occur after an abrasion, puncture, or with any wound of the hand that has been inadequately immobilized or neglected, and is commonly seen in

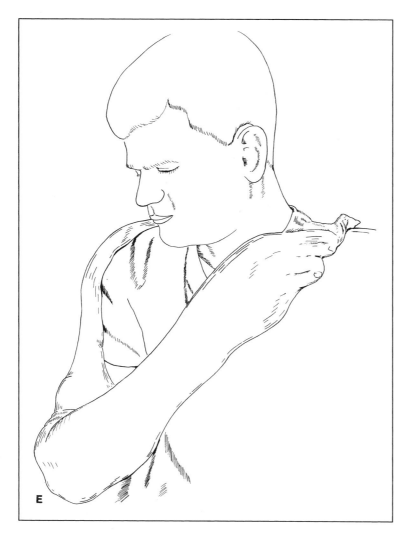

E

Figure 9–47. (*Cont.*) The stockinette is fitted onto the upper extremity and the ends are then tied together as shown (***E***). The ends can be tied together to maintain elevation of hand or distal end can be tied to "lamp post" when patient is seated to maintain elevation at home.

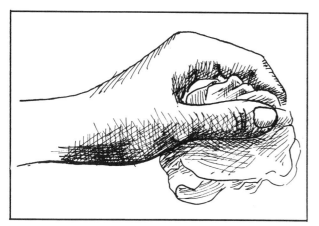

Figure 9–48. The optimal position of immobilizing the hand.

addicts. The cellulitis may develop rapidly or slowly depending on the offending agent.[64] The hand should be immobilized to control congestion, and the limb elevated. In cases where the cellulitis is progressing rapidly over a period of hours, fasciotomy must be considered because of the likelihood of a necrotizing hemolytic streptococcal infection. This type of cellulitis requires immediate decompression and debridement as well as large doses of antibiotics.[50] Patients with cellulitis of the hand of any degree that is compromising function should be admitted. All diabetics with this condition should be admitted.[48]

☐ Infections about the Nail
☐ *Paronychia and Eponychia*

A paronychia is an inflammatory involvement of the fold of the nail on the radial or ulnar side. Eponychia is involvement of the basal fold of the nail. These may be associated with cellulitis when the infection extends proximally into the tissues around the nail fold. The typical patient comes into the emergency department with an abscess well localized around the nail fold or at the base of the nail. Most of these are due to staphylococcal infection and are treated by incision and drainage as shown (Fig. 9–49). An 11 scalpel is used and the "incision" is carried out by holding the blade against the nail and entering the abscess through the nail fold to the pus.

TABLE 9–1. ANTIBIOTIC USE IN HAND INFECTIONS

Infection	Antibiotic	Most Likely Organism	Notes
Felon	1st-generation cephalosporin	S aureus	PO treatment usually adequate, consider herpetic whitlow
Flexor tenosynovitis	Ampicillin/Sublactum 3q IV q 6h	S aureus, streptococci, gram-negative bacteria	Consider disseminated gonorrhea, treat with ceftriaxone
Herpetic whitlow	None, unless secondary bacterial contamination	Herpes simplex 1 and 2	Consider acyclovir for prophylaxis against recurrence
Deep-space abscess	Nafcillin 2gm IVPB q6h and Gentamycin 1.5mg/Kg	S aureus, gram-negative bacteria, anaerobes	
Cellulitis/Lymphangitis	Inpatient: Nafcillin 2gm I.V. q 4h Outpatient: Dicloxacillin 500mg q6h	Streptococcus spp	Slow infusion, observe for "Red Man" syndrome
Hand infection in intravenous drug abuser	Vancomycin	Methicillin-resistant S aureus	
Human bite	Amoxicillin/Clavulanate 500mg p.o. tid	S aureus, Eikenella corrodens, anaerobes	This treatment is effective for dog or cat bites.
Animal bite	Same as for human bite	Pasteurella, gram-positive cocci, anaerobes	Clindamycin is an alternative in allergic patients.

From Hausman MR, Lisser SP: Hand infections. *Orthop Clin North Am* **1**:171–183, 1992, p 172.

The nail fold is simply uplifted off of the nail and drainage occurs. An incision is usually not necessary except for large abscesses. The patient should be advised to continue warm soaks. If cellulitis is present proximally, the patient is given systemic antibiotics.[65]

□ *Subungual Abscess and Subeponychial Abscess*

A subungual abscess floats the fingernail off its bed and is drained by removing only the base of the fingernail. The distal nail plate is not usually excised. A tiny loose pack of fine meshed gauze is inserted to separate the matrix from the eponychial fold for a few days. This should be done under digital or metacarpal block anesthesia. In

patients with a subeponychial abscess usually resulting from a splinter or puncture wound, the treatment is to excise a small notch directly over the abscess at the nail's distal end.[65] A foreign body should be looked for in these infections.

□ SPACE INFECTIONS

□ Felon

Felons are pulp space infections of the distal phalangeal area. Incision and drainage should be at the *point of maximum tenderness* in these infections. The best incision is the longitudinal midline incision directly over the abscess which spares the flexion creases (Fig. 9–50). This avoids injury to the vessels and the digital nerves. Many other incisions for this common problem have been advocated (fish-mouth, through-and-through, and lateral), all of which invoke necrosis and ischemia and lead to anesthesia of the tip of the digit as well as producing a more painful scar than the midline incision.

□ Web Space

Web space infections usually are caused by a puncture wound to the web space; an abscess usually points dorsally. Drainage is by a dorsal incision between the fingers, which should be longitudinal (at the thumb web it should be zigzag to avoid contracture). This infection often leads to stiffness at the MCP joint unless treated early with incision and drainage elevation and antibiotics.

□ Midpalmar Space

Infection here is secondary to extension of an infection from the adjacent flexor sheaths or to a puncture wound

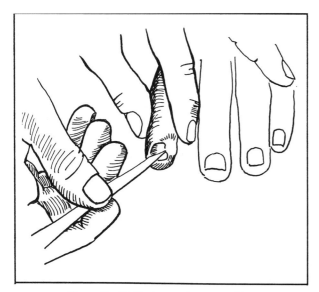

Figure 9–49. Drainage of a paronychia.

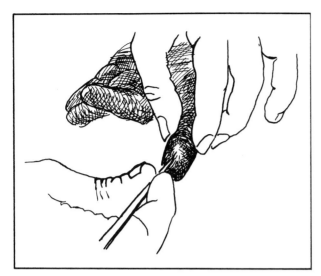

Figure 9–50. Drainage of a felon should be with an incision over the point of maximal fluctuance in a vertical direction.

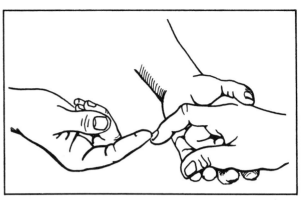

Figure 9–51. Testing for acute suppurative flexor tenosynovitis. Uplifting the nail of the involved digit without palpating the tendon causes exquisite pain.

of the palm of the hand. The palmar fascia is under great tension and maximal edema forms over the dorsum of the hand. However, the point of maximal tenderness is the midpalm. This abscess requires immediate drainage in the operating room.

☐ Dorsal Subaponeurotic Space and Subcutaneous Space

The dorsum of the hand is covered by loose, redundant skin permitting significant edema to accumulate from any of the infections occurring elsewhere in the hand. This dorsal edema must be differentiated from infections of the subcutaneous spaces and aponeurosis along the dorsum of the hand and the long extensor tendons, respectively. Infection is accompanied by tenderness which is not present with simple dorsal edema. These infections usually require drainage through multiple incisions and should be referred.

☐ Septic Tenosynovitis

The flexor and extensor tendon bursas may be infected by puncture wounds and lacerations, especially those occurring at the joint creases where the tendon and its surrounding sheath are in close proximity to the skin. *S aureus* and *Streptococcus* are the most common infecting agents. Because there is no obstruction to spread of the infection, usually the entire tendon sheath becomes involved.

The diagnosis can be made by stretching the involved synovial sac, which is best done by avoiding palpation over the tendon itself or actively or passively stretching the finger. The diagnosis can be made by extending the finger by lifting up on the nail alone, which produces exquisite pain along the course of the flexor tendon (Fig. 9–51). Kanavel (in Burkhalter's article[11])

describes four cardinal signs of acute flexor tenosynovitis that are usually present.

1. Excessive tenderness over the course of the tendon sheath, limited to the sheath
2. Symmetric enlargement of the whole finger
3. Excruciating pain on passively extending the finger, along the entire sheath
4. Flexed resting position of the finger

These patients should be admitted for splinting, elevation, and appropriate antibiotics. Cases that do not resolve promptly require surgical decompression.

☐ Human Bites

A human bite wound is a very serious injury,[44] especially when it occurs over poorly vascularized tissues such as the ligaments, joints, or tendons in the hand.[18] Although a variety of organisms are involved, the prime pathogen is anaerobic streptococcus.[27] *S aureus* is also common, however, and the cephalosporins are a good choice.[47] Wounds around the knuckles occurring from fist fights are self-sealing and when the anaerobe from a tooth inflicting the wound is sealed into the joint or around the capsule, a serious infection ensues that leads to stiffness and destruction of the joint. The same is true when a tooth-inflicted wound occurs in the proximity of a tendon sheath. These wounds should be treated with the utmost expediency and should never be closed, but debrided and irrigated thoroughly, immobilized, elevated, systemic antibiotics administered, and the patient hospitalized.

☐ Animal Bites

The most common organism in cat bites is *Pasteurella multocida*, which responds well to penicillin or erythromycin.[27,80] Up to 50 percent of infections are caused by this agent in dog bites, and 95 percent of the infections respond to penicillin.[12]

☐ Lymphangitis and Lymphadenitis

Lymphangitis can occur from any open wound and is diagnosed by the presence of a red streak on the dorsum of the hand extending proximally over the volar surface of the forearm. The onset is usually rapid, within hours, and is almost always streptococcal in origin. In more advanced cases, lymph nodes may be palpated near the elbow or at the axilla. The treatment involves rest, elevation, immobilization in a position of function, and antibiotics. The infection may be accompanied by edema and swelling over the dorsum of the hand.

REFERENCES

1. Adams KM, Thomson ST: Continuous passive motion use in hand therapy. *Sports Medicine* 12(1):109–127, 1996.
2. Allieu Y, et al: External fixation for treatment of hand infections. *J Bone Joint Surgery* 9(4):675–682, 1993.
3. Arrington ED, Miller MD: Skeletal muscle injuries. *Emerg Med Clinics of North America* 26:3, 1995.
4. Belsole RJ, Hess A: Concomitant skeletal muscle injuries. *Orthopedic Clinics of North America* 24:2, 1993.
5. Blair WF, Steyers CM: Extensor tendon injuries. *Orthop Clin North Am* 1:141, 1992.
6. Boles CA, et al: Imaging of orthopedic hardware hand and wrist. *Orthopedic Surgery* 33:2, 1995.
7. Bowers W, et al: Gamekeeper's thumb. *J bone Joint Surg* 59(4):519, 1977.
8. Brand PW, et al: Tendon and pulleys at the meacarpophalangeal joint of the finger. *J Bone Joint Surg* 57(6):779, 1975.
9. Browne EZ, Ribik CA: Early dynamic splinting for extensor tendon injuries. *J Hand Surg* 14A:72, 1989.
10. Burke ER: Ulnar neuropathy in bicyclists. *Phys Sports Med* (9)53, 1981.
11. Burkhalter WE: Deep space infections. *Hand Clin* (5)553, 1989.
12. Callahan MC: Treatment of common dog bites. *JACEP* 7(3):83, 1978.
13. Caputo AE, et al: Scaphoid nonunion in a child. A case report. *J Hand Surg* 20(2):243–245, 1995.
14. Carrol RE, Lakin JF: Fracture of the hook of the hamate: Acute treatment. *J Or Trauma* 34:6, 1993.
15. Carroll E: Ring injuries in the hand. *Clin Orthop* 104:175, 1974.
16. Chin, HW, Visotsky J: Ligamentous wrist injuries. *Hand EM* 11:3, 1993.
17. Chin, HW, Visotsky, J: Wrist fractures. *Hand EM* 11:3, 1993.
18. Chuinard RG, et al: Human bite infections of the hand. *J Bone Joint Surg* 59(3):416, 1977.
19. Corley FG Jr, Shenck RC Jr: Fracture of the hand. *Hand Surg* 23:3, 1996.
20. Crenshaw AH (ed): *Campbell's Operative Orthopedics*, 8th ed. St. Louis: Mosby, 1992.
21. David AM, Taiwo OA: Bartenders hand: An unusual form of occupational cumulative trauma disorder. *Alerts, Notices and Case Report* 164:4, 1996.
22. Dellaero DT, Levin S: Compartment syndrome of the hand. Etiology, diagnosis, and treatment. *Am J Orthope* 25(6):404–408, 1996.
23. Eaton RG, et al: Antibiotic guidelines for hand infections. *Surg Gynecol Obstet* 12:119, 1970.
24. Freiberg AM, Levine R: Nonoperative treatment of trigger fingers and thumbs. *J Hand Surg* 14A:553, 1989.
25. Gelberman RH, et al: High pressure injection injuries of the hand. *J Bone Joint Surg* 57(7):935, 1975.
26. Gilbert TJ, Cohen M: Imaging of acute injuries to the wrist and hand. *Imaging Orthop Trauma* 35:3, 1997.
27. Goldstein EJ, et al: Bacteriology of human and animal bite wounds. *J Clin Microbiol* 8(6):667, 1978.
28. Grossman JAI, Adams JP, Kunter J: Prophilactic antibiotics in simple hand laceration. *JAMA* 254:1055, 1981.
29. Gupta A, et al: Evaluating the injured hand. *Occup Dis Hand* 9(2):195–212, 1993.
30. Hainline B: Nerve injuries. *Sports Med* 78(2), 1994.
31. Halikis M, Taleisnik J: Soft tissue injuries of the wrist. *Clin Sports Med* 15:2, 1996.
32. Harris C Jr, et al: The functional anatomy of the extention mechanism of the finger. *J Bone Joint Surg* 54(4):713, 1972.
33. Hart RG, Kutz JE: Extensor tendon injuries of the hand. *Emerg Med Clin North Am* 11:3, 1993.
34. Hart RG, Kutz JE: Flexor tendon injuries of the hand. *Emerg Med Clin North Am* 11:3, 1993.
35. Harvey FJ, Harvey PM, Horsley MW: De Quervain's disease: Surgical or nonsurgical treatment. *J Hand Surg* 15A:83, 1990.
36. Haughey RE, Lammers RL, Wagner DK: Use of antibiotics in the initial management of soft tissue hand wounds. *Am Emer Med* 10:187, 1981.
37. Hausman MR, Lisser SP: Hand infections. *Orthop Clin North Am* 1:171, 1992.
38. Hayeems EB, Schemitsch EH: Volar trasscaphoid perlunate fracture dislocation. *Orthop Surg Toronto* 40:6, 1996.
39. Howse C: Wrist injuries in sports. *Sport Med* 17(3):163–175, 1975.
40. Herndon JH, et al: Management of painful neuromas of the hand. *J Bone Joint Surg* 58(3):369, 1976.
41. Hoffman DF, Schaffer TC: Management of common finger injuries. *Am Fam Phys* 5:1594, 1991.
42. Jebson JL, et al: Dislocation and fracture–dislocation of the carpometacarpal joints
. Orthopedic review. *Aspects Trauma Suppl.* 19–28 Rev, 1994.
43. Johnson SL: Therapy of the occupationally injured hand and upper extremity. *Hand Clin* 9:2, 1993.
44. Kilgore ES Jr, Graham WP III: *The Hand*. Philadelphia: Lea & Febiger, 1977.
45. Leibovic SJ, Geissler WB: Treatment of complex intraarticular distal radius fractures. *Orthop Clin North Am* 25:4, 1994.
46. Lindscheid RL, Dobyns JH: Treatment of scapholunate dissociation: Rotary subluxation of the scaphoid. *Hand Clin* 8:645, 1992.
47. Malinowski RWW, et al: The management of human bite injuries of the hand. *Emerg Med Clinics of North America* 19(9):655, 1979.
48. Mann RJ, et al: Hand infections in patients with diabetes mellitus. *Trauma* 17(5):376, 1977.

49. Mann RJ, et al: Human bites of the hand. *J Hand Surg* **2**(2):97, 1977.
50. McConnell CM, et al: Two-year review of hand infections at a municipal hospital. *Am Surg* **61**:643, 1979.
51. McCoy RL II, et al: Common injuries in the child or adolescent athlete. *Primary Care* **22**:1, 1995.
52. McCue FC, et al: Athletic injuries of the proximal joint requiring surgical treatment. *J Bone Surg* **52**:937, 1970.
53. McCue FC III, Meister K: Common sports hand injuries. *Sports Med* **15**(4):281–289, 1993.
54. McElfresh EC, et al: Management of fracture-dislocations of the proximal interphalangeal joints by extenstion-block splints. *J Bone Joint Surg* **54**(8):1705, 1972.
55. Meldon SW, Hargarten SW: Ligamentous injuries of the wrist. *J Emer Med* **13**(2):217–225, 1995.
56. Metz VM, Gilula LA: Imaging techniques for distal radius fractures and hand injuries. *Orthop Clin North Am* **24**:2, 1993.
57. Morgan RL, Linder MM: Common wrist injuries. *Am. Fam Phys* **55**:3, 1997.
58. Murray PM, Cooney WP: Golf-induced injuries of the wrist. *Clin Sports Med* **15**:1, 1996.
59. Nelson DL: Additional thoughts on the physical examination of the wrist. *Hand Clin* **13**:1, 1997.
60. Newport ML, Lane LB, St Chin SA: Treatment of trigger finger by steroid injection. *J Hand Surg* **15A**:748, 1990.
61. Overton DT, Uehara DT: Evaluation of the injured hand. *Emerg Med Clin North Am* **11**:3, 1993.
62. Pichora DR, McMurtry RY, Bell MJ: Gamekeeper's thumb: A prospective study of functional bracing. *Hand Surg* **14A**:567, 1989.
63. Proust AF: Special injuries of the hand. *Emerg Med Clin North Am* **11**:3, 1993.
64. Resnick D: Osteomyelitis and septic arthritis complicating hand injuries and infections. *J Can Assoc Radiol* **27**:21, 1976.
65. Rhode CM: Treatment of hand infections. *Am surg* **27**(2):85, 1961.
66. Russell RC, Williams DA, Sullivan JW, et al: Detection of foreign bodies in the hand. *J Hand Surg* **16A**:2, 1991.
67. Shrewburry M, et al: The faccia of the fistal phalanx. *J Bone Joint Surg* **57**(6):784, 1975.
68. Siegel S, et al: Magnetic resonance imaging of the musculoskeletal system. *Clin Orthop Rel Res* (332):281–300, 1996.
69. Sloan EP: Nerve injuries in the hand. *Emerg Med Clin North Am* **11**:3, 1993.
70. Smith R: Post-traumatic instability of the metacarpophalangeal joint of the thumb. *J Bone Joint Surg* **59**(1):14, 1977.
71. So YC, Chow SP, Pun WK, et al: Evaluation of results in flexor tendon repair: A critical analysis of five methods in ninety-five digits. *J Hand Surg* **15A**:258, 1990.
72. Spinner M: Anterior dislocations of the proximal intephalangeal joint. *J Bone Joint Surg* **52**(7):1329, 1970.
73. Steffanich RJ, Peimer CA: Longitudinal incision for trigger finger release. *J Hand Surg* **14A**:316, 1989.
74. Stein A, Lemos M, Stein S: Clinical evaluation of flexor tendon function in the small finger. *Am Emerg Med* **19**:991, 1990.
75. Steinbach, G. et al: Magnetic resonance imaging of muscle injuries. *Orthop Muscle Injuries* **17**:11, 1994.
76. Stern PJ: Tendinitis, overuse syndromes and tendon injuries. *Hand Clin* **3**:467, 1990.
77. Strickland LW, Rettig AC: *Hand Injuries in Athletes.* Philadelphia: WB Saunders, 1990.
78. Taras JS, et al: Complications of flexor tendon injuries. *Hand Clin* **10**:1, 1994.
79. Uriburn IJF, et al: Compression syndrome of the deep motor branch of the ulnar nerve. *J Bone Joint Surg* **58**(1):145, 1976.
80. Veitch J, Omer C: Treatment of cat bite injuries of the hand. *J Trauma* **19**(9):655, 1979.
81. Verdon ME: Overuse syndromes of the hand and wrist. *Orthop Primary Care* **23**:2, 1996.
82. Wang AW, Gupta A: Early motion after flexor tendon surgery. *Hand Clin* **12**:1, 1996.
83. Watson HK, Weinzweig J: The natural progression of scapoid instability. *Hand Clin* **13**:1, 1997.
84. Watson HK, Weinzweig J: Physical examination of the wrist. *Hand Clin* **13**(1):17–30, 1997.
85. Wells SA Jr: Hand injuries. *Curr Probl Surg* August 1993.
86. Witt J, Pess G, Gelberman RH: Treatment of De Quervain tenosynovitis. *J Bone Joint Surg* **73A**:219, 1991.
87. Wojtys EM, et al: Electrical stimulation of soft tissues. rehabilitation (chap. 44). Principles and Practice of Emergency Medicine. Mosby.
88. Yu JS: Magnetic resonance imaging of the wrist. *Orthopedics MRI* **17**:11, 1994.

BIBLIOGRAPHY

Andrew L, Eiken O: Arthrographic studies of wrist ganglions. *J Bone Joint Surg* **53**(2):300, 1971.
Chanfers GH, et al: Treatment of dog bite wounds. *Minn Med* **11**:427, 1969.
Kettlekamp DB, et al: Traumatic dislocations of the long-finger extension tendon. *J Bone Joint Surg* **53**(2):229, 1971.
Nelson CL, Sawmiller S: Ganglions of the wrist and hand. *J Bone Joint Surg* **54**:1671, 1972.

10
CHAPTER

FRACTURES OF THE RADIUS AND ULNA

PROXIMAL FOREARM FRACTURES

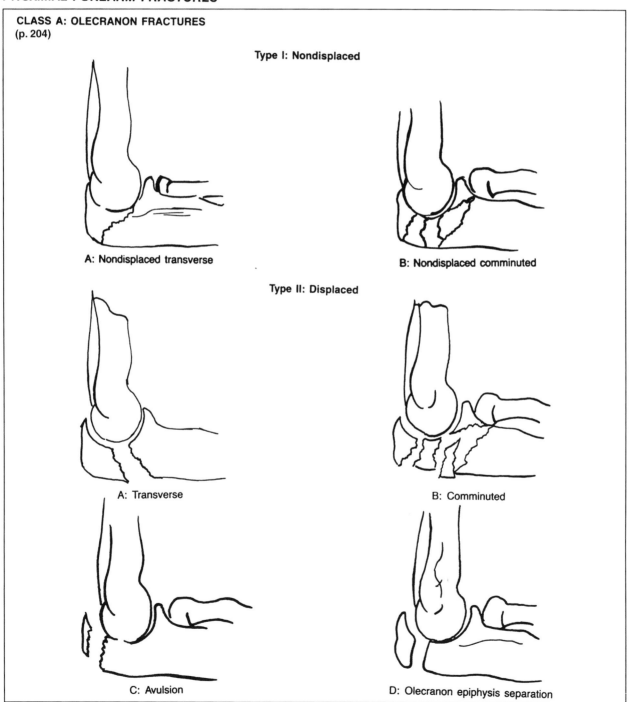

CLASS A: OLECRANON FRACTURES
(p. 204)

Type I: Nondisplaced

A: Nondisplaced transverse

B: Nondisplaced comminuted

Type II: Displaced

A: Transverse

B: Comminuted

C: Avulsion

D: Olecranon epiphysis separation

PROXIMAL FOREARM FRACTURES (cont.)

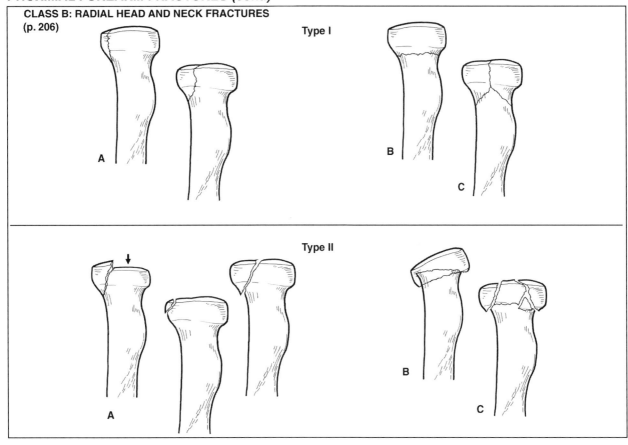

CLASS B: RADIAL HEAD AND NECK FRACTURES
(p. 206)

Type I

A

B

C

Type II

A

B

C

CLASS B: RADIAL HEAD AND NECK FRACTURES (EPIPHYSEAL FRACTURES IN CHILDREN) (p. 206)

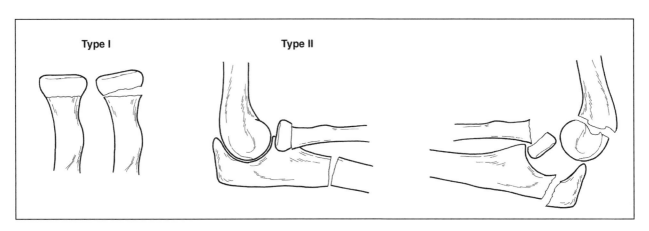

Type I   Type II

CLASS C: CORONOID PROCESS FRACTURES
(p. 212)

Type I

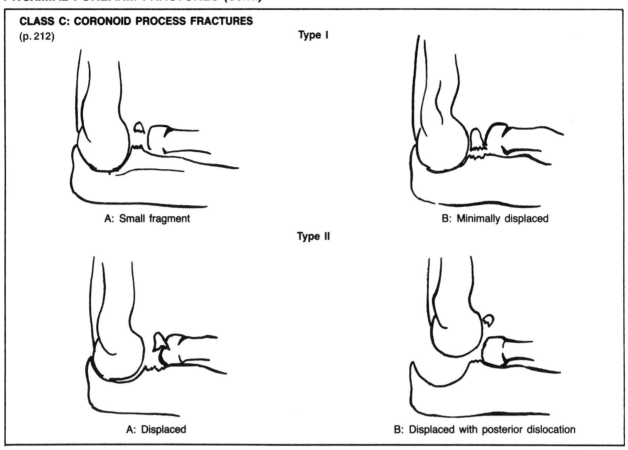

A: Small fragment

B: Minimally displaced

Type II

A: Displaced

B: Displaced with posterior dislocation

SHAFT FRACTURES

CLASS A: RADIAL FRACTURES
(p. 213)

Type I

Type II

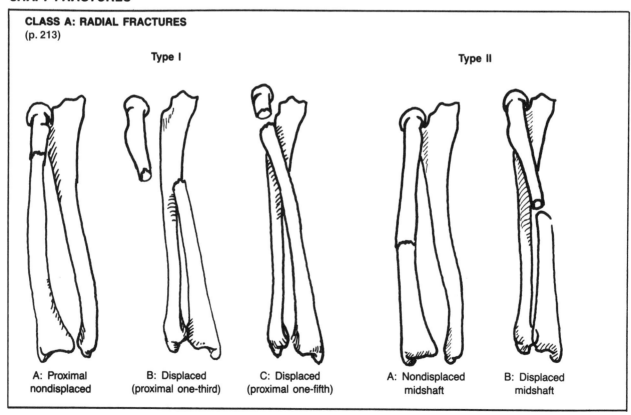

A: Proximal nondisplaced

B: Displaced (proximal one-third)

C: Displaced (proximal one-fifth)

A: Nondisplaced midshaft

B: Displaced midshaft

CLASS A: RADIAL FRACTURES (cont.)
(p. 213)

Type III

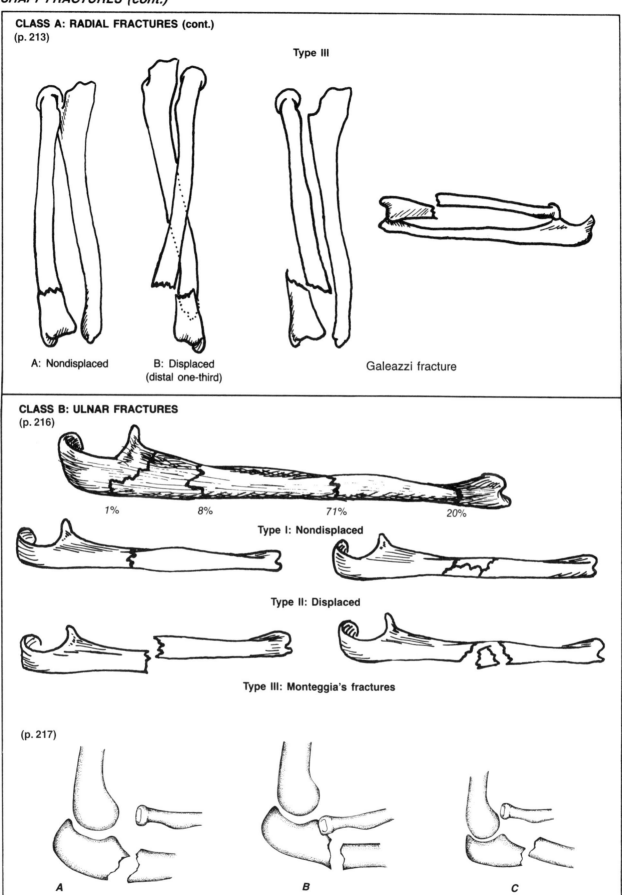

A: Nondisplaced

B: Displaced
(distal one-third)

Galeazzi fracture

CLASS B: ULNAR FRACTURES
(p. 216)

1%   8%   71%   20%

Type I: Nondisplaced

Type II: Displaced

Type III: Monteggia's fractures

(p. 217)

A   B   C

SHAFT FRACTURES (cont.)

CLASS C: COMBINED RADIAL AND ULNAR FRACTURES
(p. 219)

Type I

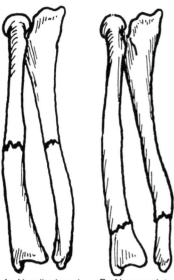

A: Nondisplaced   B: Nonangulated

Type II

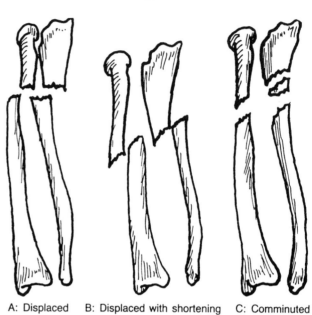

A: Displaced   B: Displaced with shortening   C: Comminuted

Type III

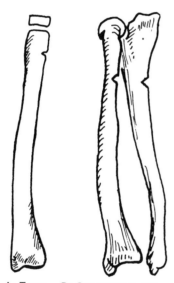

A: Torus   B: Greenstick (>15° angulation)

Type IV: Combined proximal one-third radius and ulna with anterior dislocation of the radial head

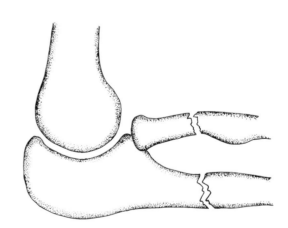

CLASS A: EXTENSION TYPE (COLLES' FRACTURE)
(p. 222)

Type I

A: Extra-articular radial fracture

B: Extra-articular radial and ulnar fracture

Type II

A: Distal radial fracture with radiocarpal joint involvement

B: Distal radial and ulnar fractures with radiocarpal joint involvement

Type III

A: Distal radial fracture with radioulnar joint involvement

B: Distal radial and ulnar fractures with radioulnar joint involvment

Type IV

A: Distal radial fracture with radiocarpal and radioulnar joint involvement

B: Distal radial and ulnar fractures with radiocarpal and radioulnar joint involvement

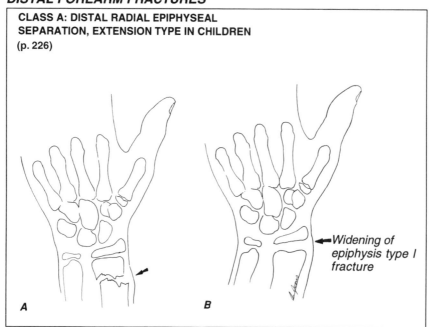

CLASS A: DISTAL RADIAL EPIPHYSEAL
SEPARATION, EXTENSION TYPE IN CHILDREN
(p. 226)

Widening of
epiphysis type I
fracture

A   B

DISTAL FOREARM FRACTURES

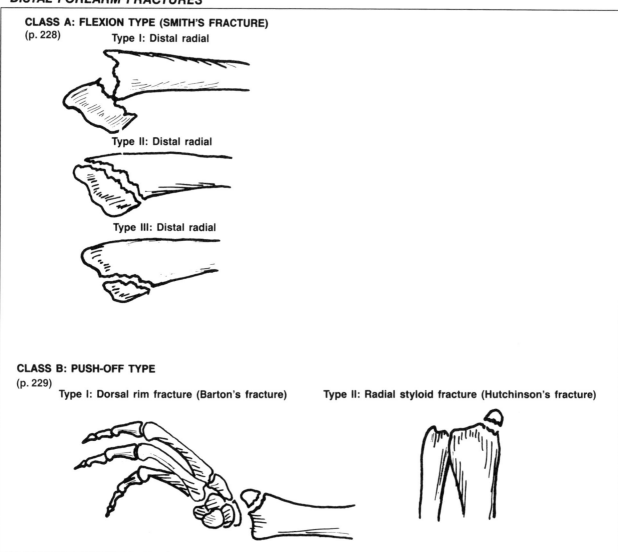

CLASS A: FLEXION TYPE (SMITH'S FRACTURE)
(p. 228)
Type I: Distal radial

Type II: Distal radial

Type III: Distal radial

CLASS B: PUSH-OFF TYPE
(p. 229)
Type I: Dorsal rim fracture (Barton's fracture)   Type II: Radial styloid fracture (Hutchinson's fracture)

Essential Anatomy

The radius and the ulna can be thought of conceptually as two cones lying next to each other but pointing in opposite directions as shown in Figure 10–1. The radius and the ulna lie parallel to each other and are invested at their proximal ends with a relatively large muscle mass. Because of their close proximity, injurious forces typically disrupt both bones and their ligamentous attachments.

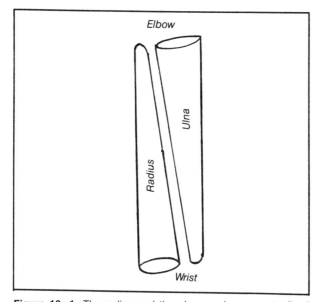

Figure 10–1. The radius and the ulna can be conceptualized as two cones that come together at the ends, thus permitting supination and pronation as the radius "rolls" around the ulna.

Axiom: *A fracture of one of the paired bones, especially when angulated or displaced, is usually accompanied by a fracture or dislocation of its "partner."*

The essential ligamentous attachments of the radius and the ulna are shown in Figure 10–2. These bones are bound together by joint capsules at the elbow and the wrist. Additionally, they are attached at their proximal ends by the anterior and posterior radioulnar ligaments. Distally, the radioulnar ligaments form a joint that contains a fibrocartilaginous articular disk. Throughout the midshaft of both bones is a strong interconnecting fibrous interosseous membrane.

Simply speaking the radius and the ulna are surrounded by four primary muscle groups whose pull frequently results in fracture displacement or nullification of an adequate reduction. As shown in Figures 10–3 and 10–4 these groups are:

1. *Proximal:* The biceps brachia and the supinator insert on the proximal radius and exert a supinating force.
2. *Shaft:* The pronator teres inserts on the radial shaft and exerts a pronating force.
3. *Distal:* Two groups of muscles insert on the distal radius.
   a. The pronator quadratus exerts a pronating force and displacement.
   b. The brachioradialis and abductor pollicis longus and brevis produce deforming forces as shown in Figure 10–4. Of these, the brachioradialis exerts the predominant displacing force.

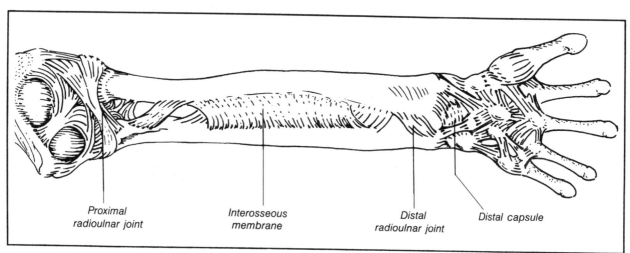

Figure 10–2. The radius and the ulna are joined together by the capsules at either end of the wrist and elbow joints. The interosseous membrane joins the two bones together throughout shafts.

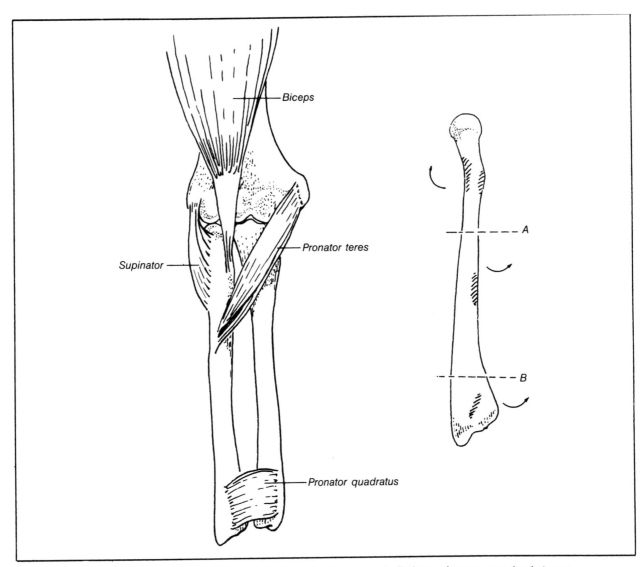

Figure 10–3. Note the important muscle attachments to the radius that serve to displace a fracture occurring between them. The arrows indicate the direction in which the radius will displace due to the muscular contraction when a fracture occurs at point A and at point B.

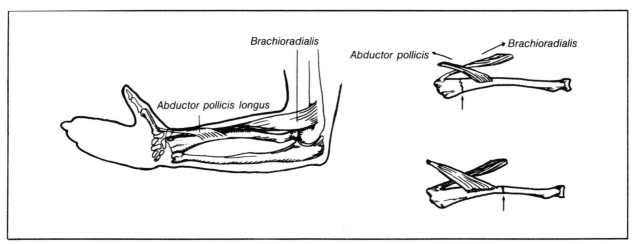

Figure 10–4. The brachioradialis and the abductor pollicis longus produce deforming forces that tend to displace fractures occurring in the distal radius. The brachioradialis exerts the predominant displacing force.

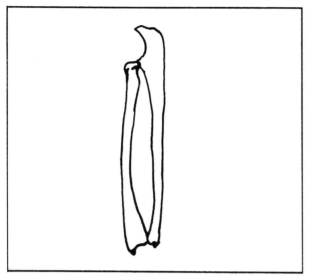

Figure 10–5. The lateral bow of the radius must be preserved to allow full pronation and supination to occur.

When considering treatment of these fractures, careful attention must be paid to the maintenance of length and alignment. Also, the *lateral bow* of the radius as shown in Figure 10–5 must be preserved to allow full pronation and supination after healing.

Classification of Radial and Ulnar Fractures

The classification system used is based on anatomic as well as therapeutic considerations.

PROXIMAL FOREARM FRACTURES

- ☐ Class A: Olecranon fractures (Fig. 10–6)
- ☐ Class B: Radial head and neck fractures (Figs. 10–7, 10–8)
- ☐ Class B: Radial head and neck fractures (epiphyseal fractures in children)
- ☐ Class C: Coronoid process fractures (Fig. 10–15)

SHAFT FRACTURES

- ☐ Class A: Radial fractures (Fig. 10–16)
- ☐ Class B: Ulnar fractures (Figs. 10–18, 10–19)
- ☐ Class C: Combined radial and ulnar fractures (Fig. 10–21)

DISTAL FOREARM FRACTURES

- ☐ Class A: Extension type (Colles' fractures) (Fig. 10–23, 10–28A)
  Distal radial epiphyseal separation, extension type in children (Fig. 10–28B)
  Flexion type (Smith's fracture) (Fig. 10–30)
- ☐ Class B: Type I push-off dorsal rim fracture (Barton's fracture) (Fig. 10–32)
  Type II push-off radial styloid fractures (Hutchinson's fracture) (Fig. 10–32)

PROXIMAL FOREARM FRACTURES

☐ CLASS A: OLECRANON FRACTURES (FIG. 10–6)

All fractures of the olecranon should be considered as intra articular and to have disrupted the integrity of the joint. Because of this, it is essential that near perfect anatomic reduction be achieved to ensure full range of motion.

Mechanism of Injury

Olecranon fractures are usually the result of one of two mechanisms. A fall or direct blow to the point of the el-

PROXIMAL FOREARM FRACTURES

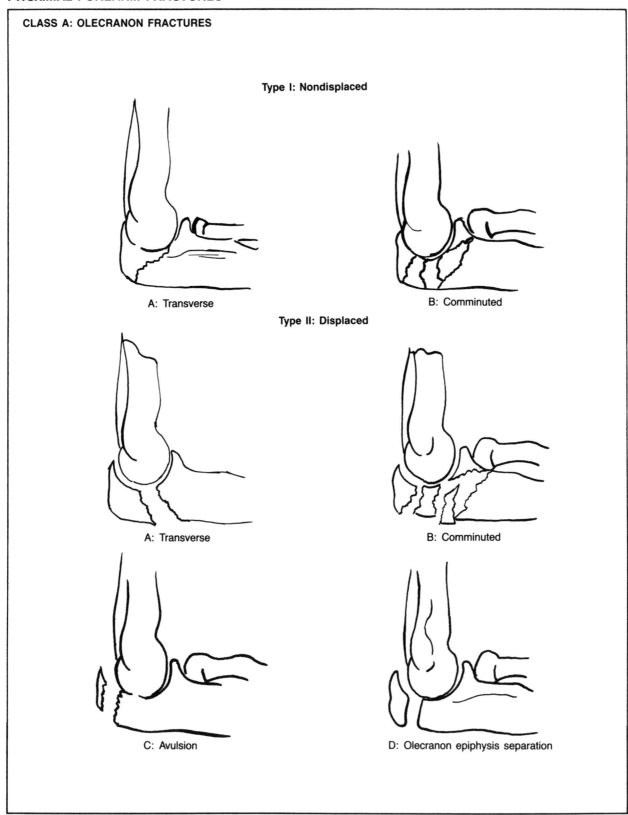

Figure 10–6.

bow may result in a comminuted fracture. The amount of triceps tone and the integrity of the triceps aponeurosis determines if the fracture will be type I or II. (Type I fractures have little or no displacement; type II are displaced.)

Indirectly, a fall on the outstretched hand with the elbow flexed and the triceps contracted may result in a transverse or oblique fracture (type IA or IIA). The amount of displacement is contingent on the tone of the triceps, the integrity of the triceps aponeurosis, and the integrity of the periosteum.

Axiom: *All type II olecranon fractures have either a rupture of the triceps aponeurosis or the periosteum.*

Examination
The patient will present with a painful swelling over the olecranon and a hemorrhagic effusion. The patient will be unable to actively extend the forearm against gravity or resistance due to the inadequacy of the triceps mechanism. It is of critical importance that the initial examination include documentation of *ulnar nerve* function. It is not uncommon for comminuted fractures to result in the compromise of ulnar nerve function.[24]

X Ray
Radiographically a lateral view with the elbow in 90 degrees of flexion is best for demonstrating olecranon fractures and displacement. Type I fractures are not displaced, and, therefore, the triceps aponeurosis and periosteum are intact. Absence of displacement on extension views is not considered definite proof of a type I injury. Separation of the fragments by more than 2 mm is indicative of a type II injury.

In children, the olecranon epiphysis ossifies at 10 years of age and fuses by the age of 16. Interpretation of fractures in children may be difficult and comparison views should be used whenever doubt exists. In addition, the presence of a posterior fat pad or a bulging anterior fat pad should be regarded as indicative of a fracture.

Associated Injuries
Frequently seen associated injuries include ulnar nerve injury, elbow dislocation or anterior dislocation of the radioulnar joint, or other fractures including radial head, shaft, and distal humeral.

Treatment
☐ Class A: Type IA (Nondisplaced Transverse)

  Type IB (Nondisplaced Comminuted)

Treatment begins with immobilizing in a long arm cast (see Appendix) with the elbow flexed at 50 to 90 degrees and the forearm in a neutral position. The cast should be well molded posteriorly and supported with a collar and cuff. Finger and shoulder range of motion exercises should be started as soon as possible with a repeat radiographic examination in 5 to 7 days to exclude displacement. Union is complete in 6 to 8 weeks but the cast may be removed as early as 1 week in adults for motions as tolerated.

An alternate program used in *stable fractures* is the initial application of a posterior long arm splint with the elbow in 90 degrees of flexion (see Appendix). Supination and pronation exercises can be initiated in 3 to 5 days with flexion extension exercises at 1 to 2 weeks. The protective splint is used until healing is complete (usually 6 weeks).

☐ Class A: Type IIA (Displaced Transverse)

  Type IIB (Displaced Comminuted)

  Type IIC (Displaced Avulsion)

  Type IID (Displaced Olecranon Epiphysis Separation)

Patients with these fractures require open reduction with internal fixation, and, therefore, emergent orthopedic referral is indicated. Initial emergency management includes splinting in 50 to 90 degrees of flexion with the application of ice, analgesics, and elevation.

Complications
The most common complication is the development of shoulder arthritis and inhibition of shoulder mobility. There is a small incidence (5 percent) of nonunion.[10]

☐ CLASS B: RADIAL HEAD AND NECK FRACTURES (FIGS. 10-7 AND 10-8)

Radial head and neck fractures are relatively common in adults. Smooth motion of the radial head is essential for full and painless pronation and supination. With fragmentation or displacement, arthritis with restricted motion may result. When selecting a therapeutic program the primary intention must focus on the restoration and retention of full motion. The classification system that follows is therapeutically oriented. In general, type I injuries are treated closed (at least initially) whereas in most cases type II injuries require open reduction. There is some controversy in the management of these fractures particularly in the postinjury mobilization phase. As before, the authors will make every effort to present both positions where legitimate controversy exists.

Mechanism of Injury
The most common mechanism is a fall on the outstretched hand (indirect). With the elbow in extension the force drives the radius against the capitellum resulting in a marginal or radial neck fracture. As the force-

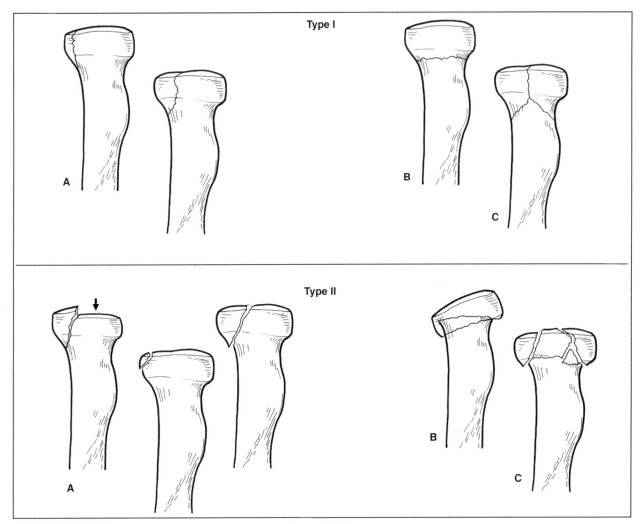

Figure 10-7.

PROXIMAL FOREARM FRACTURES

CLASS B: RADIAL HEAD AND NECK FRACTURES (EPIPHYSEAL FRACTURES IN CHILDREN)

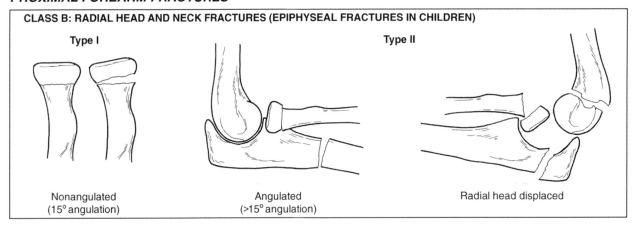

Type I		Type II
Nonangulated (15° angulation)	Angulated (>15° angulation)	Radial head displaced

Figure 10-8.

increases, comminution, dislocation, or displaced fragments may result. The fracture pattern in adults and children is variable due to differences in strength of the proximal radius. In adults, marginal or comminuted fractures of the radial head or neck with articular involvement are common. In children, displacement through the plate or neck of the radial epiphysis is common whereas articular involvement is rarely seen.

Similarities between adults and children do exist as in both groups a valgus strain often results in medial collateral ligament sprain or rupture. In addition, avulsion of the medial epicondyle or injury to the capitellum is often seen in both groups.

X Ray

Radial head and neck fractures often require oblique views for radiographic visualization. Impact fractures of the neck are best seen on the lateral projection. If a radial head fracture is suspected, but not seen, additional views in varying degrees of radial rotation should be obtained. In addition, the radiocapitellar line should be evaluated in attempting to diagnose occult fractures or radial head dislocations.

A line drawn through the midportion of the radius normally passes through the center of the capitellum (Fig. 10–9A) on the lateral view of the elbow. This is called the *radiocapitellar line*. In a subtle fracture at the epiphysis of the radial head in children (Fig. 10–9C), this line will be displaced away from the center of the capitellum. This may be the only finding suggesting a fracture in a child.

The presence of a bulging anterior fat pad or a posterior fat pad sign is indicative of significant joint capsule distension. (See Fig. 10–10.)

Axiom: *In a traumatized elbow where a fracture is not seen radiographically, the presence of a fat pad sign strongly suggests a radial head fracture.*

Examination

There will be tenderness over the radial head with swelling secondary to a hemarthrosis. Pain is exacerbated with supination and associated with reduced mobility. Children with epiphyseal injuries may have very little swelling, but pain will be elicited with palpation or motion. If the patient has associated wrist pain, disruption of the distal radioulnar joint should be suspected, and urgent orthopedic referral is recommended (Essex-Lopresti fracture).

Axiom: *Wirst pain associated with a fracture of the radial head suggests disruption of the distal radialulnar joint and the radioulnar interosseous membrane (Essex-Lopresti fracture–dislocation).*

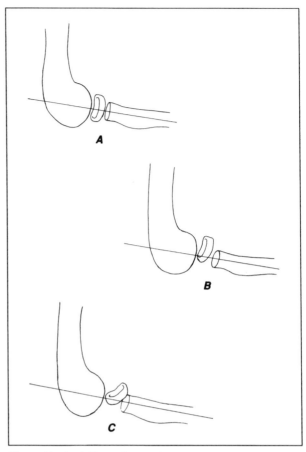

Figure 10–9. A. The radiocapitellar line drawn through the center of the radius should pass through the center of the capitellum of the humerus on the lateral view. **B.** In patients with a fracture of the radial neck in whom the epiphysis has not closed this is useful in making the diagnosis. **C.** This is true particularly when a subtle fracture exists as shown here.

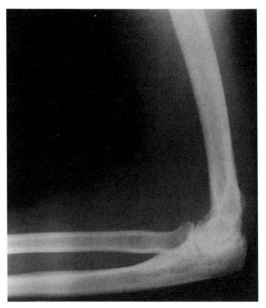

Figure 10–10. Anterior fat pad sign is shown.

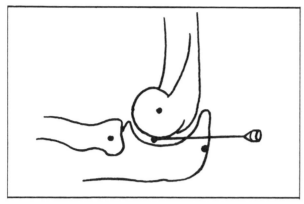

Figure 10–11. The safest place to aspirate the elbow is in the center of a triangle produced by connecting the lateral epicondyle of the humerus, the olecranon, and the radial head. Aspiration should be performed by inserting the needle through the center of this triangle under which is the anconeus muscle and then the joint cavity.

Associated injuries of the capitellum should be suspected in all proximal radial fractures.

Axiom: *In all radial head or neck fractures closely examine the capitellum for any evidence of fracture.*

Treatment

Early aspiration of the joint serves to reduce pain and facilitate early mobilization and is recommended by several authors.[12,20,21] The technique as shown in Figure 10–11 is as follows:

1. The skin of the lateral elbow should be prepped using sterile technique.
2. An imaginary triangle should be constructed over the lateral elbow connecting the *radial head*, the *lateral epicondyle*, and the *olecranon*. The joint capsule in this area is covered only by skin and the anconeus muscle, and there are no significant neurovascular structures in the area.
3. The skin should be anesthetized with lidocaine.
4. Using a 20-mL syringe and an 18-gauge needle the joint capsule should be penetrated by directing the needle medially and perpendicularly to the skin. When the capsule is entered, the blood is aspirated (usually 2 to 4 mL).

☐ Class B: Type IA   (Nondisplaced Marginal) (Fig. 10–12)

When dealing with radial head fractures in which less than one third of the articular surface is involved or with displacement of less than 1 mm (marginal fractures or minimal depression fractures), the treatment is a long arm posterior splint or cast (see Appendix). Early motion exercises as allowed for by pain are recommended.

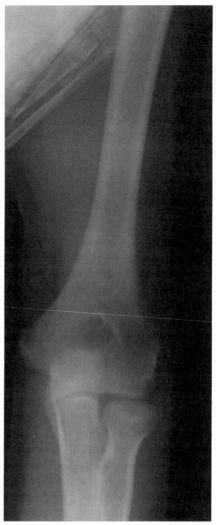

Figure 10–12. Nondisplaced marginal fracture of the radial head.

☐ Class B: Type IB   (Nonangulated Neck) Type IC   (Comminuted Head)

Neck fractures with angulation of less than 30 degrees are treated with immobilization in a long arm posterior splint and referral (see Appendix) and with urgent orthopedic referral. This therapy is controversial, and some surgeons would recommend surgical excision. An attempt should be made to reduce the angle in type IB fractures whereas type IC fractures can be treated conservatively.

☐ Class B: Type IIA   (Displaced)

Displaced fractures with less than one third of the articular surface involved should be reduced and followed by early motion (Fig. 10–13).

When there is displacement over 1 mm or depression of over 3 mm with over one third of the articular surface involved, excision is the recommended mode of therapy. Excision is, however, controversial, and the authors recommend that the initial emergency department

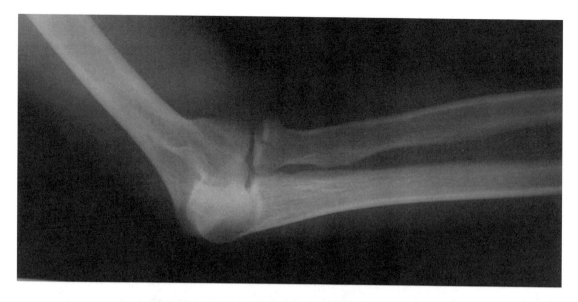

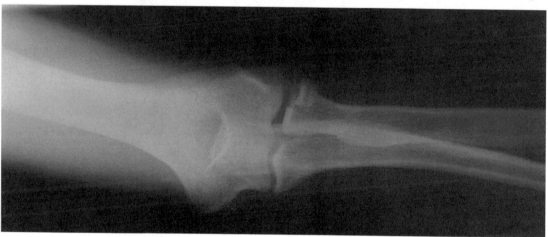

Figure 10–13. A displaced fracture of the radial head class B type IIA.

management include aspiration and a long arm posterior splint with the elbow in 90 degrees of flexion and the forearm neutral (see Appendix). Early referral is indicated for all of these fractures.

☐ Class B: Type IIB   (Displaced)
                  Type IIC   (Comminuted)
                        (Fig. 10–14A,B)

With angulation over 30 degrees or severe comminution of the head, early excision (within 5 days) is recommended.

☐ CLASS B: RADIAL HEAD AND NECK FRACTURES (EPIPHYSEAL FRACTURES IN CHILDREN)

☐ Class B: Type I   (Nonangulated)

Fractures with angulation of less than 15 degrees are best treated with immobilization for 2 weeks in a long arm posterior splint (see Appendix). This should be followed

by active exercises with a sling for support. Remodeling will generally correct this degree of angulation.

☐ Class B: Type II   (Angulated)

With angulation of over 15 degrees, the arm should be immobilized in a posterior splint, and the patient admitted for reduction under general anesthesia. Reduction attempts in children without good anesthesia are difficult to perform and fraught with complications.

Angulation of over 60 degrees is regarded as complete displacement and usually requires open reduction. Limited success has been achieved with manipulative reductions.

Complications

These fractures are frequently associated with debilitating complications.

1. Radial head or neck fractures accompanied by an elbow dislocation require early referral as bone fragments lying over the brachialis muscle may re-

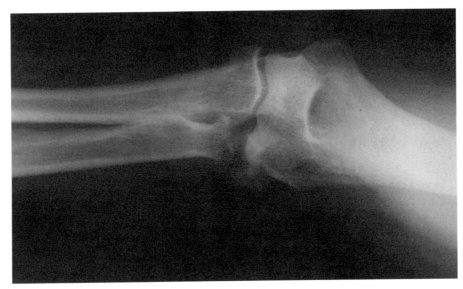

Figure 10–14A. Comminuted fractures of the radial head and neck. (*Cont.*)

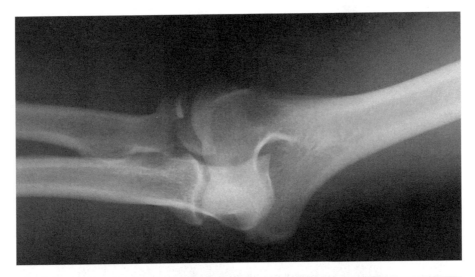

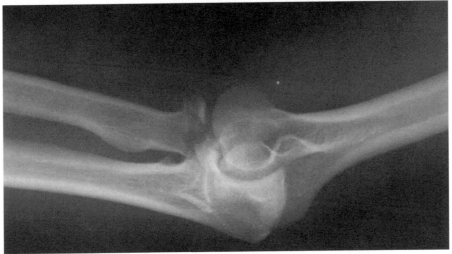

Figure 10–14B. (*Cont.*) Comminuted fractures of the radial head and neck.

sult in *myositis ossificans* with restricted painful motion.

2. Early motion should be limited strictly to only *slow active exercises*. Passive stretching or intense exercise are contraindicated because this often results in increased edema and more extensive adhesions with secondary joint stiffness.

3. Malunion can result from an inadequate reduction or inadequate immobilization and frequently results in restricted motion.

4. The valgus deforming force often leads to medial collateral ligamentous injury with subsequent recurrent dislocations.

5. Capitellum injuries are associated frequently with radial head fractures.

6. Pain and subluxation of the distal radioulnar joint can be seen in up to 50 percent of patients with radial head excisions.

7. In children, avulsion of the medial epicondyle secondary to the valgus stress is not an uncommon injury.

8. Nerve injuries are rare complications. The radial nerve is more often involved than are the ulnar or median nerves.

□ CLASS C: CORONOID PROCESS FRACTURE (FIG. 10–15)

These fractures are rarely seen as isolated injuries and are noted more commonly with posterior dislocations of the elbow.

PROXIMAL FOREARM FRACTURES

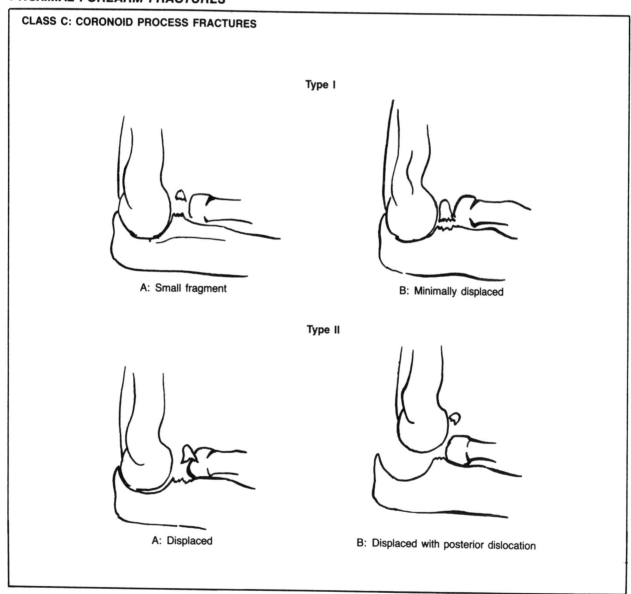

CLASS C: CORONOID PROCESS FRACTURES

Type I

A: Small fragment

B: Minimally displaced

Type II

A: Displaced

B: Displaced with posterior dislocation

Figure 10–15.

Mechanism of Injury

Isolated coronoid process fractures are thought to be due to hyperextension with joint capsular tension and subsequent avulsion. When coronoid fractures are associated with posterior dislocations the mechanism is a "push-off" injury by the distal humerus.

Examination

Tenderness and swelling over the antecubital fossa is noted frequently.

X Ray

The coronoid fragment is best visualized on a lateral radiograph although oblique views may be necessary. The fragment may be displaced as with an avulsion fracture or impacted against the trochlea as is frequently noted with dislocation fractures.

Treatment

This fracture is commonly associated with elbow dislocations and a more detailed discussion of treatment can be found in that section.

☐ Class C: Type IA   (Small Fragment)
            Type IB   (Minimally Displaced)

Isolated nondisplaced fractures are treated with a long arm posterior splint (see Appendix). The elbow should be in over 90 degrees of flexion and the forearm in supination. This should be followed by active exercises with sling support. The treatment of these fractures is controversial and early referral is strongly urged.

☐ Class C: Type IIA   (Displaced)

Displaced fractures require emergent orthopedic referral. Fragment fixation is recommended if the ulno-humeral joint is unstable. Some authors recommend stabilization using a distraction device.

☐ Class C: Type IIB   (Displaced with
                         Posterior Dislocation)

Fracture dislocations will be discussed under elbow dislocations.

Complications

Coronoid process fractures are only infrequently associated with the development of osteoarthritis.

SHAFT FRACTURES

Shaft fractures can occur anywhere along the length of the radius or ulna except in those areas encompassed by joint capsules or ligaments. These fractures are divided into three separate classes: class A and B fractures are single bone fractures whereas class C includes combined fractures. The Monteggia and Galeazzi fractures are classified under their respective single bone fractures.

☐ CLASS A: RADIAL FRACTURES
(FIG. 10–16)

Radial shaft fractures can be divided into three groups on the basis of muscular attachments and therefore fragment displacement after a fracture. The first group includes the proximal one third of the radial shaft just distal to the insertion of the supinator and the biceps

SHAFT FRACTURES

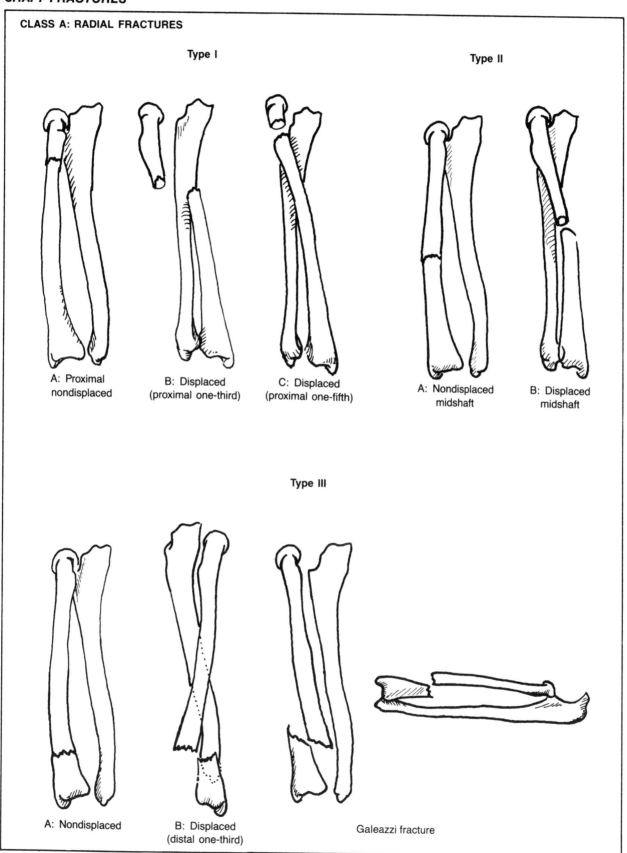

CLASS A: RADIAL FRACTURES

Type I

A: Proximal nondisplaced

B: Displaced (proximal one-third)

C: Displaced (proximal one-fifth)

Type II

A: Nondisplaced midshaft

B: Displaced midshaft

Type III

A: Nondisplaced

B: Displaced (distal one-third)

Galeazzi fracture

Figure 10–16.

brachia. Both of these muscles exert a supinating force or displacement on the proximal radius. The second group includes the middle one third of the radial shaft where the pronator teres exerts a pronating force. The third group includes the distal one third of the radius. In this area the pronator quadratus both inserts and exerts a pronating force on the fracture fragment.

Radial shaft fractures are most commonly seen at the junction of the middle and distal one third. It is at this point that the bone is enshrouded with a minimum of muscle mass and therefore exposed to a greater amount of direct trauma.

Mechanism of Injury
The most common mechanism is a direct blow to the radial shaft.

Examination
There is tenderness along the fracture site that can be elicited with direct palpation or longitudinal compression. Tenderness over the distal radioulnar joint may be secondary to subluxation or dislocation.

X Ray
Routine anteroposterior (AP) and lateral views are usually adequate. Radial shaft fractures are associated frequently with serious but often occult elbow and wrist injuries.

Axiom: *Distal radial shaft fractures are commonly associated with distal radioulnar dislocations.*

There are four reliable radiographic signs of rupture of the distal radioulnar joint capsule:

1. Fracture of the base of the ulnar styloid
2. On the AP view widening of the distal radial ulnar joint space
3. On lateral view dislocation of the distal radius relative to the ulna
4. Shortening of the radius by more than 5 mm[18]

Associated Injuries
A distal shaft fracture associated with a distal radioulnar dislocation is commonly referred to as a *Galeazzi fracture*. High-energy impact injuries or those with extensive soft tissue injuries may be associated with an acute compartment syndrome.[3]

Treatment
☐ Class A: Type IA (Proximal Nondisplaced)
These fractures are rare and require urgent orthopedic referral. Emergency department management should include the application of a long arm cast or anterior posterior splints (see Appendix). The elbow should be in 90 degrees of flexion with the forearm in supination. Follow-up radiographs to detect displacement are essential.

☐ Class A: Type IB (Displaced Proximal One Third)
Emergent referral is indicated as the treatment of choice is open reduction and internal fixation. Emergency management should include immobilization in a long arm posterior splint (see Appendix) with the forearm in supination and the elbow in 90 degrees of flexion.

☐ Class A: Type IC (Displaced Proximal One Fifth)
Consultation is indicated as the treatment of these fractures is controversial. Because of the small size of the proximal fragment, internal fixation is difficult. Most patients are treated with a manipulative reduction and immobilization in a long arm cast or anteroposterior splints (see Appendix). The elbow should be in 90 degrees of flexion and the forearm in supination.

☐ Class A: Type IIA (Nondisplaced Midshaft)
Referral is indicated after immobilization in a long arm cast or anterior posterior splints (see Appendix). The elbow should be in 90 degrees of flexion and the forearm in moderate supination. Follow-up radiographs are strongly encouraged.

☐ Class A: Type IIB (Displaced Midshaft)
Emergent referral is indicated as the treatment of choice is open reduction and internal fixation. Initially, immobilize with 90 degrees of elbow flexion and moderate forearm supination.

☐ Class A: Type IIIA (Nondisplaced)
This fracture may be associated with subluxation of the distal radioulnar joint. Referral is indicated after immobilization in a long arm cast or anterior posterior splints (see Appendix). The elbow should be in 90 degrees of flexion and the forearm in pronation.

☐ Class A: Type IIIB (Displaced Distal One Third and Galeazzi Fracture) (Fig. 10–17)
These fractures are commonly seen and require emergent referral as open reduction with internal fixation is the treatment of choice. The fracture line is typically transverse or oblique, noncomminuted, with angulation of the distal radial segment dorsally. Galeazzi fractures

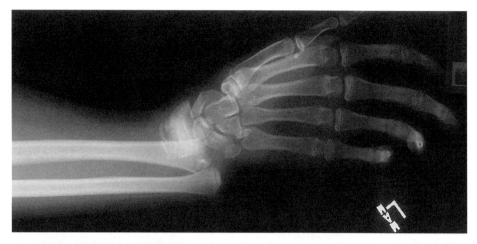

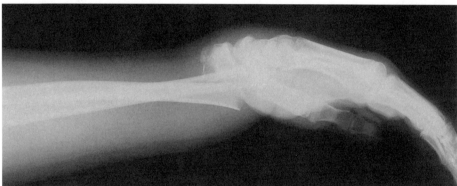

Figure 10–17. Fractured distal radius—severe displacement.

are fractures of the distal one third of the radius associated with instability of the distal radioulnar joint. Galeazzi fractures should be suspected if distal radial ulnar joint tenderness or ulnar head prominence are present.[1]

Axiom: *Galeazzi fractures are commonly associated with distal radioulnar subluxations (acute or delayed).*

Complications
Radial shaft fractures are often associated with several complicating factors.

1. Nondisplaced fractures may undergo delayed separation due to muscular traction despite immobilization. Follow-up radiographs to ensure proper positioning are essential.
2. Malunion or nonunion may be secondary to inadequate reduction or immobilization.
3. Rotational deformities must be detected and treated early in managing of these fractures.
4. Distal radioulnar joint subluxation or dislocation is associated frequently with radial shaft fractures.

5. Neurovascular injuries are uncommonly seen with radial shaft fractures.

☐ CLASS B: ULNAR FRACTURES (FIG. 10–18)

Ulnar shaft fractures can be classified into three groups. Type I fractures are nondisplaced whereas type II fractures are displaced (5 mm or greater). Type III shaft fractures are displaced fractures of the proximal one third that are associated with radial head subluxation or dislocation. Type III fractures are also known as *Monteggia's fractures* and will be discussed separately at the end of this section.

Mechanism of Injury
There are two mechanisms that frequently result in fractures of the ulna. A direct blow is the most common mechanism and the resulting fracture is often referred to as a "nightstick fracture." This mechanism involves a direct blow to the forearm that has been elevated to a defensive position of protecting the face. This mechanism and subsequent fracture is seen commonly after automobile accidents or fights.

Excessive pronation or supination can also result in ulnar shaft fractures.

SHAFT FRACTURES

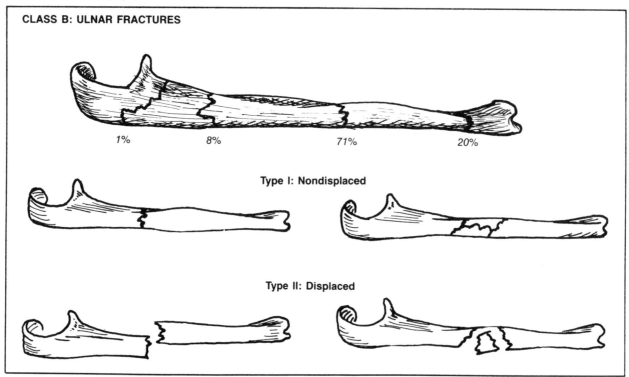

CLASS B: ULNAR FRACTURES

1%   8%   71%   20%

Type I: Nondisplaced

Type II: Displaced

Figure 10–18.

Examination
There is swelling and tenderness to palpation over the fracture site. Percussion of the ulna will elicit pain localized to the fracture site.

X Ray
AP and lateral views will generally demonstrate the fracture. If there is significant displacement elbow and wrist views should be included to exclude articular damage or subluxation.

Associated Injuries
A fracture of the distal two thirds of the ulnar shaft is rarely accompanied by associated injuries. Infrequently, paralysis of the deep branch of the radial nerve can occur; however, function usually returns without treatment. High-energy impact injuries or those with extensive soft tissue injuries may be associated with an acute compartment syndrome.

Treatment
☐ Class B: Type I (Nondisplaced)
The recommended therapy is not without controversy. Traditionally, immobilization in a long arm cast with the elbow in 90 degrees of flexion and the forearm neutral (see Appendix) was recommended. Cast sup-

port of proximal one-third fractures is limited owing to the large amount of soft tissue surrounding the bone in this region. Because of this lack of support, open reduction and internal fixation is recommended for proximal one-third fractures of the ulna. Emergent orthopedic referral for these fractures is recommended.[27]

The remaining nondisplaced distal two-third fractures of the ulna can typically be treated emergently with a long arm splint.

Some authors have recommended that after 1 week the splint or cast be replaced by a prefabricated functional brace. The prefabricated functional brace allows for an earlier return to work and better wrist mobility when compared to the use of a long arm cast.[13]

☐ Class B: Type II (Displaced)
Referral after immobilization is indicated as most orthopedic surgeons prefer open reduction with internal fixation in the management of these fractures.

Axiom: *Displaced ulnar fractures are associated frequently with radial fractures or dislocations of the radial head.*

□ CLASS B: ULNAR FRACTURES, TYPE III (MONTEGGIA'S FRACTURES) (FIGS. 10–19, 10–20)

Monteggia's fractures are of the proximal one third of the ulnar shaft combined with a radial head dislocation. Radial head dislocations can only occur if there is complete rupture of the annular ligament. Monteggia's fractures are classified into four types.

□ Class B: Type IIIA
This group includes fractures of the ulnar shaft (usually the proximal one third) combined with an anterior dislocation of the radial head. There is usually anterior angulation of the distal fragment. *Sixty percent of Monteggia's fractures are type A.*

□ Class B: Type IIIB
Ulnar shaft fractures with posterior or posterior lateral dislocation of the radial head are responsible for *15 percent of Monteggia's fractures.*

□ Class B: Type IIIC
Ulnar metaphyseal fractures with lateral or anterolateral dislocation of the radial head are responsible for *20 percent of Monteggia's fractures.*

□ Class B: Type IIID
This is the most rare (5 percent) of the Monteggia's fractures. It is characterized by a fracture of both the ulna and radius at the proximal one third of the forearm and the anterior dislocation of the radial head.[19]

Mechanism of Injury
□ Class B: Type IIIA
A direct blow to the posterior lateral ulnar may result in a fracture. Forceful pronation with external rotation as during a fall may also result in a fracture.

□ Class B: Type IIIB
The mechanism is similar to that encountered with a posterior dislocation of the elbow. In this case, however, the ulnar–humeral ligaments are stronger than the bone resulting in fracture with radial head dislocation.

□ Class B: Type IIIC
This is a common childhood fracture resulting from a direct blow to the inner elbow.

□ Class B: Type IIID
The mechanism of injury here is similar to that for a type IIIA fracture.

SHAFT FRACTURES

CLASS B: ULNAR FRACTURES

Type III: Monteggia's fractures

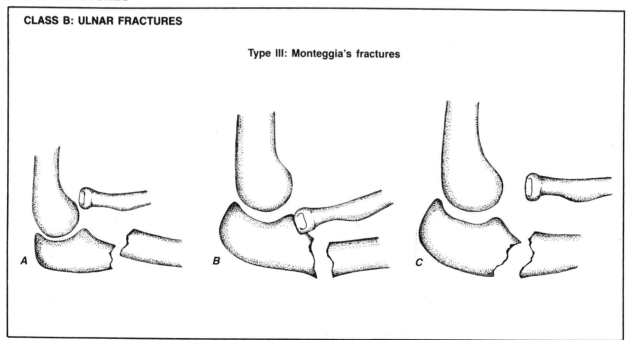

Figure 10–19.

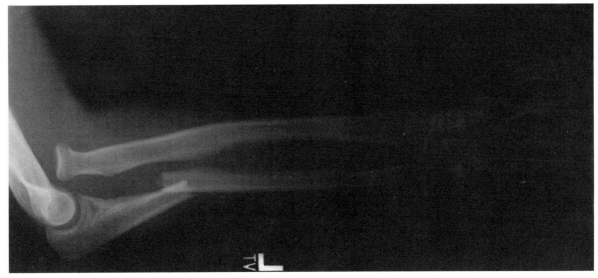

Figure 10–20. Monteggia's fracture. (*Courtesy of Scott Bingham—Cook County Hospital.*)

Examination

Type A fractures reveal shortening of the forearm due to angulation along with a palpable radial head in the antecubital fossa secondary to the anterior dislocation. Types B and C may also be associated with forearm shortening. Pain and tenderness will occur in all type III fractures over the upper ulna. Pain is exacerbated with flexion, extension, pronation, and supination. This is in contradistinction to type I and II fractures where moderate pronation and supination are only mildly painful.

X Ray

AP and lateral views usually demonstrate the fracture. Elbow and wrist views must be included to exclude articular damage or subluxation.

Associated Injury

Paralysis of the deep branch of the radial nerve is frequent. It is usually secondary to a contusion and function returns without treatment.

Treatment

In children, emergency management includes immobilization in a posterior long arm splint (see Appendix) and emergent referral. Closed reduction of the ulnar fracture is then typically carried out under general anesthesia followed by relocation of the radial head by direct pressure during supination of the forearm. Interposition of the annular ligament may impede radial reduction necessitating a surgical repair.[2]

In adults, the extremity should be immobilized in a long arm posterior splint and the patient referred for emergent evaluation (see Appendix). Most orthopedic surgeons prefer surgical correction.[4]

Complications

Monteggia's fractures require emergent referral because of a high incidence of complications.

1. Paralysis of the deep branch of the radial nerve is usually secondary to a contusion and typically heals without treatment.
2. Nonunion may be due to an inadequate reduction or may be secondary to inadequate immobilization.
3. Recurrent dislocation or subluxation of the radial head is a common sequela after closed reductions secondary to the unrepaired tear in the annular ligament.

☐ CLASS C: COMBINED RADIAL AND ULNAR FRACTURES (FIG. 10–21)

These fractures are most commonly seen in children. Only two fractures will be discussed, *torus* and *greenstick*, as the remainder of these fractures require emergent referral for reduction under general anesthesia.

Mechanism of Injury

There are two mechanisms that result in fractures of the forearm shaft. A direct blow as during a vehicular accident is the most common mechanism encountered. Indirectly, falls exerting longitudinal compression forces may result in combined shaft fractures.

Examination

Pain, swelling, and loss of function of the hand and forearm are usually encountered. Deficits of the radial, median, and ulnar nerves are uncommonly seen, but must be excluded by careful physical examination and documentation.

SHAFT FRACTURES

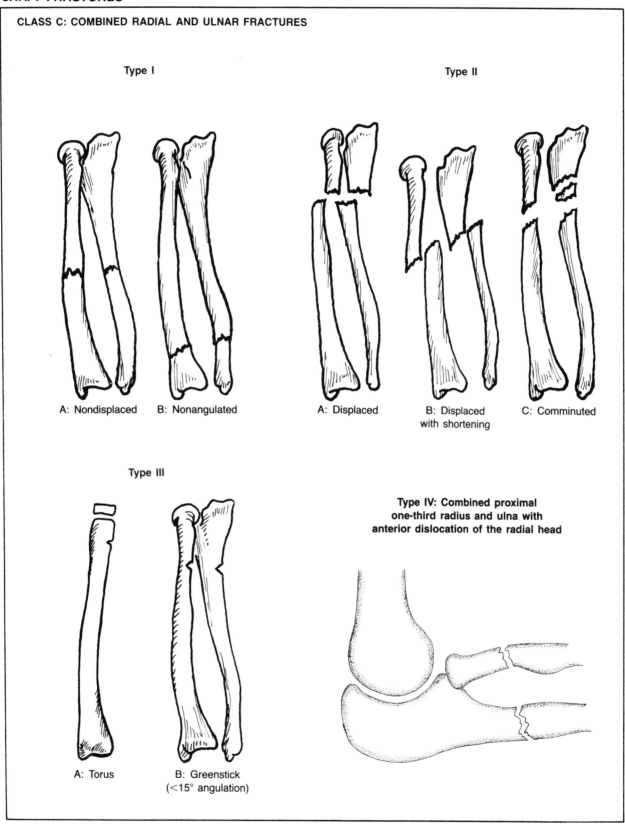

CLASS C: COMBINED RADIAL AND ULNAR FRACTURES

Type I

A: Nondisplaced   B: Nonangulated

Type II

A: Displaced   B: Displaced with shortening   C: Comminuted

Type III

A: Torus   B: Greenstick (<15° angulation)

Type IV: Combined proximal one-third radius and ulna with anterior dislocation of the radial head

Figure 10–21.

X Ray

AP and lateral views are adequate for defining the fracture fragments. Wrist and elbow views should also be obtained and evaluated for articular damage, dislocation, or subluxation.

Associated Injury

Neurovascular involvement is uncommon in closed injuries to the forearm. Documentation of function, however, must be considered an essential part of the physical examination of all forearm fractures. High-energy impact injuries or those with extensive soft tissue injuries may be associated with an acute compartment syndrome.

Treatment

☐ Class C: Type IA   (Nondisplaced)
                   Type IB   (Nonangulated)

This is an uncommon injury treated with a well-molded long arm cast or anteroposterior splints, with the elbow in 90 degrees of flexion and the forearm neutral (see Appendix). *Caution:* Repeated x ray examinations are required as delayed displacement is seen frequently. Urgent orthopedic follow-up is indicated in all cases.

☐ Class C: Type IIA   (Displaced)
                   Type IIB   (Displaced with
                                   Shortening)
                   Type IIC   (Comminuted)

Emergency department management includes immobilization and emergent referral for surgical reduction. Closed reductions are generally inadequate in achieving and maintaining proper alignment and rotational corrections (Fig. 10–22).

☐ Class C: Type IIIA   (Torus)
                   Type IIIB   (Greenstick)

Torus fractures are treated with immobilization in a long arm cast for 4 to 6 weeks (see Appendix). Greenstick fractures with less than 15 degrees of angulation may be treated with immobilization in a long arm cast for 4 to 6 weeks. With angulation of greater than 15 degrees, orthopedic referral for completion of the fracture with reduction is indicated.

☐ Class C: Type IV   (Combined Proximal
                                   One Third Fractures
                                   with Anterior
                                   Dislocation of the
                                   Radial Head)

These fractures require open reduction and internal fixation.

Axiom: *Combined shaft fractures of the proximal one third of the radius and the ulna are commonly associated with an anterior dislocation of the radial head.*

Complications

Combined shaft fractures of the radius and the ulna are associated with numerous complications.

1. Infection is commonly seen with open fractures but may also be associated with closed injuries.
2. Nerve damage is uncommon in closed injuries but is frequently seen with open fractures. There is an equal frequency of involvement between the radial, ulnar, and median nerves.
3. Vascular injuries are an uncommon complication because of the presence of arterial collaterals.
4. Nonunion or malunion may be secondary to inadequate reduction or inadequate immobilization.
5. Compartment syndromes including both anterior and posterior can be associated with combined shaft fractures. It is important to recognize that distal pulses may remain intact despite elevated compartment pressures and compromised capillary flow.

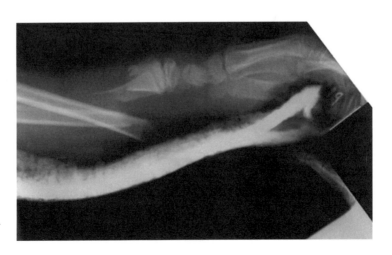

Figure 10–22. Displaced open fracture of the distal radius and ulna.

CLASS A: EXTENSION TYPE (COLLES' FRACTURE)

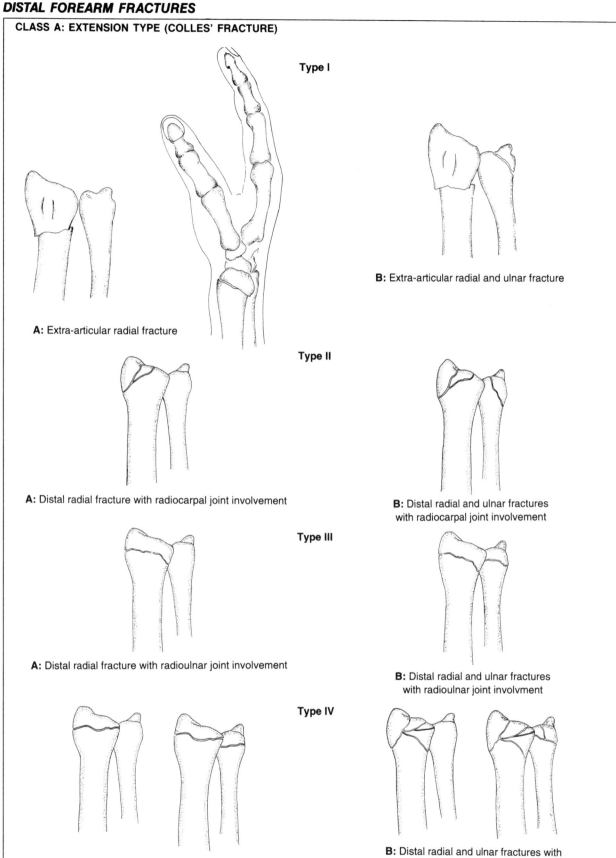

Type I

A: Extra-articular radial fracture

B: Extra-articular radial and ulnar fracture

Type II

A: Distal radial fracture with radiocarpal joint involvement

B: Distal radial and ulnar fractures with radiocarpal joint involvement

Type III

A: Distal radial fracture with radioulnar joint involvement

B: Distal radial and ulnar fractures with radioulnar joint involvment

Type IV

A: Distal radial fracture with radiocarpal and radioulnar joint involvement

B: Distal radial and ulnar fractures with radiocarpal and radioulnar joint involvement

Figure 10-23.

The diagnosis is strongly suggested on the basis of three points:

a. diminished sensation in the fingers,
b. decreased function of the forearm muscles,
c. deep boring forearm pain. The treatment is emergent referral for *fasciotomy*.

6. Synostosis of the radius and the ulna may complicate the management of combined shaft fractures.
7. Pronation and supination may be impaired if fractures are poorly managed.

DISTAL FOREARM FRACTURES

☐ CLASS A: EXTENSION TYPE (COLLES' FRACTURES) (FIG. 10–23)

Distal forearm fractures can be classified into three main groups: extension fractures (Colles'), flexion fractures (Smith's), and push-off fractures (Hutchinson's and Barton's). There are many classification systems used for extension fractures of the distal radius. The most practical in the authors' opinion is the Frykman system.[11] Under this system, extension fractures of the distal radius are classified in the following manner:

- **Type IA:**   Extra-articular radial fracture
- **Type IB:**   Extra-articular radial and ulnar fracture
- **Type IIA:**   Distal radial fracture with radiocarpal joint involvement
- **Type IIB:**   Distal radial and ulnar fractures with radiocarpal joint involvement
- **Type IIIA:**   Distal radial fracture with radioulnar joint involvement
- **Type IIIB:**   Distal radial and ulnar fractures with radioulnar joint involvement
- **Type IVA:**   Distal radial fracture with radiocarpal and radioulnar joint involvement
- **Type IVB:**   Distal radial and ulnar fractures with radiocarpal and radioulnar joint involvement

Approximately 60 percent of distal radius extension fractures are associated with ulnar styloid fractures (type B), and 60 percent of ulnar styloid fractures are associated with fractures of the ulnar neck.

Essential Anatomy
The normal radiocarpal joint is angled from 1 to 23 degrees in a palmar (ventral) direction as shown in Figure 10–24. Fractures associated with ventral angulation generally result in good functional recovery whereas fractures associated with dorsal angulation of theradiocarpal joint will have a poor functional recovery ifreduction is not accomplished. Figure 10–25 demonstrates the normal ulnar

angulation of 15 to 30 degrees of the radiocarpal joint. The evaluation of this angulation is essential when treating fractures of the distal forearm because failure or incomplete reduction with loss of this angulation will result in an inhibition of ulnar hand motion.

Mechanism of Injury
Most distal forearm fractures are the result of a fall on the outstretched hand (indirect mechanism). The amount of comminution and location of the fracture line is dependent on the force of the fall and the brittleness (age) of the bone. A supinating force often results in an associated ulnar fracture.

Examination
Examination typically reveals pain, swelling, and tenderness of the distal forearm. The displaced angulated fracture typically resembles a dinner fork as shown in Figure 10–26. Documentation of the neurologic status with special emphasis on the median nerve should be stressed. Elbow pain may be indicative of the proximal radioulnar joint subluxation or dislocation.

X Ray
AP and lateral views are usually sufficient for demonstrating the fracture fragments. When evaluating these fractures the physician must answer the following questions:

1. Is there an associated ulnar styloid fracture (60 percent incidence) or ulnar neck fracture?
2. Does the fracture involve the radioulnar joint?
3. Does the fracture involve the radiocarpal joint?

The lateral radiograph should be evaluated for evidence of distal radioulnar subluxation. In addition, the radiocarpal and radioulnar angles must be evaluated before reduction to ensure a complete return of function. Computed tomography (CT) or magnetic resonance imaging (MRI) may be helpful in delineating the extent of radiocarpal or radioulnar involvement.[17,29]

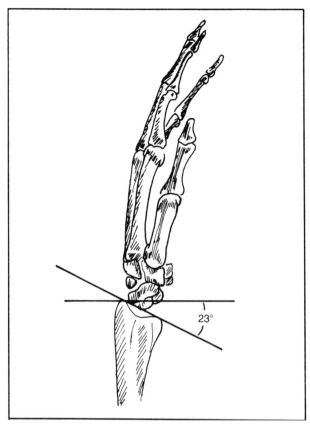

Figure 10-24. The normal radiocarpal joint is at an angle of 23 degrees in the ventral direction as shown in the lateral view.

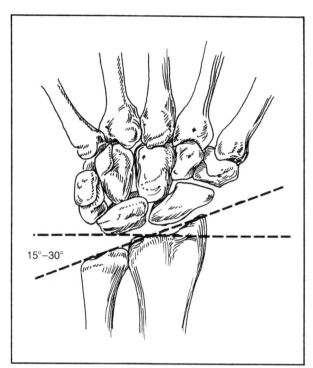

Figure 10-25. The normal angulation of the ulna in relation to the radiocarpal joint is 15 to 30 degrees.

Associated Injuries

Extension fractures of the distal radius are often associated with several significant injuries.

1. Sixty percent of distal radial extension fractures are accompanied by ulnar styloid fractures.
2. Fractures of the ulnar neck infrequently accompany extension fractures of the radius.
3. Carpal fractures can be associated with these fractures.
4. Distal radioulnar subluxation may be associated with distal radial extension fractures.
5. Flexor tendon injuries may accompany these fractures.
6. Median or ulnar nerve injury must be excluded in all distal forearm injuries. If the median nerve function is abnormal, carpal canal pressures should be documented to distinguish an acute carpal tunnel syndrome versus a median nerve contusion.[26]

Treatment

Colles' fractures, even when managed appropriately, result frequently in long-term complications.[7] For this reason it is the authors' belief that only type IA or B or type IIA fractures should be treated initially by the emergency physician. These fractures can typically be treated with dorsal and palmar long arm splints with the wrist in 15 degrees of flexion and 15 degrees of ulnar deviation. Urgent orthopedic referral is strongly recommended.[26] All other distal

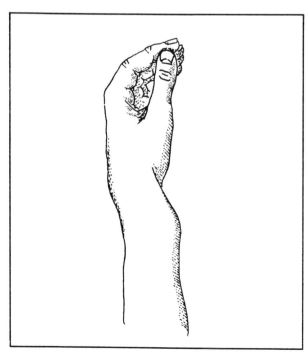

Figure 10-26. The dinner fork deformity described at the distal radius in a Colles' fracture.

forearm fractures should be referred for emergent treatment and follow-up. Unstable fractures may require percutaneous pinning or external fixation.[8,15,22,26]

All Colles' fractures should be followed by an orthopedic specialist.

In treating distal forearm fractures three principles must be remembered:

1. The extensors of the hand have a tendency to exert dorsal traction resulting in fragment displacement.
2. The normal radiocarpal joint varies from 1 to 23 degrees in a palmar direction. Dorsal angulation is not acceptable.
3. The normal radioulnar angulation is from 15 to 30 degrees. The angle is easily achieved with reduction but difficult to maintain during the healing phase unless positioned properly.

If emergent orthopedic referral is not available, reduction can be carried out in the following manner as shown in Figure 10–27.

1. The optimal method of anesthesia is regional block. A less effective but acceptable method is to aspirate the hematoma surrounding the fracture and to inject 5 to 10 mL of lidocaine into the area.
2. The recommended method of reduction is with traction followed by manipulation. The fingers should be placed in Chinese finger traps and the elbow elevated in 90 degrees of flexion. Eight to ten pounds of weight is then suspended from the elbow for a period of 5 to 10 minutes or until the fragments disimpact.
3. After disimpaction and continuance of traction, pressure is applied over the distal fragment in a volar direction with the thumbs, and dorsally directed pressure over the proximal segment with the fingers. When proper positioning has been achieved the traction weight is removed.
4. The forearm should be immobilized in a position of slight supination or midposition with the wrist in 15 degrees of flexion and with 20 degrees of ulnar deviation. It should be noted that many orthopedic surgeons prefer to immobilize the patient in pronation.[7] The position of the forearm is controversial, and before treatment is undertaken consultation with the orthopedist who is to follow the patient is recommended.
5. The forearm should be wrapped in one layer of Webril followed by the application of anteroposterior long arms splints (see Appendix). Short arm splints may be used in an impacted fracture where reduction is not necessary; or in a fracture in an elderly patient who will not exercise the involved extremity.
6. Postreduction radiographs must be obtained to ensure proper positioning. In addition, after reduction the function of the median nerve must be documented.
7. After reduction, the arm should remain elevated for 72 hours to keep swelling at a minimum. Finger and shoulder exercises should begin immediately and radiographs for documentation of proper positioning should be obtained at 3 days and 2 weeks postinjury. Nondisplaced fractures should remain immobilized for 4 to 6 weeks whereas displaced fractures require 6 to 12 weeks of immobilization.

Complications

Complications associated with wrist fracture are being reported with increasing frequency now of between 20 and 31 percent.[16] Early adequate reduction of the fracture is the most important means of avoiding complications. In addition, the principle of early exercise must be stressed to avoid secondary joint stiffness. The two categories of complications frequently seen are early and late.

Early Complications

1. The patient with median nerve compression will usually complain of pain and paresthesias over the distribution of the median nerve. If casted, the cast and Webril should be split and the arm elevated for 48 to 72 hours. If the symptoms persist, a carpal tunnel syndrome should be suspected, and surgical relief is then indicated. *Caution:* The function of the median nerve in distal forearm fractures should always be documented. Persistent pain should be regarded assecondary to median nerve compression until proven otherwise.
2. Tendon damage secondary to trauma may complicate the management of these fractures.
3. Ulnar nerve contusion or compression must be diagnosed early.
4. Postreduction swelling with secondary compartment syndromes may accompany distal forearm fractures.
5. Fragment displacement with loss of reduction after casting can be diagnosed with follow-up radiographs.

Late Complications

1. Stiffness of the fingers, shoulder, or radiocarpal joint may result from distal forearm fractures.
2. The shoulder–hand syndrome may be associated with distal forearm fractures.
3. Cosmetic defects may follow displaced distal forearm fractures.
4. Rupture of the extensor pollicis longus has been noted after distal radial extension fractures.
5. Malunion or nonunion are usually secondary to inadequate immobilization or incomplete reduction.
6. Flexor tendon adhesions secondary to trauma and immobilization can be a debilitating complication.
7. Chronic pain over the radioulnar joint with supination may be associated with these fractures.

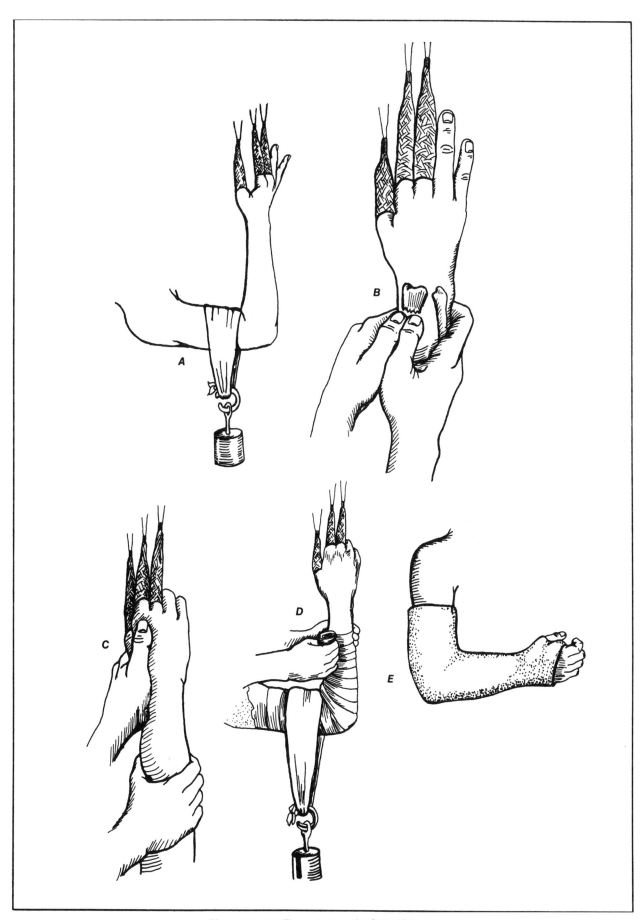

Figure 10–27. The reduction of a Colles' fracture.

II. FRACTURES AND RHEUMATOLOGY

DISTAL FOREARM FRACTURES

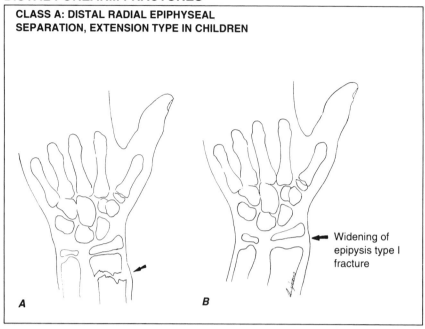

CLASS A: DISTAL RADIAL EPIPHYSEAL
SEPARATION, EXTENSION TYPE IN CHILDREN

Widening of
epipysis type I
fracture

A   *B*

Figure 10–28.

Childhood Distal Radial Fractures (Fig. 10–28A)

It is essential to exclude the diagnosis of an epiphyseal slip (see next section). It is the authors' recommendation that all of these patients require emergent referral for reduction under general anesthesia (see Fig. 10–29).

☐ CLASS A: DISTAL RADIAL EPIPHYSEAL SEPARATION, EXTENSION TYPE IN CHILDREN (FIG. 10–28B)

This injury usually results from a fall on the outstretched hand with forced dorsiflexion of the hand and epiphyseal plate. The typical result is a Salter type 1 or 2 fracture of the epiphysis. Growth arrests are uncommon but may occur and therefore all of these fractures require orthopedic referral.

In treating these injuries, more angulation and displacement can be accepted. Reduction must be implemented for angulation greater than 25 degrees or displacement of over 25 percent of the radial diameter. Immobilization can be accomplished by one of two means. For stable fractures, the physician should apply short arm anteroposterior splints (see Appendix) with the forearm in supination and the wrist in slight extension. For unstable fractures, the authors recommend immobilization in long arm anteroposterior splints (see Appendix) with the forearm in supination and the wrist in flexion. Some authors advocate placing the wrist in extension in managing these fractures.[5,6,9,14,25,28] Others[23] feel that extension of the wrist should be avoided as it places a volar distracting force

against the fracture. If the fracture is unstable after a closed reduction, pin fixation or open reduction with internal fixation is advocated.

☐ CLASS A: FLEXION TYPE (SMITH'S FRACTURE) (FIGS. 10–30, 10–31)

This fracture has often been described as a reverse Colles' fracture. It is an uncommon fracture and it rarely involves the distal radioulnar joint. The classification system used here involves both therapeutic and prognostic implications and was developed by Thomas.[28]

Mechanism of Injury

There are two mechanisms that result in distal forearm flexion fractures. A flexion fracture may result from a fall on the supinated forearm with the hand in dorsiflexion. Also, a punch with the clenched fist and the wrist slightly flexed may result in a flexion fracture. A direct blow to the dorsum of the wrist or distal radius with the hand flexed and the forearm in pronation may result in a flextion fracture.

Examination

There will be pain and swelling over the ventral aspect of the wrist. The presence and function of the radial artery and median nerve should be examined and documented.

X Ray

Routine AP and lateral views are adequate for demonstrating this fracture.

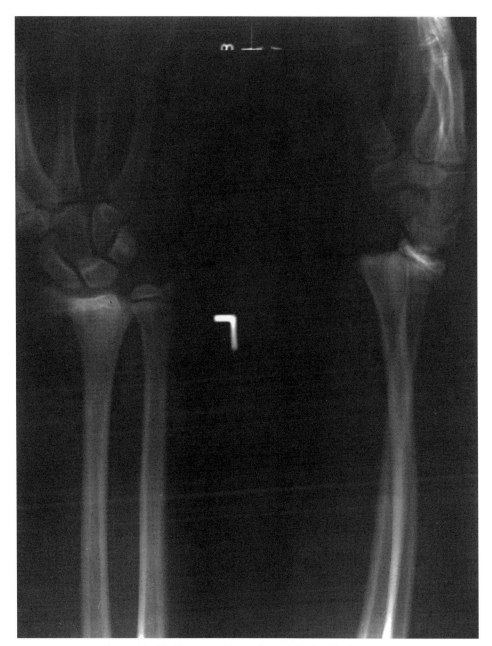

Figure 10–29. Fracture of the radius epiphysis with slippage.

Associated Injuries
Carpal fractures or dislocations are uncommonly associated with these fractures.

Treatment
In the child, general anesthesia is preferred whereas adults require regional block anesthesia.

☐ **Class A: Type I   (Distal Radial)**
Type II   (Distal Radial)
These fractures require emergent orthopedic referral for reduction. If orthopedic referral is unavailable, the fracture may be reduced as follows. Traction is applied using Chinese finger traps with 8 to 10 pounds of weight at the flexed elbow. The wrist is then pronated and flexed until the fragments are disimpacted. With the thumbs against the distal fragment dorsal pressure is applied with supination until the fragments are properly positioned. The forearm should be immobilized in a well-molded long arm cast or long arm anteroposterior splint (see Appendix). Postreduction radiographs for documentation of reduction should be obtained.

☐ **Class A: Type III   (Distal Radial)**
These patients require emergent referral for pinning of the bony fragment.

Complications
Complications are only seen infrequently with these fractures and include tendon damage and the development of

DISTAL FOREARM FRACTURES

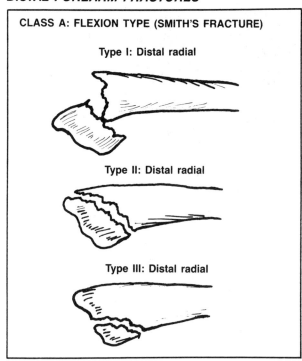

CLASS A: FLEXION TYPE (SMITH'S FRACTURE)

Type I: Distal radial

Type II: Distal radial

Type III: Distal radial

Figure 10–30.

osteoarthritis. Acute injuries of the epiphyses of the wrist may result in traumatic joint arrest with subsequent radioulnar joint incongruity.[23]

□ CLASS B: TYPE I PUSH-OFF DORSAL RIM FRACTURE (BARTON'S FRACTURE) (FIG. 10–32)

This fracture involves the dorsal rim of the distal radius and typically a triangular fragment of bone is noted on x ray.

Mechanism of Injury
Extreme dorsiflexion of the wrist accompanied by a pronating force may result in this intra-articular fracture.

Examination
The distal dorsal radius is tender and swollen. Occasionally radial nerve sensory branches may be compromised and present as paresthesias in the area of distribution.

X Ray
Lateral radiographs are best in demonstrating the fracture fragment and the amount of displacement.

Associated Injuries
Carpal bone injury or dislocations along with damage to the sensory branches of the radial nerve are uncommon injuries.

Treatment
The therapy selected depends on the size of the fracture fragment and the amount of displacement.

□ Class B: Type I   (Nondisplaced Barton's Fracture)
A short arm cast (see Appendix) with the forearm in a neutral position is the recommended mode of therapy.

□ Class B: Type I   (Displaced Barton's Fracture)
A large displaced fragment with subluxation or dislocation of the carpal bones requires regional anesthesia followed by a closed manipulative reduction. If the fracture is stable and in a good position, a short arm cast (see Appendix) with the forearm in a neutral position is recommended. If the fracture is unstable or reduced inadequately open reduction with internal fixation is indicated. A small fragment may be reduced and fixed by the placement of a percutaneous pin.

Complications
Frequent complications include arthritis secondary to intra-articular involvement as well as those associated with Colles' fractures.

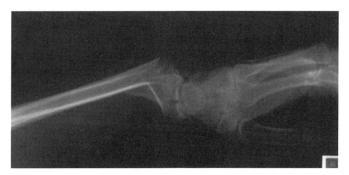

Figure 10–31. Severely displaced Smith's fracture.

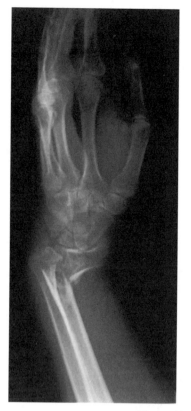
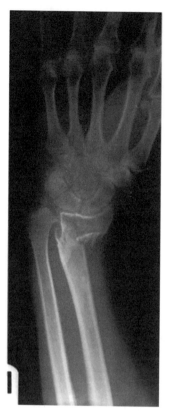

Figure 10–31. *(Continued)*

□ CLASS B: TYPE II PUSH-OFF RADIAL STYLOID FRACTURES (HUTCHINSON'S FRACTURE) (FIG. 10–32)

Mechanism of Injury
The mechanism involved is similar to that seen in a scaphoid fracture. Here, the force is transmitted from the scaphoid to the styloid resulting in a "push-off" fracture.

Examination
Pain, tenderness, and swelling are noted over the radial styloid.

X Ray
AP films of the wrist best demonstrate this fracture.

Associated Injuries
Fractures of the scaphoid as well as scapholunate disruption may be associated with these fractures.[26]

Treatment
The forearm should be immobilized in a posterior splint (see Appendix) with ice and elevation. These patients re-

DISTAL FOREARM FRACTURES

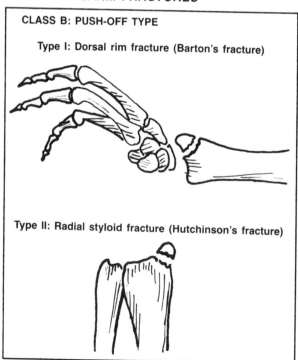

CLASS B: PUSH-OFF TYPE

Type I: Dorsal rim fracture (Barton's fracture)

Type II: Radial styloid fracture (Hutchinson's fracture)

Figure 10–32.

quire urgent orthopedic referral as percutaneous fixation is indicated for unstable fractures.

Complications

Complications are rarely encountered although a full neurovascular examination with documentation is indicated to exclude acute complications.

REFERENCES

1. Aulicino PL, Siegle JL: Acute injuries of the distal radioulnar joint. *Hand Clin* 7(2):283–293, 1991.
2. Boyd HB: The Monteggia lesion. *Clin Orthop* **66:**94, 1969.
3. Brostrom L, Stark A, Svartengren G: Acute comartment syndrome in forearm fractures. *Acta Orthop Scand* **61**(1):50–53, 1990.
4. Bruce HE, et al: Monteggia fracture. *J Bone Joint Surg* **56:**1563, 1974.
5. Caldwell JA: Device for making traction on the fingers. *JAMA* **96:**1226, 1931.
6. Carothus RG, Benning DD: Colles' fracture. *Am J Surg* **80:**626, 1950.
7. Cooney W: Management of Colles' fractures (editorial). *J Hand Surg* [Br] **14**(2):137–139, 1989.
8. Edwards GS Jr: Intra-articular fractures of the distal part of the radius treated with the small AO external fixator: *J Bone Joint Surg* **73-A**(8):1241–1250, 1991.
9. Ellis J: Smith's and Barton's fractures: A method of treatment. *J Bone Joint Surg* [Br] **47:**724, 1965.
10. Eriksson E, et al: Late results of conservative and surgical treatment of fractures of the olecranon. *Acta Chir Scand* **113:**153, 1957.
11. Frykman G: Fractures of the distal radius including sequelae. *Acta Orthop Scand* **108:**1, 1967.
12. Gaston SR, et al: Adult injuries of the radial head and neck. *Am J Surg* **78:**631, 1949.
13. Gebuhr P, Holmich P, Orsnes T, Soelberg M, Krashenin-

14. Iversen LD, Clawson DK: *Manual of Acute Orthopaedic Therapeutics*. Boston Little, Brown, 1977.
15. Jakim I, Pieterse HS, Sweet MBE: External fixation for intra-articular fractures of the distal radius. *J Bone Joint Surg* **71-B**(3):302–306, 1991.
16. Kozin SH, Wood MB: Early soft-tissue complications after fractures of the distal part of the radius. *J Bone Joint Surg* **75-A**(1):144–153, 1993.
17. Metz VM, Gilula LA: Imaging techniques for distal radius fractures and related injuries. *Orthop Clin North Am* **24**(2):218–228, 1993.
18. Moore EM, Klein JP, Patzakin MJ, et al: Results of compression-plating of closed Galeazzi fractures. *J Bone Joint Surg* [Am] **67:**1015–1021, 1985.
19. Morgan WJ, Breen TF: Complex fractures of the forearm. *Hand Clin* **10**(3):375–390, 1994.
20. Pike W: Fractures of the head of the radius. *J Bone Joint Surg* [Br] **51:**198, 1969.
21. Pinder IM: Fracture of the head of the radius in adults. *J Bone Joint Surg* [Br] **51:**386, 1969.
22. Rayhack JM: The history and evolution of percutaneous pinnig of displaced distal radius fractures. *Orthop Clin North Am* **24**(2):287–300, 1993.
23. Rockwood CA, Green DP: Fractures. Philadelphia: Lippincott, 1975.
24. Smith F: Surgery of the Elbow. Philadelphia: Saunders, 1972.
25. Steiner C, et al: Fracture of the shaft of the radius and ulna. *Surg Clin North Am* **20:**1669, 1940.
26. Szabo RM: Comminuted distal radius fractures. *Orthop Clin North Am* **23**(1):1–5, 1992.
27. Szabo RM, Skinner M: Isolated ulnar shaft fractures. *Acta Orthop Scand* **61**(4):350–352, 1990.
28. Thomas FB: Reduction of Smith's fracture. *J Bone Joint Surg* [Br] **39:**463, 1957.
29. Williams RL, Haddad FS, Lavy CBD: Current management of fractures of the distal radius and ulna. *Brit J Hosp Med* **55**(6):320–328, 1996.

nikoff M, Kjersgaard AG: Isolated ulnar shaft fracture. *J Bone Joint Surg* [Br] **71:**757–759, 1992.

11
CHAPTER
FRACTURES OF THE DISTAL HUMERUS

HORIZONTAL DISTAL HUMERAL FRACTURES

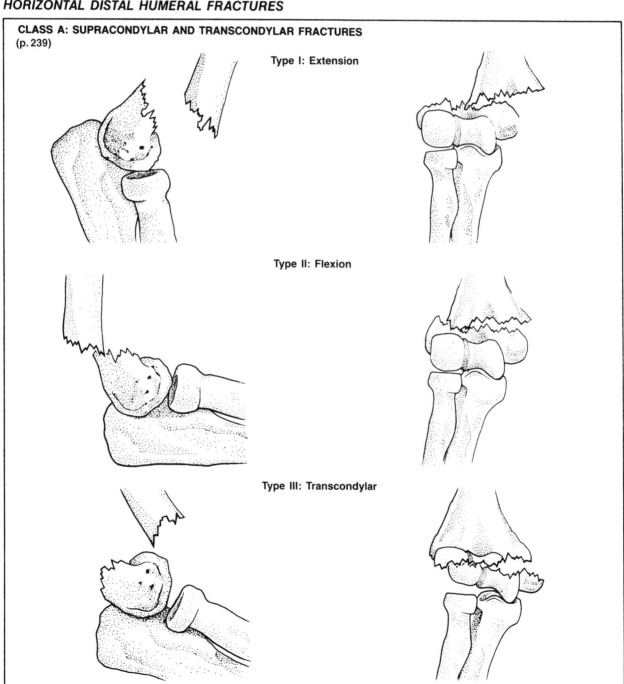

CLASS A: SUPRACONDYLAR AND TRANSCONDYLAR FRACTURES
(p. 239)

Type I: Extension

Type II: Flexion

Type III: Transcondylar

CLASS B: INTERCONDYLAR FRACTURES
(p. 245)

Type I   Type II   Types III and IV

T fracture   *T fracture*

T fracture
Alternate fracture patterns
(not considered in classification)

CLASS C: CONDYLAR FRACTURES
(p. 246)

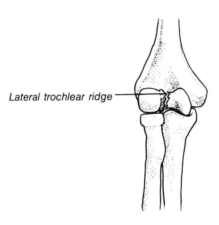

Lateral trochlear ridge

Type I: Lateral trochlear ridge stays with the humerus   **Type II: Lateral trochlear ridge stays with the fragment**

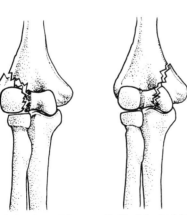
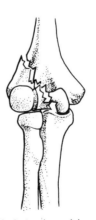
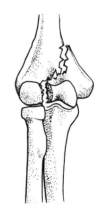

A: Lateral condylar   B: Medial condylar   A: Lateral condylar   B: Medial condylar
     fracture   fracture   fracture   fracture

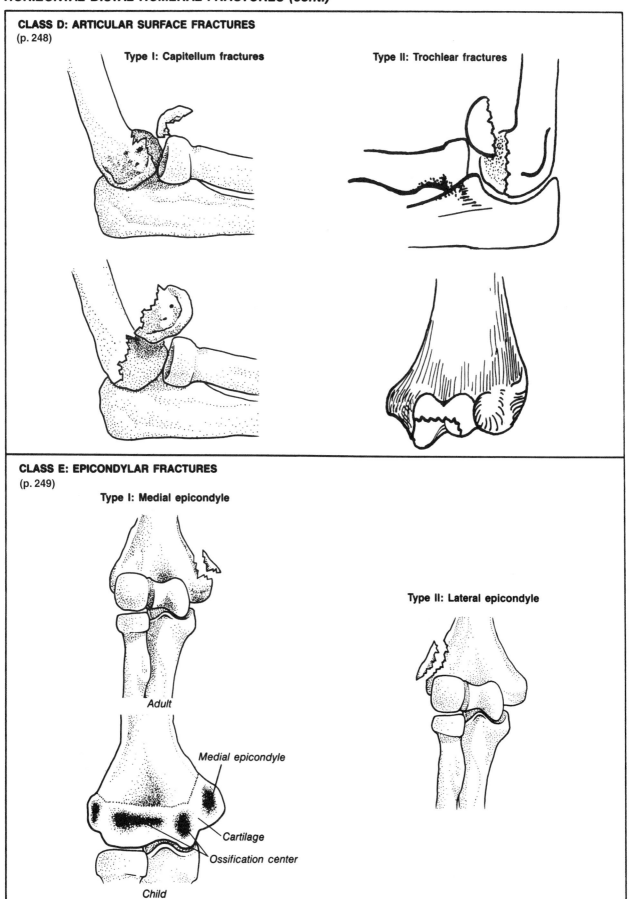

CLASS D: ARTICULAR SURFACE FRACTURES
(p. 248)

Type I: Capitellum fractures

Type II: Trochlear fractures

CLASS E: EPICONDYLAR FRACTURES
(p. 249)

Type I: Medial epicondyle

Type II: Lateral epicondyle

Adult

Medial epicondyle

Cartilage

Ossification center

Child

Distal humeral fractures are most commonly seen in children between the ages of 3 and 11 or in adults over the age of 50. In children, 60 percent of all elbow fractures are supracondylar; in the older age group, these fractures are often comminuted.

Essential Anatomy (Fig. 11–1)

The distal humerus consists of two columns of bone whose terminal ends make up the condyles. The coronoid fossa is the area of very thin, sometimes transparent bone that connects the two condyles of the distal humerus. The articular surface of the medial condyle is called the *trochlea* whereas the lateral surface is the *capitellum*. The nonarticular portions of the condyles are called *epicondyles* and serve as points of attachment for the muscles of the forearm. Those muscles concerned with forearm flexion insert on the medial epicondyle whereas those of extension insert on the lateral epicondyle. Just proximal to either epicondyle are the supracondylar ridges that also serve as points of attachment for the forearm muscles. The bone distal to and including the supracondylar ridges is anatomically defined as the distal humerus.

The muscles surrounding the distal humerus are depicted in Figures 11–2 and 11–3. With a fracture, continual traction by these muscles results in displacement of the fragments and on occasion nullification of an adequate reduction. A more inclusive description of muscular traction will be incorporated in the discussion of specific fractures.

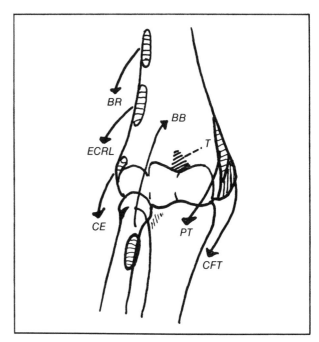

Figure 11–2. The muscles surrounding the distal humerus are demonstrated. These muscles act to displace fractures occurring at their attachments. BR = bracheoradialis; ECRL = extensor carpi radialis longus; CE = common extensor tendon; PT = pronator teres; CFT = common flexor tendon; BB = biceps brachia; T = triceps.

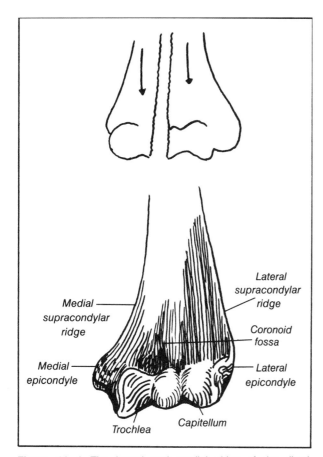

Figure 11–1. The lateral and medial sides of the distal humerus can be conceptualized as two columns running down to form the articulations with the radius and the ulna. The bone between these condyles is very thin.

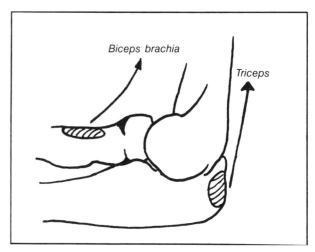

Figure 11–3. The triceps and the biceps act to pull the radius and the ulna proximally and thus cause overriding of distal humeral fractures.

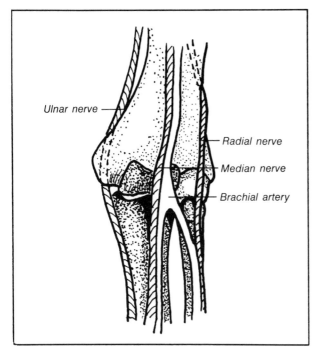

Figure 11-4. The neurovascular structures at the distal humerus.

The neurovascular structures of the distal humerus are diagrammed in Figure 11-4. The assessment of these neurovascular bundles is of critical importance when evaluating and treating distal humeral fractures. Further discussion will be included under the management of specific fractures.

Mechanism of Injury

There are two mechanisms that result in fractures of the distal humerus. With the elbow in flexion, a direct blow can result in a distal humeral fracture as shown in Figure 11-5. The position of the fragments is dependent on the magnitude and direction of force as well as the initial position of the elbow and the forearm (eg, flexion and supination) along with the muscular tone.

The indirect mechanism involves a fall on the outstretched hand as shown in Figure 11-6. As before, the magnitude and direction of force as well as the position of the elbow and the muscular tone determines the position of the fracture fragments.

Over 90 percent of distal humeral fractures are secondary to the indirect mechanism. Typically, the fracture is an extension fracture where the distal humeral fragment is displaced posteriorly. Flexion fractures, where the distal humeral fragment is displaced anteriorly, account for only 10 percent of humeral fractures. Either the direct or indirect mechanism can result in a flexion fracture.

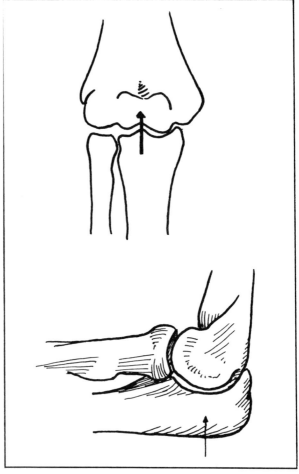

Figure 11-5. With the elbow in flexion a direct blow to the olecranon can result in a distal humeral fracture.

X Ray

The initial radiographic examination should include anteroposterior (AP) and lateral views. In the AP film, the forearm should be supinated and the elbow in as much extension as possible. The lateral film should be taken with the elbow in 90 degrees of flexion. Additional oblique views with the elbow in extension may be helpful in diagnosing occult fractures of the radial head, coronoid fossa, and even small condylar fractures.

The fat pad signs seen on elbow radiographs are often helpful in diagnosing occult fractures. The normal elbow joint capsule is covered with a thin layer of fat. When the capsule becomes distended with blood secondary to trauma the distention and displacement of the fat shadows can be readily seen (Fig. 11-7).

Anterior Fat Pad Sign. The anterior fat pad is over the coronoid fossa and is seen occasionally as a thin radiolucent line just anterior to the fossa in many normal radiographs. With a fracture, the joint capsule will be distended with blood and the anterior fat pad will be displaced anteriorly away from the coronoid fossa.

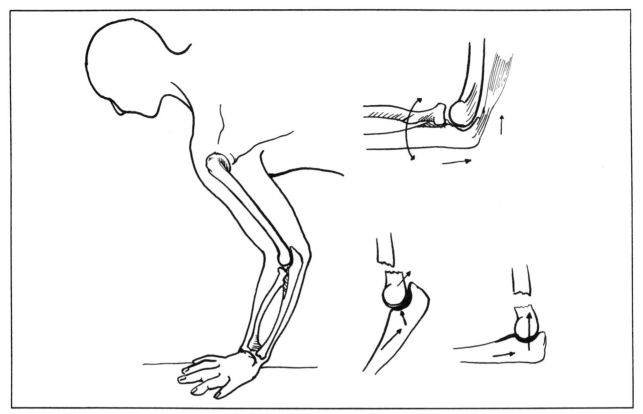

Figure 11–6. The indirect mechanism of producing a supracondylar fracture involves a fall on the outstretched hand. Two forces are transmitted to the elbow, one is a longitudinal force that will cause either forward or backward displacement of the distal fragment depending on the degree of flexion at the elbow and the other is a horizontal force that accounts for the horizontal fracture line noted. A vertical force will result in an intercondylar or condylar fracture.

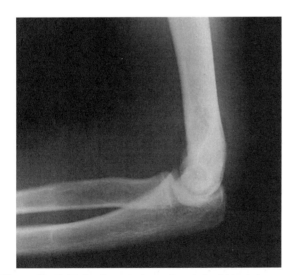

Figure 11–7. Notice the anterior and posterior fat pad sign.

Posterior Fat Pad Sign. The posterior fat pad lies over the olecranon fossa. Because the olecranon fossa is much deeper, the posterior fat pad is never visualized on normal radiographs. Only with joint capsule distention, as with an intra-articular fracture with a capsular hematoma, will the posterior fat pad be visualized. In the child, where cartilaginous growth and various centers of ossification make fracture identification difficult, the detection of a posterior fat pad can be regarded as diagnostic of an intra-articular fracture.

Axiom: *A posterior fat pad sign in the child or adolescent indicates a fracture or dislocation of the elbow. Therapy must be initiated until fracture or dislocation is absolutely ruled out.*

In the child or adolescent the distal humerus has four centers of ossification. Their locations and the age ranges when they are most commonly seen are listed in Table 11–1. Whenever a fracture is suspected in a child

TABLE 11–1. CENTER OF OSSIFICATION IN CHILDREN

	First Appears*	Fuses at Age (Yr)
Capitellum	3–6 mo	14–16
Medial epicondyle	5–7 yr	18–20
Trochlea	9–10 yr	14–16
Lateral epicondyle	9–13 yr	14–16

*Centers appear earlier in girls.

or adolescent comparison radiographs with similar positioning must be obtained.

Treatment

With distal humeral fractures, the distal segment may be displaced from the proximal bone resulting in various deformities. The following deformities may be present singly or in combination:

1. Anterior or posterior displacement
2. Medial or lateral displacement
3. Medial or lateral rotation
4. Medial or lateral angulation

In addition, it must be remembered that the humeral condyles act through the same horizontal plane forming a *center of articulation* as shown in Figure 11–8. Realignment of fractures must take this into consideration as malalignment will result in limited extension and flexion.

Axiom: *Rotation and angulation deformities must be corrected in the child or adolescent. Remodeling will often correct for some displacement but will not correct for angulation or significant rotation.*

Before a radiographic examination, the emergency physician must complete a careful physical examination with special attention to and documentation of the brachial, radial, and ulnar pulses along with the median, radial, and ulnar nerves. Comparison with the uninjured extremity should be a routine part of each examination. Frequently, these fractures are associated with extensive hemorrhage and swelling, which, in some instances, may compromise arterial flow and venous return.

The therapy for distal humeral fractures is divided into three basic modes:

1. Closed reduction with casting or splinting
2. Open reduction with internal fixation.[1]
3. Olecranon pin traction or skin traction (Dunlop's traction) with later casting

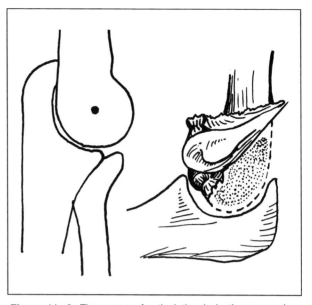

Figure 11–8. The center of articulation is in the same plane normally for the capitellum and the trochlea. In some fractures of the condyles, displacement or rotation malalignment results. If this persists therse will be limitation of flexion and extension. This malalignment must be corrected.

Each therapeutic modality has its indications and contraindications although in many instances the appropriate therapy remains controversial. Each therapeutic modality will be discussed under the management of specific fractures and the authors will make every effort to present both positions where a legitimate controversy exists.

Classification

In the following discussion, distal humeral fractures are classified on the basis of anatomy. These five fracture categories represent a simplistic approach when compared with many orthopedic texts. The authors sought a classification that encompasses a holistic approach where fractures that are anatomically and therapeutically similar are classified in the same category. The five classes of distal humeral fractures are:

HORIZONTAL DISTAL HUMERAL FRACTURES

☐ Class A: Supracondylar and transcondylar fractures   (Figs. 11–11 through 11–17)

☐ Class B: Intercondylar fractures, including the T and Y types   (Fig. 11–18)

☐ Class C: Condylar fractures   (Fig. 11–19)

☐ Class D: Articular surface fractures of the capitellum and trochlea   (Fig. 11–20)

☐ Class E: Epicondylar fractures, which are for the most part avulsion fractures   (Fig. 11–22)

HORIZONTAL DISTAL HUMERAL FRACTURES

☐ CLASS A: SUPRACONDYLAR AND
TRANSCONDYLAR FRACTURES

Horizontal fractures of the distal humerus can be divided into two broad categories: supracondylar and transcondylar. The supracondylar fractures are further subdivided, based on the position of the distal humeral segment, into extension type I (posterior displacement) or flexion type II (anterior displacement) fractures. Transcondylar fractures involve the joint capsule and may be of the flexion or extension type.

Supracondylar fractures are generally extra-articular and are most commonly seen in children between the ages of 3 and 11 years. The vast majority (95 percent) of displaced supracondylar fractures are of the extension type; 20 to 30 percent of supracondylar fractures will have little or no displacement. In those fractures that are posteromedially displaced, associated neural compromise is more likely to occur.[5] In children, 25 percent of supracondylar fractures are of the greenstick type. Radiographic diagnosis in these cases may be exceedingly difficult. Subtle changes, such as the presence of a posterior fat pad or an abnormal *anterior humeral line*, may be the only radiographic clues to the presence of a fracture. The anterior humeral line (Fig. 11–9) is a line drawn on a lateral radiograph along the anterior surface of the humerus through the elbow. Normally, this line transects the middle third of the capitellum. With a supracondylar extension fracture, this line will either transect the anterior third of the capitellum or pass entirely anterior to it.

Another diagnostic aid in evaluating radiographs of suspected supracondylar fractures in children is to determine the carrying angle. As shown in Figure 11–10, the intersection of a line drawn through the midshaft of the humerus and a line through the midshaft of the ulna on an AP extension view determines the carrying angle. Normally the carrying angle is between 0 and 12 degrees. Traumatic or asymmetric carrying angles of greater than 12 degrees are often associated with fractures.

☐ Class A: Type I (Supracondylar
Extension Fractures)
(Fig. 11–11)
Mechanism of Injury

The most common mechanism encountered is a fall on the outstretched arm with the elbow in extension (indirect mechanism). In children the surrounding anterior capsule

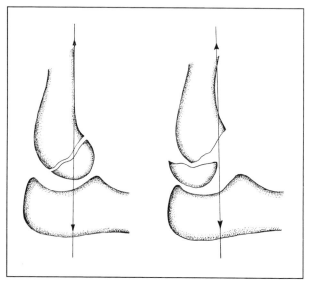

Figure 11–9. The anterior humeral line is a line drawn on the lateral radiograph along the anterior surface of the humerus through the elbow. Normally this line transects the middle of the capitellum. With an extension fracture of the supracondylar region this line will either transect the anterior third of the capitellum or pass entirely anterior to it.

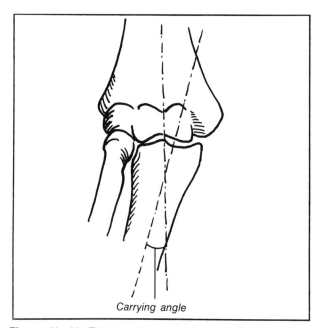

Carrying angle

Figure 11–10. The carrying angle demonstrated by a line drawn through the midshaft of the ulna and another line through the midshaft of the humerus. The normal carrying angle is between 0 and 12 degrees. A carrying angle of greater than 12 degrees is often associated with fractures of the distal humerus.

HORIZONTAL DISTAL HUMERAL FRACTURES

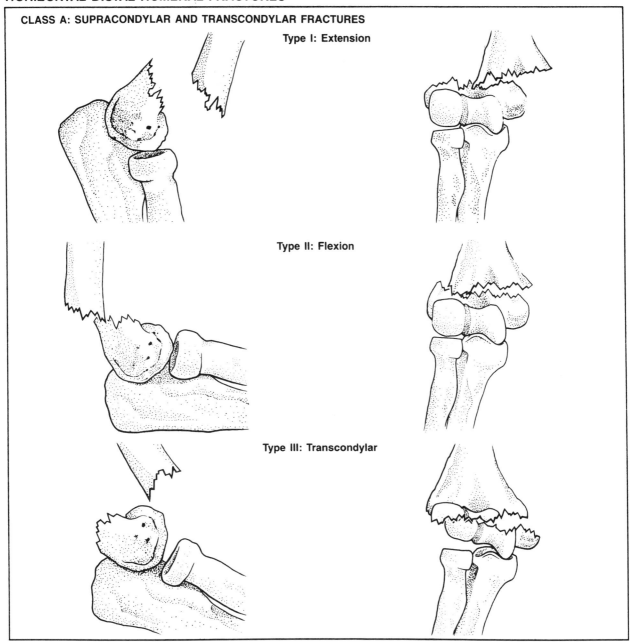

CLASS A: SUPRACONDYLAR AND TRANSCONDYLAR FRACTURES

Type I: Extension

Type II: Flexion

Type III: Transcondylar

Figure 11–11.

and collateral ligaments are stronger than the bone, and fractures rather than ligamentous tears usually result.[6] After the age of 20, ligamentous tears without fractures are more commonly seen.[4] A second mechanism involves a direct blow to the elbow (direct mechanism).

Examination

Recent injuries typically demonstrate little swelling with severe pain. The displaced distal humeral fragment can often be palpated posteriorly and superiorly because of the pull of the triceps muscle. As swelling increases, this injury can easily be confused with a posterior dislocation of the elbow resulting from the prominence of the olecranon and the presence of a posterior concavity. In addition, the involved forearm may appear shorter when compared with the uninvolved side.

(Fig. 11–12)

Routine views must include AP and lateral projections with comparison to the uninvolved extremity in children. The presence of a posterior fat pad, abnormal anterior humeral line, or a carrying angle of over 12 degrees

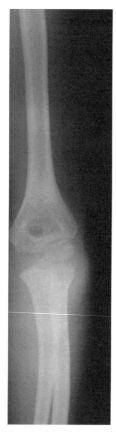

Figure 11–12. Supracondylar fracture.

strongly suggests an occult fracture. Oblique views should be obtained under these circumstances.

Associated Injuries

Distal humeral fractures are associated frequently with neurovascular complications even in the absence of displacement. The most commonly injured structures are the median nerve and the brachial artery. The physician must initially document the presence and strength of the radial, ulnar, and brachial pulses. A pulse oximeter could be applied to measure the pulse rate as well as the hemoglobin saturation. It must be noted that this apparatus should only be used to confirm already established clinical findings.[2] The presence of a pulse, however, does not exclude a significant arterial injury, of which there are three types: arterial wall contusion, intimal tear, and laceration or severing of the artery. The physician must also examine and document the motor and sensory components of the radial, ulnar, and median nerves. The three types of nerve injuries are contusion, partial severance, and complete severance. *Caution:* The physician must always assume that there is neurovascular compromise until a physical examination has excluded this threat. Subsequent manipulation may result in serious neurovascular compromise.

Treatment

All class A fractures require emergent consultation with an experienced orthopedic surgeon. Manipulative reductions are at times difficult to perform and fraught with complications. Emergent reduction by the emergency specialist is indicated only when the displaced fracture is associated with vascular compromise, which immediately threatens the viability of the extremity. Supracondylar fractures, whether displaced or not, require hospitalization. Delayed swelling with subsequent neurovascular compromise is noted frequently following these fractures.

☐ *Class A: Type I   (Nondisplaced with Less than 20 Degrees Posterior Angulation) (Fig. 11–13)*

1. The extremity must be immobilized in a posterior long arm splint extending from the axilla to a point just proximal to the metacarpal heads. The splint should encircle three quarters of the circumference of the extremity (see Appendix).
2. The elbow should be in over 90 degrees of flexion. The distal pulses should be checked and, if absent, the elbow is to be extended 5 degrees to 15 degrees or until the pulses return.
3. A sling for support and ice to reduce swelling are applied.
4. The patient should be hospitalized as frequent examinations of the neurovascular status are essential.

Axiom: *A cylinder cast should never be applied initially on any supracondylar fracture.*

☐ *Class A: Type I   (Nondisplaced with More than 20 Degrees Posterior Angulation) (Fig. 11–14)*

The emergency management includes immobilization in a similar splint as previously described, ice, elevation, and emergent referral for reduction under general or regional anesthesia. Some authors recommend pin fixation for all supracondylar fractures that require an anesthetic for reduction.[7] Excessive swelling may impede a complete stable closed reduction thus necessitating either percutaneous pin fixation or open reduction with internal fixation. Skin traction as shown in Figure 11–15 is an uncommonly utilized treatment option that may be a viable alternative in the absence of orthopedic surgical backup.

☐ *Class A: Type I   (Posterior Displacement) (Fig. 11–16)*

With an intact neurovascular status reduction of these fractures should be attempted by an experienced orthopedic surgeon. Fractures associated with limb-threatening vascular compromise where emergent orthopedic

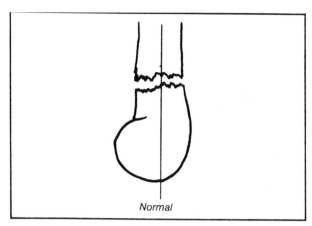

Figure 11-13. Posterior angulation of less than 20 degrees with a nondisplaced supracondylar fracture.

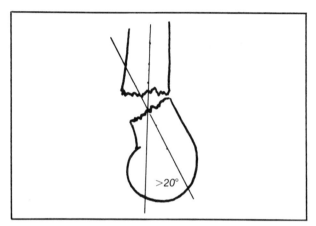

Figure 11-14. Posterior angulation of greater than 20 degrees with a nondisplaced supracondylar fracture.

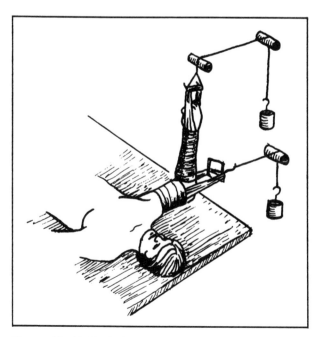

Figure 11-15. Dunlop's skin traction used in supracondylar fractures.

consultation is not available should be reduced by the emergency medicine specialist.

1. The initial step is to apply an axillary block of the entire extremity along with administering a skeletal muscle relaxant or general anesthesia. (The latter is preferred in the child.)
2. While an assistant immobilizes the arm proximal to the fracture site the physician holds the forearm at the wrist exerting longitudinal traction until the length is near normal as shown in Figure 11-16A.
3. The physician now slightly hyperextends the elbow to unlock the fracture fragments while he or she applies pressure in an anterior direction against the distal humeral segment (Fig. 11-16B). At this point, medial and lateral angulation should be corrected. The assistant simultaneously exerts a gently posteriorly directed force against the proximal humeral segment.
4. To complete reduction, the elbow is flexed to maintain the proper alignment and posterior pressure is applied to the distal fragment (Fig. 11-16C). The elbow should be flexed to the point where the pulse diminishes and then extended 5 to 15 degrees and the pulses rechecked and documented.
5. The extremity is immobilized in a long arm posterior splint (see Appendix). Controversy exists about the position of the forearm. In the child, if there is medial displacement of the distal fragment the forearm should be immobilized in pronation. With lateral displacement, the forearm should be immobilized in supination. Adults are generally immobilized in a neutral position or in slight pronation.
6. A sling should be supplied for support and ice to reduce swelling.
7. Postreduction x rays for documentation of position are essential.
8. Hospital admission for close follow-up of neurovascular status is mandatory.
9. X rays should be repeated in 7 days to ensure proper positioning of the distal fragment.

Caution: Only one attempt should be made at a manipulative reduction due to the proximity of neurovascular structures and the likelihood of injury with repeated attempts.

Alternate methods of treatment are available, including open reduction with internal fixation or overhead (overface) olecranon traction. *Overhead olecranon traction* is used for the following indications:

1. Failure of manipulative reduction
2. Excessive swelling with secondary circulation impairment
3. Failure to maintain reduction
4. Associated injuries including compound fractures, nerve paralysis, or additional comminuted fractures

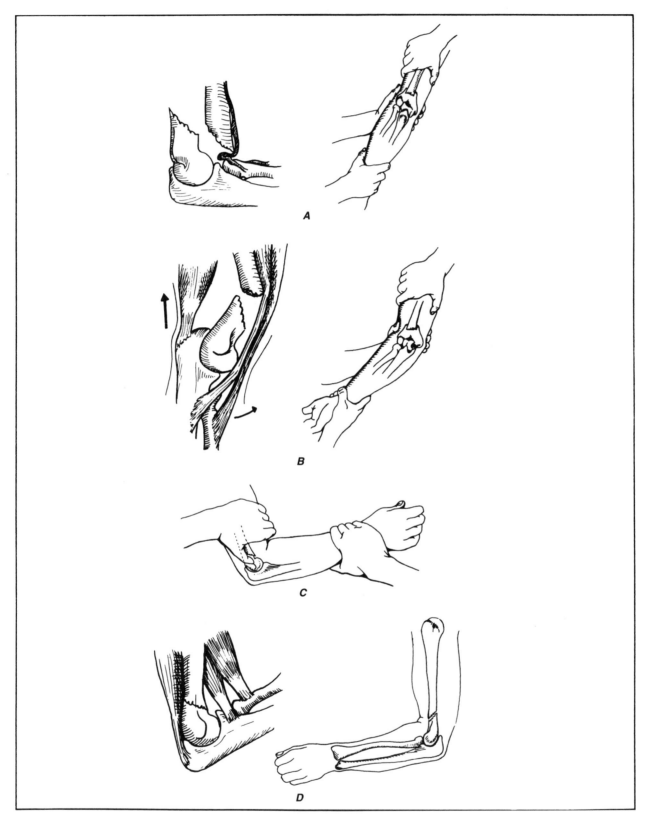

Figure 11–16. Reduction of a supracondylar fracture.

Open reduction with internal fixation is indicated under the following circumstances:

1. Inability to achieve a satisfactory closed reduction
2. Complicating fractures of the forearm
3. Inability to maintain a closed reduction
4. Vascular compromise where repair is indicated

Complications

Class A, type I supracondylar fractures are associated with several complications:

1. Neurovascular injuries may present acutely or with delayed symptoms. In all cases where vascular injury is suspected, the consideration of urgent arteriography should be discussed with the consulting orthopedic surgeon. Volkmann's ischemic contracture or an ulnar nerve palsy are delayed complications.
2. Cubitus varus and valgus deformities are commonly seen in children. Malposition of the distal humeral fragment after reduction is the most frequent cause.
3. Stiffness and loss of elbow motion are common complications in adults secondary to prolonged immobilization. After a stable reduction, pronation and supination exercises should be initiated in 2 to 3 days. Within 2 to 3 weeks the posterior splint may be removed for fixation-extension exercises. Unstable reductions, as noted above are best treated with overhead olecranon traction.

☐ Class A: Type II (Supracondylar Flexion Fractures) (see Fig. 11–11)

Supracondylar flexion fractures are usually the result of a direct blow against the posterior aspect of the flexed elbow as shown in Figure 11–5. The indirect mechanism (fall on the outstretched arm) only uncommonly results in a flexion fracture.

Examination

The elbow is usually carried in flexion, and there is a loss of the olecranon prominence.

X Ray

AP and lateral views without obvious fracture lines should be evaluated for the presence of a posterior fat pad sign. The anterior humeral line and the carrying angle should be calculated to exclude an occult fracture.

Associated Injuries

Neurovascular injury is an uncommon complication. The examiner must, however, document the presence of adequate distal pulses and nerve function before manipulation.

Treatment
☐ *Class A: Type II (Displaced)*

An experienced orthopedic surgeon should be consulted for reduction of these fractures. Pinning of the fracture is a frequently utilized treatment modality for these injuries.[7] Where there is limb-threatening neurovascular compromise and an emergent orthopedic consultation is not available, reduction may be carried out by an experienced emergency medicine specialist.

1. The initial step is to apply an axillary nerve block of the entire extremity and skeletal muscle relaxants or general anesthesia.
2. With the elbow in flexion, longitudinal traction is applied to the distal fragment while an assistant exerts countertraction on the proximal humerus.
3. The physician then exerts gentle posteriorly directed pressure over the distal fragment.
4. When the fragment is in position, the elbow is extended and maintained in extension.
5. The extremity is immobilized with a long arm posterior splint (see Appendix). It is the authors' preference to position the elbow at 35 degrees short of full extension to avoid the development of delayed elbow stiffness. Some authors recommend splinting with the elbow in full extension.
6. The patient should be hospitalized and treated with elevation, ice, and analgesics.

Operative reduction of supracondylar flexion fractures is indicated when there is a failure of one attempt at manipulative reduction or unstable fracture fragments except in extreme extension.

Complications

Class A, type II flexion fractures are associated with serious complications:

1. Stiffness and loss of elbow motion are more fre-quently seen in patients immobilized in full extension.
2. Neurovascular injuries including Volkmann's ischemic contracture and ulnar nerve palsy are infrequently seen delayed complications.
3. Deformity and reduced range of motion may occur secondary to inadequate reduction.

☐ Class A: Type III (Transcondylar Fractures) (Fig. 11–11)

The fracture line transects both condyles and lies within the joint capsule. This fracture is most often seen in patients over the age of 50. The distal humeral segment may be positioned anterior (flexion) or posterior (extension) to the proximal humeral segment. Therefore, the mechanisms, x ray, and treatment are identical to those of the supracondylar extension or flexion fractures. This fracture results frequently in the deposition of callus within the olecranon and coronoid fossas with subsequent diminished range of motion. All transcondylar fractures require an urgent consultation with an orthopedic surgeon and are best managed initially in an inpatient setting.

☐ Class A: Type III (Posadas Fracture)
(Fig. 11–17)

Mechanism of Injury

The most common mechanism is a direct blow with the elbow in flexion displacing the condylar fragments anteriorly.

Examination

In addition to pain and swelling, there is loss of the olecranon prominence with fullness in the antecubital fossa.

X Ray

Undisplaced fractures of the transcondylar type are more commonly seen than displaced fractures. The Posadas fracture is a flexion fracture with the condyles displaced anterior to the proximal humeral segment.

Associated Injuries

This fracture is always associated with a posterior dislocation of the radius or the ulna.

Treatment

The emergency management is to splint the fracture *without repositioning the arm* because flexion or extension of the joint may result in serious limb-threatening vascular compromise. These fractures are difficult to treat, and an emergent orthopedic consult should be obtained. If there is vascular compromise initially, traction with an olecranon pin is the treatment of choice.

Complications

Class A, type III: Posadas fractures are associated with several complications:

1. Neurovascular compromise may be acute or delayed.
2. Diminished range of motion may be secondary to inadequate reduction or callus formation within the joint.

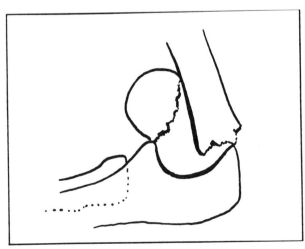

Figure 11–17. Posadas fracture.

☐ CLASS B: INTERCONDYLAR FRACTURES (FIG. 11–18)

Intercondylar fractures occur generally in patients over the age of 50. This is actually a supracondylar fracture with a vertical component. The terms *T* and *Y* indicate the direction of the fracture line. T fractures have a single transverse line whereas Y fractures present with two oblique fracture lines through the supracondylar humeral column. Classification is based on the amount of separation between the fracture fragments.

Mechanism of Injury

The most common mechanism is a direct blow driving the olecranon into the distal humerus at the trochlea. The position of the elbow at the time of impact determines whether there will be extension or flexion displacement of the fragments. Extension or posterior displacement of the fragments is more commonly seen. Rotation frequently accompanies these fractures because of the pull of the muscles inserting on the epicondyles. The condyles may separate from each other and from the humeral shaft. The degree of separation is dependent on the direction and force of injury along with the muscular tone.

Examination

On examination there is shortening of the forearm. With extension fractures, there is a concavity of the posterior arm with prominence of the olecranon. All of these fractures are grossly unstable with the exception of type I.

X Ray

AP and lateral views may demonstrate comminution and interpretation may be difficult due to overlapping bony edges. Classification of intercondylar fractures is based on the displacement of the humeral condyles from each other and from the proximal humeral shaft. Generally, larger condylar displacements are associated with greater offending forces.

☐ Class B: Type I (Nondisplaced)
There is no displacement between the capitellum and the trochlea.

☐ Class B: Type II (Separation)
There is separation between the capitellum and the trochlea without rotation in the frontal plan. This indicates that the capsular ligaments are intact and holding the fragments in their normal position.

☐ Class B: Type III (Separation with Rotation)
There is separation between the capitellum and the trochlea combined with rotation of the fragments. Rotation

HORIZONTAL DISTAL HUMERAL FRACTURES

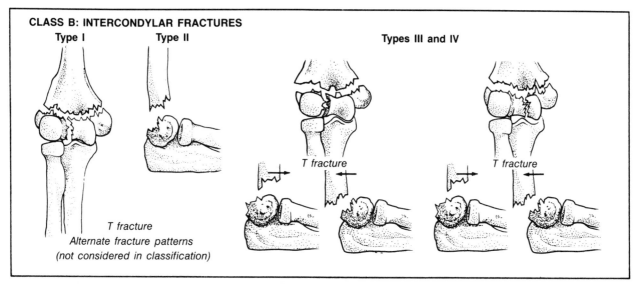

Figure 11–18. Four types of intercondylar fractures of the distal humerus are described. Type I (undisplaced) is a fracture between the capitellum and the trochlea with no displacement. Type II fractures are those in which the trochlea and the capitellum are separated but not rotated in the frontal plane. Type III fractures demonstrate separation and rotation of the fragments. In type IV fractures, there is severe comminution of the articular surface and wide separation of the condyles.

is secondary to the pull of the muscles inserting on the epicondyles.

☐ Class B: Type IV (Severe Comminution and Separation)

There is severe comminution of the articular surface and wide separation of the humeral condyles.

Associated Injuries

Neurovascular injuries are infrequently associated with these fractures.

Treatment

It is the authors' recommendation that all patients with class B intercondylar fractures be admitted to the hospital for observation and treatment.

☐ Class B: Type I (Nondisplaced Fractures)

This is a stable fracture and can be initially treated with a long arm posterior splint with the forearm in a neutral position (see Appendix). Sling and elevation with ice packs should be used early. Active motion exercises can be started within 2 to 3 weeks.

☐ Class B: Type II–IV (Displaced or Rotated)

These fractures are uncommonly seen, difficult to treat, and require an emergent orthopedic consultation. The treatment varies from the use of a collar and cuff (elderly patients) to the insertion of a prosthesis. The therapeutic program selected depends on the type of fracture, the activity level of the patient, and the judg-

ment and past experiences of the consulting orthopedic surgeon. Emergency care involves splinting the fracture in the position of presentation and applying ice. Surgical fixation and traction are the two most commonly selected therapeutic modalities.

Complications

Class B fractures may be associated with several complications:

1. The most common complication is loss of elbow joint function.
2. Neurovascular complications are rare.
3. Malunion and nonunion are uncommon complications.

☐ CLASS C: CONDYLAR FRACTURES

The humeral condyle includes both an articular portion and a nonarticular epicondylar portion. Condylar fractures, therefore, incorporate both the articular and the nonarticular portion of the condyle into the fracture fragment. Class D fractures involve only the articular components of the condyles.

Condylar fractures are classified into two types.[3] Type I fractures as shown in Figure 11–19 may involve either the medial or lateral condyle, but the *lateral trochlear ridge* remains attached to the proximal humeral segment. In type II fractures, as shown in Figure 11–19, the *lateral trochlear ridge* is incorporated

HORIZONTAL DISTAL HUMERAL FRACTURES

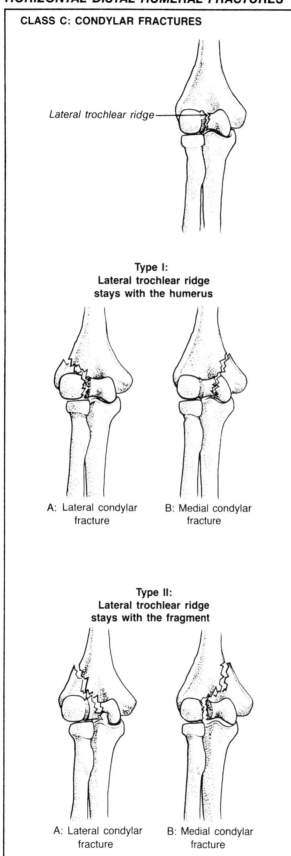

CLASS C: CONDYLAR FRACTURES

Lateral trochlear ridge —

Type I:
Lateral trochlear ridge
stays with the humerus

A: Lateral condylar   B: Medial condylar
   fracture   fracture

Type II:
Lateral trochlear ridge
stays with the fragment

A: Lateral condylar   B: Medial condylar
   fracture   fracture

Figure 11–19.

into the distal humeral segment. Type II fractures demonstrate medial and lateral instability of the elbow, radius, and ulna.

☐ Class C: Type IA and IIA   (Lateral
                               Condylar
                               Fractures)
                               (Fig. 11–19)

Mechanism of Injury

There are two mechanisms that result in class C lateral condylar fractures. First, the lateral condyle is anatomically more exposed and thus predisposed to fracture. With the elbow in flexion a direct force applied to its posterior aspect may result in a fracture.

Second, with the elbow in extension, a force causing adduction and hyperextension may result in a fracture. In children, rotation of the fracture fragment is secondary to the pull of the extensor muscles. Fragment rotation is uncommon in adults.

Examination

Physical examination typically reveals tenderness and swelling over the involved condyle.

X Ray

AP and lateral views typically reveal widening of the intercondylar distance. The fractured segment may be displaced proximally, but generally it will be seen posterior and inferior to its normal position. Type II fractures may result in a translocation of the ulna. In children in whom ossification is incomplete, comparison views must be obtained.

Associated Injuries

None are commonly seen.

Treatment

Because of the high rate of complications, all lateral condylar fractures require urgent orthopedic evaluation and follow-up.

☐ *Class C: Type IA (Nondisplaced)*

The arm should be immobilized in a long arm posterior splint with the elbow in flexion, the forearm in supination, and the wrist in extension to minimize distraction by the pull of the extensor muscles (see Appendix). The arm should be elevated with a sling and x rays repeated in 2 days to ensure proper positioning. A long arm cast can be applied when the swelling is reduced (see Appendix).

☐ *Class C: Type IA (Displaced)*

Emergent orthopedic consultation should be obtained. If unavailable, reduction can be carried out by the emergency department specialist. After the use of analgesics and skeletal muscle relaxants, the forearm is extended and direct pressure is placed over the fracture fragment. Supination combined with an adduction force may also facilitate the reduction. Postreduction radiographs, ice, elevation, immobilization, and hospital admission are indicated. Many orthopedic surgeons prefer open reduction with internal fixation for these fractures.

☐ Class C: Type IIA   (Nondisplaced)

Initial therapy includes the application of anterior and posterior long arm splints (see Appendix). The elbow should be in over 90 degrees of flexion with the forearm supinated and the wrist extended. X rays should be repeated in 2 or 3 days to ensure proper positioning and a long arm cast applied (see Appendix).

☐ Class C: Type IIA   (Displaced)

All of these fractures should be referred immediately to an experienced orthopedic surgeon. These fractures are best treated with open reduction and internal fixation. Closed manipulative reductions often result in cubitus valgus deformities.

Complications

Types I and II lateral condylar fractures may result in several complications:

1. Cubitus valgus deformity
2. Lateral transposition of the forearm
3. Arthritis due to joint capsule and articular disruption
4. Tardy ulnar nerve palsy
5. Overgrowth with subsequent cubitus varus deformity in children

☐ Class C: Type IB and IIB   (Medial Condylar Fractures) (Fig. 11–19)

These fractures are less common than lateral condylar fractures.

Mechanism of Injury

There are two mechanisms that result in class C medial condylar fractures. First, a direct force applied through the olecranon in a medial direction may fracture the medial condyle. Second, abduction with the forearm in extension may result in a fracture of the medial condyle.

Examination

Tenderness over the medial condyle with painful flexion of the wrist against resistance is frequently noted.

X Ray

Similar findings as with the lateral condylar fractures are noted except the distal fragment tends to be pulled anteriorly and inferiorly by the flexor muscles.

Associated Injuries

No associated injuries are commonly seen.

Treatment

☐ Class C: Type IB   (Nondisplaced)

A long arm posterior splint is applied with the elbow flexed, the forearm in pronation, and the wrist in flexion (see Appendix). Orthopedic follow-up with repeated radiographs to exclude delayed displacement is strongly urged.

☐ Class C: Type IB   (Displaced)

Emergency management includes immobilization, ice, and elevation with emergent referral for surgical fixation.

☐ Class C: Type IIB   (Displaced)

Emergency management includes immobilization, ice, elevation, and emergent referral for surgical fixation.

Complications

Types I and II medial condylar fractures are associated with the following complications:

1. Posttraumatic arthritis
2. Malunion with subsequent cubitus varus deformity
3. Ulnar nerve palsy

☐ CLASS D: ARTICULAR SURFACE FRACTURES

These fractures are limited to the capitellum and the trochlea and are very uncommon as isolated injuries. They are often seen in conjunction with posterior dislocations of the elbow. Capitellum fractures may be either type A or type B. Type A fractures result in a small distal bony fragment whereas type B fractures are associated with a larger distal capitellar fragment.

☐ Class D: Type I   (Capitellum Fractures) (Fig. 11–20)

Mechanism of Injury

The fracture mechanism is usually the result of a blow inflicted on the outstretched hand. The force is transmitted up the radius to the capitellum. The capitellum has no muscular attachments, and, consequently, the fragment may be nondisplaced. In some circumstances, secondary displacement occurs from elbow motion.

Examination

Initially, there may be a silent interval where there is an absence of signs and symptoms. Later, as blood distends the joint capsule, pain and swelling may become quite severe. Anterior displacement of the fracture fragment into the radial fossa may result in incomplete painful flexion. With posterior displacement, the range of motion is complete; however, there is increased pain with flexion.

HORIZONTAL DISTAL HUMERAL FRACTURES

CLASS D: ARTICULAR SURFACE FRACTURES

Type I: Capitellum fractures

Type II: Trochlear fractures

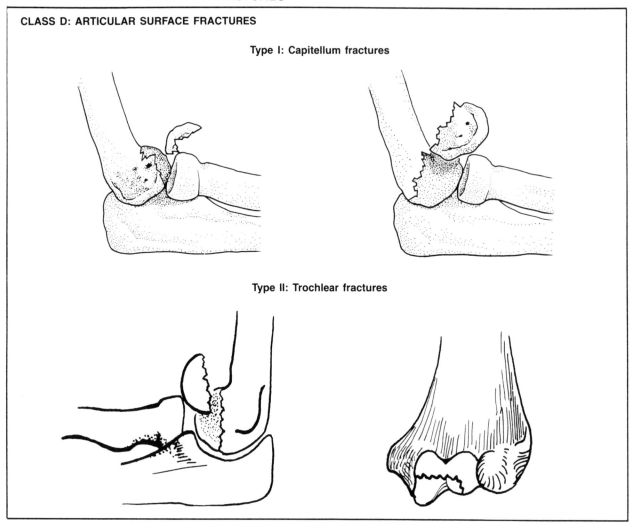

Figure 11–20.

X Ray
The lateral view usually demonstrates the fragment lying anterior and proximal to the main portion of the capitellum. Radial head fractures are frequently associated with this lesion.

Associated Injuries
Radial head fractures are commonly seen with class D fractures.

Treatment
☐ *Class D: Type IA*
Surgical excision of the fragment is the treatment of choice. Emergency management consists of immobilization in a posterior splint, ice, elevation, and analgesics.

☐ *Class D: Type IB*
Emergent orthopedic consultation for reduction is indicated. An accurate reduction is imperative to ensure normal motion of the radial humeral joint.

Complications
Class D fractures are associated with the following complications:

1. Posttraumatic arthritis
2. Avascular necrosis of the fracture fragment
3. Restricted range of motion

☐ Class D: Type II (Trochlear Fractures) (Fig. 11–20)
These fractures are extremely rare and require emergent orthopedic evaluation and treatment.

☐ CLASS E: EPICONDYLAR FRACTURES (FIG. 11–21)

Epicondylar fractures are most commonly seen in children. Medial epicondylar fractures are more common than are lateral. The ossification center for the medial

HORIZONTAL DISTAL HUMERAL FRACTURES

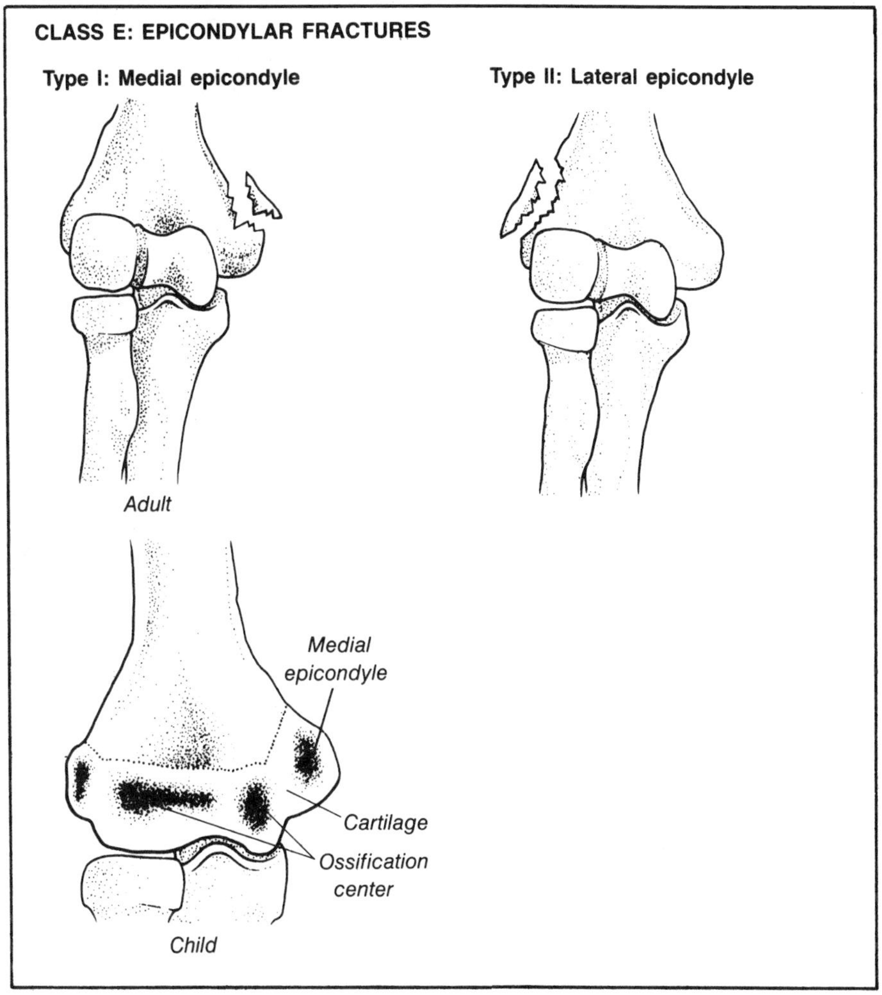

CLASS E: EPICONDYLAR FRACTURES

Type I: Medial epicondyle

Type II: Lateral epicondyle

Adult

Medial epicondyle

Cartilage

Ossification center

Child

Figure 11–21.

epicondyle appears by age 5 to 7 and fuses to the distal humerus by approximately age 20. Medial epicondylar displacement as an isolated injury is uncommon. More commonly seen is the palpable avulsion fracture associated with a posterior dislocation of the elbow.

□ Class E: Type I (Medial Epicondylar)
(Fig. 11–22)

Mechanism of Injury

There are three mechanisms commonly associated with fractures of the medial epicondyle.

1. The more common avulsion fracture is associated with childhood or adolescent posterior dislocations. This fracture is rarely associated with posterior dislocations over the age of 20.

2. The flexor pronator tendon is attached to the medial epicondylar ossification center. Repeated valgus stress on the elbow may result in a fracture with fragment displacement distally. This is commonly seen in adolescent baseball players and is called "little league elbow."

3. Isolated medial epicondylar fractures in adults are usually due to a direct blow.

Examination

If this fracture is associated with a posterior dislocation, the elbow will be in flexion and there will be a prominence of the olecranon. Isolated fractures produce localized pain over the medial epicondyle. Pain is increased with flexion of the elbow and the wrist or with pronation of the forearm. *Caution:* When assessing this fracture the physician must examine and document ulnar nerve function before initiating therapy.

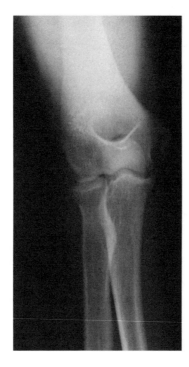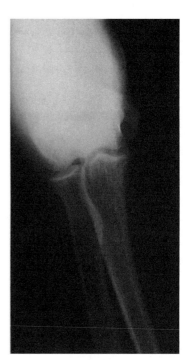

Figure 11–22. Epicondylar fracture involving the medial epicondyle of the humerus. A transcondylar fracture of the humerus is shown.

(Fig. 11–23)

Comparison views bare essential in children and adolescents. Displaced fragments may migrate and become intra-articular. *Caution:* Radiographically, if the fragment has migrated to the joint line it should be considered intra-articular.

Treatment

☐ *Class E: Type I (Dislocation)*

The elbow dislocation is reduced (refer to section on elbow dislocations) and fracture fragments assessed. If the epicondyle is within the joint, open reduction is indicated.

☐ *Class E: Type I (Nondisplaced)*

Fragments that are displaced less than 4 mm, as determined by measuring the clear space between the fracture fragment and the humerus, can be immobilized in a long arm posterior splint (see Appendix). The elbow and the wrist should be flexed with the forearm pronated. The splint should remain in place for 7 to 10 days.

Complications

Class E medial epicondylar fractures are associated with two main complications.

1. Persistent displacement may result in ulnar nerve bony intrapment.
2. For those fractures associated with the dislocation refer to the section on elbow dislocation in Chapter 12.

☐ Class E: Type II (Lateral Epicondylar) (Fig. 11–21)

This is an exceedingly rare injury that usually is the result of a direct blow. It is much more common for the condyle to fracture than the epicondyle. Most fractures are nondisplaced and can be treated similar to lateral condylar fractures.

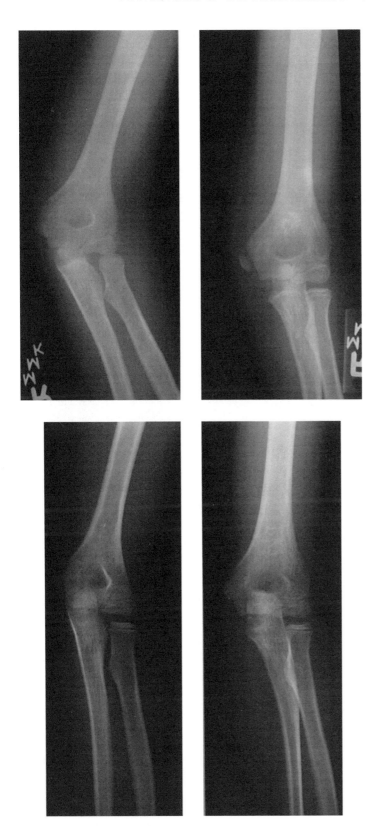

Figure 11–23. A medial epicondylar fracture is shown in a child. Notice the displacement in (**A**) which is difficult to recognize without the comparison views (**B**).

REFERENCES

1. Anderson L: Fractures. In Crenshaw AH (ed): *Campbell's Operative Orthopeadics*, 5th ed. St Louis: Mosby, 1971.
2. Best CJ, Woods KR: An aid to the treatment of supracondylar fractures of the Humerus: Brief report. *J Bone Joint Surg* [Br] **1:**141, 1989.
3. Brown RF, Morgan RG: Intercondylar T-shaped fractures of the humerus. *J Bone Joint Surg* [Br] **53:**426, 1971.
4. Bryan RS, Bickel WH: "T": Condylar fractures of distal humerus. *J Trauma* **11:**830, 1971.
5. Culp RW, Osterman AL, Davidson RS, Skirven T, Bora FW: Neural injuries associated with supracondylar fractures of the humerus in children. *J Bone Joint Surg* **8:**1211–1215, 1990.
6. Garceau GJ: Fractures of the lower end of the humerus. *JAMA* **112:**623, 1939.
7. Minkowitz B, Busch MT: Supracondylar humerus fractures. *Orthop Clin North Am* **25**(4):581–594, 1994.

BIBLIOGRAPHY

Charnley J: *The Closed Treatment of Common Fractures*, 3rd ed. Baltimore: Williams & Wilkins, 1972, p 99.

Conner AN, Smith MGH: Displaced fractures of the lateral humeral condyle in children. *J Bone Joint Surg* [Br] **52:**460, 1970.

Fowles JV: Displaced supracondylar fractures of the elbow in children. *J Bone Joint Surg* [Br] **56**(3):490, 1974.

Knight RA: Fractures of the humeral condyles in adults. *South Med J* **48:**1165, 1955.

Koen-Cohen BT: Fractures at the elbow. *J Bone Joint Surg* **48:**1623, 1966.

Ladd WE: Fractures of the lower end of the humerus. *Boston Med Surg J* **175:**220, 1916.

Lee WE, Summey TJ: Fracture of the capitellum of the humerus. *Ann Surg* **99:**497, 1934.

Norell HG: Roentgenologic visualization of extracapsular fat: Its importance in the diagnosis of trsaumatic injuries to the elbow. *Acta Radiol* **42:**205, 1964.

Patrick J: Fracture of the medial epicondyle with displacement into the elbow joint. *J Bone Joint Surg* **28:**143, 1935.

Quigley KTB: Aspiration of the elbow joint in treatment of fractures of the head of the radius. *N Engl J Med* **240:**915, 1949.

Riseborough EJ, Radin EL: Intercondylar T-fractures of the humerus in the adult. *J Bone Joint Surg* **51:**1130, 1969.

Siris IE: Supracondylar fracture of the humerus. *Surg Gynecol Obstet* **68:**201, 1939.

Smith JEM: Deformity following supracondylar fracture of the humerus. *J Bone Joint Surg* **27:**623, 1945.

12
CHAPTER

SOFT TISSUE INJURIES, DISLOCATIONS, AND DISORDERS OF THE ELBOW AND FOREARM

The elbow is a hinge joint that provides for good inherent stability. This joint is composed of three articulations located between the distal humerus and the ulna, at the radiohumeral, and at the radioulnar articulation. The distal humerus is divided into two condyles above which are the epicondyles. These provide the surface for the tendinous attachments of the flexors of the hand and the wrist medially and the extensors laterally. There are four ligamentous structures of importance in considering injuries to the elbow: radial collateral ligament, ulnar collateral ligament, annular ligament, and anterior capsule (Fig. 12–1). Three bursae are of clinical significance around the elbow: one between the olecranon and

the triceps, another between the radius and the insertion of the biceps tendon, and finally the olecranon bursa, which lies between the skin and the olecranon process. The olecranon bursa is the one most often involved in bursitis about the elbow (Fig. 12–2).

Elbow injuries are most often caused by valgus stress from throwing or axial compression, resulting in increased force absorbed by the medial elbow. With repetitive valgus stress, patients may develop chondromalacia, loose bodies in the posterior or lateral compartments, injury to the ulnar collateral ligament, tenderness injury of the flexor pronator muscle group, or osteochondritis dissecans and ulnar neuritis.[30]

ELBOW INJURIES

The majority of elbow injuries occur from chronic use, particularly in athletes. A valgus stress from throwing in axial compression causes increased force on the medial elbow, as indicated above. A number of conditions will

be discussed in detail in this chapter. First, however, a general discussion as to how to approach patients with elbow pain is warranted.

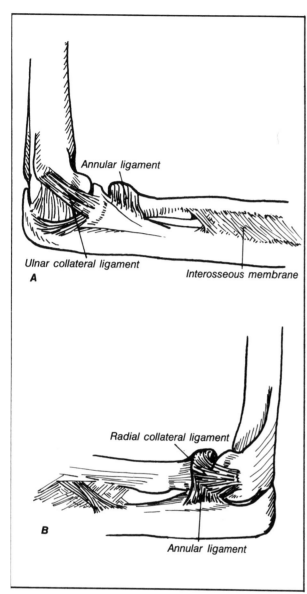

Figure 12–1. Note the ulnar collateral ligament (**A**). The annular ligament holds the radial head in position. The radial collateral ligament is broader and blends with the annular ligament (**B**).

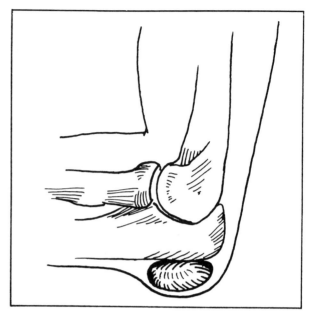

Figure 12–2. Olecranon bursitis.

Anterior elbow pain is a common presenting problem, particularly in the young athlete. This is usually caused by a stretch or tear of the anterior capsule, distal biceps, or brachialis tendons with or without dislocation. This injury can be from a fall of the extended elbow. Climber's elbow is defined as a strain of the brachialis tendon.[30] Ectopic bone may deposit after a traumatic blow to the anterior arm. This usually occurs within the brachialis muscle 3 weeks after the injury. Prevention with indomethicin and early range of motion is of paramount importance. Anterior elbow pain may result from median nerve entrapment such as with the pronator syndrome and annular ligament injury secondary to radial head subluxation or dislocation.

Medial elbow pain may result from a variety of conditions and is much more common. Medial epicondylar fracture or stress fracture can occur. Medial epicondylitis can be due to tendonitis of the flexor or pronator muscle group. An unusual condition called snapping elbow syndrome occurs when the ulnar nerve snaps out of the cubital tunnel. Medial elbow pain may result from instability caused by acute or chronic ulnar collateral ligament disruption. Ulnar neuritis is the common cause of medial elbow pain in athletes because of the ulnar nerve's superficial location at the cubital tunnel and its unfavorable response to valgus stresses. Compression can occur proximal to the cubital tunnel because of a tight intramuscular septum. The earliest symptom is medial joint line pain, clumsiness, or heaviness of the hand, fingers, or both. This is associated with or exacerbated by throwing or overhead activity and may manifest as numbness and tingling in the little and ring fingers.[30]

Posterior elbow pain is less common than medial or lateral elbow pain but more common than anterior pain. Abnormal stresses may cause triceps pain at its attachment or olecranon apophysis injuries, which may present in a similar fashion to Osgood-Schlatter disease.[30] Triceps tendonitis is an uncommon cause of posterior elbow pain and is treated with rest. Triceps tendon rupture is one of the most uncommon tendon ruptures. Stress fracture of the olecranon is also an uncommon cause of elbow pain that occurs in athletes who throw. Olecranon bursitis, discussed below, is by far the most common condition in this group.

Lateral elbow pain is the most common location of elbow pain in the general population. Lateral epicondylitis, discussed below, is the most common cause.

Osteochondritis dissecans is another problem, occasionally called "Little League elbow," and is a focal lesion of the lateral elbow that occurs in young throwers. This is discussed below. Radial nerve entrapment at the elbow can occur alone or in conjunction with lateral epicondylitis.[30]

☐ TENNIS ELBOW (EPICONDYLITIS)

Tennis elbow is a chronic disabling disorder of unknown cause seen commonly in patients who have occupations requiring rotary motion at the elbow, such as pipefitters, tennis players, and carpenters.[2,3] The pain usually originates from either the radiohumeral region or the lateral epicondyle (epicondylitis). It is usually called by the nondescriptive term of *tennis elbow* because the origin is not clear.[22] Many entities have been implicated as the cause of tennis elbow including arthritis of the radiohumeral joint, radiohumeral bursitis, traumatic synovitis of the radiohumeral joint, and periostitis of the lateral epicondyle; however, at present none of these can be implicated as the sole cause of this condition.[2,22] The underlying feature is the presence of tears in the aponeurosis of the extensor tendons.[5] Many patients with tennis elbow have microavulsion fractures of the lateral epicondyle in addition to possible microscopic tears in the tendon proper.[5]

The patient usually presents with a history of a gradual onset of a dull ache along the outer aspect of the elbow referred to the forearm. The pain increases with *grasping* and *twisting* motions.[2] Tenderness is localized over the lateral epicondyle or the radiohumeral articulation. Although most cases involve the lateral epicondyle, involvement of the medial epicondyle can occur. A reliable test for tennis elbow is elicited by the following maneuver: Ask the patient to extend the elbow and to actively attempt to dorsiflex the wrist and supinate the forearm against resistance (Fig. 12–3). In patients with tennis elbow, this maneuver intensifies the discomfort.[2] The neurologic examination should be normal. Magnetic resonance imaging (MRI) is helpful in identifying areas of inflammation and lateral epicondylitis.[4]

The treatment of this condition is to splint the elbow in a flexed position with the forearm supinated and the wrist extended. The patient should be advised to apply heat to the elbow and rest. Anti-inflammatory agents, such as phenylbutazone or ibuprofen (Motrin) are of value. Caution should be exercised in prescribing anti-inflammatory medications because of their common side effects of gastrointestinal upset and increased bleeding problems. Corticosteroids injections are useful. Up to three injections is considered appropriate; after that, one should be cautious in the amount of steroids injected. Counterforce bracing or "tennis elbow bands" are quite effective in reducing the symptoms and allowing the individual to continue normal activity[4] (Fig. 12–4).

Medial epicondylitis, which is inflammation at the origin of the wrist flexors, is characterized by pain over the medial epicondyle and medial pain on forced flexion of the wrist[4] (Fig. 12–5). The treatment of medial epicondylitis is similar to that of lateral epicondylitis. Because of the close proximity of the ulnar nerve, local anesthetic that is used with the corticosteroid may cause a temporary paralysis of the ulnar nerve when treating this problem.[4]

As a last resort, surgical intervention may be necessary for the treatment of these conditions.

☐ OSTEOCHONDRITIS DISSECANS

Osteochondritis dissecans occur in young athletes who overload and hyperextend the elbow. Gymnasts are constantly loading their elbows as they balance on

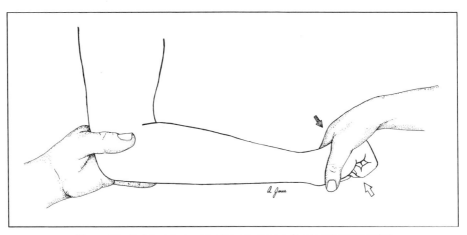

Figure 12–3. A test for tennis elbow is shown. See text for discussion.

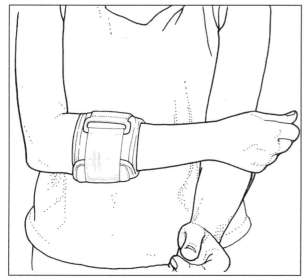

Figure 12–4. Placement of a tennis elbow band. The proximal edge of the band should be placed 2 to 3 cm distal to the lateral epicondyle, over the bulk of the extensor muscles.

osteochondritis dissecans. MRI is often helpful in suspicious cases where the x ray is negative.

Treatment is conservative unless there are loose bodies within the joint that require mechanical removal. Conservative treatment for acute exacerbations consists of splinting the elbow for 3 to 4 days, anti-inflammatory medications, and the application of heat.[4] If mechanical symptoms occur and persist, arthroscopic intervention to remove and debride loose bodies is necessary.[4]

"Little league elbow" occurs when young throwers have repetitive microtrauma at the ossification center along the radial head. Osteochondral changes in the capitellum, premature proximal radial epiphyseal closure, and fragmentation of the medial epicondyle are collectively known as Little League elbow. The condition is predominantly a result of forces applied during a late phase of throwing causing a valgus strain of the elbow.[10] Comparison views on x rays show that the apophysis has become separated. Bony fragments can ultimately lodge in the joint and require open reduction and removal. Loss of extension occurs as a result of tightening of the ulnar collateral ligament, producing pain and unvalgus stress. Ulnar neuritis may present due to subluxation or compression of the fascial planes. Treatment often requires arthroscopy, if a fragment is noted, as well as drilling of the subchondral bone.

beams and high bars and are particularly susceptible to this condition. The symptoms that occur are locking, giving way, and crepitus on range of motion. X rays may reveal a loose body within the joint or demonstrable

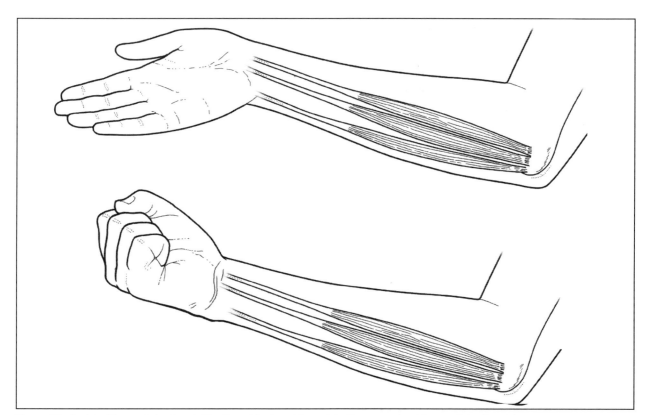

Figure 12–5. A test for medial epicondylitis. Forced flexion of the wrist will cause pain of the medial epicondyle.

□ SUBLUXATION OF THE RADIAL HEAD IN CHILDREN

This is the most common injury occurring in children between the ages of 2 and 5 years and represents 27.5 percent of all elbow injuries in young children.[8,19,33] Other names for this condition are "nursemaid's elbow," "pulled elbow," and "temper tantrum elbow."[31] The annular ligament provides support for the radial head maintaining the head in its normal relationship with the humerus and the ulna.[21] In children there is little structural support between the radius and the humerus. With sudden traction of the hand or the forearm, such as occurs when a parent pulls a child up by the arm to prevent a fall, the annular ligament is pulled over the radial head and is interposed between the radius and the capitellum.

The patient presents with the arm dangling to the side and held in *flexion* at the elbow and *pronation*. The child resists any motion involving *supination*, which is quite *painful*. Flexion and extension are limited with a sensation of a "block" in the normal range of motion on examination.[8,19] The three most common problems during initial evaluation are pain, loss of motion of the elbow, and deformity due to prominence of the radial head.[1]

To reduce the subluxation thumb pressure is applied over the forearm in the region of the radial head. The elbow is slowly supinated and extended (Fig. 12–6). A sudden release of resistance accompanied by a click

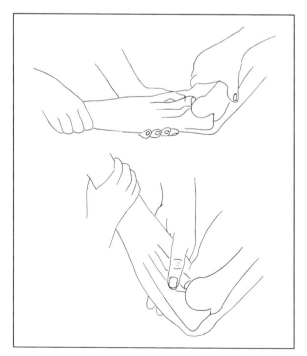

Figure 12–6. Reducing subluxation is accomplished by compressing the radial head while supinating the elbow and then flexing.

signifies reduction. Reduction can also be accomplished by supination and flexion.[31] Studies indicate that supination-flexion maneuver was actually more successful than the supination-extension maneuver with 80.4 percent success with flexion versus 68 percent with extension.[31] Roentgenograms should always be taken before any attempts at reduction. After reduction, if the child is less than 2 years of age he or she should be allowed to rest the arm for 30 minutes prior to use. If the child is older than 2 years of age, the child should be allowed to use the arm soon after reduction.

□ DISLOCATION OF THE ELBOW

Elbow dislocations are among the most commonly seen dislocations in the body, second in frequency only to dislocations of the shoulder and the fingers. The mechanism by which most dislocations of the elbow occur is secondary to a fall on the extended and abducted arm. This causes the most common dislocation, a posterior dislocation of the joint.[18,28]

Types of Dislocations (Fig. 12–7)
Posterior dislocations account for the majority of dislocations seen at the elbow in which the ulnar olecranon is displaced posteriorly in relation to the distal humerus.[18] *Anterior dislocations* are far less common, occurring from a blow to the flexed elbow that drives the olecranon forward. Lateral and medial dislocations have been described; however, these are often seen in combination with either of the above dislocations or with fractures and are not discussed separately here.[8,19]

□ Posterior
Patients with posterior dislocations present to the emergency department with the limb held in flexion at 45 degrees. The olecranon is prominent posteriorly, and there is usually moderate swelling and deformity at the joint. Swelling may make the diagnosis difficult, and the differentiation between dislocation and supracondylar fracture can also be difficult.[8] If one palpates the two epicondyles and the tip of the olecranon in patients with a supracondylar fracture they will be on the same plane whereas with dislocations, the olecranon will be displaced from the plane of the epicondyles on palpation.

After roentgenographic confirmation of the dislocation an examination of the peripheral nerves and the distal pulses should be completed. Early reduction is advocated as delay may damage the articular cartilage or result in excessive swelling or circulatory compromise. Reduction is accomplished after administering an analgesic and a muscle relaxant. The reduction technique preferred by the authors is a modification of the Stimson technique used in shoulder reductions (Fig. 12–8).

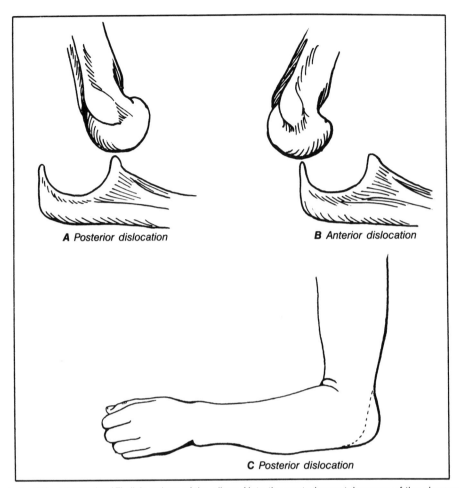

Figure 12–7. Posterior (**A**) and anterior (**B**) dislocations of the elbow. Note the posterior protuberance of the olecranon in a posterior dislocation (**C**).

The patient should be placed in the prone position with the dislocated elbow hanging perpendicular to the table, as shown in Figure 12–8. A small pillow or folded sheet should support the humerus just proximal to the elbow joint. Weights are then suspended from the wrist with the elbow flexed approximately 30 degrees from the extended position. Over a period of several minutes the patient's elbow dislocation will reduce. The authors prefer beginning with approximately 5 pounds of weight, and this could be increased if needed. After reduction of the elbow, the ligaments are stress tested and the elbow is immobilized in a posterior splint or a sling at 90 degrees.[29] This allows for early flexion but restricts extension. One must be careful to avoid forceful manipulation during reduction and in the rehabilitation period, which can result in myositis ossificans.

Commonly associated injuries are to the peripheral nerves, especially the ulnar nerve, and this should be checked before and after reduction.[23] Neurovascular injury of which the ulnar nerve lesion is the most common occurs in 8 to 21 percent of patients with posterior elbow dislocations.[29] A fractured medial epicondyle can

sometimes become entrapped in the joint requiring open reduction.[7] Fractures of the coronoid process are common associated injuries and usually will come into near normal opposition once reduction occurs. Large fragments that are displaced may require operative fixation. Injury to the brachial artery has also been described with posterior dislocations of the elbow.[20] Median nerve entrapment may also occur in patients with posterior dislocations.[32]

□ Anterior

Anterior dislocations are far less common than posterior dislocations as has been previously mentioned (see Fig. 12–7). These injuries occur from a blow to the flexed elbow driving the olecranon anteriorly. Associated injuries to vessels and nerves around the joint are much more common with anterior dislocations making this a more serious dislocation.

On examination, the arm appears shortened and the forearm is elongated and held in supination. The elbow is usually held in full extension. The olecranon fossa is often palpable posteriorly.

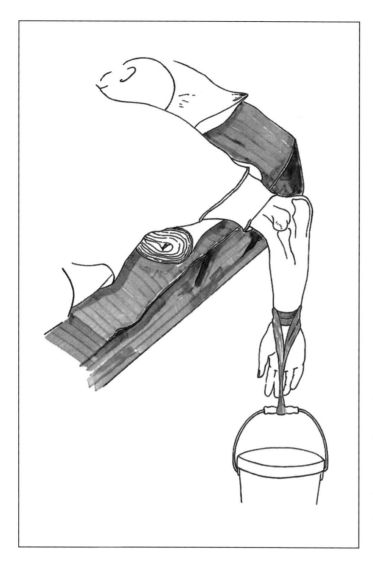

Figure 12–8. A reduction technique for posterior dislocation of the elbow is shown. In this technique weights are suspended from the wrist while the arm is held over the edge of the bed as shown. A folded sheet can be placed under the arm to allow free movement of the forearm as the reduction occurs. With proper muscle relaxation, reduction usually occurs within a period of 5 to 10 minutes. If using a bucket of sand, weights can be added as needed.

All of these patients should be splinted, and the vascular and neurologic status assessed. They should be referred for immediate reduction. Many of these dislocations are open and vascular damage is quite common. Complete avulsion of the triceps mechanism is another commonly associated soft tissue injury.

□ BURSITIS

Bursitis can occur in any of the bursae surrounding the elbow as shown in Figure 12–2 and present with the same symptoms as bursitis elsewhere in the body. Olecranon bursitis is the most common form seen in the emergency department and is secondary to either a single traumatic blow to the point of the elbow or repeated episodes of minor trauma such as occurs when a patient leans on the elbow for prolonged periods of time.[17]

On examination of the patient with olecranon bursitis, one will note swelling in the posterior aspect of the elbow with slight restriction of flexion due to the inflamed bursa.[17] In patients with bursitis caused by gout or infectious processes, there will be surrounding inflammatory reaction and pain with minimal motion of the elbow. The bursa will be hot and tender to palpation.

Olecranon bursitis is treated by aspiration and application of a compressive dressing with local heat and preventive measures directed at the inciting cause. In cases of purulent bursitis, patients should have the bursa incised and drained in the operating room and appropriate antibiotics begun in the emergency department.

Recently it has been shown that many cases of olecranon bursitis are, in fact, septic. Septic bursitis is often misdiagnosed as nonseptic. In a recent study, *Staphylococcus aureus* was identified in a large number of cases in which patients with olecranon or prepatellar bursitis had fluid aspirated and studied. Seventy-six percent of the organisms were resistant to penicillin. The recommendation of the authors was to use intravenous antibiotics and to drain the bursal fluid, which was uniformly successful.[12]

☐ INJURIES TO THE LIGAMENTS OF THE ELBOW

In sports, sprains occur involving the ulnar and radial collateral ligaments of the elbow. These injuries are of less consequence and of little problem as compared with other disorders described above. They are diagnosed by appropriate stress testing of the involved ligaments and treated with immobilization of the elbow in a flexed position (Fig. 12–9). When there is opening of the joint on a stress examination one must always assess the neurologic status to be certain there is no accompanying neurologic deficit.[9]

☐ Ulnar Collateral Ligament Injury

Ulnar collateral ligament injury is a common problem. Point tenderness inferior and distal to the medial epicondyle is present. Posterior medial joint line tenderness is also present, and one must examine the ulnar nerve and the ulnar groove as this may sometimes be involved in the injury.[15]

The most significant ligament injury of the elbow occurs in this ulnar collateral ligament (UCL). Studies have shown that a sprain or rupture here compromises medial stability in the elbow joint.[25] It has been found that the anterior oblique portion of the UCL is a primary stabilizer of the elbow, and that trauma to this ligament may significantly hinder normal elbow function. Thus, an accurate diagnosis indicating the degree of tear is important to determine appropriate treatment.[25] In severe cases, surgical intervention may be necessary to reestablish valgus stability where complete rupture has made the medial elbow unstable.[25]

The patient with significant opening should be placed in a posterior mold with the elbow in 90 degrees of flexion and referred. Because the elbow is a hinge joint, opening indicates a significant disruption of the joint capsule. When medial joint opening occurs, there may be an associated injury (stretch) of the brachial artery and this should always be checked.

The history and examination are crucial to diagnosing ulnar collateral ligament insufficiency in that there is usually tenderness medially over the ligament. The valgus stress test may demonstrate instability. Routine x rays may show calcification within the UCL or chronic traction spurs from repetitive stresses. As indicated, rest, ice, and anti-inflammatory medications are the mainstay of therapy.[27] In unusual cases, UCL may require repair and reconstruction.

☐ Distal Radioulnar Joint Injury

The primary function of the distal radioulnar joint is one of rotation.[6] Inflammatory disease of this joint is usually associated with generalized conditions such as rheumatoid arthritis or other collagen vascular diseases. Trauma can cause radioulnar joint subluxation or ligamentous tears, which may lead to instability. If the joint is unstable the distal radioulnar ligaments should be repaired and the joint should be immobilized with Kirschner-wire fixation.[33] In fractures of the distal radius and ulna which are complex (high-grade Colle's fractures) we recommend computed tomography (CT) scan and closed reduction with internal fixation or a limited open reduction with internal fixation and short-term external fixation if necessary.[6]

☐ Proximal Radioulnar Joint Injury

The mechanism for this injury has not been clearly defined with the exception of those which are related to proximal ulnar fractures. With severe radioulnar joint dysfunction, excision of the radial head has produced excellent long-term results in patients with radial head problems, but not radioulnar dissociation.[33] Unfortunately, patients who have had this procedure may experience instability of the distal radioulnar joint which presents with severe pain at the wrist. Thus, the authors recommend early referral of patients with proximal radioulnar joint dysfunction whether it be related to a

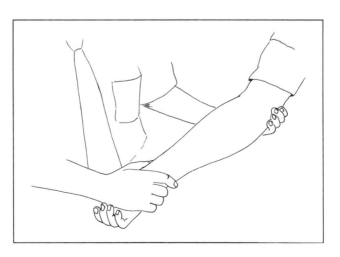

Figure 12–9. Stress test of the collateral ligaments of the elbow is shown.

traumatic event or otherwise as this is a complicated problem that requires careful evaluation and follow-up.[33]

☐ NEUROPATHIES

Compressive neuropathies can be subtle and are often overlooked in the upper extremity. These nerve injuries, as indicated in the Chapter 9, are classified into three types: neuropraxia, axonotmesis, and neurotmesis. Few of the lesions ever fit exclusively into one category.

Neuropraxia is the mildest form, which is characterized by reduced function but anatomic continuity within the nerve. This injury is caused by loss of axon excitability or segmental demyelination. This is the most common nerve injury. In axonotmesis, there is axonal injury and distal degeneration, with the connective tissue supporting the nerve structure remaining intact. In neurotmesis, there is complete disruption of the nerve.

☐ High Radial Nerve Palsy
Injury to the nerve above the elbow is unusual and usually secondary to trauma such as humeral fractures, crutch use, tourniquets, and so on. "Saturday night palsy" and other sources of traction or tortional injury cause this problem. Compression or injury in the spiral groove may be seen in injuries from gymnastics or wrestling. Compression may occur at the fibrous area around the origin of the lateral head of the triceps or at the intermuscular septum. In this compressive injury, a mixed motor and sensory involvement occurs. Conservative treatment will often result in complete recovery although the time required varies.[26] Surgical exploration of the radial nerve is indicated only when symptoms persist or there is evidence of degeneration.

☐ Radial Tunnel Syndrome
This is the most common compressive neuropathy of the radial nerve. There are five sites for compression, however afound the elbow only one is discussed, compression in the radial tunnel, including the fibrous band that lies at the entrance of the tunnel at the vessels that supply the brachioradialis, and a number of other sites. This condition can often be confused with lateral epicondylitis. These patients often complain of soreness and aching just distal to the lateral epicondyle over the extensor muscle mass. There is a chronic deep ache that is common at night. There is no true sensor involvement. Motor weakness is uncommon. What differentiates this from lateral epicondylitis is that in the patients with epicondylitis the pain is sharp and knifelike, whereas with radial tunnel syndrome the pain is a dull ache.[26] The patient with radial tunnel syndrome often exhibits pain with resisted supination of the extended forearm, which is made worse with wrist flexion.

Treatment consists of rest, anti-inflammatory drugs, and splinting for 3 to 6 months. If there is no improvement, surgical decompression may be indicated.

☐ Median Nerve Syndrome
There are a number of median nerve syndromes that occur in the forearm, only a few of which will be discussed here.

In *pronator syndrome*, there is a compression of the median nerve at any one of several sites at the elbow and proximal forearm. The first area is beneath the bicipital aponeurosis as the fascia is confluent with the pronator teres. The second site is at the level of the pronator teres as the nerve passes between the humeral and ulnar heads where fibrous bands within the muscle may cause the compression. This compression occurs where the median nerve passes below the thickened fibrous arch of the flexor digitorum superficialis.[26] This syndrome is seen in athletes whose sports require repetitive forceful pronation and gripping. Several clinical indicators help confirm the diagnosis of a pronator syndrome. Pain with resisted pronation when the elbow is extended and the wrist flexed to eliminate flexor digitorum superficialis suggests localization of compression within the pronator teres. One of the most sensitive tests for pronator syndrome is deep, direct palpation of the proximal forearm over the pronator teres with reproduction of symptoms. The workup should include x rays to look for a supercondylar process or electrodiagnostic studies. Initial management is rest of the muscles, especially from weight training, anti-inflammatory drugs, and occasional splinting. Surgical treatment is only necessary when the symptoms are refractory for 6 months or more.

Anterior interosseous nerve syndrome is uncommon and may present clinically as a vague pain or with activity-related proximal forearm pain with atrophy but no sensory changes. Motor weakness usually begins within a day after the pain is noted. Discussion of this and other uncommon syndromes is beyond the scope of this book. *Carpal tunnel syndrome* is discussed in Chapter 9.

☐ Ulnar Nerve Neuropathies
Cubital tunnel syndrome is an ulnar nerve entrapment syndrome near the elbow and is the second most common compressive neuropathy in the upper extremity. The nerve is vulnerable to compression, traction, and friction. Entrapment can occur in three areas. The first is within structures approximately 8 cm proximal to the medial epicondyle. A second area is in the ulnar groove of the medial epicondyle. The third, and most common, site is the cubital tunnel forearm distal to the medial epicondyle as the nerve passes between the two heads of the flexor carpi ulnaris. The act of throwing is often responsible for ulnar nerve entrapment at the elbow in the athlete. Cubital

tunnel syndrome is more often found in the throwing athlete but can be seen in a number of other sports injuries. Patients classically present with medial elbow and foream pain and paresthesias radiating into the ring and little fingers Motor findings are subtle. The patient may not a weak grip or early fatigue of the hand. the elbow flexion test may be used for reproducing symtpoms. [30] Nonoperative treatment consist of rest, ice, anti-inflammatory medications, and night splinting iwht the elbow at 45 degrees at flexion and the forearm in the neutral position. If this treatment regimen is unsuccessful, or test demonstrate a significant neuropathy, surgery may be indicated.

Ulnar tunnel syndrome is a compression of the ulnar nerve at the level of the wrist that may occur as the nerve enters the ulnar tunnel or as the deep branch curves around the hook of the hamate in the palm. The predominant mechanism is direct compression. This injury occurs in cyclers and others who have compression in this area. This lesion represents a motor, sensory, and mixed palsy. Fixed deficits are rare but the characteristic lesion is an ulnar claw hand. Treatment is usually nonsurgical, involving adjusting hand positions with the sport, splinting, and anti-inflammatory drugs.

FOREARM INJURIES

Most injuries of the forearm involve the elbow or the wrist and the hand (see Chap. 9) and are discussed in those sections. The forearm functions as a conduit on which the muscles of the hand course.

☐ CONTUSIONS

The tendons of the lower forearm are close to the skin and *traumatic tenosynovitis* can occur after a direct blow. The treatment for this condition is simple immobilization. Contusions of the upper forearm are treated the same as contusions elsewhere.

☐ STRAINS

The muscles of the forearm are closely interconnected in the same sheath and a strain of one muscle often causes discomfort with motion of other nearby muscles, making it difficult to isolate individual strains. This is usually due to overuse.[13, 16] On examination, the patient will demonstrate swelling and inflammation of the tendon, which is painful to stress and tender to palpation. The treatment consists of ice compresses followed by local heat and immobilization.

☐ COMMON COMPARTMENT SYNDROMES

The leg is by far the most common site of compartment syndromes in athletes and following injuries. The thigh, forearm, and foot are the next most common sites. It is of critical importance that emergency physicians be aware of this problem in the upper extremity.

The mechanism of injury that leads to the development of compartment syndromes can vary. Anything that causes swelling and edema within a compartment space can cause compartment syndrome. The fascia enveloping the compartment has limited space for expansion and swelling causes intercompartmental pressure to rise. Common causes are tight dressings, localized external pressure, and application of excessive traction to a fractured limb.[24] All of these lead to a decrease in the compartment space. Causes associated with an increase in compartment space include bleeding, postischemic swelling, intense use of muscles following exercise, seizures, trauma from a fracture or contusion, and reduction and fixation of fractures. Exercise can lead to increased capillary pressure and may also lead to this syndrome.[14]

Clinical Presentation

Knowledge of the anatomical compartments and their components is essential to make the diagnosis. The following listing gives the physician critical information about the upper extremity:

- Deltoid muscle—posterior humeral circumflex artery and axillary nerve
- Volar forearm—flexor carpi ulnaris, flexor carpi radialis, pronator teres, flexor digitorum superficialis and profundus, flexor pollicis longus, and pronator lquadratus; radial and ulnar artery and medial and ulnar nerve
- Dorsal forearm—extensor digitorum communis, extensor carpi ulnaris, abductor pollicis longus, extensor pollicis longus, extensor pollicis brevis; no artery; radial nerve

The clinical presentation involves the following sequence:

1. *Severe pain* is the first and most important symptom to occur. The pain is usually out of proportion to the severity of the injury.
2. Intercompartmental pressure will rise and lead to a palpably tense compartment. This is one of the earliest objective signs.
3. Pain with passive stretch may be present but can be confusing depending upon the injury or problem. This is also accompanied by pain on active movement of the muscles within the compartment.
4. Paresis and parethesias develop later in the syndrome. By this time, often some element of muscle necrosis may have begun.
5. Pulses may be reduced or absent. This is an ominous finding that occurs late in the development of this syndrome.

Ultimately, the diagnosis of compartment syndrome is confirmed by measuring intercompartmental pressures. The best way to do this with items that are readily available in any emergency department is discussed in Chapter 8. There are also other devices readily available in many hospitals to measure compartment pressures rapidly. The normal intercompsart- mental pressure is between 0 and 8 mm Hg. The level of elevated pressure considered significant and demanding immediate surgical intervention is debated in the literature.[14] However, most authors agree that a pressure is greater than 30 mm Hg, is quite significant. Some feel that a pressure of between 40 to 55 mm Hg is necessary before surgical intervention should be considered.[14]

Treatment

Surgical and nonsurgical treatments are considered. In an acute compartment syndrome, complete opening of all tight fascial envelopes is necessary. All restricted clothing, braces, and casts, should be removed. The extremities should not be elevated but rather placed at heart level to optimize arterial pressure and venous drainage.[14] When measuring compartmental pressures, the white sides techniques is quick and easy and can be performed with equipment readily available in any emergency department. This technique is discussed in detail in Chapter 28, as indicated above.

REFERENCES

1. Bell SN, Morrey BF, Bianco JR, Shounfield AJ: Chronic posterior subluxation and dislocation of the radial head. *J Bone Joint Surg* **73A**(3):154, 1991.
2. Boyd HB, McLeod AD: Tennis elbow. *J Bone Joint Surg* **55**(6):1183, 1973.
3. Coonrad RW, Hooper WR: Tennis elbow: Its course, natural history conservative and surgical management. *J Bone Joint Surg* **55**(6):1177, 1973.
4. Curl WW: Office treatment of elbow injuries in the athlete. In: Sports, Exercise, Overuse Injuries. *Instr Course Lect* **43**:55–61, 1995.
5. Doran A, Gresham GA, Rushton N, et al: Tennis elbow. *Acta Orthop Scand* **61**(6):535, 1990.
6. Drobner WS, Hausman MR: The distal radioulnar joint: Ligament injuries in the wrist and hand. *J Emerg Med* **8**(4), 1992.
7. Duringm, et al: The operative treatment of elbow dislocation in the adult *J Bone Joint Surg* **61**(2):239, 1979.
8. Ellman H: Anterior angulation deformity of the radial head. *J Bone Joint Surg* **57**(6):776, 1975.
9. Field LD, Altchek DW: Elbow injuries. *Clin Sports Med* **14**:1, 1995.
10. Gill TJ, Micheli LJ: The immature athlete: Common injuries and overuse syndromes of the elbow and wrist. *Clin Sports Med* **15**:2, 1996.
11. Griggs SM, et al: Bony injuries of the wrist, forearm, and elbow. *Clin Sports Med* **15**:2, 1996.
12. Ho G, Tice A: Septis bursitis in the prepatellar and olecranon bursae *Ann Intern Med* **89**:21, 1978.
13. Hotchkiss RN: Injuries to the interosseous ligament of the forearm. *Hand Clin* **10**:3, 1994.
14. Johnston J, et al: Elbow injuries to the throwing athlete. *Clin Sports Med* **15**:2, 1996.
15. Kibler WB: Pathophysiology of overload injuries around the elbow. *Clin Sports Med* **14**:2, 1995.
16. Kohn HS: Prevention and treatment of elbow injuries in golf. *Clin Sports Med* **15**:1, 1996.
17. Leach RE, Wasilewski S: Olecranon bursitis. *J Sports Med* **7**(5):299, 1979.
18. Linscheild RI, Wheeler DK: Elbow dislocations. *JAMA* **1949**(11):806, 1969.
19. Lloyd R, Bucknill TM: Anterior dislocation of the radial head in children. *J Bone Joint Surg* [Br] **59**(4):402, 1977.
20. Louis DS, et al: Arterial injury: A complication of posterior elbow dislocation. *J Bone Joint Surg* **56**(8):1631, 1974.
21. Moray FR: Passive motion of the elbow joint. *J Bone Joint Surg* **58**(4):501, 1976.
22. Nirschl RP, Pettrone FA: Tennis elbow. *J Bone Joint Surg* **61**(6):832, 1979.
23. Omer GE: Injuries to nerves of the upper extremity. *J Bone Joint Surg* **56**(8):1615, 1974.
24. Patten RM: Overuse syndromes and injuries involving the elbow: MR imaging findings. *AJR* **164**:1205–1211, 1995.
25. Pincivero DM, et al: Medical elbow stability: Clinical implications *Sports Med* **18**(2):141–148, 1994.
26. Plancher KD, et al: Compressive neuropathies and tendinopathies in the athletic elbow and wrist. *Clin Sports Med* **15**:2, 1996.
27. Rettig AC, Patel DV: Epidemiology of elbow, forearm, and wrist injuries in the athlete. *Clin Sports Med* **14**:2, 1995.
28. Roberts PH: Dislocation of the elbow. *J Bone Joint Surg* [Br] **56**(11):806, 1969.
29. Royle SG: Posterior dislocation of the elbow. *Clin Orthop* **269**(8):201, 1991.
30. Safran MR: Elbow injuries in athletes: A review. *Clin Orthop Rel Res* **310**:257–277, 1995.

31. Schunk JE: Radial head subluxation: Epidemiology and treatment of 87 episodes. *Ann Emerg Med* **19**(9):1019, 1990.
32. Sofia IM: Radiological sign of entrapment of the median nerve in the elbow joint after posterior dislocation. *J Bone Joint Surg* [Br] **58**(3):353, 1976..
33. Trousdale RT, Amadio PC, Cooney WP, et al: Radioulnar dissociation. *J Bone Joint Surg* **74A:**1486, 1992.

BIBLIOGRAPHY

Amir D, Frankl U, Pogrund H (Eng.): Pulled elbow and hyper-mobility of joints. *Clin Orthop* **257:**94–99, 1990.
Braun, RM: The distal joint of the radius and ulna (diagnostic studies and treatment rationale). *J Bone Joint Surg* **74A:**74–78, 1992.

13
CHAPTER

FRACTURES OF THE HUMERAL SHAFT

HUMERAL SHAFT FRACTURES

CLASS A: NONDISPLACED OR MINIMALLY DISPLACED FRACTURES
(p. 269)

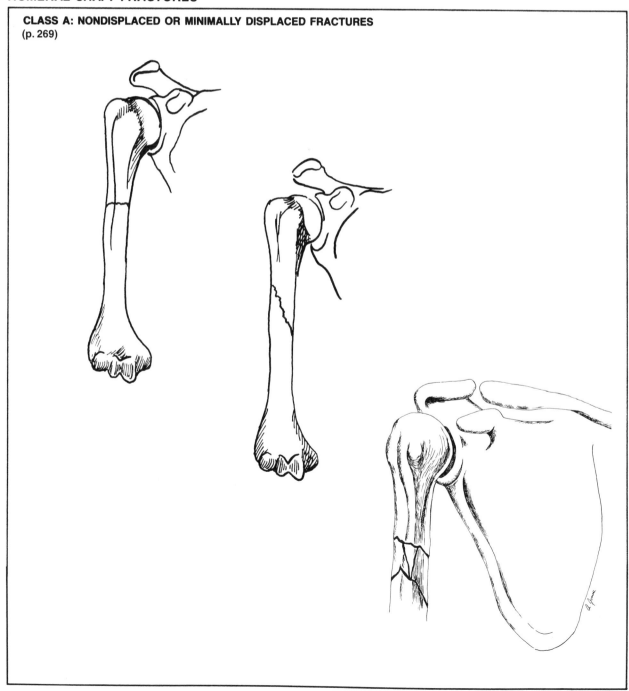

CLASS B: DISPLACED OR ANGULATED FRACTURES
(p. 271)

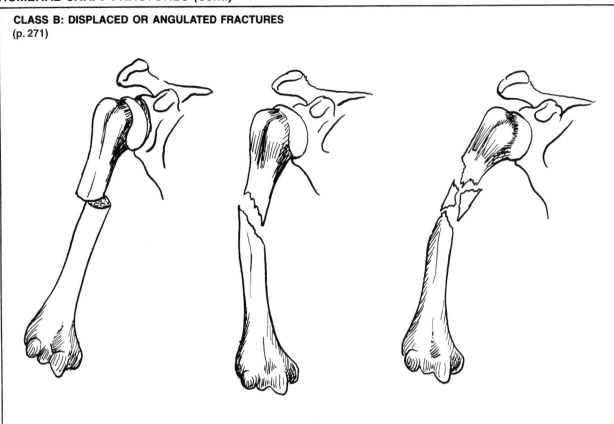

CLASS C: SEVERELY DISPLACED FRACTURES OR ASSOCIATED WITH NEUROVASCULAR DAMAGE
(p. 271)

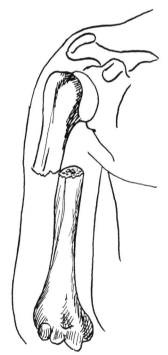

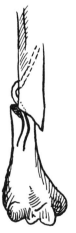

Displaced with
soft tissue interposed

Spiral fracture of
the distal one-third
with radial nerve injury

The humeral shaft extends from the insertion of the *pectoralis major* to the *supracondylar ridges*. Humeral shaft fractures are most frequently seen in patients more than 50 years of age and usually involve the middle third of the shaft. There are four basic patterns commonly seen with humeral shaft fractures.

1. Transverse
2. Oblique
3. Spiral
4. Comminuted

The type of fracture is dependent on the mechanism of injury, the force of injury, the location of the fracture, and the muscular tone at the time of injury. Each of the above fracture patterns may be further classified based on the amount of displacement.

Essential Anatomy

The extensive musculature surrounding the humeral shaft may result in distraction and displacement of the bony fragments after a fracture. As shown in Figure 13–1, the deltoid inserts along the anterolateral humeral shaft, whereas the *pectoralis major* inserts on the medial inter-tubercular groove. The supraspinatus inserts into the greater tuberosity of the humeral head, resulting in abduction and external rotation. The *biceps* and the *triceps* insert distally and tend to displace the distal fragment superiorly. A fracture proximal to the pectoralis major insertion may be accompanied by abduction and external rotation of the humeral head because of the action of the supraspinatus. A fracture between the insertion of the pectoralis major and the deltoid will usually result in adduction of the proximal fragment secondary to the pull of the pectoralis major. Fractures distal to the deltoid insertion usually result in abduction of the proximal fragment secondary to the pull of the deltoid muscle.

The neurovascular bundle, which supplies the forearm and the hand, extends along the medial border of the humeral shaft.[11] Although it is true that any of these structures may be injured with a fracture, the most commonly injured is the *radial nerve*.[6,11] As shown in Figure 13–2, the radial nerve lies in close proximity to the humeral shaft at the junction of its middle and distal third. Fractures in this area are often accompanied by radial nerve impairment.

Mechanism of Injury

There are several mechanisms that result in humeral shaft fractures. The most common mechanism of injury

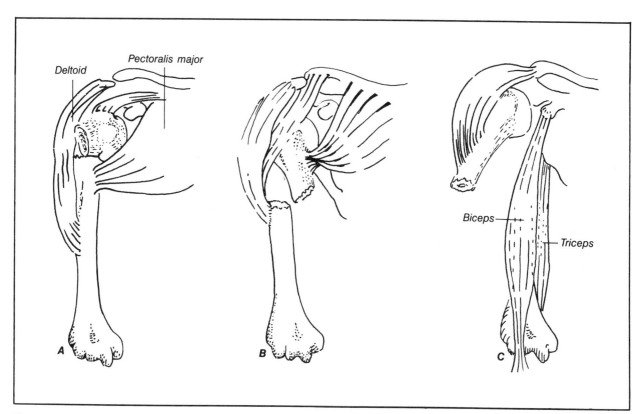

Figure 13–1. In humeral shaft fractures, the muscles of the proximal humerus cause displacement of the fracture fragments. Five muscles play a major role in displacing fractures in this region: the deltoid, supraspinatus, pectoralis major, biceps, and triceps. **A.** In fractures between the rotator cuff and the pectoralis major, abduction and rotation of the proximal fragment occur. **B.** Fractures occurring between the pectoralis major insertion and the insertion of the deltoid are associated with adduction deformity of the proximal fragment. **C.** Fractures occurring below the deltoid insertion are associated with abduction of the proximal fragment.

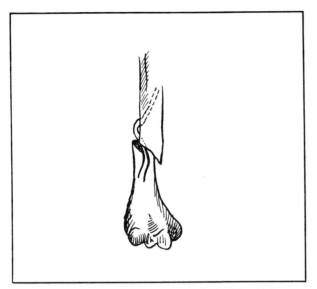

Figure 13-2. The radial nerve courses in the lateral intermuscular septum along the lateral aspect of the humerus and can be involved in fractures of the shaft.

is direct force usually resulting from a fall or direct blow as during an automobile accident.[2] Typically, a transverse fracture is diagnosed.

An indirect mechanism involves a fall on the elbow or outstretched arm. In addition, a violent contraction in an area of pathologically weakened bone may result in a fracture. The indirect mechanism usually results in a spiral fracture.[3,10]

Recent studies have revealed a third cause of humeral shaft fractures. This involves overzealous reaming or impaction during the secure fitting of a humeral prosthesis.[1]

Examination

The patient will present with pain and swelling over the area of the humeral shaft. On examination, shortening, obvious deformity, or abnormal mobility with crepitation may be detected. It is imperative that a thorough neurovascular examination accompany the initial assessment of all humeral shaft fractures. The examination should emphasize the function of the radial nerve and document the time of onset should neurovascular damage be detected.[6]

1. Damage at the time of injury is usually a neurapraxia, which is usually treated with a suspension splint and close follow-up.
2. Damage detected after manipulation or immobilization may lead to axonotmesis if the pressure is not relieved.
3. Damage detected during healing is typically due to a slowly progressive axonotmesis.

X Ray

Perpendicular anteroposterior (AP) and lateral views of the entire humerus are essential. Shoulder and elbow views should be included to exclude accompanying injuries.

Associated Injuries

Humeral shaft fractures may be associated with several significant injuries:[2,3,8,11]

1. Brachial artery damage
2. Neural damage (radial, ulnar, or median)
3. Associated shoulder or distal humeral fracture

Treatment

Humeral shaft fractures may be treated by several methods depending on the type of fracture, the amount of displacement, and the presence of associated injuries.[9,10] If the brachial plexus is injured, the soft tissue sleeve surrounding the muscles of the arm will lose its stability.[5] It will now become difficult to maintain an alignment since gravity will distract the ends of the fracture.[2] Therefore, consultation with an orthopedic surgeon early in the management of these fractures is strongly recommended. Humeral shaft fractures generally take from 10 to 12 weeks for healing. Spiral fractures generally heal faster than transverse fractures because of the larger surface area. Fractures close to the elbow or the shoulder are associated with longer healing periods and poorer results.

Classification

Nondisplaced and displaced fractures of the humeral shaft.

HUMERAL SHAFT FRACTURES

☐ Class A: Nondisplaced or minimally displaced fractures (Fig. 13-3)

☐ Class B: Displaced or angulated fractures (Fig. 13-5)

☐ Class C: Severely displaced fractures with interposed soft tissues or associated with neurovascular damage (Fig. 13-6)

□ CLASS A: NONDISPLACED OR MINIMALLY DISPLACED FRACTURES (FIG. 13–3)

The emergency management of these fractures includes ice, analgesics, and application of a coaptation splint with early referral (Fig. 13–4).[9,10] The splint is applied by first applying tincture of benzoin followed by padding to the arm. Next, U-shaped splints extending from the axilla to the elbow to the acromion process are applied and secured with a kling dressing. A collar and cuff or sling and swathe support is then applied. A hanging cast should not be used as the weight of the plaster might result in distraction of the fragments.

□ CLASS B: DISPLACED OR ANGULATED FRACTURES (FIG. 13–5)

The emergency management of these fractures includes ice, analgesics, immobilization, and emergent referral.

The therapy selected is controversial and varies from a hanging cast to olecranon pin traction.[7–10] If there is no accompanying neurovascular damage and the patient is ambulatory without other fractures, the authors prefer a hanging cast for the management of these injuries.[4,7] If emergent orthopedic referral is not available, the cast may be applied by the emergency physician. The cast should extend only 1 inch proximal to the fracture line and should be lightweight, using only two rolls of 4-inch plaster. The forearm should be in a neutral position with the elbow in 90 degrees of flexion. The cast is suspended from the neck in a collar and cuff fashion. The loop's position is determined by the angulation, which must be corrected. Lateral angulation requires placement of the loop on the dorsum of the wrist, whereas medial angulation requires that the loop be placed on the volar aspect of the wrist. Posterior angulation is corrected by lengthening the sling. The correction of anterior angulation requires shortening of the sling.[4,7] The arm must remain dependent at all times requiring the patient to sleep in a semirecumbent position. The patient should begin

HUMERAL SHAFT FRACTURES

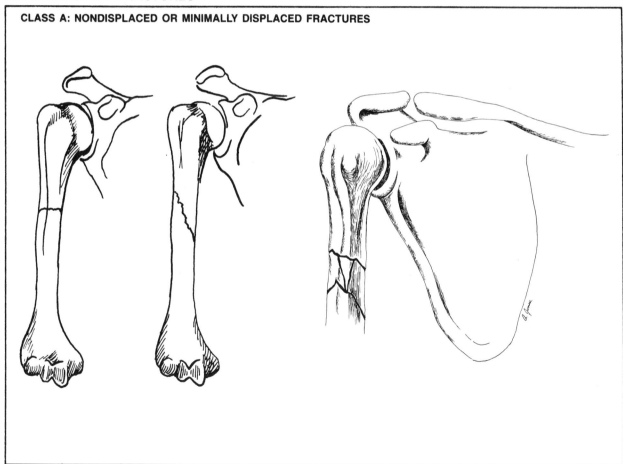

CLASS A: NONDISPLACED OR MINIMALLY DISPLACED FRACTURES

Figure 13–3.

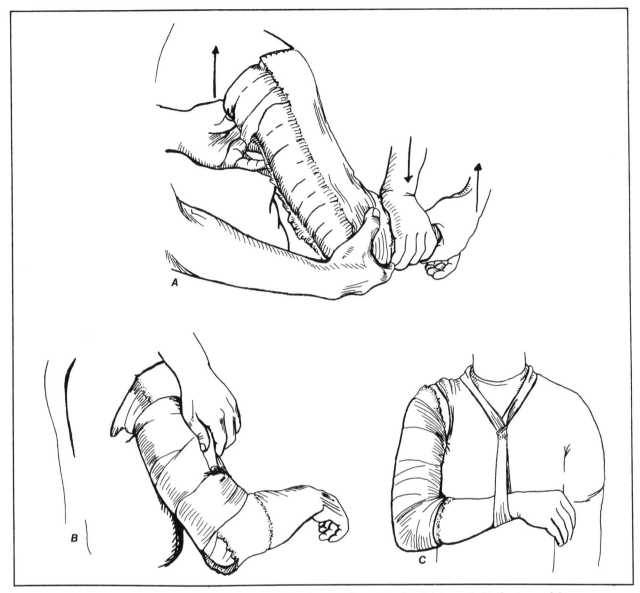

Figure 13–4. A U-shaped coaptation splint, sometimes re-ferred to as a "sugar-tong" splint, is applied to fractures of the humeral shaft to maintain reduction. The arm is then suspended at the wrist from the neck in a collar and cuff apparatus.

hand exercises immediately with shoulder circumduction ex-ercises as soon as pain permits.

□ CLASS C: SEVERELY DISPLACED FRACTURES OR FRACTURES ASSOCIATED WITH NEUROVASCULAR DAMAGE (FIG. 13–6)

The emergency management of these fractures includes ice, analgesics, immobilization, and emergent referral. Operative management of humeral shaft fractures is indicated under the following circumstances:[4,9,10]

1. Humeral shaft fracture with vascular compromise

2. Spiral fracture of the distal third with a radial nerve palsy
3. Associated fractures that require early mobilization such as an elbow fracture
4. The presence of interposed soft tissues that cannot be reduced by other means
5. Injuries to the ipsilateral brachial plexus that require compression plating

Complications
Humeral shaft fractures may be followed by the development of several significant complications.

1. The development of shoulder adhesive capsulitis may be prevented by early circumduction exercises.

HUMERAL SHAFT FRACTURES

CLASS B: DISPLACED OR ANGULATED FRACTURES

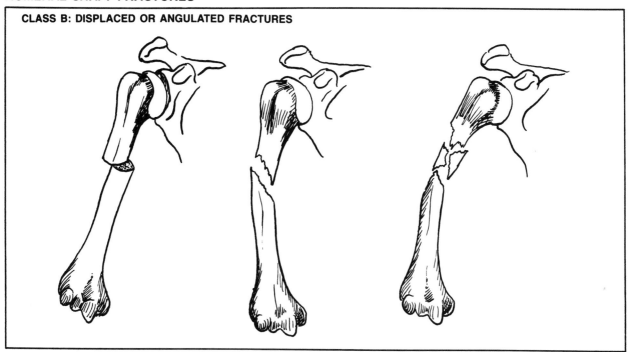

Figure 13-5.

HUMERAL SHAFT FRACTURES

CLASS C: SEVERELY DISPLACED FRACTURES OR FRACTURES ASSOCIATED WITH NEUROVASCULAR DAMAGE

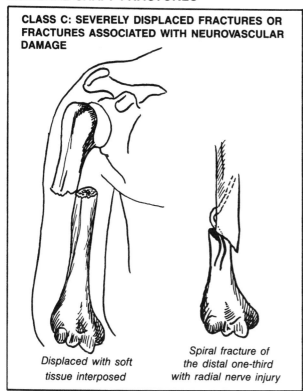

Displaced with soft
tissue interposed

Spiral fracture of
the distal one-third
with radial nerve injury

Figure 13-6. Displaced fractures of the humeral shaft may have soft tissue interposed between the fracture fragments. A spiral fracture of the distal third may have radial nerve entrapment, and this must be examined for before any manipulation.

2. Myositis ossificans of the elbow may develop. This can be avoided by using active routine exercises and not passive stretching.
3. The delayed development of radial nerve palsies complicates 5 to 10 percent of all humeral shaft fractures. This is especially common in spiral fractures of the distal third.
4. Nonunion or delayed union may complicate the management of these fractures.

REFERENCES

1. Bonutti PM, Hawkins RJ: Fracture of the humeral shaft associated with total replacement arthroplasty of the shoulder. *J Bone Joint Surg* **4:**617–618, 1992.
2. Brien WW, Gellmann H, Becker AM, et al: Management of fractures of the humerus in patients who have an injury of the ipsilateral brachial plexus. *J Bone Joint Surg* **8:**1208–1210, 1990.
3. Charnley J: *The Closed Treatment of Common Fractures*, 3rd ed. Baltimore: Williams & Wilkins, 1972.
4. Christensen S: Humeral shaft fractures, operative and conservative treatment. *Acta Chir Scand* **133:**455, 1967.
5. Holm CL: Management of humeral shaft fractures. Fundamentals of non operative techniques. *Clin Orthop* **71:**132, 1970.
6. Holstein A, Lewis GB: Fractures of the humerus with radial nerve paralysis. *J Bone Joint Surg* **45:**1382, 1963.
7. Hudson RT: The use of the hanging cast in treatment of fractures of the humerus. *South Surgeon* **10:**132, 1941.

8. Mann R, Neal EG: Fractures of the shaft of the humerus in adults. *South Med J* **58:**264, 1965.

9. Stewart MJ, Handley JM: Fractures of the humerus. A comparative study of methods in treatment. *J Bone Joint Surg* **37:**681, 1955.

10. Stewart MJ, Hawkins RJ: Fractures of the humeral shaft. In Adams JP (Ed.): *Current Practice in Orthopaedic Surgery.* St Louis: Mosby, 1964.

11. Whitson RO: Relation of the radial nerve to the shaft of the humerus. *J Bone Joint Surg* **36:**85, 1954.

14
CHAPTER
FRACTURES OF THE PROXIMAL HUMERUS

SURGICAL NECK FRACTURES

CLASS A: IMPACTED FRACTURES WITH ANGULATION
(p. 285)

Type I: Minimal angulation (<45°)

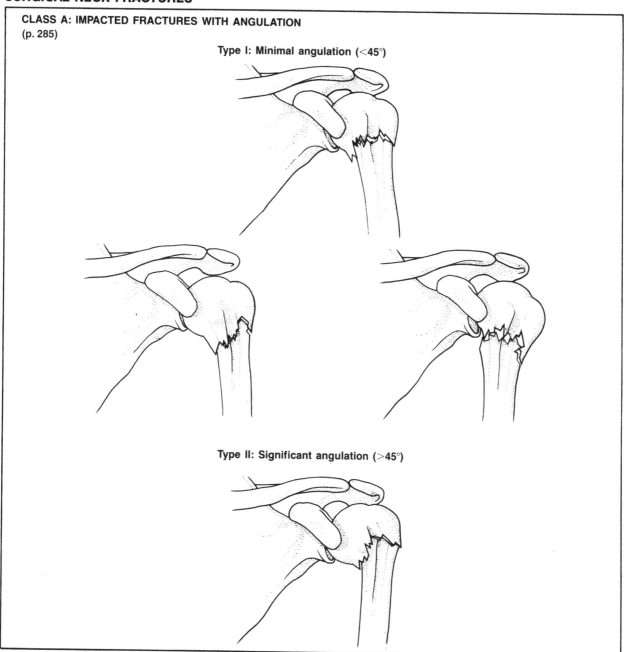

Type II: Significant angulation (>45°)

SURGICAL NECK FRACTURES (cont.)

CLASS B: DISPLACED FRACTURES
(p. 286)

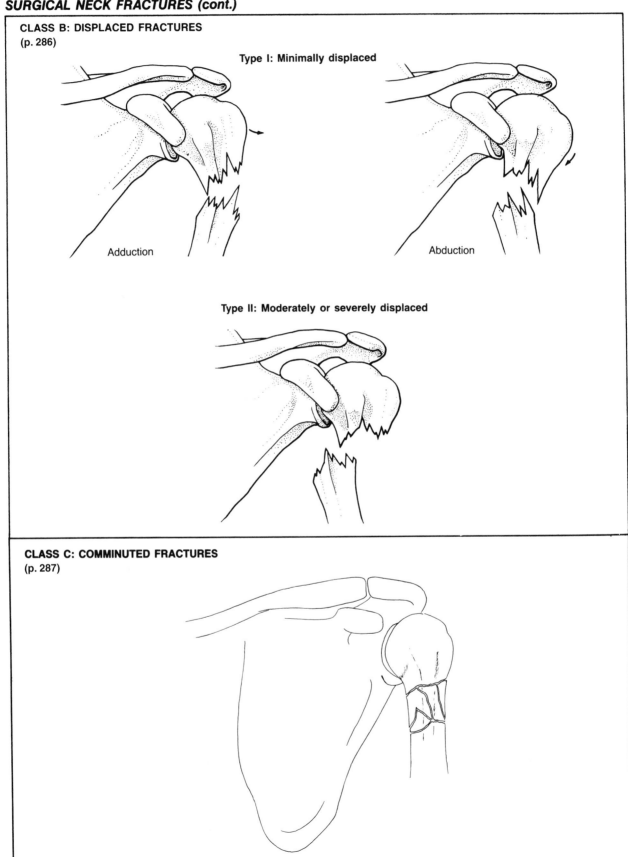

Type I: Minimally displaced

Adduction

Abduction

Type II: Moderately or severely displaced

CLASS C: COMMINUTED FRACTURES
(p. 287)

ANATOMIC NECK FRACTURES (EPIPHYSIS)

CLASS A: NONDISPLACED FRACTURE
(p. 289)

CLASS B: DISPLACED FRACTURE

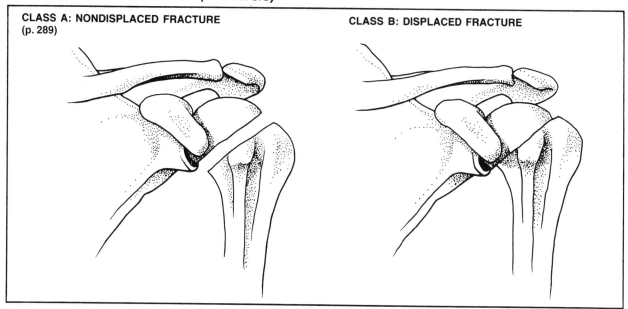

GREATER TUBEROSITY FRACTURES

CLASS A: NONDISPLACED FRACTURES
(p.290)

Type I: Compression fracture

Type II: Nondisplaced fracture

CLASS B: DISPLACED FRACTURES

Type I

Type II

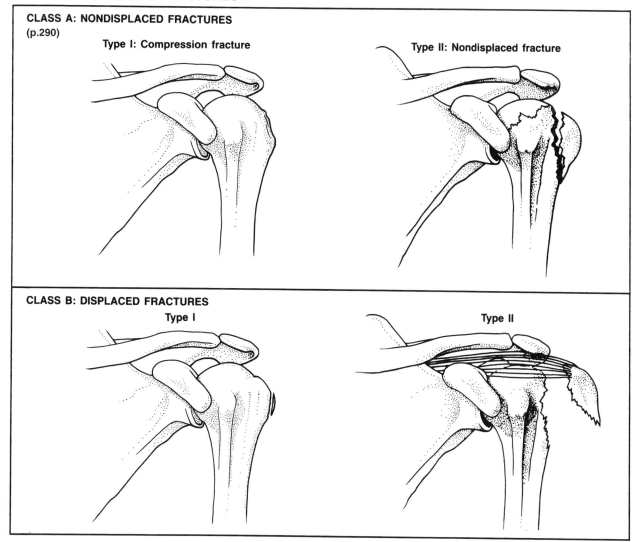

LESSER TUBEROSITY FRACTURES

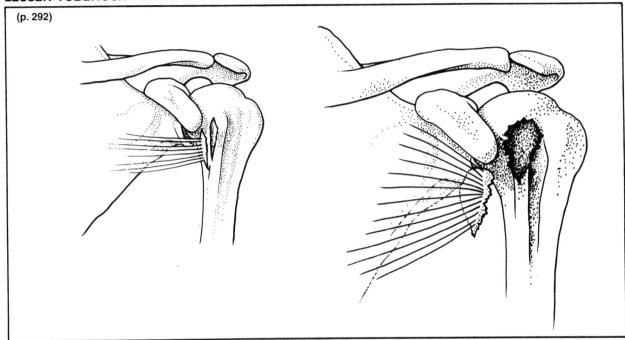

(p. 292)

COMBINATION FRACTURES

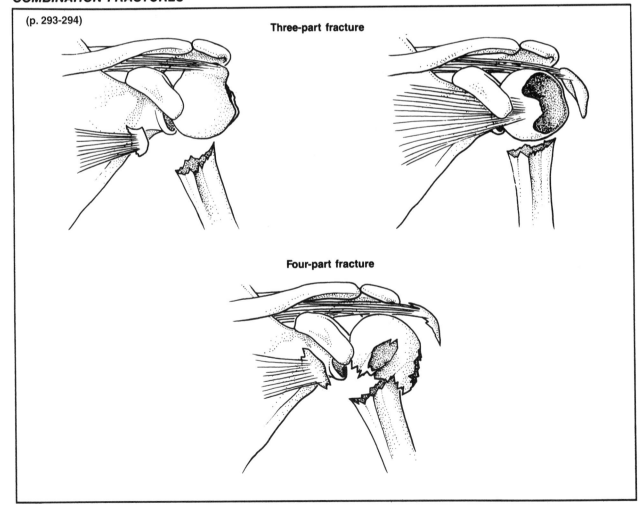

(p. 293-294)

Three-part fracture

Four-part fracture

ARTICULAR SURFACE FRACTURES

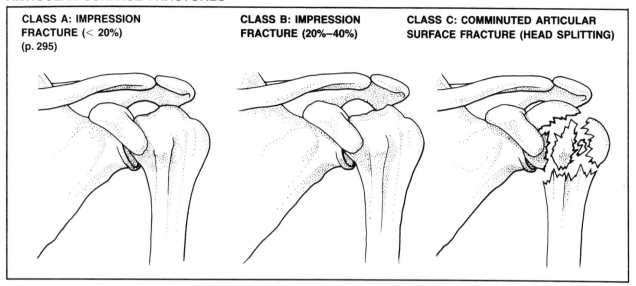

| CLASS A: IMPRESSION FRACTURE (< 20%) (p. 295) | CLASS B: IMPRESSION FRACTURE (20%–40%) | CLASS C: COMMINUTED ARTICULAR SURFACE FRACTURE (HEAD SPLITTING) |

Proximal humeral fractures account for 5 percent of all fractures and are most commonly seen in the elderly patient.[7] Anatomically, proximal humeral fractures include all humeral fractures proximal to the surgical neck. The classification system used in this text was developed by Neer.[4,5] Using the Neer system the proximal humerus is divided into four segments (Fig. 14–1):

1. Greater tuberosity
2. Lesser tuberosity
3. Anatomic neck
4. Surgical neck

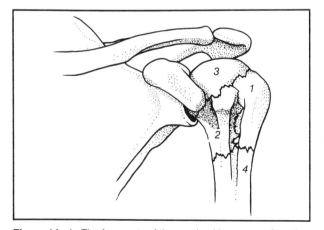

Figure 14–1. The four parts of the proximal humerus referred to in the Neer classification of fractures of this region, which include the greater tuberosity (1), lesser tuberosity (2), anatomic neck (3), and surgical neck (4). Fractures are classified according to displacement of one or more of the "parts" from the remainder. Displacement is defined as separation of greater than 1 cm from the humerus or angulation of the part greater than 45 degrees.

This classification system has both prognostic and therapeutic implications and is dependent only on the relationship of the bone segments involved and their displacement.

After injury, if all of the proximal humeral fragments are nondisplaced and without angulation the injury would be classified as a *one-part fracture*. If a fragment has more than 1 cm of displacement or angulation of over 45 degrees from the remaining intact proximal humerus the fracture is classified as a *two-part fracture*. If two fragments are individually displaced from the remaining proximal humerus the fracture is classified as a *three-part fracture*. Finally, if all four fragments are individually displaced, the fracture is a *four-part fracture*. A fragment of bone containing two segments that is displaced from the proximal humerus would be classified as a *two-part fracture*. It is important to recall that displacement is based on the separation of fragments by more than 1 cm or angulation of over 45 degrees. Figures 14–2 and 14–3 diagrammatically summarize the Neer classification system of proximal humeral fractures. Note that three- and four-part fractures are often associated with a dislocation. Articular surface fractures are not included in the Neer system and will be discussed separately at the end of the chapter.

Nearly 80 percent of all proximal humeral fractures are one-part fractures.[4] The humeral fragments are held in place by the periosteum, the rotator cuff, and the joint capsule. The initial stabilization and management of these fractures should be initiated by the emergency physician. The remaining 20 percent of proximal humeral fractures are typically two-, three-, or four-part fractures.[4,5] These fractures require reduction and may remain unstable after reduction.

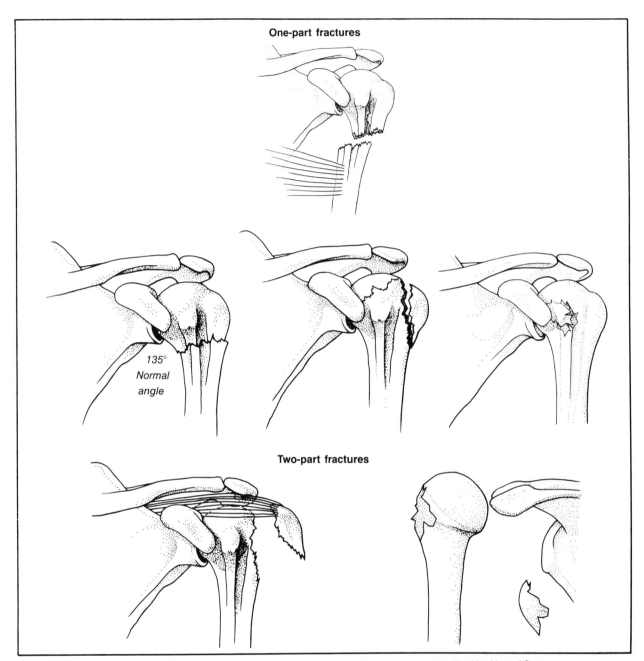

Figure 14–2. Examples of one-, two-, three-, and four-part fractures as described by Neer. (*Cont.*)

Essential Anatomy

To understand the mechanism of proximal humeral fractures and their displacement tendencies, a knowledge of the essential anatomy is necessary.

The bony anatomy of the proximal humerus is illustrated in Figure 14–3. The *articular surface* articulates with the glenoid forming the *glenohumeral joint*.

The articular surface ends at the *anatomic neck*; therefore, fractures located proximal to the anatomic neck are considered articular surface fractures. The surgical neck is the narrowed portion of the proximal humerus distal to the anatomic neck. The *greater* and *lesser tuberosities* are bony prominences located just distal to the anatomic neck.

There are several muscles that insert on and surround the proximal humerus. The muscles of the *rotator cuff* include the *supraspinatus*, the *infraspinatus*, and the *teres minor*. The musculature of the rotator cuff inserts on the greater tuberosity. Rotator cuff muscles tend to pull fracture fragments in a superior direction with some anterior rotation. The *subscapularis* muscle inserts on the *lesser tuberosity*. This muscle tends to pull fracture fragments in a medial direction with posterior rotation. The *pectoralis major* muscle inserts on the

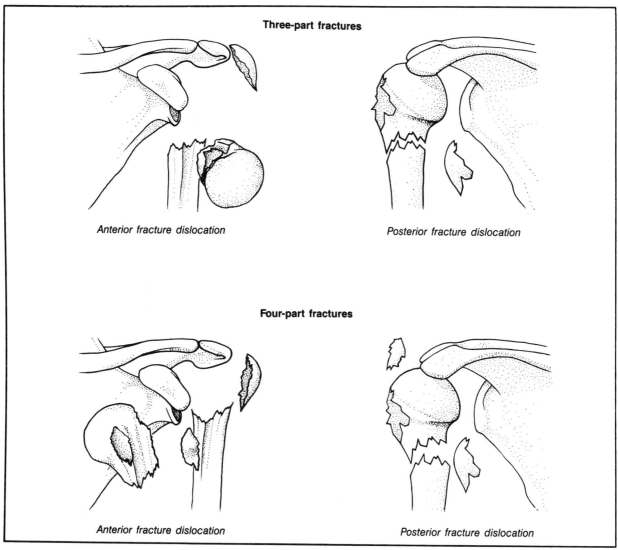

Figure 14-2. (*Cont.*)

lateral lip of the intertubercular groove whereas the *deltoid muscle* inserts on the *deltoid tubercle*. Both insert distal to the surgical neck and, therefore, are not part of the proximal humerus. These muscles tend to exert medial and superior forces, respectively, on the shaft after proximal humeral fractures.

The neurovascular structures of the proximal humerus are diagrammed in Figure 14-4. It is important to note the close relationships between the *brachial plexus*, the *axillary nerve*, and the *axillary artery* to the proximal humerus. Neurovascular injuries frequently accompany proximal humeral fractures.

Mechanism of Injury

There are two mechanisms that commonly result in proximal humeral fractures. A direct blow on the lateral aspect of the arm such as during a fall may result in a fracture. The indirect mechanism is more common

and is usually secondary to a fall on the outstretched arm.[1]

The position of the humeral shaft after an indirect fracture is dependent on the position of the arm before the fracture. Abduction fractures, where the distal humeral segment is abducted, occur after a fall on the outstretched abducted arm. Adduction fractures, where the distal humeral segment is adducted, occur after a fall on the outstretched adducted arm. The position and type of fracture of the proximal fragments is dependent on four factors:

1. The fracture force determines the severity of the fracture and to some extent its displacement.
2. Humeral rotation at the time of impact determines the fracture type.
3. The muscular tone and balance at the time of impact determine the amount of displacement.

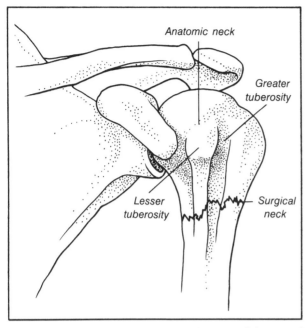

Figure 14–3. Anatomy of the proximal humerus. A fracture of the surgical neck is shown.

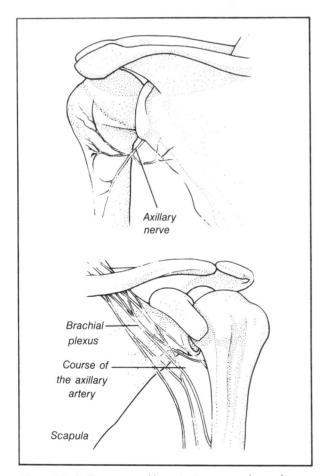

Figure 14–4. The course of important nerves and vessels considered in discussions of fractures of the proximal humerus.

4. The age of the patient determines the location of the fracture.
   a. Young children with *open epiphyses* usually suffer epiphyseal separation rather than fractures.
   b. Adolescents with *ossified epiphyses* have very strong bones and, thus, have a tendency to develop dislocations sometimes accompanied by fractures.
   c. Elderly patients have weak bones and have a tendency to suffer fractures.

X Ray (Fig. 14–5)

The *trauma series* recommended by Neer[4] is very helpful in evaluating proximal humeral trauma (Fig. 14–6). In addition, the authors recommend an anteroposterior (AP) internal rotation view as well as an axillary projection (Fig. 14–7). These four views permit full evaluation of the shoulder and the proximal humerus including the articular surface. These films may be obtained with the patient supine, standing or sitting, although the authors recommend the sitting position.

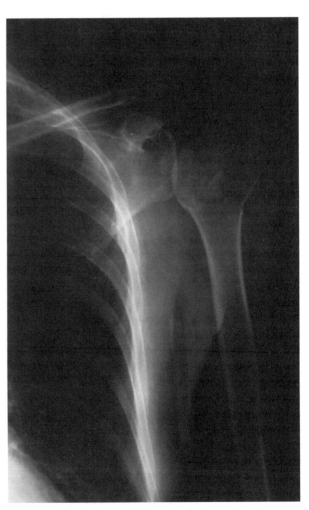

Figure 14–5. Comminuted fracture of the proximal humerus without displacement.

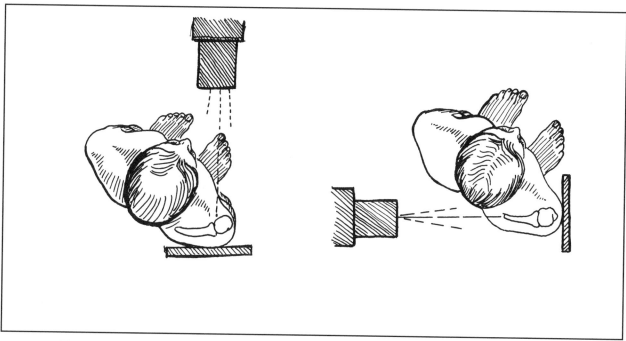

Figure 14–6. The trauma series recommended by Neer is very helpful in evaluating proximal humeral trauma.

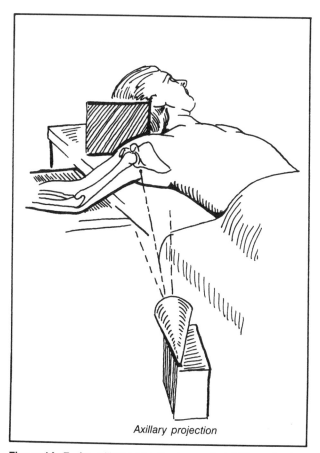

Axillary projection

Figure 14–7. An axillary projection is very helpful in evaluating the shoulder and the proximal humerus including the articular surface. The x ray tube is near the hip area and the film is held above the patient's shoulder.

Intra-articular fractures are associated with a hemarthrosis that may displace the humeral head inferiorly. Radiographically this is referred to as a *pseudosubluxation*, indicating the presence of an intra-articular fracture.

An additional radiographic sign indicating an intra-articular fracture is the presence of a *fat fluid line*.

Treatment

The therapy for proximal humeral fractures may vary depending on the age of the patient and his or her life style.

Axiom: *Successful treatment of proximal humeral fractures is dependent on early mobility. A compromise in anatomic reduction may be accepted so that prolonged immobilization can be avoided.*

One-part fractures which comprise 80 percent of all proximal fractures, may be treated with a *sling and swathe* (Fig. 14–8). Early passive exercises, as shown in Figure 14–9 are generally recommended. Active exercises are recommended during the later stages of healing.

Classification

Proximal humeral fractures are classified on the basis of anatomic as well as therapeutic principles.

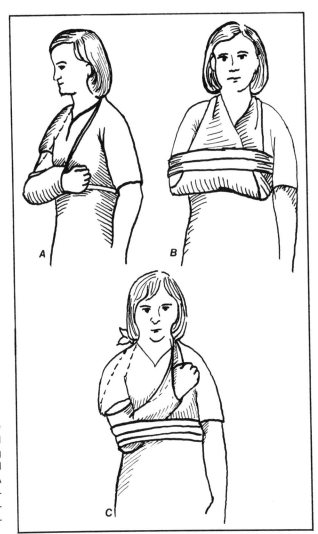

Figure 14-8. *A.* A sling and swathe manufactured for proximal humeral fracture immobilization. ***B.*** A sling and swathe made with a commercial sling and an elastic bandage. ***C.*** A Valpeau and swathe used for unstable surgical neck fractures. This position permits relaxation of the pectoralis major.

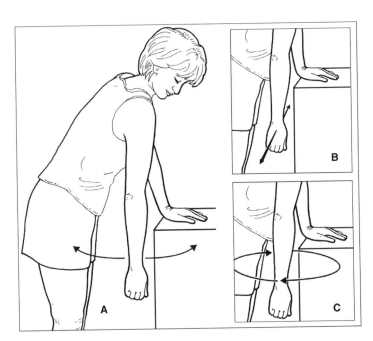

Figure 14-9. Codman exercises are used especially in the elderly with proximal humerus fractures.

SURGICAL NECK FRACTURES

CLASS A: IMPACTED FRACTURES WITH ANGULATION

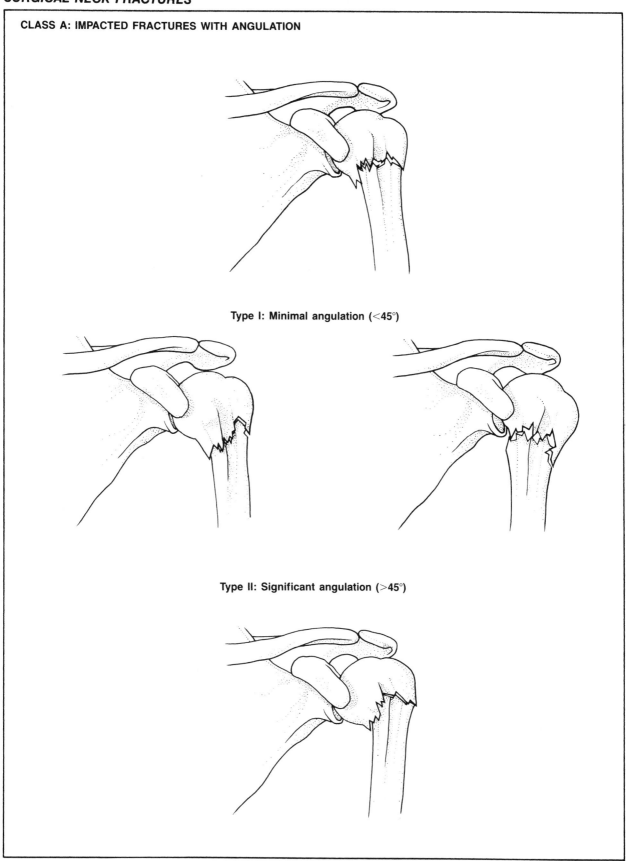

Type I: Minimal angulation (<45°)

Type II: Significant angulation (>45°)

Figure 14–11.

SURGICAL NECK FRACTURES

☐ Class A: Impacted fractures   (Fig. 14–11)
             with angulation
☐ Class B: Displaced   (Fig. 14–12)
             fractures
☐ Class C: Comminuted   (Fig. 14–14)
             fractures

ANATOMIC NECK FRACTURES (EPIPHYSIS)

☐ Class A: Nondisplaced   (Fig. 14–16A)
             including
             epiphyseal
             injuries
☐ Class B: Displaced fractures (Fig. 14–16B)

GREATER TUBEROSITY FRACTURES

☐ Class A: Nondisplaced   (Fig. 14–17)
             fractures
☐ Class B: Displaced   (Fig. 14–18)
             fractures

LESSER TUBEROSITY   (FIG. 14–19)
FRACTURES

COMBINATION FRACTURES   (FIGS. 14–20, 14–21)
(THREE- AND FOUR-PART
FRACTURES)

ARTICULAR SURFACE   (FIG. 14–22)
FRACTURES

SURGICAL NECK FRACTURES

The angle between the humeral head and the shaft is normally 135 degrees as shown in Figure 14–10. It is imperative that the physician treating proximal humeral fractures measure this angle. An angle of 90 degrees or less or 180 degrees or more is considered significant and, depending on the age and activity of the patient, may require reduction. Surgical neck fractures can be divided into three classes.

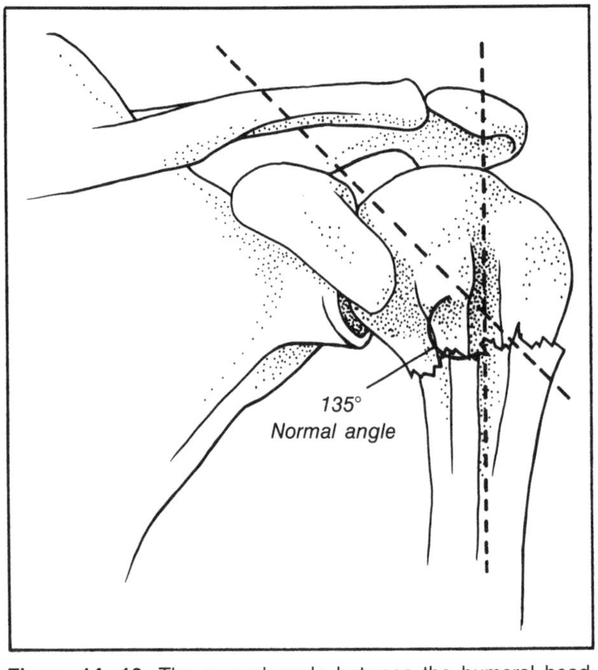

☐ CLASS A: IMPACTED FRACTURES WITH ANGULATION (FIG. 14–11)

The angulation may vary from less than 45 degrees requiring no reduction to over 45 degrees, which may require reduction depending on the age and activity of the patient.

☐ CLASS B: DISPLACED FRACTURES (FIGS. 14–12, 14–13)

Fragments separated by more than 1 cm are considered displaced. These fractures can be further subdivided into abduction or adduction injuries, depending upon the position of the humeral shaft.

☐ CLASS C: COMMINUTED FRACTURES (FIG. 14–14)

Comminution does not usually result in the shattered appearance shown in Figure 14–14.

Mechanism of Injury

There are two mechanisms that result in surgical neck fractures of the proximal humerus. The most common

Figure 14–10. The normal angle between the humeral head and shaft is 135 degrees. An angle of 90 degrees or less, or greater than 180 degrees, is significant and may require reduction, depending on the age and activity of the patient.

mechanism is indirect and is due to a fall on the outstretched arm. If the arm was abducted during the fall an abduction fracture will occur. If, however, the arm was adducted during the fall an adduction fracture will occur although rarely an abduction injury may be seen.

Direct trauma, which often is minimal in the elderly, may result in a surgical neck fracture.

Examination

The patient will present with tenderness and swelling over the upper arm and shoulder. If on presentation the arm is held in adduction the incidence of brachial plexus and axillary arterial injury is low. If the patient presents with the arm abducted, the incidence of neurovascular injury is much more significant.

Axiom: *A patient with a suspected surgical neck fracture who presents with the arm abducted should have the extremity immobilized in the position of presentation. These patients may have a class B, type II fracture and adduction may result in permanent neurovascular damage. Radiographs should be obtained in the position of presentation.*

Before the radiologic examination the physician must document the presence of distal pulses and sensory function.

X Ray

The trauma series, as discussed earlier and shown in Figures 14–6 and 14–7, with an AP view is usually adequate in demonstrating these fractures.

Associated Injuries

Class A surgical neck fractures may be associated with a contusion or tear of the axillary nerve. Class B and class C fractures are commonly associated with axillary neurovascular injuries and even brachial plexus injuries.

Treatment
☐ Class A: Type I (Minimal Angulation [<45°]) (Fig. 14–11)

This fracture is a one-part fracture. Sling and swathe (see Fig. 14–8) is the recommended mode of therapy. Ice, elevation, and analgesics with hand exercises should be initiated soon after injury. Circumduction exercises should begin as soon as tolerated and be followed by elbow and shoulder passive exercises at 2 to 3 weeks. Shoulder motion exercises can usually be started within 3 to 4 weeks.

☐ Class A: Type II (Significant Angulation [>45°]) (Fig. 14–11)

These injuries are classified as two-part fractures and require reduction. A portion of the periosteum remains intact and will aid in the reduction. The emergency department management consists of immobilization in a sling and swathe (see Fig. 14–8), analgesics, and emergent referral for reduction under regional or general anesthesia.

☐ Class B: Type I (Minimally Displaced) (Fig. 14–12)

In type I injuries, there is contact between the humeral shaft and the fragment although there is displacement of over 1 cm. Closed reduction under regional or general anesthesia is preferred followed by immobilization with a sling and swathe. If the reduction is unstable, overhead olecranon pin traction may be employed. An alternate method of reduction is the *hanging cast*. A plaster cast extending from the metacarpals to above the elbow is applied and suspended from the neck with the elbow in 90 degrees of flexion. This traction device must remain in place for at least 6 weeks with the patient cautioned never to recline more than 45 degrees.

☐ Class B: Type II (Moderately or Severely Displaced) (Fig. 14–12)

The emergency management of these fractures includes immobilization, ice, analgesics, and emergent referral. If emergent referral is not available in a situation of limb-threatening vascular compromise, reduction under general anesthesia can be carried out by the following method (Fig. 14–15):

1. With the patient supine or at 45 degrees upright, the physician should apply steady traction to the arm along the long axis of the humerus.
2. While maintaining traction the arm is brought across the anterior chest and flexed slightly.
3. While traction is maintained to distract the fragments, the other hand of the physician is placed along the fractured medial border of the humerus. The fragments are manipulated manually back into position, and the traction is gradually released.
4. A complete neurovascular examination must be documented after any attempt at a manipulative reduction. After this, a sling and swathe dressing should be applied.

If limb-threatening vascular compromise is not present, an alternative mode of reduction is olecranon pin traction.

SURGICAL NECK FRACTURES

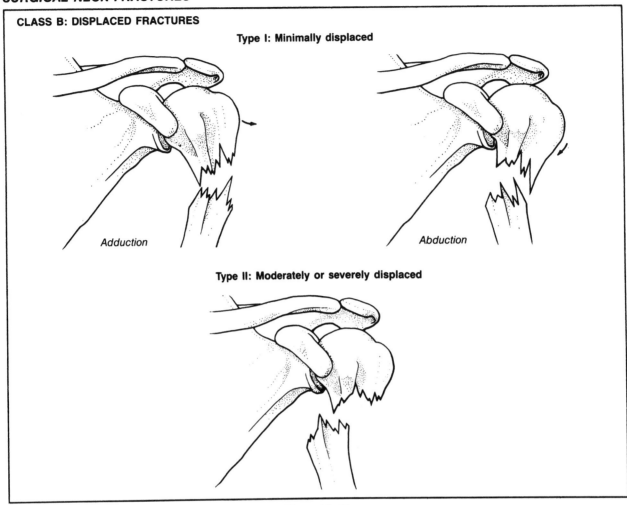

CLASS B: DISPLACED FRACTURES

Type I: Minimally displaced

Adduction

Abduction

Type II: Moderately or severely displaced

Figure 14–12.

□ Class C: (Comminuted Fractures)
(Fig. 14–14)

The emergency management of these fractures includes immobilization, ice, analgesics, and emergent referral. The therapeutic alternatives include a hanging cast, internal fixation, or overhead olecranon pin traction.

Complications

Surgical neck fractures are associated with several significant complications.

1. Joint stiffness with adhesions is a frequent complication that can be avoided or minimized with early motion exercises.
2. Malunion is common after displaced fractures. Fortunately, the normal shoulder has such a wide range of motion that this complication results in little debility.
3. Myositis ossificans that clears spontaneously in most instances may complicate the management of these fractures.

ANATOMIC NECK FRACTURES (EPIPHYSIS)

Anatomic neck fractures are essentially through the area of the epiphysis (Fig. 14–16) and can be divided into adult or childhood injuries. Adult injuries may be classified as nondisplaced (class A) or displaced (greater than 1 cm of separation, class B). Childhood injuries are generally limited to the 8- to 14-year-olds.

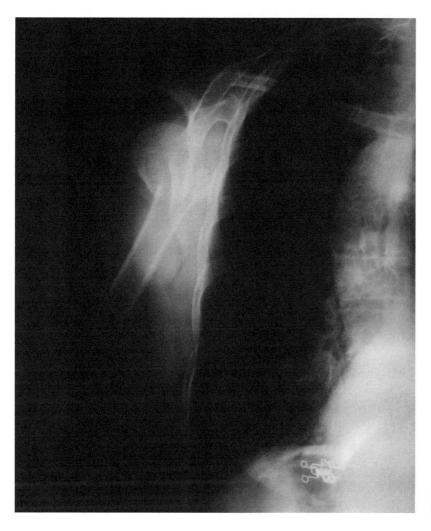

Figure 14–13. Displaced fracture of the surgical neck of the humerus.

Mechanism of Injury
The usual mechanism of injury is a fall on the outstretched arm in both the child and the adult.

Examination
There will be swelling and tenderness to palpation in the shoulder area. Pain will be increased with any shoulder motion.

X Ray
Routine radiographic views are generally adequate for demonstrating the fracture. In children, a Salter class 2 injury is usually apparent.

Associated Injuries
Anatomic neck fractures are usually not associated with any serious surrounding injuries.

Treatment
The emergency management of these fractures includes immobilization, ice, analgesics, and early referral. Class A fractures may be treated with a sling and

SURGICAL NECK FRACTURES

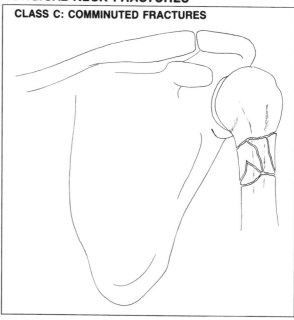

CLASS C: COMMINUTED FRACTURES

Figure 14–14.

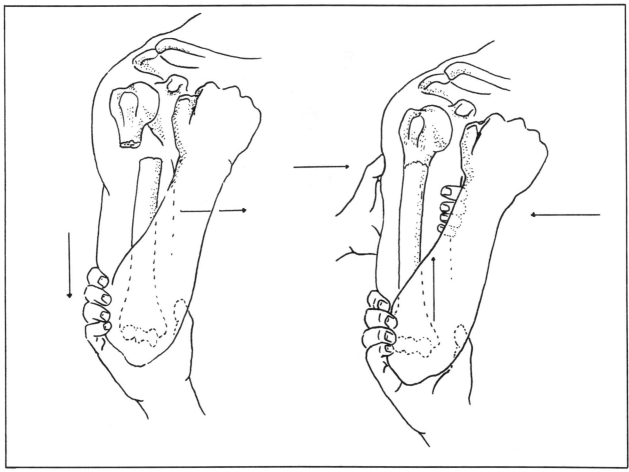

Figure 14–15. The method for reducing a displaced fracture of the proximal humerus. Distraction followed by repositioning of the distal fragment is vital in all reductions.

swathe (see Fig. 14–8) with referral to follow-up. Class B injuries may be immobilized in a sling and swathe with emergent referral for reduction and follow-up.

Childhood anatomic neck fractures are referred to as *proximal humeral epiphyseal* injuries. Again, ice, immobilization, analgesics, and emergent referral are recommended strongly. After reduction under general anesthesia a shoulder spica should be applied for 4 to

6 weeks followed by a sling and swathe with shoulder circumduction exercises.

Complications

Anatomic neck injuries are often complicated by the development of *avascular necrosis*. It is the authors' recommendation that physicians treating anatomic neck fractures consult with an orthopedic surgeon before therapy and refer all patients for follow-up.

GREATER TUBEROSITY FRACTURES

The supraspinatus, the infraspinatus, and the teres minor insert on the greater tuberosity and, when fractured, cause upward displacement of the fragment. This superi-

orly displaced tuberosity will mechanically block the abduction of the shoulder.[2] There are two types of greater tuberosity fractures: nondisplaced class A and

ANATOMIC NECK FRACTURES
(EPIPHYSIS)

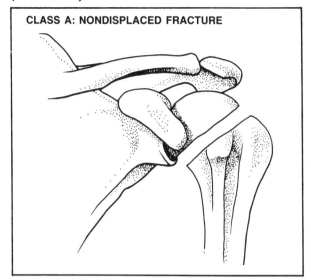

CLASS A: NONDISPLACED FRACTURE

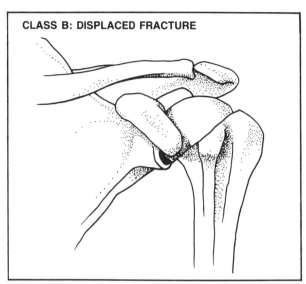

CLASS B: DISPLACED FRACTURE

Figure 14–16.

displaced class B (Figs. 14–17 and 14–18). Class A fractures may be further classified as type I compression fractures or type II nondisplaced fractures.[3] Furthermore, class B injuries may be type I where a thin cortical fragment is displaced or type II where the entire greater tuberosity is fractured and displaced.

A fracture of the greater tuberosity with displacement of over 1 cm is often associated with a tear of the rotator cuff. Also, the external rotation of the shoulder may be inhibited if a posteriorly displaced tuberosity impinges against the posterior glenoid.[2]

Axiom: *Displaced greater tuberosity fractures are always associated with a longitudinal tear of the rotator cuff.*

Greater tuberosity fractures are seen in approximately 15 percent of all anterior shoulder dislocations.[2,6]

Mechanism of Injury
There are two mechanisms that result in greater tuberosity fractures. Class A, type I fractures are usually the result of a direct blow to the upper humerus as during a fall. The elderly are particularly susceptible to these injuries due to atrophy and weakening of the surrounding musculature. Class A, type II fractures are only infrequently associated with this mechanism.

Class A, type II injuries usually result from a fall on the outstretched arm (indirect). Class B fractures typically are secondary to a fall on the outstretched arm with external rotator contraction resulting in displacement.

Examination
The patient will complain of pain and swelling over the greater tuberosity. The patient will be unable to abduct the arm and will note increased pain with external rotation.

X Ray
AP and outlet radiographs are able to assess a superior displacement, but often fail to demonstrate precisely the amount of posterior retraction and overlap of the fragment with the articular surface. However, standard or Velpeau axillary radiographs can be used to assess the amount of posterior retraction. Therefore, if AP and outlet radiographs are used alone, the posterior displacement will be underestimated as well as the number of two-part displaced fractures.[2]

Associated Injuries
Neurovascular injuries are rarely associated with these injuries. Greater tuberosity fractures are commonly associated with anterior shoulder dislocations and rotator cuff tears. Both of these injuries are more common with class B fractures.

GREATER TUBEROSITY FRACTURES

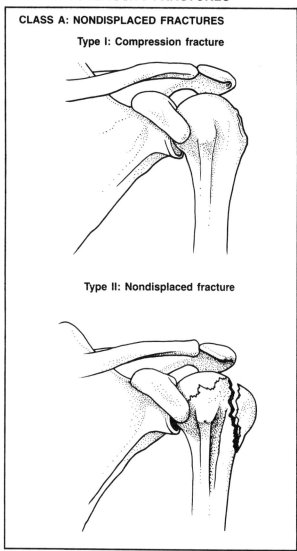

Figure 14-17.

GREATER TUBEROSITY FRACTURES

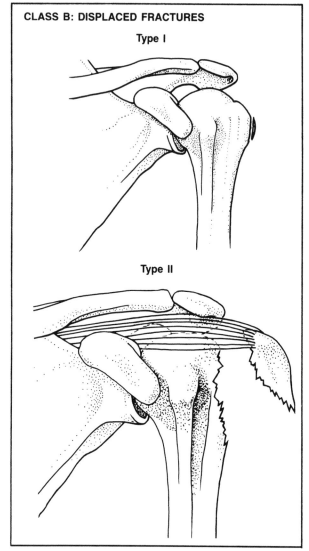

Figure 14-18.

Treatment

☐ Class A: Type I   (Compression)
             Type II (Nondisplaced)

The emergency management consists of ice, analgesics, sling, and swathe immobilization (see Fig. 14–8) and early referral because of the high incidence of complications (see below).

☐ Class B: Type I   (Displaced)
             Type II (Displaced)

The management of these injuries is dependent on the age and activity of the patient. Young patients require internal fixation or excision of the fragment with repair of the torn rotator cuff. Good bone stock must be present for fixation with screws, but is frequently lacking in these types of fractures.[2] Older patients are usually not

candidates for surgical repair and require ice, immobilization with a sling and swathe (see Fig. 14–8), analgesics, and early referral. Early mobilization in the elderly patient is essential.

Complications

Greater tuberosity fractures may be associated with several complications:

1. Compression fractures are often complicated by impingement on the long head of the biceps resulting in chronic tenosynovitis and eventually tendon rupture.
2. Nonunion may complicate the management of greater tuberosity fractures.
3. Myositis ossificans may develop; however, it usually disappears with the implementation of early motion.

LESSER TUBEROSITY FRACTURES

Lesser tuberosity fractures (Fig. 14–19) commonly occur in conjunction with posterior shoulder dislocations. These fractures are less common than are greater tuberosity fractures.

Mechanism of Injury
Lesser tuberosity fractures are usually associated with an indirect mechanism of injury such as a seizure or a fall on the adducted arm. Both of these situations result in an intense contraction of the subscapularis muscle and an avulsion of the lesser tuberosity.

Examination
There will be tenderness to palpation over the lesser tuberosity. Pain will be increased with active external rotation or adduction against resistance. In addition, passive external rotation will exacerbate the pain.

X Ray
Routine shoulder views are generally adequate in demonstrating this fracture.

Associated Injuries
Posterior dislocations of the shoulder are commonly associated with these injuries. In addition, nondisplaced surgical neck fractures may be associated with these fractures. Neurovascular injuries are rarely associated with lesser tuberosity fractures.

Treatment
The emergency management of lesser tuberosity fractures includes ice, analgesics, sling and swathe immobilization (see Fig. 14–8), and orthopedic consultation. Most orthopedic surgeons recommend sling immobilization for 3 to 5 days followed by gradually increasing range of motion exercises. Some surgeons prefer surgical fixation and, therefore, early consultation is advised.

Complications
These fractures usually heal without complications because of compensation by the surrounding shoulder musculature. Some surgeons feel that this fracture can lead to a weakening of the anterior capsular support that may predispose to the development of recurrent anterior dislocations.

COMBINATION FRACTURES

Combination fractures (Figs. 14–20 and 14–21) refer to *Neer fractures that are classified as three- or four-part injuries* (a displaced fracture with three or more parts). These fractures are usually the result of severe injury forces, and are often associated with dislocations and are best treated surgically.

Mechanism of Injury
The most common mechanism is a hard fall on the outstretched arm. The segments involved and the amount of displacement are dependent on the force of the fall and the muscular tone at the time of injury.

Examination
There will be diffuse pain and swelling of the proximal humerus and the patient will resist all motion.

X Ray
The routine trauma series (see Fig. 14–6) is generally adequate in delineating these fractures.

Associated Injuries
Combined proximal humeral fractures are associated with several significant injuries.

1. Shoulder dislocations are common with these injuries.
2. Rotator cuff injuries are commonly seen in conjunction with these injuries.
3. Injury to the brachial plexus, axillary vessels, axillary and musculocutaneous nerves are occasionally associated with combined proximal humeral fractures.

LESSER TUBEROSITY FRACTURES

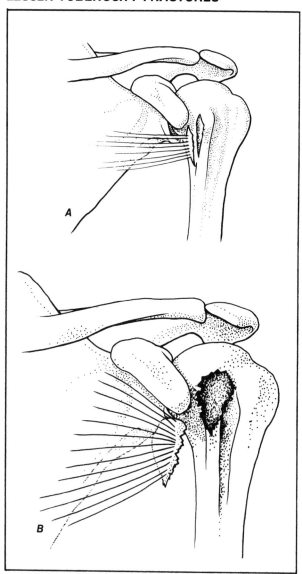

Figure 14–19. *A* = small fragment avulsed; *B* = fragment more than 1 cm avulsed.

Treatment
Emergency management includes ice, analgesics, sling immobilization, and emergent referral usually necessitating admission. Virtually all combined fractures require surgical repair and, in some instances, the insertion of a prosthesis (four-part fractures).

Complications
As noted earlier, neurovascular injuries may complicate the management of these fractures. Four-part fractures are complicated by a high incidence of avascular necrosis of the humeral head secondary to a compromised blood supply.

COMBINATION FRACTURES

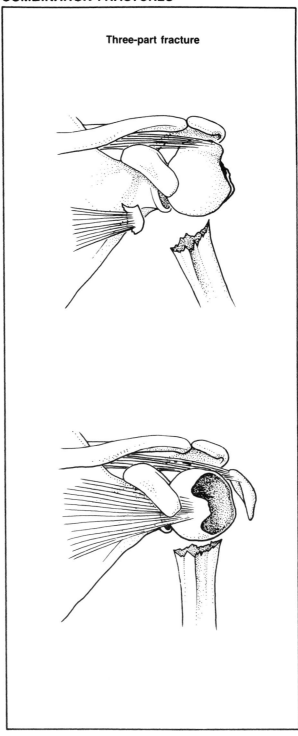

Three-part fracture

Figure 14–20.

COMBINATION FRACTURES

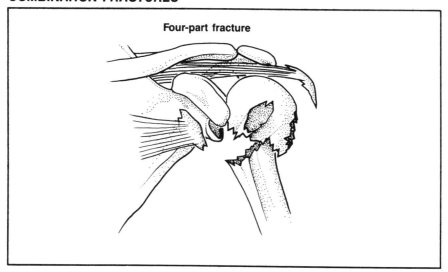

Four-part fracture

Figure 14–21.

ARTICULAR SURFACE FRACTURES

Articular surface fractures (Fig. 14–22) are referred to as *impression fractures* by some authors. These fractures may be classified as follows:

- **Class A:** Impression fracture with less than 20 percent involvement
- **Class B:** Impression fracture with 20 to 40 percent involvement
- **Class C:** Comminuted articular surface fracture (head splitting)

Mechanism of Injury
Class A and B fractures are usually secondary to a direct blow to the lateral arm as during a fall. Anterior shoulder dislocations may be associated with an impression fracture and are referred to as a *Hill-Sacks fracture*.[8]

Examination
Impression fractures are associated with only minimal pain with humeral motion. Comminuted fractures are associated with severe pain.

X Ray
Typically, AP views with internal and external rotation are best for visualization of the fracture lines. Impression fractures are often difficult to define and frequently secondary signs of fracture are employed in making the correct diagnosis. The presence of a *fat fluid level* on the AP upright film is indicative of an articular surface fracture. In addition, inferior pseudosubluxation of the humeral head secondary to a hemarthrosis is often seen in conjunction with impression fractures.

Associated Injuries
Articular surface fractures are often associated with anterior or posterior shoulder dislocations.

Treatment
The emergency management of these fractures includes ice, analgesics, sling and swathe immobilization (see Fig. 14–8), and early referral. Class A injuries are immobilized in external rotation whereas class B and C injuries require surgical repair or the insertion of a prosthesis. Because elderly patients require early mobility, surgical repair may not be elected.

Complications
Articular surface fractures may be complicated by:

1. Joint stiffness
2. Arthritis
3. Avascular necrosis (seen most frequently with class C fractures)

ARTICULAR SURFACE FRACTURES

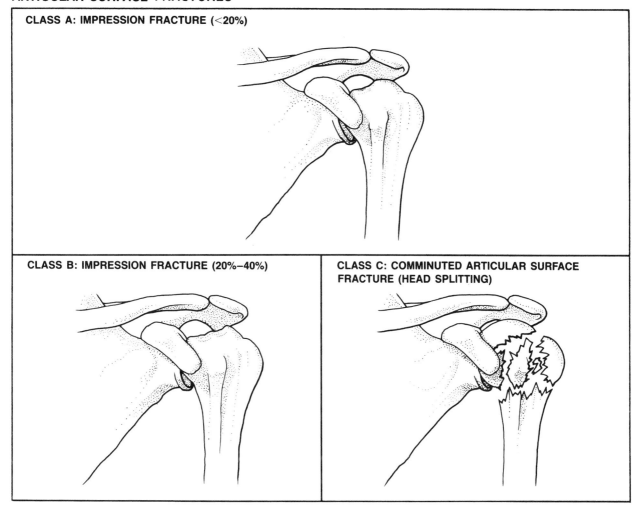

Figure 14–22.

REFERENCES

1. Dehne E: Fractures of the upper end of the humerus. A classification based on etiology of trauma. *Surg Clin North Am* **25:**28, 1945.
2. Flatlow EL, Cuomo F, Maday MG, et al: Open reduction and internal fixation of two-part displaced fractures of the greater tuberocity of the proximal part of the humerus. *J Bone Joint Surg* **8:**1213–1218, 1991.
3. Hill H, Sachs MD: The grooved defect of the humeral head. *Radiology* **35:**690, 1940.
4. Neer CS II: Displaced proximal humeral fractures. Part I. Classification and evaluation. *J Bone Joint Surg* **52:**1077, 1970.
5. Neer CS II: Fractures about the shoulder. A classification. *J Bone Joint Surg* **52:**1081, 1970.
6. Rockwood CA, Green DP (Eds.): *Fractures.* Philadelphia: Lippincott, 1975.
7. Stimson BB: *A Manual of Fractures and Dislocations*, 2nd ed. Philadelphia: Lea and Febiger, 1947.
8. Turek SL: *Orthopedics*, 2nd ed. Philadelphia: Lippincott, 1967.

15
CHAPTER

FRACTURES OF THE CLAVICLE

CLAVICULAR FRACTURES

CLASS A: MIDDLE THIRD FRACTURES
(p. 298)

Type II: Displaced in children and in adults

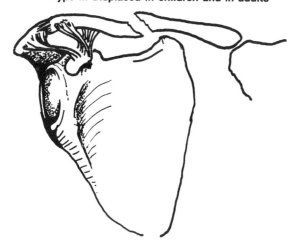

CLASS B: DISTAL THIRD FRACTURES
(p. 301)

Type I: Nondisplaced, with ligaments intact

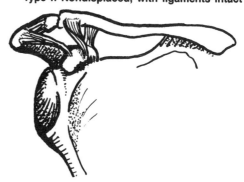

Type II: Displaced, with ligaments ruptured (unstable)

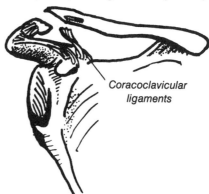

Coracoclavicular ligaments

CLASS C: MEDIAL THIRD FRACTURES
(p. 302)

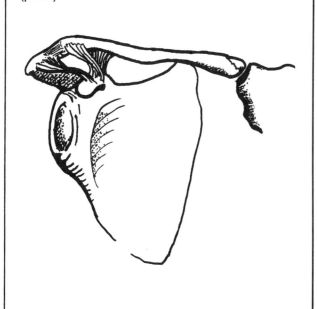

Type III: Articular surface involvement of the acromioclavicular joint

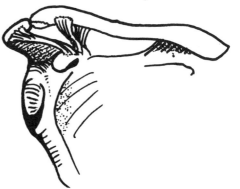

Clavicular fractures are the most common of all child-hood fractures. These fractures are often encountered in newborn infants secondary to birth trauma. Overall, clavicular fractures account for 5 percent of all the fractures seen for all age groups. Eighty percent of all clavicular fractures occur in the middle one third whereas 15 percent occur in the distal one third and the remaining 5 percent in the medial one third.[3]

Essential Anatomy

The clavicle is an oblong bone the middle portion of which is tubular and the distal portion, flattened. The clavicle is anchored to the scapula by the *acromioclavicular* and the *coracoclavicular* ligaments. The *sternoclavicular* and the *costoclavicular* ligaments anchor the clavicle medially as shown in Figure 15–1. The clavicle serves as points of attachment for both the sternocleidomastoid and the subclavius muscles. The ligaments and the muscles act in conjunction to anchor the clavicle and thus maintain the width of the shoulder and serve as the attachment point of the shoulder to the axial skeleton.

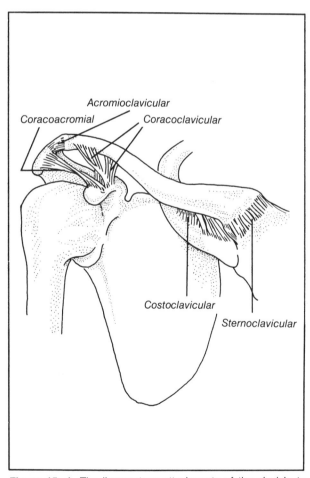

Figure 15–1. The ligamentous attachments of the clavicle to the sternum medially and the acromion laterally.

Both the subclavian vessels and the brachial plexus lie in close proximity to the clavicle. Displaced clavicular fractures can be associated with injuries to these vital structures.

Examination

The clavicle is the point of attachment of the upper extremity to the axial skeleton. Clavicular fractures often present with pain and swelling over the injury associated with inferior and anterior displacement of the shoulder secondary to the loss of support. If severe displacement is present that is associated with the tearing of the soft tissues, the ecchymosis may be present.[9]

X Ray

The routine clavicular radiograph (anteroposterior [AP] view of the upper thorax) is generally adequate in defining these fractures. Occasionally, special views may be necessary to delineate medial clavicular fractures. These views will be discussed under the appropriate section when indicated.

Treatment

Childhood clavicular fractures generally require little treatment with only a figure-of-eight clavicular strap, as rapid healing with remodeling and full return of function is the usual outcome. Adult clavicular fractures are associated with more serious complications and therefore require a more accurate reduction and closer follow-up to ensure a full return of function. Adult fractures may be complicated by excessive callus formation with neurovascular compromise secondary to compression against the first rib.

Classification

Clavicular fractures can be divided into three groups on the basis of anatomy, therapy, and incidence.[1] *Class A* fractures involve the middle one third of the clavicle whereas *class B* and *C* fractures involve the distal and medial thirds, respectively. Each class is associated with a particular deformity along with specific injuries to surrounding neurovascular and ligamentous structures.

CLAVICULAR FRACTURES

☐ Class A: Middle third fractures   (Fig. 15–2)
☐ Class B: Distal third fractures   (Fig. 15–5)
☐ Class C: Medial third fractures   (Fig. 15–6)

☐ CLASS A: MIDDLE THIRD FRACTURES (FIG. 15–2)

The majority of these fractures occur at the junction of the middle and outer thirds of the clavicle, medial to the coracoclavicular ligaments. Type I fractures are nondis-

CLAVICULAR FRACTURES

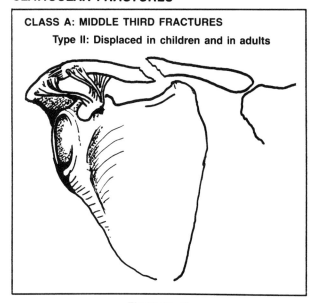

CLASS A: MIDDLE THIRD FRACTURES

Type II: Displaced in children and in adults

Figure 15–2.

placed whereas type II fractures are displaced. Typically, the proximal fragment is displaced upward because of the pull of the sternocleidomastoid.

Mechanism of Injury

There are two mechanisms commonly responsible for clavicular fractures.[3,4,7] A direct blow to the clavicle may result in a fracture. A posteriorly directed force may result in a single fracture. Neurovascular damage may be associated with these fractures. If the force is directed inferiorly, the resulting fracture is often comminuted. Neurovascular damage is more likely with inferiorly directed forces.

The indirect mechanism is a force typified by a fall on the lateral shoulder. The force is transmitted via the acromion to the clavicle. The clavicle usually fractures in the middle one third as the natural "S" shape of the clavicle has a tendency to focus the indirect force at this point.

Examination

The clavicle is subcutaneous over nearly its entire extent and therefore fractures can be easily diagnosed on the basis of examination. Most patients will have swelling and tenderness over the fracture site. Middle third clavicular fractures usually result in a downward and inward slump of the involved shoulder due to loss of support. Patients will usually carry their arm adducted against the chest wall and will resist motion of the extremity.

All clavicular fractures require examination and documentation of the neurovascular function distal to the injury.[8] If severe displacement is present that is associated with the tearing of the soft tissues, the ecchymosis may be present.[9]

X Ray

Routine AP views are usually adequate in demonstrating the fracture and any displacement if present (Fig. 15–3). An AP view with the tube directed 45 degrees cephalad is often useful in defining these fractures (apical lordotic).

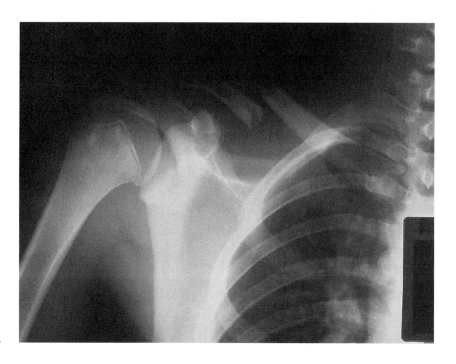

Figure 15–3. Mid-clavicular fracture.

Associated Injuries

Middle third clavicular fractures may be associated with neurovascular injuries. Subclavian vascular injuries are not uncommon, especially with displaced clavicular fractures. Whenever a vascular injury is suspected angiographic studies are strongly recommended. Neurologic damage may involve either contusion or avulsion of the nerve roots. A meticulous neurologic examination of cranial nerve roots IV through VIII should accompany the diagnosis of any displaced clavicular fracture.[3,4]

Treatment

Figure of 8 clavicular straps are often used in managing these fractures. Commercial devices are available and if applied properly they will be useful in children over the age of 10. The literature shows no real difference between patients treated with a sling or placed in a figure of 8. However many orthopedic surgeons still prefer these. The family should be instructed by the physician in the proper application and adjustment of this device (Fig. 15–4).

1. Pull both shoulders backward tightly as if standing in a military position.
2. Apply the commercial splint and tighten while in this position.

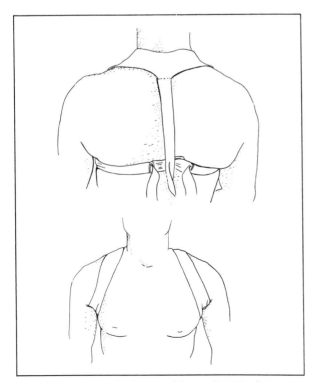

Figure 15–4. Application of figure-of-eight splint.

3. Examine the patient for neurovascular compromise and educate the family as to the worrisome symptoms of this complication.
4. Instruct the family in the method of daily tightening the splint as it comes loose.

Roentgenograms should be taken on the seventh and fourteenth days after manipulation of a fracture to be certain that the positions of the fracture fragments are satisfactory.[9]

In children under the age of 10, commercial straps are generally too large for a secure fit.[4,7] Tubular stockinette can be used in making a custom figure-of-eight splint. Both splints will require frequent tightening and should be worn until the patient can abduct the extremity without pain. Children generally require 3 to 5 weeks of immobilization whereas adults usually require 6 weeks or more.[7]

If children using a figure-of-eight splint complain of swelling or tingling in the hands, then the children should (1) hold their hands on their hips with the arms abducted from the body, (2) lie back with their arms outward toward the overhead position, or (3) hold their hands clasped on top of their heads. These techniques will help minimize the compression of the arterial circulation against the hard edge of the splint in the axilla.[9]

Recent studies have shown that newborns who have sustained a fractured clavicle during birth should be treated with gentle care and rest. Figure-of-eight clavicular straps are not necessary because healing occurs easily within 2 weeks without additional treatment.[9]

☐ Class A: Type I (Nondisplaced in Children)

The authors recommend a figure-of-eight splint for 10 days followed by a sling. Active children may displace these fractures if a figure-of-eight splint is not applied.

☐ Class A: Type I (Nondisplaced in Adults)

Nondisplaced fractures have an intact periosteum and therefore only a sling for support with ice is necessary in the management of these fractures. Repeat radiographs at 1 week to ensure proper positioning are indicated.

☐ Class A: Type II (Displaced in Children)

A properly applied figure-of-eight splint that is adjusted frequently is the treatment of choice. The patient needs to be seen frequently in follow-up to ensure proper reduction and maintenance of positioning. If the child or family is uncooperative and will not use the figure-of-eight splint properly, referral for a shoulder spica is indicated. Neurovascular compromise, excessive skin tenting, and open fractures require emergent referral.

☐ Class A: Type II   (Displaced in Adults)

A commercially available figure-of-eight splint can be used for reduction and maintenance of position. If after 1 week the fracture is not reduced, the patient should be referred to an orthopedic surgeon for consideration of a shoulder spica cast. If the patient is uncooperative initially and will not properly wear a figure-of-eight splint, referral for a shoulder spica is indicated.[7] Neurovascular compromise, excessive skin tenting, and open fractures require emergent referral.

Complications

Middle third clavicular fractures may be associated with several complications.

1. Malunion is primarily a complication of adult fractures. In children, malunion is uncommon due to the extensive remodeling that normally accompanies these fractures.
2. Excessive callus formation may occur resulting in a cosmetic defect or neurovascular compromise.
3. Nonunion is a rare complication that is usually associated with those fractures treated with open reduction and internal fixation.

☐ CLASS B: DISTAL THIRD FRACTURES (FIG. 15–5)

Class B fractures occur distal to the coracoclavicular ligaments. Distal third clavicular fractures can be divided into three types. Type I fractures are nondisplaced with *intact ligaments* whereas type II fractures are displaced with *rupture of the coracoclavicular ligaments*.[1,2] Typically, the proximal clavicular segment will be pulled upward secondary to the sternocleidomastoid. Type III fractures involve the *articular surface of the acromioclavicular joint* and may be diagnosed clinically as most of these fractures are difficult to delineate radiographically.

Mechanism of Injury

Class B fractures are usually the result of direct trauma. A blow from above directed downward to the lateral third of the clavicle may result in a type I or type II fracture. Type III fractures usually result from a blow to the outer aspect of the shoulder (a fall) or a compression force.

Examination

The patient will complain of pain over the involved area and will carry the arm in adduction. The pain will be increased with palpation or with attempted abduction.

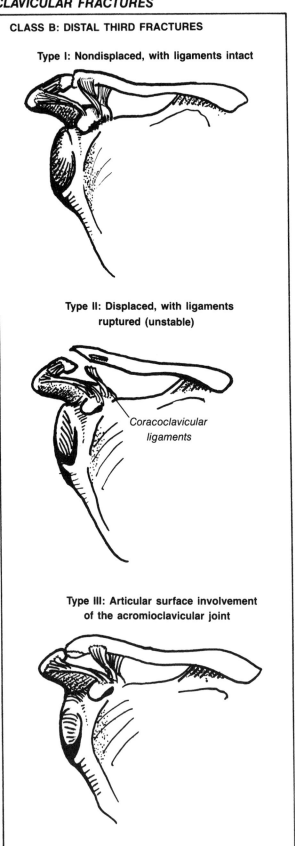

CLAVICULAR FRACTURES

CLASS B: DISTAL THIRD FRACTURES

Type I: Nondisplaced, with ligaments intact

Type II: Displaced, with ligaments ruptured (unstable)

Coracoclavicular ligaments

Type III: Articular surface involvement of the acromioclavicular joint

Figure 15–5.

Type II fractures may have palpable displacement on examination.

X Ray
Routine views are generally adequate in demonstrating type I or type II fractures. Type III, articular surface fractures, may be difficult to detect radiographically. Special techniques such as cone views, lateral views, or weightbearing (10 pounds) films may be necessary for accurate delineation of this fracture.

Associated Injuries
Coracoclavicular ligament damage may accompany these fractures.

Axiom: *All displaced lateral third clavicular fractures (class B, type II) are associated with coracoclavicular ligament rupture and should be treated similar to an acromioclavicular joint dislocation.*

Acromioclavicular joint subluxation or dislocation may accompany any class B clavicular fracture.

Treatment
☐ Class B: Type I (Nondisplaced)
Nondisplaced class B fractures are splinted by the surrounding intact ligaments and muscles and are usually treated symptomatically with ice, analgesics, and early motion.

☐ Class B: Type II (Displaced)
The emergency management of these fractures includes sling immobilization, ice, analgesics, and orthopedic referral for internal fixation and reduction.[5,6]

☐ Class B: Type III (Articular Surface Involvement)
These patients should be treated symptomatically with ice, analgesics, and a sling for support. Early motion is strongly urged to prevent the development of degenerative arthritis.

Complications
Class B clavicular fractures are associated with two major complications.[10]

1. Delayed union is frequently associated with type II fractures treated conservatively.
2. Degenerative arthritis may be noted after type III injuries.

CLAVICULAR FRACTURES

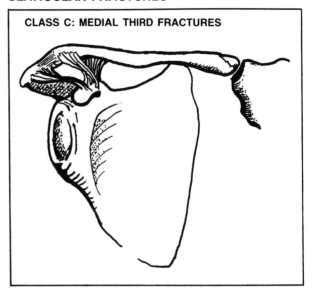

CLASS C: MEDIAL THIRD FRACTURES

Figure 15–6. Fracture of the inner aspect of the clavicle involving the sternoclavicular joint. Tomograms may be necessary to visualize this.

☐ CLASS C: MEDIAL THIRD FRACTURES (FIG. 15–6)

Medial third clavicular fractures are uncommon, representing only 5 percent of all clavicular fractures. Considerably strong injury forces are required to fracture the clavicle in this area and therefore, a diligent search for associated injuries should accompany all of these fractures.

Mechanism of Injury
A direct blow to the medial clavicle may result in a fracture. An indirect mechanism is a blow to the lateral shoulder that may compress the clavicle against the sternum and result in a fracture. A fall on the abducted outstretched arm may indirectly compress the clavicle against the sternum resulting in a fracture.

Examination
There will be tenderness and pain over the sternoclavicular joint. Pain will be exacerbated with abduction of the arm.

X Ray
An AP view with the tube directed 45 degrees cephalad (apical lordotic) is usually adequate for demonstrating these fractures (Fig. 15–7). At times, cone views, upper

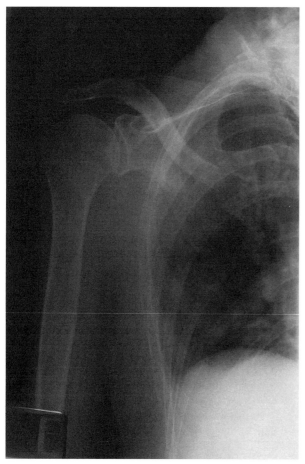

Figure 15–7. Medial clavicular fracture.

rib radiographs, or tomograms may be necessary to adequately delineate the fracture.

Associated Injuries

These fractures are usually secondary to severe forces, and may be associated with significant underlying organ damage. Intrathoracic injury must be excluded early in the management of all class C clavicular fractures. Sternal fractures or subluxation of the sternoclavicular joint may be associated with these fractures.

Treatment

The emergency management includes ice, analgesics, and a sling for support. All patients should have the threat of underlying intrathoracic damage excluded early in their evaluation. Displaced fractures require orthopedic referral for reduction.

Complications

Degenerative arthritis frequently accompanies these fractures.

REFERENCES

1. Allman FL: Fractures of the distal third of the clavicle. *Clin Orthop* **58:**43, 1968.
2. Allman FL: Fractures and ligamentous injuries of the clavicle and its articulation. *J Bone Joint Surg* **49:**774, 1967.
3. Conwell HE: Fractures of the clavicle. *JAMA* **90:**838, 1928.
4. Kini MG: A simple method of ambulatory treatment of fractures of the clavicle. *J Bone Joint Surg* **23:**795, 1941.
5. Lee HG: Treatment of fracture of the clavicle by internal nail fixation. *N Engl J Med* **234:**222, 1946.
6. Moore TO: Internal pin fixation for fracture of the clavicle. *Am Surg* **17:**580, 1951.
7. Packer BD: Conservative treatment of fracture of the clavicle. *J Bone Joint Surg* **26:**770, 1944.
8. Peen I: The vascular complications of the fractures of the clavicle. *J Trauma* **4:**819, 1964.
9. Post M: Current concepts in the treatment of fractures of the clavicle. *Clin Orthop* **245:**89–101, 1989.
10. Worcester JN, Green DP: Osteoarthritis of the acromioclavicular joint. *Clin Orthop* **58:**69, 1968.

16
CHAPTER

FRACTURES OF THE SCAPULA

- *SCAPULAR FRACTURES*

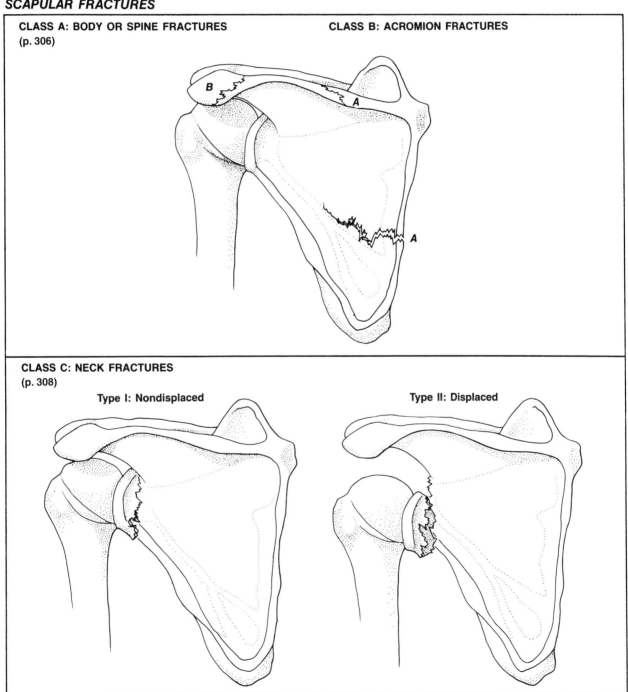

CLASS A: BODY OR SPINE FRACTURES
(p. 306)

CLASS B: ACROMION FRACTURES

CLASS C: NECK FRACTURES
(p. 308)

Type I: Nondisplaced

Type II: Displaced

SCAPULAR FRACTURES (cont.)

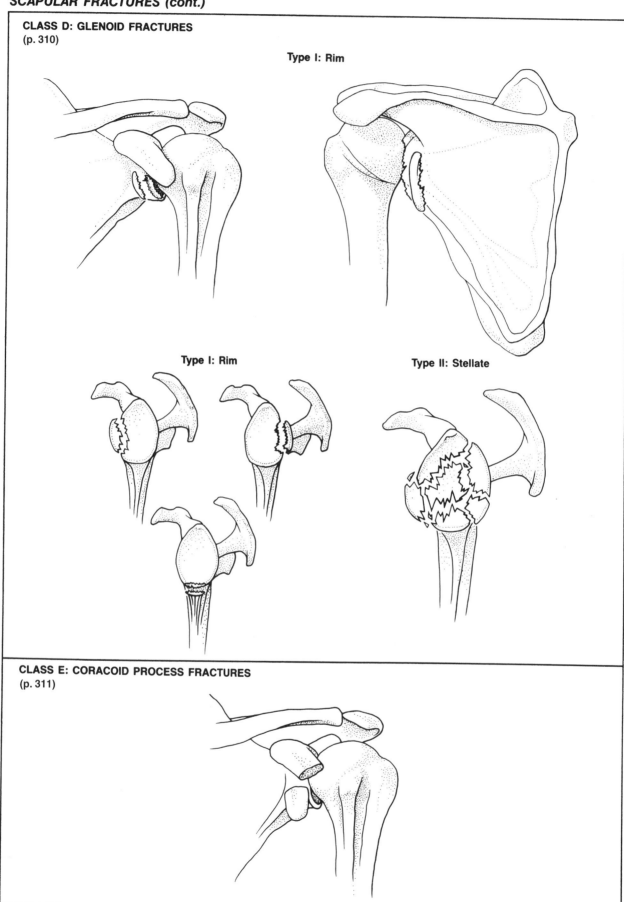

CLASS D: GLENOID FRACTURES
(p. 310)

Type I: Rim

Type I: Rim

Type II: Stellate

CLASS E: CORACOID PROCESS FRACTURES
(p. 311)

Scapular fractures are relatively uncommon injuries that generally occur in patients between 40 and 60 years of age.[4] This type of injury represents only 1 percent of all fractures and 5 percent of fractures involving the shoulder.[7] There are a multiplicity of fracture patterns associated with the scapula. Frequently, scapular fractures are associated with dislocations, as for example, a shoulder dislocation with a posterior glenoid rim fracture.[1]

Essential Anatomy

The scapula is covered with thick muscles over its entire body and spine. The supraspinatus muscle covers the fossa superior to the spine whereas the infraspinatus muscle covers the fossa below the spine. The anterior surface of the scapula is separated from the rib cage by the subscapularis muscle. These muscles offer protection and support for the scapula. The scapula is connected to the axial skeleton only by way of the acromioclavicular joint. The remainder of the scapular support is by way of the thick investing musculature surrounding its surface.

Other muscles insert on the scapula and may initiate displacing forces when fractures are encountered. The triceps inserts in the inferior rim of the glenoid fossa whereas the short head of the biceps, the coracobrachialis, and the pectoralis minor insert on the coracoid process.

X Ray

Routine scapular radiographs should include an anteroposterior (AP) frontal along with a transcapular lateral view.[7] On occasion, computed tomography (CT) scanning may be helpful in precisely defining the full extent of the fracture.

Classification

Scapular fractures are classified anatomically and further subdivided based on the amount of displacement or comminution as follows:

SCAPULAR FRACTURES

☐ Class A: Body or spine fractures   (Fig. 16–1)
☐ Class B: Acromion fractures   (Fig. 16–1)
☐ Class C: Neck fractures   (Fig. 16–3)
☐ Class D: Glenoid fractures   (Fig. 16–6)
☐ Class E: Coracoid process fractures   (Fig. 16–7)

☐ CLASS A: BODY OR SPINE FRACTURES (FIG. 16–1)

Mechanism of Injury

The mechanism involved is usually a direct blow over the involved area.[8] A great deal of force is necessary to fracture the body or the spine and associated injuries may complicate or mask these fractures.[7] Typically, there is little displacement due to the support of the investing muscles and the periosteum.

Examination

The patient will present with pain, swelling, and ecchymosis over the involved area. The involved extremity will be held in adduction, and the patient will resist abduction. Abduction past the first 90 degrees is largely the result of scapular motion and, thus, will exacerbate painful scapular fractures.[4]

X Ray (Fig. 16–2)

Routine AP and transcapular views are generally adequate in defining these fractures. Tangential oblique views may be helpful in defining small body fractures.

Associated Injuries

Scapular fractures involving the body or the spine are usually the result of large blunt forces and are associated with several life-threatening injuries.[1,8]

1. The diagnosis of pneumothorax must be considered whenever a scapular fracture is suspected.
2. Rib fractures or vertebral compression fractures are often associated with these injuries.
3. Both upper and lower extremity fractures are frequently seen in association with scapular fractures.
4. Injuries to the axillary artery, nerve, or the brachial plexus are rarely associated with these fractures.

SCAPULAR FRACTURES

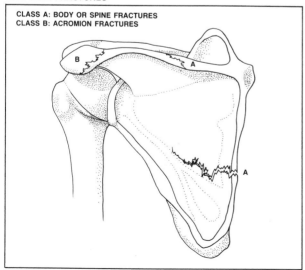

CLASS A: BODY OR SPINE FRACTURES
CLASS B: ACROMION FRACTURES

Figure 16–1.

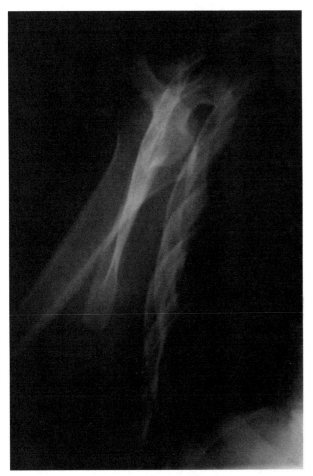

Figure 16–2. Scapular body fracture.

Treatment

The emergency management of these fractures includes sling or sling and swathe immobilization with ice and analgesics. It is essential to exclude the possibility of life- or limb-threatening injuries early when managing these fractures. Early limited exercise is strongly recommended. After about 2 weeks, limited activity as tolerated is advised. Significantly displaced fractures with functional impairment should have an emergent referral for consideration of open reduction and internal fixation (ORIF.[5])

Complications

Neurovascular or visceral injuries as mentioned earlier may complicate the management of these fractures.

□ CLASS B: ACROMION FRACTURES (FIG. 16–1)

Mechanism of Injury

Acromion fractures are usually the result of a direct down ward blow to the shoulder. The force required is generally large and associated injuries often complicate the management of these fractures. Superior dislocation of the shoulder may result in a displaced fracture (superior) of the acromion.

Examination

Tenderness and swelling will be maximal over the acromion process. The pain will be exacerbated with deltoid stressing.

X Ray

Routine scapular radiographs are generally adequate in defining the fracture. On occasion, CT scanning may be helpful in precisely defining the full extent of the fracture.

Associated Injuries

Acromion process fractures may be associated with several significant injuries.

1. Brachial plexus injuries must be suspected whenever acromion fractures are encountered.
2. Acromioclavicular joint injuries or lateral clavicular fractures are often associated with these fractures.
3. Rotator cuff tears typically occur in conjunction with superior shoulder dislocations.

Treatment

Nondisplaced fractures can be treated with sling immobilization. In addition, an elastic circular dressing that pushes the elbow upward and the lateral clavicle downward should be used for the first 4 weeks of management. Range of motion exercises should be started early in the management of these fractures (see Fig. 17–31).

Displaced fractures often require internal fixation to avoid compromise of the subacromial space resulting in a restricted range of motion. Also, recent studies have shown that internal fixation is necessary if both the clavicle and scapula are injured together.[7]

Complications

The most frequent complication of acromion fractures is bursitis. Bursitis is most often seen in association with fractures with inferior displacement.

□ CLASS C: NECK FRACTURES (FIG. 16–3)

Scapular neck fractures are uncommon injuries that are often associated with humeral fractures.

Mechanism of Injury

An anterior or posterior force directed against the shoulder is the usual mechanism of injury. In most patients, the glenoid will be impacted; however, if displaced, typically the fragment will be anterior.[2]

SCAPULAR FRACTURES

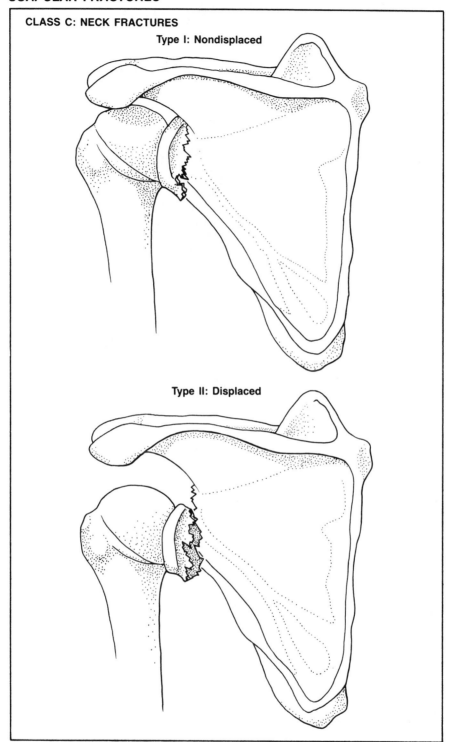

CLASS C: NECK FRACTURES

Type I: Nondisplaced

Type II: Displaced

Figure 16–3.

Examination

The patient will present with the arm held in adduction and will resist all movement of the shoulder. Medial pressure over the lateral humeral head will exacerbate the patient's pain.[3]

X Ray (Figs. 16–4, 16–5)

AP and tangential views are generally adequate in defining the fracture. Axillary views may be helpful in delineating displaced fractures. On occasion, CT scanning may be helpful in precisely defining the full extent of the fracture.

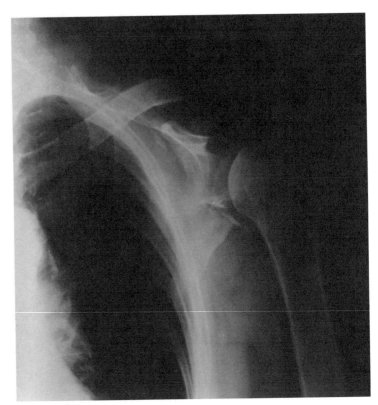

Figure 16–4. A fracture of the base of the glenoid.

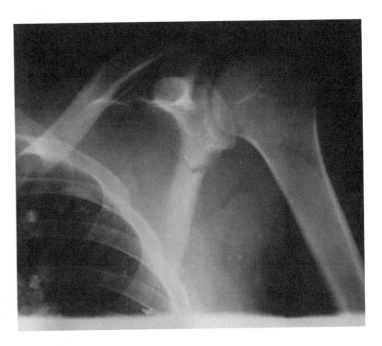

Figure 16–5. Comminuted fracture of the neck of the glenoid with displacement.

Associated Injuries

Proximal humeral fractures or shoulder dislocations are often noted in conjunction with these fractures. Also, an associated fracture of the ipsilateral clavicle may occur.[7]

Treatment
□ Class C: Type I (Nondisplaced)

The emergency management of these fractures includes sling immobilization, ice, and analgesics. Passive exercise should be started at 48 hours graduating to active exercise as tolerated.[2,3]

□ Class C: Type II (Displaced)

Emergent orthopedic consultation is advised for these patients. Although many modes of therapy are acceptable most orthopedic surgeons prefer reduction with skeletal traction.[2,3] If the associated clavicle is fractured, internal fixation of the clavicle should be performed as soon as possible. This procedure will prevent the malunion of the scapular neck fracture.

Complications

Frequently encountered complications include diminished shoulder mobility or the development of posttraumatic arthritis.

□ CLASS D: GLENOID FRACTURES (FIG. 16–6)

Glenoid fractures can be divided into two types. Type I fractures involve the glenoid rim and may demonstrate anterior or posterior displacement as shown in Figures 16–6A and B. In addition, glenoid rim fractures can traverse the rim and the spine as shown in Figure 16–6C. Type II fractures, as shown in Figure 16–6D, are comminuted fractures of the glenoid.

Mechanism of Injury

Two mechanisms are commonly responsible for glenoid fractures. A direct blow, usually secondary to a fall on the lateral shoulder, may result in a stellate (type II) fracture.[6]

A fall on the flexed elbow results in a force that is transmitted up the humerus and expended on the glenoid rim. This mechanism often results in a rim fracture whose displacement is dependent on the direction of force. In addition, violent contraction of the triceps may result in avulsion of the inferior glenoid rim. This mechanism is commonly seen with shoulder dislocations (20 percent associated with glenoid rim fractures).[1,6]

Examination

Avulsion fractures will often be associated with shoulder dislocations. In addition, there will be pain and weakness of the triceps with inferior rim fractures. Stellate fractures will present with swelling and pain, which is increased with lateral compression.

X Ray

Routine views as well as an axillary view are generally adequate in defining the fracture. On occasion, CT scanning may be helpful in precisely defining the full extent of the fracture.

Associated Injuries

Shoulder dislocation is commonly associated with glenoid rim fractures.

Treatment
□ Class D: Type I (Rim)

Small fragments require only sling immobilization, ice, and analgesics. Exercise (pendulum type) should be started as soon as the symptoms subside. Large or widely displaced fragments or those associated with triceps impairment may require surgical fixation. Early consultation is strongly urged. Displaced fractures associated with dislocations are often reduced simultaneously with the joint reduction.

□ Class D: Type II (Stellate)

The emergency management should include sling immobilization, ice, analgesics, and early consultation. Depressed fractures or those with large displaced fragments often require operative reduction. Many surgeons prefer skeletal traction in the management of these fractures.[8]

Complications

Glenoid fractures are frequently complicated by the development of arthritis.

□ CLASS E: CORACOID PROCESS FRACTURES (FIG. 16–7)

The muscles attaching to the coracoid process include the coracobrachialis, the short head of the biceps, and the pectoralis minor. The ligaments inserting on the coracoid process are the coracoacromial, the coracoclavicular, and the coracohumeral.

Mechanism of Injury

Two mechanisms commonly result in coracoid process fractures. A direct blow to the superior point of the shoulder may result in a coracoid process fracture.[8] Violent contraction of one of the inserting muscles may result in an avulsion fracture.

SCAPULAR FRACTURES

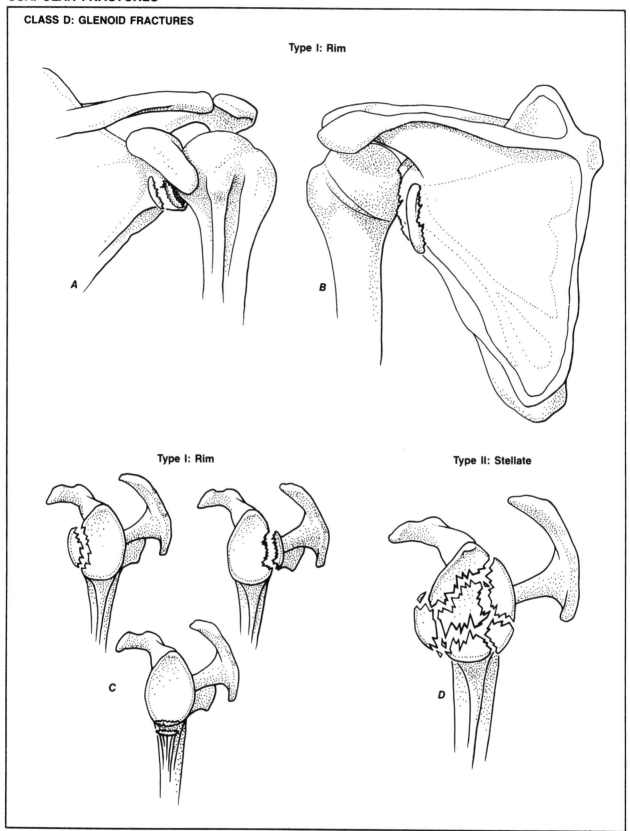

CLASS D: GLENOID FRACTURES

Type I: Rim

Type I: Rim

Type II: Stellate

Figure 16–6. Fractures of the rim of the glenoid. **A.** A small fragment from the anterior rim. **B.** A large fragment from the posterior rim of the glenoid. **C.** A variant of glenoid rim fractures. **D.** Severely comminuted fractures of the glenoid.

SCAPULAR FRACTURES

CLASS E: CORACOID PROCESS FRACTURES

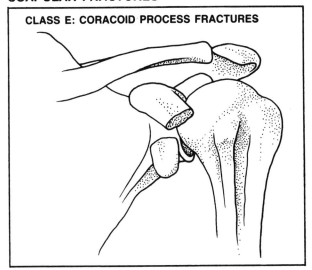

Figure 16-7.

Examination

The patient will present with tenderness to palpation anteriorly over the coracoid process. In addition, there will be pain with forced adduction and with flexion at the elbow.[3]

X Ray

Routine radiographs of this fracture-should include an axillary lateral view for delineation of any displacement (usually downward and medially) of the fragment. On occasion, CT scanning may be helpful in precisely defining the full extent of the fracture.

Associated Injuries

Brachial plexus injuries along with acromioclavicular dislocations or clavicular fractures are often associated with coracoid fractures.

Treatment

Coracoid process fractures are usually treated symptomatically. The patient should be given a sling, ice, analgesics, and instructions to begin early motion as tolerated. Associated injuries must be excluded before discharge from the emergency department.

Complications

None are commonly seen after these injuries.

REFERENCES

1. Aston JW, Gregory CF: Dislocation of the shoulder with significant fracture of the glenoid. *J Bone Joint Surg* **55**:1531–1533, 1973.
2. Charlton MR: Fractures of the neck of the scapula. *Northwest Med* **37**:18, 1938.
3. Cotton FJ, Brickley WJ: Treatment of fracture of neck of scapula. *Boston Med Surg J* **185**:326, 1921.
4. Findlay RT: Fractures of the scapula. *Ann Surg* **93**:1001, 1931.
5. Goss TP: The scapula: Coracoid, acromial, and avulsion fractures. *Am J Orthop* February 1996.
6. Harmon PH, Baker DR: Fractures of the scapula with displacement. *J Bone Joint Surg* **25**:834, 1943.
7. Herscovici D, Finnes AG, Allgower M, Ruedi TP: The floating shoulder: Ipsilateral clavicle and scapular neck fractures. *J Bone Joint Surg* [Br] **3**:362–364, 1992.
8. Rowe CR: Fractures of the scapula. *Surg Clin North Am* **43**:1565, 1963.

17
CHAPTER

SOFT TISSUE INJURIES, DISLOCATIONS, AND DISORDERS OF THE SHOULDER AND UPPER ARM

Shoulder pain is a very common presenting complaint to the emergency department. This remarkable joint is capable of a wide, almost global, range of motion. The intricate ligamentous and muscular attachments make it a complex joint and render differential diagnosis of single pathologic entities difficult. The tendons are close to the capsule and in part actually adhere to the capsule. The muscles, tendons, and ligaments provide support for the shoulder and maintain the humerus in its position within the glenoid against gravity. Gravity actually acts against shoulder stability and pulls the humerus downward out of the glenoid fossa. The humeral head has very little contact with the shallow glenoid fossa. Because of this close association of various structures, many conditions occur together and are hard to differentiate.

Functional Anatomy

The shoulder joint is actually composed of three joints: the sternoclavicular, the acromioclavicular, and the glenohumeral; and one articulation, the scapulothoracic (Figs. 17–1 and 17–2). These joints are intricately involved in the motions of the shoulder and are common sites of pathologic conditions that present with shoulder pain. Figures 17–1 and 17–2 provide the essential anatomy, both osseous and ligamentous, which must be understood to comprehend the disorders involving the shoulder. Superficial to the ligaments shown in Figure 17–2 are the muscles that support the shoulder and provide for its global range of motion. The rotator cuff surrounds the glenohumeral joint and is composed of the teres minor, infraspinatus, and supraspinatus muscles attaching to the greater tuberosity and the subscapularis

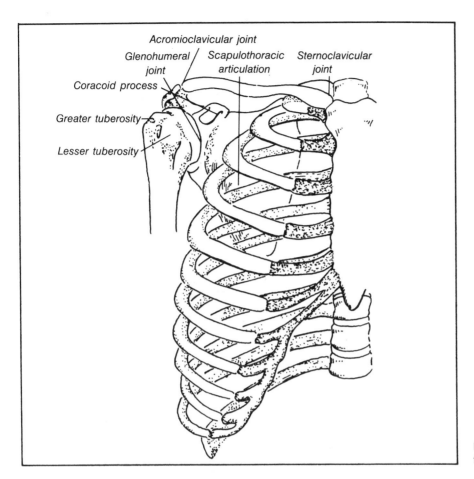

Figure 17-1. The essential anatomy of the shoulder.

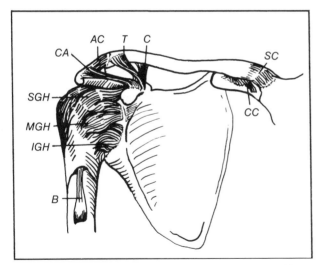

Figure 17-2. The ligaments around the shoulder. B = biceps tendon; IGH = inferior glenohumeral ligament; MGH = middle glenohumeral ligament; SGH = superior glenohumeral ligament; CA = coracoacromial arch; AC = acromioclavicular ligament; T = trapezoid; C = conoid; SC = sternoclavicular; CC = costoclavicular ligaments.

muscle attaching to te lesser tuberosity (see Fig. 17–25). Superficial to these muscles is the deltoid, which func-

tions to elevate the head of the humerus, impinging it under the coracoacromial arch, and is an abductor of the shoulder.

The Arm–Trunk Mechanism

The glenonumeral joint and scapulothoracic articulation function as a unit in abducting the humerus. The ratio of scapular to glenohumeral movement is 1:2; therefore, for every 30 degrees of abduction of the arm, the scapula moves 10 degrees and the glenohumeral joint moves 20 degrees (Fig. 17–3). If the glenohumeral joint is completely immobilized, the scapulothoracic articulation is capable of providing 65 degrees of abduction on its own. This is called the "shrugging" mechanism. This mechanism is important for the emergency physician to be aware of in assessing the movements at the shoulder joint that are hampered by certain pathologic entities.

At the sternoclavicular joint, the clavicle is elevated 4 degrees during shoulder abduction for every 10 degrees in the first 90 degrees of abduction. Beyond 90 degrees, movement at this joint is nil. The range of motion at the acromioclavicular joint is approximately 20 degrees. This motion occurs during

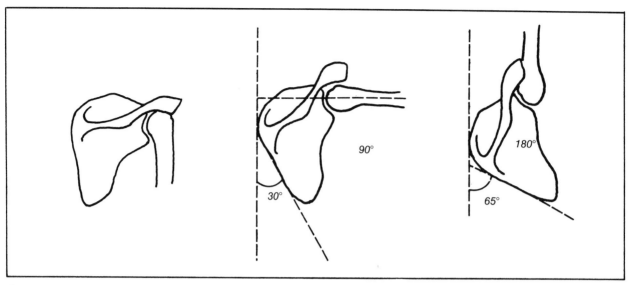

Figure 17–3. The ratio of glenohumeral to scapulothoracic motion is 2:1. At 90 degrees of abduction, 60 degrees occurs at the glenohumeral joint and 30 degrees at the scapulothoracic articulation. With the shrugging mechanism one can abduct the shoulder 65 degrees because of scapulothoracic movement even though there is no motion at the glenohumeral joint.

the first 30 degrees and after 100 degrees of abduction. During abduction of the arm, the clavicle rotates on its long axis.

Essential Surface Anatomy

A number of structures can be palpated easily around the shoulder and are important for the emergency physician to be cognizant of as they are common sites of pathology. If one palpates the suprasternal notch and immediately moves it laterally, the *sternoclavicular joint* can be palpated. The clavicle is slightly superior to the manubrium, and one is actually palpating the proximal end of the clavicle at this point. The clavicle is superficial in its entire course and can be palpated easily. If one palpates the clavicle laterally, one will note that it begins to flatten out in its lateral one third, however, it retains its round contour as it protrudes slightly above the acromion.

The *acromioclavicular joint* is palpated by pushing in a medial direction against the distal end of the clavicle as it protrudes above the flattened acromion process. The acromioclavicular joint is more easily palpated if the patient is asked to move the shoulder several times while the examiner palpates the joint. The greater tuberosity of the humerus lies lateral to the acromion process and can be palpated easily by following the acromion process to its lateral edge and then sliding the fingers inferiorly. A small step-off exists between the lateral acromion border and the *greater tuberosity*. The bicipital groove is located anterior and medial to the greater tuberosity and is bordered laterally by the greater tuberosity and medially

by the lesser tuberosity. This structure can be palpated easily if the arm is rotated externally. External rotation places the groove in a more exposed position for palpation and permits the examiner to palpate the greater tuberosity first, then the *bicipital groove*, and finally, the *lesser tuberosity* by moving from a lateral to medial po-sition. The tendon of the biceps lies within this groove. The *coracoid process* can be palpated by placing the patient in a relaxed position, noting the deepest portion of the clavicular concavity that lies along its lateral third and placing the fingers inferiorly about 1 inch from the anterior edge of the clavicle. By pressing laterally and posteriorly, one will feel the coracoid process. This region is the deltopectoral triangle and by pressing into this triangle one will also feel the coracoid process. The *scapula* can be seen posteriorly and covers ribs two through seven.

The rotator cuff, although not easily palpable, must be recognized, as it is a common site of pathologic processes. Its location and position are shown in Figure 17–26. Four bursae exist around the shoulder. The most important is the subacromial or subdeltoid bursa that lies between the deltoid muscle and the rotator cuff and extends beneath the acromion and the coracoacromial arch as it separates the structures from the rotator cuff muscles (Fig. 17–4). The subcoracoid bursa is located beneath the coracoid process. The subscapularis bursa is located near the tendonous junction of the subscapularis with the lesser tuberosity. The scapular bursae are located at the superior and inferior medial borders of the scapula and are separated from the chest wall.

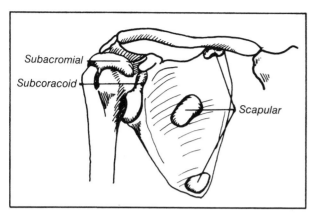

Figure 17–4. The important bursae of the shoulder.

In considering the disorders that occur around the shoulder joint, a useful categorization is to group them into three parts: disorders of the shoulder joint; disorders of the muscles, tendons, and bursae around the shoulder; and, finally, disorders of the scapulothoracic junction.

DISORDERS OF THE SHOULDER JOINT

□ ACROMIOCLAVICULAR JOINT

The acromioclavicular joint functions to elevate the arm and abduct it. Stability at this joint is provided by two ligaments: the acromioclavicular and the coracoclavicular ligaments. The coracoclavicular ligament is divided into the conoid and the trapezoid ligaments, which function together to anchor the distal clavicle to the coracoid process (see Fig. 17–2).

Acromioclavicular joint pain can occur after an old injury. The acromioclavicular stress test is performed by bringing the arm across the body approximating the elbow to the contralateral shoulder (Fig. 17–5). Localization of pain to the acromioclavicular joint confirms that this is the cause of pain. An injection of lidocaine over the joint relieves the discomfort.

□ Subluxations and Dislocations

Subluxations and dislocations of the acromioclavicular joint are common injuries presenting to the emergency department. The mechanisms by which they occur are either as a result of a direct force, usually a fall with the arm adducted to the side, or a force from above the acromion that strikes the bony prominence and dislodges it from its attachments to the clavicle.[31] An indirect mechanism by which this injury occurs is a fall on the outstretched arm with the force transmitted to the acromioclavicular joint. Most injuries of the acromioclavicular joint are caused by a direct fall onto the point of the shoulder.[46] A more horizontally directed force (ie, fall to the lateral side of the shoulder) may result in intra-articular damage with no significant injury to the ligaments. This may account for many cases of late degenerative joint disease and pain following a seemingly mild acromioclavicular sprain. This injury is divided into three basic degrees, which will be discussed separately.

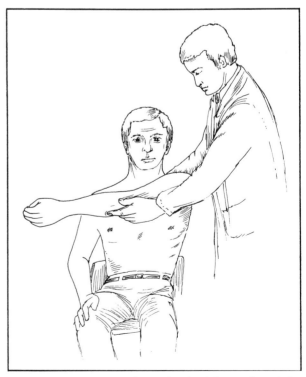

Figure 17–5. Technique for testing for inflammation of the acromioclavicular joint.

Examination and Radiographic Features

The diagnosis of acromioclavicular joint injury can be made by examining the patient in the upright position and looking for deformity at the top of the shoulder. This deformity represents a prominence of the distal clavicle indicating tear of the acromioclavicular and possible coracoclavicular ligaments. The upward displacement of the clavicle is due to downward pull of the shoulder caused by the weight of the arm and loss of the suspending coracoclavicular ligament.[11]

Stress anterior posterior radiographs using 10 to 15 pounds of weight suspended from the wrist are commonly done. This is only necessary when one cannot see the classical features of third-degree injury:

1. The inferior border of the distal clavicle is above the midpoint of the acromion.
2. The distance between the coracoid process and the inferior border of the clavicle is greater than one-half centimeter more as compared to the normal side.

If the preceding x ray features are present on an anteroposterior (AP) view, one does not need stress films. In one study, the stress films were unable to distinguish between type 2 and type 3 injuries even using 10 to 15 pounds of weight.[11]

☐ *First-degree Injury*

A first-degree injury to this joint is commonly called a sprain of the acromioclavicular ligament and involves an incomplete tear of that structure. The patient complains of tenderness over the joint; however, swelling is usually minimal. There is no subluxation involved with first-degree injuries, and the x ray is negative, even with stress films.

☐ *Second-degree Injury*

A second-degree injury involves a subluxation of the acromioclavicular joint and is always associated with disruption of the acromioclavicular ligament and a partial subluxation of the distal end of the clavicle from the acromion; however, the coracoclavicular ligament remains intact. The patient experiences tenderness to mild palpation and moderate swelling is noted. Routine roentgenograms of the shoulder are usually normal although subluxation with stress films will be noted. The *pathognomonic* x ray finding is a separation of the distal clavicle by not more than one half its diameter from the acromion on routine stress films taken of the shoulder in the AP position. Separation of the clavicle by more than one half its diameter indicates a third-degree injury. In addition, there is no increase in the distance between the coracoid and the clavicle when compared with the opposite normal shoulder on the stress film with a second-degree injury. These two findings correlate well when one is trying to separate a second-degree subluxation from a third-degree dislocation of the acromioclavicular joint.

Routine shoulder x rays in a patient whom one suspects has an acromioclavicular joint injury should include stress views. Stress views are taken in the AP position with 5 to 10 pounds of weight suspended from the arm (Fig. 17–7). A common mistake is for the radiology technician to have the patient hold the weight in the hand. This should be cautioned against because this will temper the actual degree of separation at that joint (Fig. 17–6).

☐ *Third-degree Injury*

In these patients there is a complete dislocation at the acromioclavicular joint with upward displacement of the clavicle and disruption of both the acromioclavicular and coracoclavicular ligaments (see Fig. 17–6). This can be confirmed by stress roentgenograms when one is trying to separate a second-degree from a third-degree injury.[55]

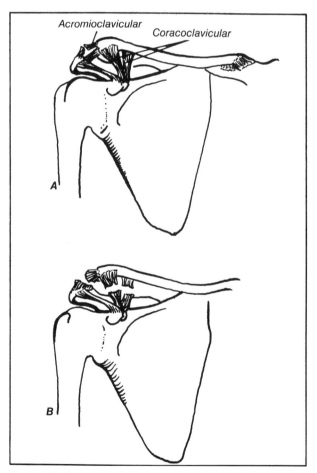

Figure 17–6. Acromioclavicular subluxation and dislocation. **A.** A grade II sprain with tear of the acromioclavicular ligament. **B.** A grade III sprain with tear of both the acromioclavicular and coracoclavicular ligaments.

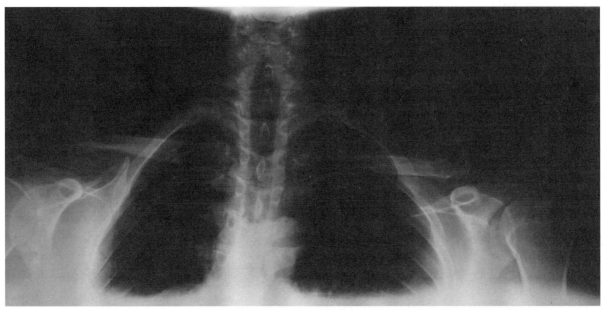

A

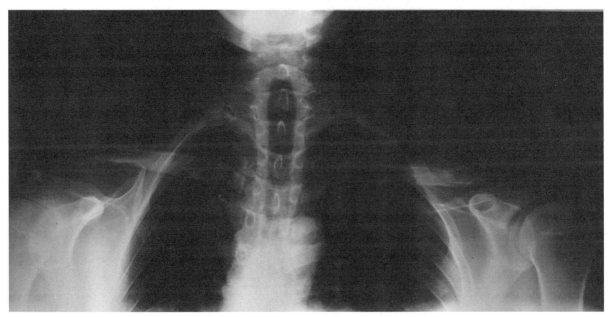

B

Figure 17–7. ***A.*** Notice that even without weights, the distance between the top of the coracoid process and the bottom of the clavicle is greater than 1 cm difference as compared with the normal side. ***B.*** With weights suspended from the arm, the distance between the coracoid process and the clavicle is increased. The key point to remember is that when one sees this separation without weights it is not necessary to then obtain a view with weights.

Treatment

In considering the treatment of acromioclavicular joint injuries one should look at a classification which has recently been introduced.[11] This assists the emergency physician making decisions regarding treatment.

Type 1   Sprain of the acromioclavicular ligaments

Type 2   Disruption of the acromioclavicular ligament with sprain of the coracoclavicular ligament

Type 3   Both acromioclavicular and coracoclavicular ligaments are disrupted

Type 4   The clavicle is displaced posteriorly into or through the trapezius muscle

Type 5   Disruption of all ligaments above the joint, and the clavicle is displaced far superiorly toward the base of the neck

Type 6   Inferior dislocation of the clavicle with the lateral end displaced down and under the acromion or the coracoid process. This is often associated with clavicle fractures, rib fractures, or brachial plexus injuries.

The treatment of type 1 injuries is rest, ice, and a sling, with early range of motion.

Type 2 injuries are treated conservatively in a similar fashion to type 1 injuries with the additional measure of reducing the clavicle and holding it in place with a brace-strap (Kenney-Howard sling), tape and sling, or other similar device. The duration of immobilization using a sling and swath has not been seen to affect the probability of recurrence, but up to 3 weeks may be necessary for comfort. A shorter immobilization period and once daily passive shoulder range of motion exercises out of the sling may help prevent the development of adhesive capsulitis.[6]

Type 3 injuries have in the past been treated surgically in young patients. Recent literature supports conservative treatment and demonstrates this as equal to or better than surgical intervention.[11] This should be treated similarly to type 2 injuries with the additional measure of early referral as late symptoms of acromioclavicular joint disease may develop. There is no definitive proof that an acromioclavicular support makes any difference in terms of long-term function as compared with a sling and ice.[42,55] There remains controversy regarding the treatment of third-degree dislocations (type 3 injuries). While some authors recommend surgical fixation, others recommend immobilization for a period of 3 weeks in the Kenney-Howard sling.[29,44] Thus, all third-degree injuries should be referred to an orthopedic surgeon for further evaluation and consultation.

Type 4, 5, and 6 injuries, all require surgical intervention.

Late symptoms of posttraumatic degenerative joint disease may occur after acromioclavicular joint injury. Excision of the distal clavicle may be necessary to avoid late degenerative joint disease and its associated pain syndrome.[11]

□ STERNOCLAVICULAR JOINT

□ Dislocation

The sternoclavicular joint is stabilized by the sternoclavicular ligament and the costaclavicular ligament (see Fig. 17–2). Maximum motion of this joint occurs with internal rotation with the arm elevated above 110 degrees. A sharp strong thrust of the arm and shoulder requires normal functioning of this joint. The most common mechanism of injury to this joint is by a force that thrusts the shoulder forward.

□ First-degree Injury

A first-degree injury is a sprain of the sternoclavicular joint and involves ligamentous tears that are incomplete

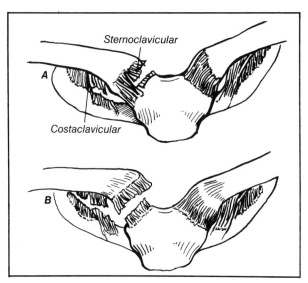

Figure 17–8. Sternoclavicular joint injuries. **A.** Grade II sprain with tear of the sternoclavicular ligament. **B.** Grade III sprain with disruption of both the sternoclavicular and costaclavicular ligaments.

of the sternoclavicular and the costaclavicular ligaments (Fig. 17–8A). The patient experiences minimal swelling and complains of tenderness over the joint. Pain is increased by elevation of the arm above 110 degrees.[44]

□ Second-degree Injury

A second-degree injury involves subluxation of the clavicle from its manubrial attachment and signifies complete rupture of the sternoclavicular ligament and partial rupture of the costaclavicular ligament. The patient experiences pain on abduction of the arm, and swelling is noted over the joint.

□ Third-degree Injury

A third-degree injury involves complete rupture of the sternoclavicular and costaclavicular ligaments (Fig. 17–8B) permitting the clavicle to dislocate from its manubrial attachment. Dislocations at this joint are either anterior or posterior. By far, the more common dislocation is an anterior dislocation of the sternoclavicular joint and is due to the same force indicated above; however, it can occur during a fall on the opposite shoulder followed by a "pile on" such as occurs during a football tackle that rolls the shoulder backward.[44] If the opposite shoulder is rolled forward during the "pile on" then a posterior dislocation will result.

On examination, the patient experiences severe pain, which is increased by any motion of the shoulder. On palpation, one will note the obvious, usually anterior, dislocation. In patients with posterior dislocations, this injury may constitute a true orthopedic emergency.[15,44] These patients may present with breathing difficulties secondary to tracheal compression, rupture, or from a pneumothorax; venous congestion may be seen, all of which are due to the posteriorly displaced clavicle compressing vital structures in the neck. This necessitates an emergency reduction by the physician in the emergency department (see discussion that follows).

Treatment

First-degree sprains of the sternoclavicular joint are treated with ice for 24 hours and a sling for 3 to 4 days.

Second-degree subluxations of the joint are treated with a figure-of-eight clavicle strap and a sling to hold the clavicle in its normal position and permit ligamentous healing. This protection should be continued for 6 weeks and the patient should be advised that he or she may later develop problems in the joint that may require operative intervention.

Third-degree dislocations are reduced as shown in Figure 17–9. A folded sheet is placed between the shoulders while the patient is supine, which serves to separate the clavicle from the manubrium. The arm is abducted and traction is applied as shown in Figure 17–9A. While traction is maintained, an assistant pushes the clavicle into its normal position. In patients with *posterior dislocations* the same maneuver is used; however, the clavicle is elevated forward while traction is maintained by grasping it as shown in Figure 17–9B and pulling it out of its posterior position.[15] In more difficult situations, a towel clip is used to grasp the clavicle (Fig. 17–10), and traction is applied in a similar manner to the grasping fingers. General anesthesia is often needed for a patient with posterior dislocation of the sternoclavicular joint.

The complications of an anterior dislocation of the sternoclavicular joint are cosmetic with chronic swelling noted around the joint. Posterior dislocations are less frequent, but are fraught with more serious complications including pneumothorax, laceration of the superior vena cava, occlusion of the subclavian artery or vein, and rupture or compression of the trachea. Approximately 25 percent of all posterior dislocations of the sternoclavicular joint are associated with tracheal, esophageal, or great vessel injury, which emphasizes the need for early reduction in the manner indicated above.

☐ ANTERIOR SHOULDER

☐ Dislocations

An anterior dislocation of the shoulder is one of the most common presenting problems to the emergency department and represents approximately 50 percent of all major joint dislocations seen by the emergency physician.[42] The mechanism by which this injury occurs is usually *abduction* accompanied by *external rotation* of the arm, which disrupts the anterior capsule and the gleno-

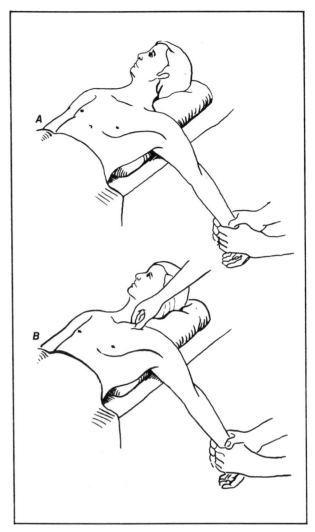

Figure 17–9. Reduction of a posteriorly displaced sternoclavicular joint injury. **A.** The arm is abducted and traction is applied. With traction maintained an assistant pushes the clavicle back into its normal position for anterior dislocations (not shown). **B.** With posterior dislocations, the clavicle is pulled back into its normal position. In difficult cases, the clavicle can be grasped with a towel clip and replaced.

humeral ligaments.[38] In the young, the common site of capsular tear is between the superior and middle glenohumeral ligaments. In addition to capsular tears, the labrum may be torn from the glenoid by the displacing humeral head. In the elderly, this dislocation is often accompanied by avulsion of the greater tuberosity. Approximately 70 percent of all anterior dislocations of the shoulder occur in patients under 30 years of age.[40,47]

There are three types of anterior dislocation: subclavicular, subcoracoid, and subglenoid (Fig. 17–11). The humeral head can interchange from one position to the next, but it usually remains in one of the three. Subcoracoid dislocations are often secondary to "hyper" external rotation. They can be seen after convulsions or a direct blow to the posterior aspect of the proximal

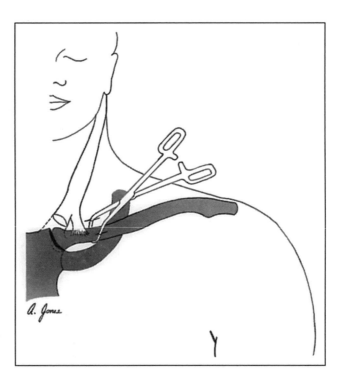

Figure 17–10. In difficult cases, the clavicle can be grasped with a towel clip and replaced.

humerus displacing it anteriorly; however, by far, the most common mechanism is that listed above.[47] Subglenoid dislocations are usually associated with more abduction than external rotation and have a higher incidence of greater tuberosity fractures and rotator cuff tears associated with them.

Clinical Presentation

The patient presents with the arms held to the side. The acromion is prominent and there is loss of the normal rounded contour of the shoulder.[40] The patient permits some abduction and external rotation of the arm and resists any attempts at internal rotation and adduction. Axillary nerve injury is the most common associated

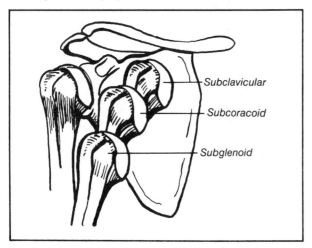

Subclavicular

Subcoracoid

Subglenoid

Figure 17–11. The three types of anterior dislocations of the shoulder.

neurologic injury in anterior shoulder dislocations occurring in approximately 12 percent of cases.[38] This is assessed by testing pinprick sensation over the lateral aspect of the arm and comparing it with the other side.[40] In addition, the radial, ulnar, and brachial pulses should be evaluated as well as the integrity of the median, ulnar, and radial nerves. The incidence of major nerve injury, in particular the axillary nerve, is 8 to 10 percent.[40] Associated fractures of the greater tuberosity are far more common in patients more than 45 years of age, occurring in approximately 40 percent of cases.

Anterior, posterior, and axillary views should be taken routinely before reduction is attempted (Fig. 17–12). If question exists, a true lateral view of the scapula will often help ascertain the extent or the type of dislocation. In evaluating the x rays of patients with suspected anterior dislocations of the shoulder, one should look for a defect in the posterior lateral portion of the humeral head called a *Hill-Sachs deformity* (ie, an impaction fracture of the humeral head). This is very common, occurring in up to 50 percent of cases, although a variable incidence has been reported.[29] The longer the humeral head is out of the glenoid fossa, the larger is the defect. The defect commonly occurs with recurrent anterior dislocations. If one suspects this, an internal rotation view can be ordered that will delineate the defect more clearly.

Treatment

Many methods have been described for reducing anterior shoulder dislocations, several of which will be

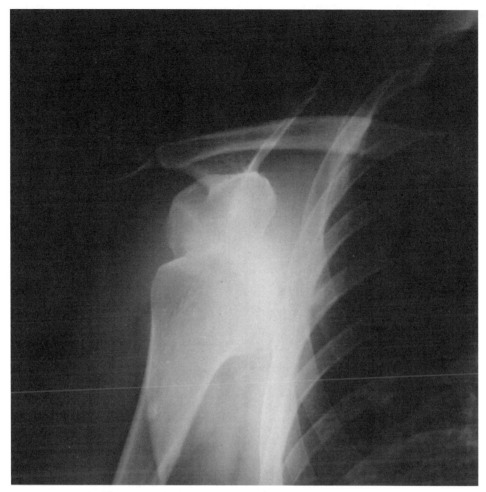

Figure 17–12. An anterior dislocation of the subcoracoid type.

discussed.[21,42,47] The authors prefer the Hennipen technique or the scapular manipulation technique as the method of first choice. In elderly patients with anterior shoulder dislocations, we recommend either the Hennipen technique or the Stimson technique. These pa-tients have a high incidence of associated injuries and thus should be carefully examined before any traction or significant manipulations are applied.

In reducing dislocations by any of the techniques, one should choose an intravenous narcotic (Demoral, morphine, Fentanyl) and a muscle relaxant (Valium, Versed), which should be administered prior to any attempt at reduction. Without adequate analgesia and muscle relaxation one cannot easily reduce the shoulder unless one sees the dislocation early enough to use the Hennipen technique, which is in essence a relaxation technique. Once muscle spasm develops one must use muscle relaxants and intravenous narcotics. Intravenous narcotics should be administered and titrated as needed. An alternate method of providing analgesia is by the suprascapular nerve block which was described by Edeland and Stefansson.[13]

Hennipen Technique. The Hennipen technique is, in the authors' opinion, the preferred technique to reduce anterior dislocations of the shoulder. This technique was popularized at Hennipen County Emergency Medicine Center. The technique requires little manipulation and permits the shoulder muscles to reduce the dislocation with little or no analgesia. In this technique, the patient is seated upright or at 45 degrees. The patient's elbow is supported by the right hand of the physician and the left hand is used to slowly and gently externally rotate the arm. The arm is externally rotated to 90 degrees as shown in Figure 17–13. If the patient experiences any discomfort during the external rotation, the examiner should stop and wait a moment until the muscles relax. During this procedure it is important that the patient be completely relaxed and that the rotation be done gradually and slowly. After reaching 90 degrees, the shoulder may have reduced spontaneously. If not, the arm is slowly elevated and the humeral head is lifted into the socket if it does not spontaneously reduce on elevation.

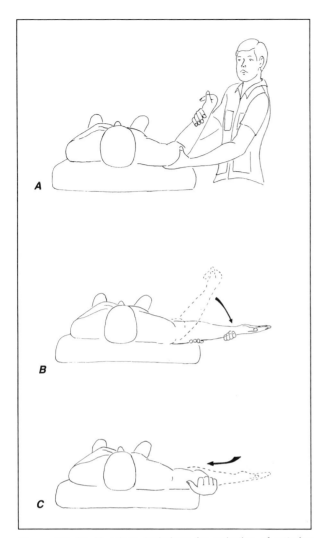

Figure 17–13. Hennipen technique for reduction of anterior dislocations of the shoulder. (***A***) Slowly rotate the arm externally to 90 degrees of external rotation. (***B, C***) After this, slowly elevate the arm until reduction is achieved.

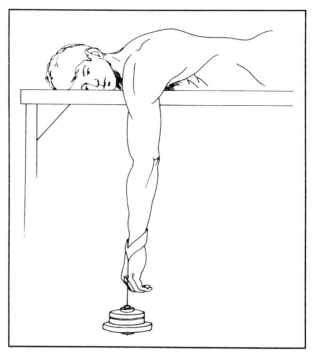

Figure 17–14. Stimson technique for reduction of anterior dislocations.

Stimson Technique. The Stimson technique is a safe procedure and the treatment of first choice to many in attempting to reduce an anterior dislocation of the shoulder.[51] The patient is placed in the prone position with the arms dependent over a pillow or folded sheets (Fig. 17–14). A strap is added to the wrist or distal forearm and weights are applied (anywhere from 10 to 15 pounds) over a period of 20 to 30 minutes.[51] This time is usually sufficient for reduction to occur. Muscle relaxation is imperative and the patient must be under constant observation by a nurse who is monitoring the patient's respiratory status and pulse. A period of 20 to 30 minutes is usually a sufficient amount of time for displacement of the humeral head and reduction. If unsuccessful, the examiner may rotate the humerus gently, externally and then internally with mild force, which usually reduces the dislocation.[51]

Scapular Manipulation Technique. The patient lies prone on the table with the affected arm hanging off of the table suspended with approximately 5 to 10 pounds of weight in a similar fashion to the Stimson technique described. The physician then pushes the tip of the scapula medially and the superior aspect of the scapula laterally. This technique is reported to have a high rate of success for reducing anterior shoulder dislocations with little associated complications.[38]

Traction and Countertraction. This method has been advocated for those anterior dislocations that are difficult to reduce by the Stimson technique (Fig. 17–15). In this method, an assistant applies countertraction with a folded sheet wrapped around the upper chest, and the examiner applies traction to the arm as indicated in the drawing. This maneuver usually dislodges the humeral head and slight lateral traction of the proximal humerus will usually reduce the dislocation.

Lateral Traction (Fig. 17–16). This maneuver is similar to the preceding one. In addition to traction as indicated in the previous section, along the longitudinal axis of the humerus a lateral force is applied to the proximal humerus by an assistant with a pillowcase folded and wrapped around the proximal humerus as far up into the axilla as possible (Fig. 17–16). The patient must have good muscle relaxation when using this maneuver to prevent avulsion injuries.

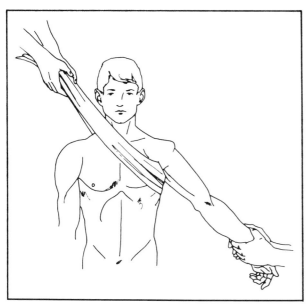

Figure 17–15. Traction-countertraction technique for reducing anterior shoulder dislocations.

The Kocher maneuver is quite dangerous and fraught with many complications and should not be used by the emergency physician in reducing anterior dislocations of the shoulder.[18] In the opinion of the authors, the Hippocratic technique should never be used under any circumstances in reducing these dislocations. Should the dislocation be irreducible by any of the above methods, then general anesthesia should be considered and reduction attempted in the operating room. Irreducible dislocations are usually due to soft tissue interposition.

Indications for Surgery with Acute Dislocations. There are several indications for surgery in an acute anterior dislocation of the shoulder beside soft tissue

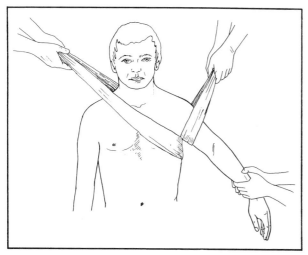

Figure 17–16. Traction and countertraction is applied to the sheet around the chest. After a few minutes the hand is disimpacted from under the glenoid and is reduced with lateral traction on the arm.

interposition (rotator cuff, capsule, biceps, tendon).[22] In a subglenoid or subclavicular dislocation there is often complete disruption of the cuff. In the young athlete repair is indicated and reduction may be attempted in the operating room at that time.[3] Another indication for surgery after reduction of an anterior dislocation is a fracture of the greater tuberosity that is displaced greater than 1 cm postreduction. Glenoid rim fractures that are displaced greater than 5 mm may require operative intervention also.

Treatment after Reduction. In patients less than 40 years of age a sling and swath are advocated or a shoulder immobilizer for 3 weeks. After this, gentle active range of motion exercises can be instituted; however, the patient should be cautioned against abduction and external rotation. External rotation and abduction should be prohibited for an additional 3 weeks after the sling and swath or shoulder immobilizer are discontinued. During the time the patient is immobilized, exercises of the wrist, hand, and elbow should be instituted.

In patients more than 30 years of age, we advocate a sling and swath for 1 week with active range of motion exercises avoiding abduction and external rotation to begin within 4 to 5 days.[30] The sling and swath should be continued for an additional week; however, the arm should be taken out of the immobilizer and circumduction exercises should be begun. The older the patient, the sooner mobilization should be instituted to avoid stiffness. When movement resumes, exercise should be performed with a pain-free range of motion. However, too little movement following a dislocation may result in severe shortening of the structures around the shoulder and prolongation of time it will take to regain full range of motion.[30]

In patients who have had an anterior shoulder dislocation or subluxation, strengthening of the subscapularis muscle is advocated. This can be done by a strengthening exercise as shown in Figure 17–17. The external rotators can be strengthened by the opposite maneuver. Thus, the capsule, which is a static stabilizer of the joint is further enhanced by the dynamic stabilizers.

Complications of an Anterior Dislocation. There are many complications of an anterior dislocation including *detachment or tear of the rotator cuff*, and an *avulsion of the greater tuberosity* that can occur in up to 38 percent of patients more than 40 years of age.[15] Brachial plexus injury or damage to the axillary nerve occurs in 5 to 14 percent of cases.[15,44] This nerve injury is usually a neuropraxia and full recovery can be expected in most instances.[15,44] Fractures of the humeral head can be seen as well as damage to the biceps tendon. The most common complication of anterior dislocation is recurrence, which is seen in 60 percent of patients less than 30 years of age

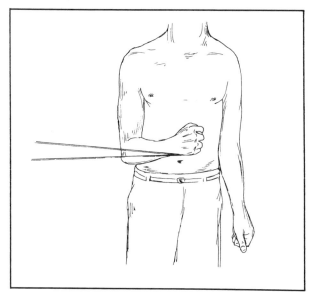

Figure 17–17. A rotator cuff strengthening exercise using rubber tubing. This strengthens the subscapularis muscle and helps prevent recurrent dislocations of the shoulder.

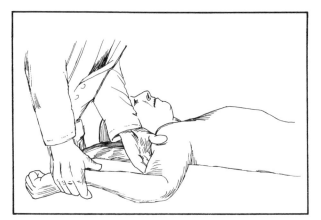

Figure 17–18. Technique for performing shoulder apprehension test.

and drops off to an incidence of approximately 10 percent in patients more than 40 years of age. Operative repair is indicated in patients who have sustained more than three dislocations. Most of the literature demonstrates that patients with recurrent dislocations have extensive capsular tears and at least partial labral detachment resulting in some instability.[23] True Bankart lesions have been found at the time of repair in 84 and 90 percent of these cases.[23]

☐ Subluxation

Anterior subluxation of the shoulder is an uncommonly diagnosed but often missed problem in the emergency department. This situation is characterized by sudden sharp pain when the shoulder is forcibly moved into external rotation during elevation. It can occur during forceful serving in a tennis match. The apprehension test is usually positive. In the shoulder apprehension test, the arm is rotated externally in a position of abduction, whereas anteriorly directed pressures are applied to the posterior aspect of the humeral head as shown in Figure 17–18. This causes sudden pain and may cause anterior displacement of the humeral head. When this is a recurrent problem the patient should be referred for further evaluation as many of these cases require surgical intervention to stabilize the shoulder.[17,41]

☐ POSTERIOR SHOULDER

☐ Dislocations

Posterior dislocations are far less common than anterior dislocations. Posterior disslocations of the shoulder are the most commonly missed major dislocations of the body. There are three types of posterior dislocations: subacromial, subglenoid, and subspinous. Ninety-eight percent of all posterior dislocations are of the subacromial type.[14] There are several mechanisms by which this injury occurs; among them being a violent internal rotational force such as would occur during a fall on the forward flexed internally rotated arm. This type of dislocation is also commonly seen after a convulsion (Fig. 17–19).[35]

Clinical Presentation

The cardinal sign of a posterior dislocation of the shoulder is that the arm is held in adduction and internal rotation with abduction severely limited. In addition, external rotation of the shoulder is blocked. On palpation of the shoulder girdle, the examiner will note a prominence in the posterior aspect of the shoulder accompanied by a flattening anteriorly of the normal shoulder contour. The coracoid process is usually more obvious than its counterpart on the normal side. Blocking of *external rotation* and *limitation of abduction* occur in all cases of posterior dislocations. In the subglenoid and subspinous type, the arm is held in 30 degrees abduction and is internally rotated.

There are two features on the routine views of the shoulder that will aid the emergency physician in suspecting this diagnosis. The first the loss of the normal elliptical pattern produced by overlap of the humeral head and the posterior glenoid rim as noted in Figure 17–20. The second is internal rotation of the greater tuberosity as shown. Internal rotation of the humeral head results on x ray in what is known as an "ice cream cone sign" (Fig. 17–21). The head appears as though it sits on top of a cone primarily made up of the greater tuberosity. The humeral head does not fill the fossa as it normally does. If there remains a question about dislocation, a true lateral view will demonstrate it quite well. This dislocation is commonly associated with fractures of the humerus and

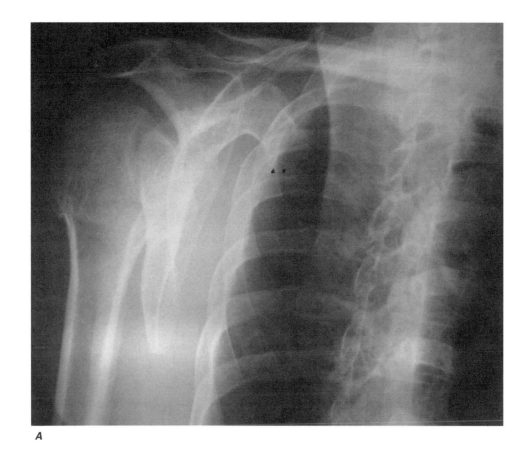

A

B

Figure 17–19. **A.** The "ice cream cone sign" is shown here. Notice that with a posterior dislocation, the greater tuberosity protrudes anteriorly as the head is rotated posteriorly. **B.** Again, a posterior dislocation of the humerus is shown with a head displaced posteriorly.

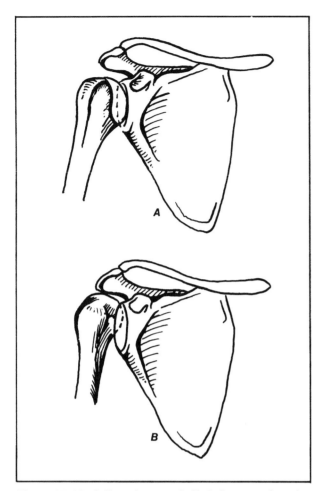

Figure 17-20. *A.* Note the normal elliptical pattern of overlap produced by the head of the humerus and the glenoid fossa. ***B.*** In the patient with a posterior dislocation, this pattern is lost, and there is also internal rotation of the greater tuberosity.

the posterior aspect of the glenoid rim. An isolated fracture of the lesser tuberosity should lead one to suspect a posterior dislocation until proven otherwise.

One of the most common physical findings in a person who has recurrent posterior dislocation with instability is a positive posterior stress test. To perform this test, the examiner stabilizes the medial border of the scapular with one hand. The other hand applies a posterially directed force to the patient's humerus, which is flexed to 90 degrees, adducted, and internally rotated (see Fig. 17-22). A positive test consists of either subluxation or dislocation with pain, or an uncomfortable sensation that reproduces a patient's symptoms during episodes of instability.[33]

Axiom: *An isolated fracture of the lesser tuberosity should lead one to suspect posterior dislocation of the shoulder until proven otherwise.*

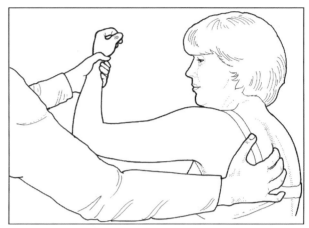

Figure 17-22. The posterior stress test to evaluate posterior shoulder instability. Stabilize the medial border of the scapula with one hand. The patient's humerus should be flexed to 90 degrees, abducted, and internally rotated. Apply a posterior force along the humerus. Subluxation, dislocation with pain, or an uncomfortable sensation that reproduces the patient's symptoms is considered a positive test.

Treatment

This injury can be reduced by applying longitudinal traction by the Stimson or some other technique to the arm and pushing the posteriorly displaced humeral head forward. In cases that are accompanied by acute pain and spasms, one may need a general anesthetic to reduce the dislocation. Most posterior dislocations should be referred as these are uncommon. Indications for surgical intervention include major displacement of the lesser tuberosity that is irreducible on reduction of the dislocation. Neurovascular complications with this injury are uncommon.

□ INFERIOR DISLOCATIONS (LUXATIO ERECTA) (FIG. 17-23)

Inferior dislocations of the shoulder are uncommon but can be quite serious injuries. Luxatio erecta has been reported almost exclusively in men.[26] The mechanism by which this injury occurs is hyperabduction. Luxatio erecta is always accompanied by detachment of the rotator cuff[24] (Fig. 17-24).

On examination, the patient complains of severe pain, and the arm is held in 180 degrees of elevation and appears to be shortened when compared with the normal side. One can feel the humeral head along the lateral chest wall. These patients usually present in significant pain and hold their arm up as if "asking a question." The patients usually have neurovascular

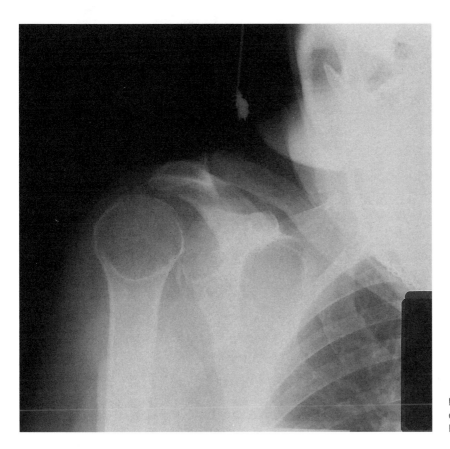

Figure 17–21. A posterior shoulder dislocation with glenoid rim fracture. Notice the "ice cream" cone sign.

compression as an involved injury; however, they practically always recover following reduction.[26] The axillary artery and brachial plexus are commonly associated with this injury because the humeral head tears through the inferior capsule rather than the anterior capsule as with the anterior dislocation of the shoulder. Vascular injury is not common, but is more common in luxatio erecta than in any of the other types of shoulder dislocation.[26] Radiological evaluation with two views at right angles of each other, a lateral view and anterior posterior view, are useful.[32] Fractures of the acromion, inferior glenoid rim, and greater tuberosity of the humerus can occur.[32]

The reduction of this type of dislocation is shown in Figure 17–25. Reduction may be difficult if the humeral head has torn a small rent in the inferior glenohumeral capsule.[26] Traction is applied by the physician as shown in the longitudinal axis of the humerus while an assistant applies countertraction with a folded sheet wrapped around the supraclavicular region. While traction is maintained, the arm is rotated inferiorly in an arch as shown. If a button hole deformity occurs in the inferior capsule, then one may have to do an open reduction.[32] Postinjury one must follow the patients closely for evidence of rotator cuff tears.[26] After reduction immobilize the shoulder for 2 to 4 weeks. Occasionally, patients may require general anesthesia to reduce the dislocation and surgical repair of the cuff may be indicated.[24]

□ ACUTE TRAUMATIC SYNOVITIS

This is common secondary to sprains of the glenohumeral ligaments or slight ears in the capsule occurring in young athletes. The patient complains of pain over the shoulder joint, and there is tenderness elicited to palpation of the capsule and motion of thes shoulder. The anterior/inferior portion of the capsule is the most commonly affected site, usually secondary to abduction ex-ternal rotation injuries. The treatment for this condition is immobilization in a sling and the application of warm moist packs. One should begin active range of motion exercises as soon as pain will permit.

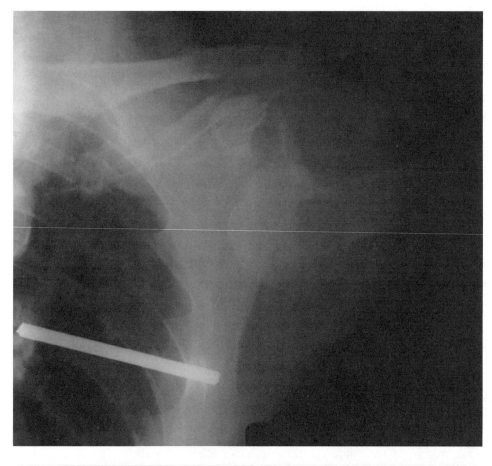

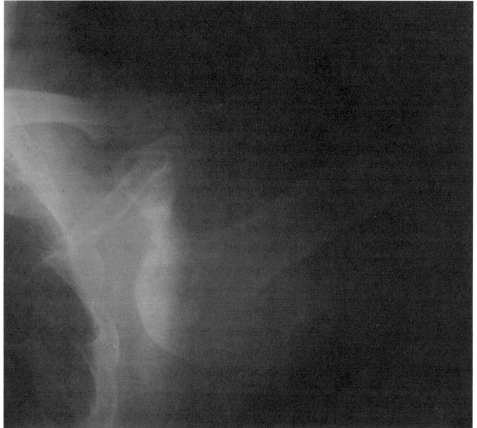

Figure 17–23. A luxatio erecta dislocation of the shoulder.

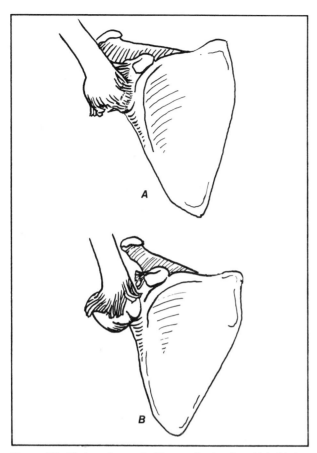

Figure 17–24. Luxatio erecta. The mechanism by which this injury occurs is hyperabduction (**A**). This is always accompanied by both disruption of the rotator cuff and tear through the inferior capsule (**B**).

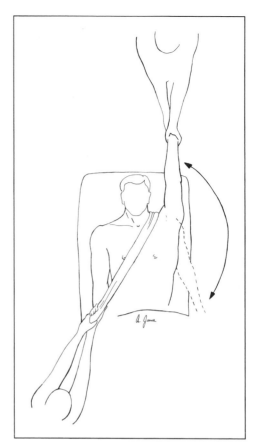

Figure 17–25. Reduction of a luxatio erecta dislocation. Traction is applied by the physician in the longitudinal axis of the humerus while an assistant applies countertraction with a folded sheet. While traction is maintained the arm is rotated inferiorly in an arc as shown.

DISORDERS OF THE MUSCLES, TENDONS, AND BURSAE AROUND THE SHOULDER

☐ ACUTE TEARS OF THE ROTATOR CUFF

Tears of the rotator cuff are more common in the elderly because of degenerative changes that occur with advancing age, particularly after the fifth decade of life.[48,50,53] When this injury is seen in the young, it requires a greater degree of trauma. Prior to the fifth decade, this injury is more likely to avulse bone.[9] The mechanism by which one disrupts the rotator cuff is a sudden powerful elevation of the arm against resistance in an attempt to cushion a fall, or it can occur secondary to heavy lifting, or a fall on the shoulder (Fig. 17–26). In the patient over 50 years of age, this may occur with minimal trauma or the patient may not report any trauma. It has been stated that the shape of the anterior acromion process has been associated with impingement, and this may cause rotator cuff tear to occur spontaneously.[54] When one looks at the anatomy of the rotator cuff, it is easy to see how eleva-

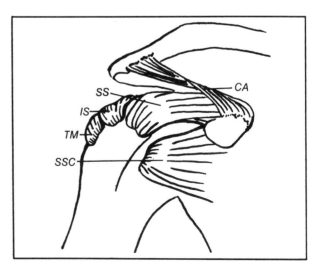

Figure 17–26. The rotator cuff. SSC = subscapularis tendon; TM = teres minor; IS = infraspinatus tendon; SS = supraspinatus tendon; CA = coracoacromial arch.

tion of the shoulder can impinge upon the acromion and the coracoacromial arch causing it to wear down with age and spontaneously rupture with minimal trauma (see Fig. 17–26).

Disruption of the rotator cuff can occur at any point; however, it is more common in the anterosuperior portion of the cuff near the attachment of the supraspinatus muscle (Fig. 17–27).[4] The tendon is worn down by compressive forces occurring between the humeral head and the coracoacromial arch. The shape of the acromion has clearly been shown to be associated with a higher incidence of tears. A hook shape underneath has been associated with a high incidence of tears both on cadaver specimens and clinically.[1,39]

Thirty percent or more of the tendon must be ruptured to produce a significant reduction of strength.[16] Conservative therapy will result in a good outcome in only 50 percent of patients.[10] The extent of the tear is directly related to the limitation of shoulder abduction.[25] Clinical examination compares favorably with arthrography and should be used instead of ultrasonography as a first-line screening test following examination.[25]

Iannotti and associates studied 127 magnetic resonance imaging (MRI) scans in 91 patients who underwent surgical intervention and in 15 volunteers. The sensitivity of MRI and the diagnosis of full-thickness rotator cuff tears was 100 percent and the specificity was 95 percent.[52] MRI was able to differentiate partial cuff tears from intact tendons with a sensitivity of 82 percent and a specificity of 85 percent. It was highly predictive of the size of the full-thickness rotator cuff tear.[19]

It is uncommon for patients who have had no previous symptoms in the shoulder to have a clear-cut history of an injury followed by immediate pain and inability to raise the arm. This type of patients in one series accounted for only 8 percent of the total patients with rotator cuff tears.

Several roentgenographic assessment methods have been advocated.[5] In addition to anteroposterior (AP) films in various positions, a special "cuff view" may also assist in viewing the humeral head. One may see signs of degenerative changes in the rotator cuff on x ray, including the following: erosion and periosteal reaction of the greater tuberosity, alterations of the inferior aspect of the acromion, and subchondral erosion in the greater tuberosity.[5]

Arthropneumotomography is an excellent modality which determines not only the extent of an established supraspinatus tear, but also the number of tendons involved. This is accomplished by filling the joint space with air and obtaining tomograms of the acromiohumeral compartment.[5] High-resolution real-time ultrasound has been shown to be a good examination technique for rotator cuff tears.[28,36]

Clinical Presentation

The patient presents with complaints of pain aggravated by activity radiating to the anterior aspect of the arm, abduction is painful and weak, and tenderness is elicited to palpation over the insertion of the greater tuberosity. Up to 40 degrees of abduction may occur by the "shrugging" mechanism alone; however, the examiner will not be fooled by this if he or she is aware of scapulothoracic

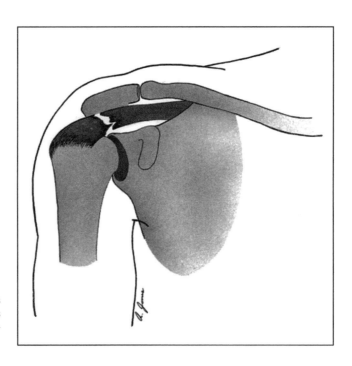

Figure 17–27. A rotator cuff tear is shown. The rotator cuff usually tears along the supraspinatus tendon insertion.

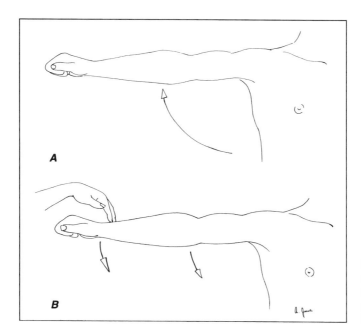

Figure 17–28. The drop arm test is shown. With minimal pressure over the abducted arm, the patient cannot sustain abduction and drops the arm to the side.

motion during the examination.[9] The patient cannot *initiate abduction* if large tears of the supraspinatus occur. The most severe pain occurs when one compresses the tendon beneath the coracoacromial arch with passive abduction between 40 and 90 degrees.[9]

The *drop arm test* (Fig. 17–28), is positive in patients with significant tears. The drop arm test is performed by laterally elevating the arm to the 90-degree position and asking the patient to hold the arm in this position. Lidocaine may be infiltrated around the cuff in patients unable to do this. A slight pressure on the distal forearm or wrist by the examiner will cause the patient to suddenly drop the arm. In addition, the patient is unable to bring the arm from the abducted position to the side in a slow fashion when asked to do so, but rather drops it suddenly. To do this examination, one may have to inject the rotator cuff with lidocaine. The strength of abduction is proportional to the size of the tear. When tears are localized to the posterosuperior aspect of the cuff, pain is elicited on abduction and internal rotation whereas tears of the anterosuperior cuff cause pain on abduction and external rotation. A defect may be palpable in early cases (ie, before swelling occurs) of acute rotator cuff rupture below the acromion. Crepitation and grating may be palpated on examination in this region. Injection is also a good technique of differentiating this condition from tendonitis of the rotator cuff.

Another diagnostic examination for rotator cuff disease in patients in whom a tear is suspected is what has been termed the near impingement test. This test is accomplished by injecting 1 percent lidocaine into the subachromial bursa space. An injection here will relieve the pain, as previously indicated. Patients with rotator cuff disease will experience restriction on forward flexion of the shoulder after injection. The test distinguishes rotator cuff disease from other sources of shoulder pain; however, it does not distinguish between a tear and early stages of inflammation and fibrosis.[49]

Treatment

Arthroscopic treatment can be done with a number of rotator cuff tears, particularly in the young. Location of the tear is more important than the size when determining outcomes for arthroscopic treatment (ie, anterior tears have better outcomes).[8,48] With arthroscopic treatment inferior tears may enlarge. If the tear involves enough of the posterior rotator cuff, then the glenohumeral fulcrum is lost, resulting in poor motion.[8] Thus, patients with massive tears in the posterior rotator cuff are bad candidates for arthroscopic treatment.[8]

In the young, early surgical repair is indicated for complete tears of the rotator cuff; however, in the elderly, with more sedentary occupations, repair is not indicated. Postoperatively, the power of the deltoid and external rotator muscles determine the success of the repair.[34] Good passive range of motion exercises should be instituted as soon as possible in elderly patients. In patients in whom there is a question as to the size of the tear or whether a tear has occurred, referral for arthrography of the shoulder is indicated.

Conservative measures remain the mainstay of initial treatment for most rotator cuff tears. It has been shown that one or two steroid injections into the subacromial space may be helpful.[7] The initial period of rest and cold followed by heat application and nonsteroidal anti-inflammatory drugs should be accompanied by modified activity and physical therapy. With partial-thickness tears, range of motion exercises are important to reduce the stiffness that occurs.[7]

☐ SUPRASPINATUS TENDONITIS AND SUBACROMIAL–SUBDELTOID BURSITIS

These conditions will be considered together because the pathologic processes are closely interrelated. Supraspinatus tendonitis is the most common cause of shoulder pain and is usually caused by degenerative changes in that tendon with advancing age. The tendons of the teres minor, infraspinatus, supraspinatus, and subscapularis muscles come together and attach on the greater and lesser tuberosities to form the rotator cuff. Tendonitis can occur in any one of these tendons but is much more common along a "critical point" where the cuff comes in close proximity with the coracoacromial arch, coinciding with the supraspinatus portion of the cuff (Fig. 17–29).

Pathogenesis

The supraspinatus tendon along with other tendons of the rotator cuff undergo degeneration with advancing age, being subject to repeated trauma. As they traverse under the acromion and the coracoacromial arch, small tears occur in these relatively avascular structures. The repair process is associated with inflammatory cells leading to a tendonitis of the supraspinatus tendon (Fig. 17–30A). The patient seen at this stage usually complains of a deep ache in the shoulder with increasing pain on abduction and internal rotation. These inflammatory cells eventually deposit fine particles of calcium within the tendon (Fig. 17–30B). This stage in the sequence is called the *silent phase* and is not visible on x ray. As the process continues, the tendon engorges as the calcium retains fluid and the inflammatory process continues. More calcium deposition ensues and the tendon swells. This is called the *engorgement phase* (Fig. 17–30C). The particles of calcium coalesce and become visible on x ray for the first time, called the *chalk phase* (Fig. 17–30D). The calcium particles absorb water from the surrounding tissue, which causes the tendon to swell and impinge on the subacromial-subdeltoid bursa that forms the roof of the supraspinatus tendon (Fig. 17–30E). This phase is called the *bulge phase*, and at this stage the tendon becomes an obstacle to pain-free abduction and the patient complains of increasing pain in the tendon. Attempts to traverse the coracoacromial arch causes severe pain at approximately 70 degrees abduction. As the process continues, the swollen tendon finally ruptures into the bursa above (Fig. 17–30F), which evokes a severe inflammatory reaction within the bursa leading to bursitis. At this stage, the patient often complains of a severe pain, before rupture, followed by a deep dull ache in the shoulder and relatively free abduction. This fluid and inflammatory transudate can swell the subacromial

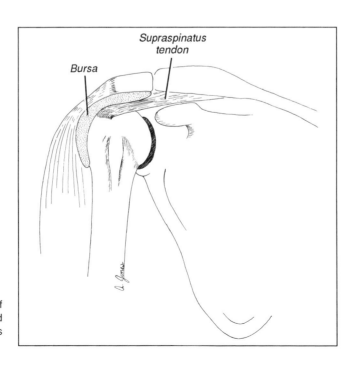

Figure 17–29. The relationship of the supraspinatus tendon and the subdeltoid-subacromial bursa is shown.

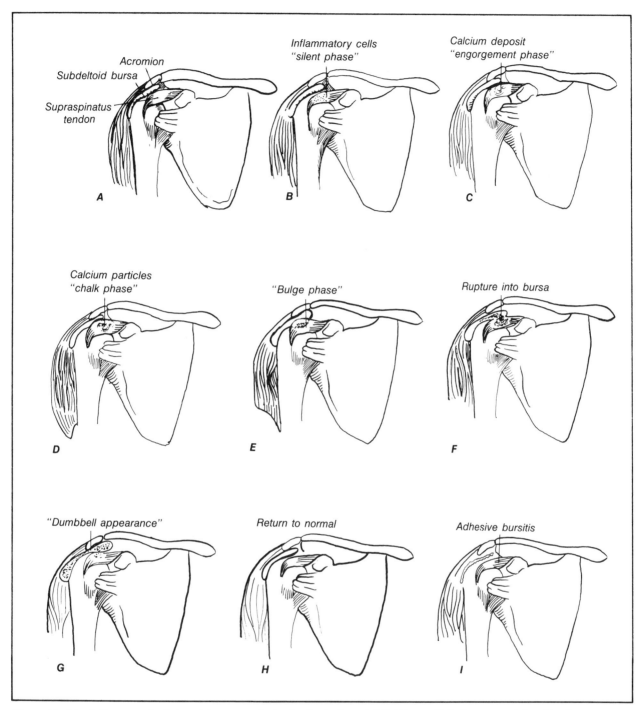

Figure 17–30. **A.** The normal relation of the supraspinatus tendon to the subdeltoid bursa. Note the cross relationship of the tendon-bursa complex to the acromion and coracoacromial arch (arch removed). **B.** Inflammatory cells invade the tendon and eventually recurrent episodes lead to deposition of calcium. **C.** Calcium deposition leads to engorgement of the tendon, called the engorgement phase. **D.** As the process continues, the calcium particles coalesce to form the "chalk phase," which is the first phase visible on x ray. **E.** The calcium takes up water and causes the tendon to bulge into the overlying bursa in the "bulge phase." **F.** As the process continues, rupture occurs into the overlying bursa and the calcium and inflammatory exudate is released into the bursa. **G.** A dumbbell appearance can result as the fluid accumulates at the ends of the bursa. **H.** Complete resolution can occur at any stage before rupture if treatment is begun early. **I.** After rupture, recurrent episodes of tendonitis and bursitis occur, leading eventually to chronic adhesive bursitis.

bursa leading to a dumbbell appearance (Fig. 17–30G), which permits partial abduction and adduction restricted by the bulging ends of the bursa, and the arm is held at approximately 30 degrees of abduction. Further adduction or abduction causes increasing pain, and the patient resists any attempt to elevate the arm beyond this point. The entire process can resolve, leading to an entirely normal tendon and bursa before the stage where rupture occurs (Fig. 17–30H). Beyond that point, although the process can resolve with treatment, the tissues never return to complete normality. The process can go on and the patient may experience a chronic bursitis leading eventually to adhesive pericapsulitis (adhesive bursitis, Fig. 17–30I).

Clinical Presentation

This condition is more common in women than in men and usually occurs between the ages of 35 and 50 years. It appears to be more common in sedentary people. Patients usually complain of a deep ache in the shoulder referred to the deltoid region and the pain may radiate to the entire limb. There is usually point tenderness at the site of the supraspinatus tendon corresponding to the critical point described earlier. The pain is increased on abduction and internal rotation of the arm. The onset is usually gradual, but may be acute after overuse of the shoulder as when the patient engages in a task requiring unaccustomed work with the arm elevated. Within 2 to 3 days the pain becomes increasingly intense at the point of the shoulder. After rupture into the bursa, the previously severe pain is followed by a dull deep ache as the material transcends laterally within the bursa, and the patient regains relatively free abduction.

In the silent and engorged phases (supraspinatus tendonitis) the roentgenograms are usually negative. Other roentgenographic findings are calcification and cystic changes along the greater tuberosity accompanied by sclerosis. These do not occur, however, until the process has become more chronic. Calcification is sometimes seen in asymptomatic patients.

Treatment

In the initial acute phase, ice packs should be applied to the shoulder for 20-minute periods to provide for adequate cooling of the deep tissues of the shoulder. The patient should be advised to immobilize the shoulder for short periods of time during the acute inflammatory phase, and salicylates or other anti-inflammatory agents should be prescribed. In severe cases, an injection with a steroid analgesic mixture (instilling a small amount every 1 to 2 mm) across the site of maximal tenderness can be used. Local corticosterid injection seems to be more effective than placebo and more effective than oral, nonsteroidal anti-inflammatory drugs.[45]

As the acute process resolves, ice can be discontinued and heat packs are advised as well as massage. Diathermy and ultrasonic heat provide the best forms of heat therapy. Circumduction exercises are recommended to all these patients and are an important part of treatment to prevent any stiffness from occurring in the shoulder (Fig. 17–31). In patients with acute calcific bursitis, aspiration of the calcium with a large-bore needle may prove fruitful if the calcium is in a fine pasty consistency. This should be followed by installation of steroids within the bursal sac. A very important part of therapy is never to place the shoulder in immobilization for any prolonged period as this will induce adhesive capsulitis in patients more than 40 years of age.

Patients with rotator cuff calcification who present for evaluation frequently have severe pain and dramatic loss of shoulder function. Initially, conservative management, including anti-inflammatory medication, physical therapy, and local injection may be helpful; however, when symptoms are refractory, surgical treatment is often the only effective alternative.[37] Arthroscopic debridement has been refined and is a good alternative in patients who have deposits located in the subscapulais tendon or other tendons that impinge shoulder movements.[37]

☐ STRAIN OR TENOSYNOVITIS OF THE LONG HEAD OF THE BICEPS

The long head of the biceps traverses between the greater and lesser tuberosities within the bicipital groove ensheathed by the capsule of the glenohumeral joint to connect to the glenoid rim (see Fig. 17–2). This position makes the long head of the biceps subject to constant trauma and irritation from motions of the shoulder. This constant motion increases the inflammatory reaction around the tendon until it slides reluctantly. This irritative process increases, especially with abduction of the shoulder when the elbow is fixed in an extended position as it occurs in some occupations such as in painters and carpenters. The tendon slides up and down in its tunnel and is subject to a reactive tenosynovitis.

Clinical Presentation

The patient complains of pain in the biceps region and anterior aspect of the shoulder joint that radiates down toward the radius. Abduction and external rotation are the most painful motions and snap extension of the elbow increases the pain markedly. On examination there is tenderness to palpation in the bicipital groove.

A reliable test for diagnosing tenosynovitis of the long head of the biceps is the Yergusons test (Fig. 17–32). In performing this test, the patient's elbow is held at 90 degrees of flexion. The patient is asked to

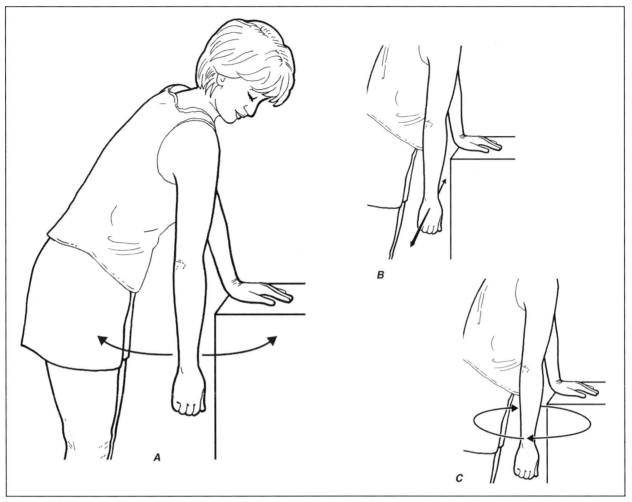

Figure 17–31. Codman exercises. **A.** The exercises begin with the patient's arm suspended and use a back-and-forth swinging movement. **B.** Next, side-to-side movement is performed in a medial-lateral direction. **C.** Finally, clockwise and counterclockwise rotational movement are performed. These three movements are repeated with the arc of movement increased daily as the patient's inflammatory condition improves.

supinate the forearm as the examiner resists this attempt. This causes pain along the intertubercular groove. This is a reliable test to distinguish tenosynovitis of the long head of the biceps from subdeltoid bursitis.

This condition may go on to complete adhesion of the tendon and either shoulder motion will be restricted or the biceps will rupture proximal to the groove.

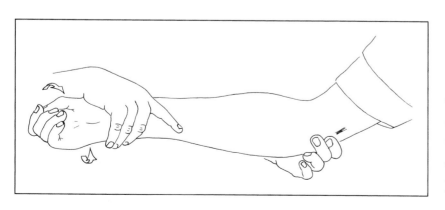

Figure 17–32. The Yergusons test is shown. Although this test was originally described for dislocation of the bicipital tendon, it can be used to diagnose tenosynovitis of the long head of the biceps as well. In doing this test, the patient is asked to supinate the forearm against resistance as the elbow is held in flexion.

Treatment

The treatment of this condition includes immobilization in a sling and injection of the bicipital canal with an anesthetic and steroid solution (Fig. 17–33). One must be careful not to inject the tendon itself. The injection is usually carried out at several points along the route of the tendon within the bicipital groove. Analgesics and anti-inflammatory agents may be administered as well as moist warm heat packs.

□ ACUTE RUPTURE OF THE LONG HEAD OF THE BICEPS

Rupture along the long head of the biceps can occur anywhere along its route. This discussion, however, will concern itself only with rupture at the proximal end. The condition often follows a chronic bicipital tenosynovitis that has left the tendon weakened. It may follow an episode where the patient admits to lifting a heavy object or having had a forceful contraction of the biceps.

Clinical Presentation

The patient usually notices an immediate sharp pain in the region of the bicipital groove and the biceps contracts within the arm.[43] There is tenderness to palpation within the bicipital groove, and the diagnosis can be confirmed by asking the patient to contract the biceps with the arm abducted and externally rotated to 90 degrees, at which point flexion at the elbow will cause the biceps to move away from the shoulder.

Treatment

Surgical reattachment to the coracoid or the bicipital groove is recommended in most active patients.[2,9] In elderly patients with the condition, repair may not be indicated. Patients with acute rupture in the belly of the biceps are treated conservatively in a Velpeau bandage with the elbow flexed 90 degrees. Acute rupture of the distal tendon of the biceps is also treated surgically with reattachment.

□ SUBLUXATION AND DISLOCATION OF THE BICIPITAL TENDON

The bicipital tendon can sublux or actually dislocate out of its groove between the greater and lesser tuberosity when there is a congenitally abnormal shallow bicipital groove that predisposes to this condition (Fig. 17–34). Tear of the cuff of the subscapularis tendon where it attaches to the lesser tuberosity and extends over the bicipital groove is another predisposing factor. The most common mechanism by which this condition occurs acutely is forced external rotation of the arm with the biceps contracted.

Clinical Presentation

The patient usually complains of a painful snap felt in the anterior aspect of the shoulder during forced external rotation of the arm while the biceps is contracted. With rotation, the tendon slips back and forth, in and

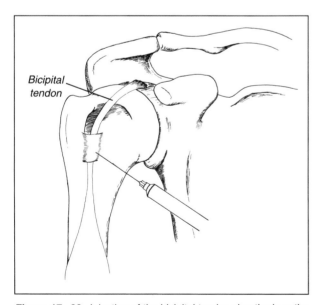

Figure 17–33. Injection of the bicipital tendon sheath along the intertubercular groove.

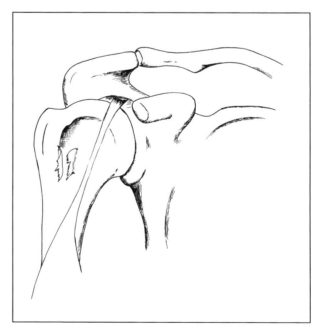

Figure 17–34. Dislocation of the bicipital tendon out of the intertubercular groove.

out of the groove. Pain is usually felt in the anterior and lateral aspect of the shoulder and is referred distally and along the anterior aspect of the arm. The pain is typically worse at night and in the acute phase, spasms of the deltoid and subscapularis muscles are common accompanying features. A reliable test that should be performed is the *Yergusons test*. This test is performed as discussed earlier. The stability of the biceps tendon is determined by subluxation of the tendon from its normal position   in the intertubercular groove. When supination against resistance is tested, the bicipital tendon will pop out of the groove and the patient will experience pain.

Treatment
Surgical transfer of the tendon is the treatment of choice in this condition.

☐ THE PAINFUL ARCH SYNDROME

The painful arch syndrome is a syndrome involving the coracoacromial arch which includes the coracoid process inferiorly, the coracoacromial ligament, and the acromion. The etiology of the painful arch syndrome involves physiologic changes in the length of the rotator cuff muscles leading to dyskinesia and abnormal thickening of the tendon of the rotator cuff.[12] When the arm is abducted the vascular supply decreases. The primary muscles involved in abducting the arm are useless without the help of the rotator cuff. The syndrome has been discussed in detail by Kessel and Watson[20] and is char-

acterized by pain that is referred to the lateral aspect of the upper arm in the region of the deltoid and its insertion. Characteristically, the pain is worse at night and is typically exacerbated within a certain arch of movement. The painful arch is between 60 and 120 degrees abduction, which indicates some disorder in the subacromial region (Fig. 17–35).[27] In situations where the pain increases at a point beyond 120 degrees of abduction up to full elevation, disorders of the acromioclavicular joints should be suspected. Although this condition has many pathologic inciting lesions, the one final common denominator is a set of symptoms and signs, usually referred to as the "painful arch syndrome." In this condition, tenderness may be maximal at the posterior, superior, or anterior aspect of the rotator cuff. Impingement on the acromion during abduction varies with rotation of the humerus and the lesion may be cleared by outward rotation of the humerus during abduction. Anterior and posterior lesions heal more readily than do superior lesions because the subscapularis tendon and the tendon of the infraspinatus are relatively well vascularized as compared with the supraspinatus tendon.

All these patients should be treated with long-acting anesthetics and steroid injections at the points of maximal tenderness along the anterior, superior, or posterior aspects of the rotator cuff. Multiple injection sites across the cuff region are recommended (Fig. 17–36). The recommended amount of steroid is 40 mg of methylprednisolone and 5 mL of 1 percent bupivacaine (Marcaine) injected at the site of maximal tenderness. The condition may require several injections before relief is obtained so the patient should be referred for continual follow-up care.

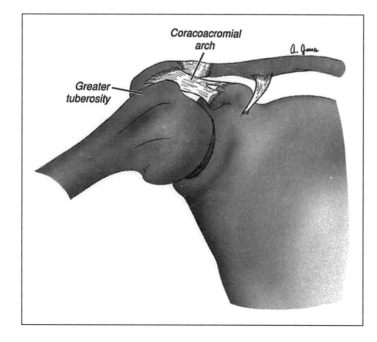

Figure 17–35. In the painful arch syndrome as the patient elevates and abducts the arm, the tuberosity encroaches upon the coracoacromial arch. This causes maximal pain between 60 and 120 degrees.

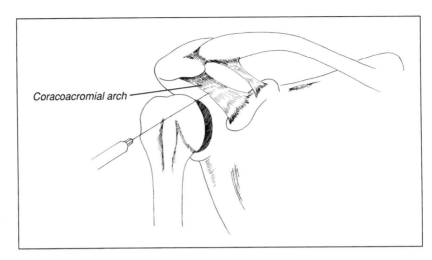

Figure 17–36. Injection along the coracoacromial arch. Injection should be concentrated under the arch which is palpable via the needle tip.

□ DIFFERENTIAL DIAGNOSIS AND SHOULDER PAIN SYNDROMES

The frequency of specific painful shoulder conditions has been ascertained from several reports.[46] The incidents of common syndromes in 160 unselected cases is as follows:

Subacromial bursitis/Supraspinatus tendonitis	60%
Bicipital tendonitis	4%
Supraspinatus tendon rupture	10%
Adhesive capsulitis shoulder	12%
Acromioclavicular joint osteoarthritis	7%
Other conditions	7%

There are a number of clinical features that help distinguish which of the syndromes described above are causing pain in the shoulder. These are described in Table 17–1.

TABLE 17–1. HELPFUL DISTINGUISHING CLINICAL FEATURES OF COMMON PAINFUL SHOULDER CONDITIONS

Referred shoulder pain from cervical area (eg, C5 radicular pain from nerve root encroachment)	Shoulder motion shows painless complete arc; no specific periarticular shoulder tender point, but muscle spasm may be present. Neck rotation or neck compression testing typically triggers radicular pain distally in C5 dermatomal distribution.	Supraspinatus tendon tear or rupture (continued)	abduction. More gradual onset of pain and weakness with tears in older patients. Anesthetic subacromial infiltration will reduce pain but absent or weak resisted abduction at 90° persists. Small tears may mimic tendinitis symptoms.
Subacromial bursitis and noncalcific supraspinatus tendonitis	Painful shoulder motion, especially between 60° and 120° of active abduction, tender subacromial region; pain may partially radiate in C5 dermatomal distribution. Anesthetic subacromial infiltration can minimize pain during movement.	Adhesive capsulitis (frozen shoulder)	Gradual onset of diffusely painful shoulder, markedly restricted passive and active motion in all planes.
		Acromioclavicular (AC) joint disorder	Shoulder arc painful but limited only during last 20° of abduction. AC joint tender and prominent compared with contralateral side if separation or osteophytes are present.
Bicipital tendonitis	Localized anterior shoulder pain over long head of biceps tendon; with forearm supination, tendon sheath is tender with thumb rolling. Shoulder motion normal.		
Supraspinatus tendon tear or rupture	Following trauma in younger patients, abrupt pain and weak or absent active	Impingement syndrome	Impingement typically begins at 60° to 70° and is maximum between 100° and 120° of abduction. Recurrent pain from compression of subacromial tissue also occurs at 90° to 100° of forward flexion.

From Smith DL, Campbell SM: Painful shoulder syndromes: Diagnosis and management. *J Gen Intern Med* **7**(May/June):328–339, 1992.

Nonoperative management of common shoulder disorders, including physical therapy and nonsteroidal anti-inflammatory drugs, as well as injection therapy, has been used extensively as described earlier.[56]

□ SCAPULOCOSTAL SYNDROMES AND BURSITIS

The syndromes in this category are a group of conditions with a common course and clinical presentation, and are usually caused by inflammations of the bursae around the scapula or muscle strains of those muscles attaching to the scapula. Pain in the scapular region is usually secondary to poor posture and occurs more commonly at the end of the day. These conditions can also be seen when the arm has not been used for a protracted length of time because of fractures or other conditions.

Clinical Presentation
The onset of bursitis and muscle strains around the scapula is usually insidious and is characterized by ex-acerbations and remissions. The most common sites for bursitidies to occur in this region are the superior and inferior angles of the scapula. The patient usually experiences pain on any motion of the scapula, and the examiner may elicit crepitation when he or she instructs the patient to bring the arm across the chest. To diagnose this condition, the physician should retract the scapula by asking the patient to place the hand on the opposite shoulder. A trigger point usually at the superior angle or near the base of the spine can be palpated. Lidocaine injection should give the patient relief if the condition is secondary to a bursitis of one of the scapular bursae.

Treatment
Local injection of a trigger point affords prompt relief and should be attempted in those cases with significant pain. Heat in the form of ultrasound bid for 20 minutes each day and diathermy affords good relief for patients with muscle strains. Patients with one of the bursitidies of the scapular region can be treated with local injection, heat, and rest.

DISORDERS OF THE SHOULDER AND UPPER ARM

□ EXTRINSIC DISORDERS PRESENTING AS SHOULDER PAIN

A number of extrinsic disorders can present as shoulder pain (Table 17–2). *Cervical spine* problems including disc degeneration, herniation, and osteoarthritis can cause shoulder pain.[57] It is important to examine the cervical spine carefully when one expects referred pain and to take radiographs of the neck.[57]

□ Brachial Plexus Neuropathy
This is an uncommon cause of shoulder pain that can present with vague symptoms that are either localized or systemic throughout the upper extremity. Brachial plexus neuropathy can occur due to allergic conditions, infectious disorders (viral syndromes), or idiopathically. The predominant symptom is pain which may be localized to the shoulder area or may be generalized. Within a few weeks, usually the patient develops weakness in the shoulder girdle. This condition usually has a good prognosis.[57]

□ Postural Pain
This is a common cause of shoulder discomfort, especially in younger patients who have desk jobs.

□ Neoplastic Disease
Neoplastic disease particularly of the apical lung may present with shoulder pain. This may involve the chest wall and brachial plexus producing local pain or radicular pain.

□ Thoracic Outlet Syndrome
This syndrome includes a number of disorders. Portions of the brachial plexus can be compressed as the plexus traverses the supraclavicular area and passes through the axilla to the arm. The structures include the scalene muscle, the first rib, the coracoid process and the tendinous insertion of the pectoralis minor muscle.[57] Patients present with symptoms of pain with certain motions. Thrusting of the shoulders back with the arms dependent at the side while the patient is taking a deep breath may produce pain. There may be signs of vascular compromise. The medial trunk of the brachial plexus is the most commonly affected by compression. Thus, pain may radiate down the forearm along the ulnar nerve distribution. The treatment for thoracic outlet syndrome consists of physical therapy and shoulder muscle strengthening which provides symptomatic relief.[57] However, occasionally surgery is necessary to relieve the area of compression.[57]

TABLE 17–2. EXTRINSIC SHOULDER DISORDERS

Disorder	Clinical Features	Laboratory and Radiographic Findings	Treatment
Cervical spine disorders	Painful restricted range of motion of the neck Range of motion may reproduce shoulder pain Pain radiates to periscapular region and into forearm and hand Neurologic findings of radiculopathy (altered sensation, diminished reflexes, motor weakness)	Cervical spine films may show degenerative changes EMG and nerve conduction study results consistent with radiculopathy Nerve encroachment confirmed by MRI or myelogram	Cervical collar, analgesics, NSAIDs, cervical traction Surgical management (discectomy, perhaps with fusion) for unresponsive, severe cases
Brachial plexus neuropathy	Diffuse shoulder pain often associated with diffuse weakness Frequently follows viral illness	EMG and nerve conduction study results are diagnostic	Supportive treatment and rehabilitation program; anticipate spontaneous resolution in 2 to 3 years in most cases
Postural pain	Associated with prolonged sitting with shoulders hunched forward Patient stands with shoulders sagging Tenderness over vertebral border of scapula Painful periscapular trigger points	Radiographs unremarkable	Postural correction exercises Trigger point injections of lidocaine (Xylocaine) or steroid for significant pain
Neoplastic disease	Fullness in supraclavicular fossa Positive Horner's sign if stellate ganglion involved History of tobacco use	Apical chest view may show mass (Pancoast's tumor)	Treatment of neoplastic disease
Thoracic outlet syndrome	Shoulder and upper extremity symptoms often vague and nonspecific Symptoms reproduced by provocative tests	Radiographs may show cervical rib, otherwise unremarkable	Shoulder girdle strengthening exercise Surgery (cervical or first rib resection or release of scalene muscle)

EMG = electromyography; MRI = magnetic resonance imaging; NSAIDs = nonsteroidal anti-inflammatory drugs.
From Zuckerman JD, Mirabello SC, Newman D, et al: The painful shoulder, Part I, Extrinsic disorders. *Am Fam Physician* **43**(1):119–128, 1991, published by the American Academy of Family Physicians.

INJURIES OF THE ARM

There is no subcutaneous bone in the arm and in all areas the skin is separated from bone by muscle.

☐ CONTUSIONS

Contusions of the triceps and biceps are common but not disabling injuries with no major complications. The treatment of these injuries is a sling and ice in the first 24 hours followed by heat. The physician should always check for fractures and injury to the radial nerve from a contusion to the lateral aspect of the distal arm.

Blockers exostosis is a contusion of the middle third of the arm over the lateral aspect at the attachment of the deltoid muscle onto the humerus. A direct blow in this region causes a contusion and a periostitis at the insertion of the deltoid tendon. The treatment for this is protective. One may later develop a spur at the site of injury and an irritative exostosis. Most of these remain asymptomatic; however, when significant discomfort occurs, the patient should be referred for consideration of excision.

Contusion of the radial nerve as it courses in close approximation to the humerus along the muscular spiral groove is an infrequent injury. As the nerve courses further it goes laterally above the lateral epicondylar ridge and is subject to contusions by a direct blow. The patient complains of a tingling sensation extending down the forearm and into the hand over the distribution of the nerve. The treatment is symptomatic.

REFERENCES

1. Altchek DW, Carson EW: Arthroscopic acromiopasty. *Orthop Clin of North Am* **28**(2):1997.
2. Archambauld R, et al: Rupture of the thoracoacromial artery in anterior dislocation of the shoulder. *Am J Surg* **97**:782, 1959.
3. Arciero RA, St. Pierre P: Acute shoulder dislocation and techniques for operative management. *Clin Sports Med* **14**(4):1995.
4. Belvins FT, et al: Biology of the rotator cuff tendon. *Orthop Clin North Am* **28**(1):1997.
5. Bernageau J: Roetgenographic assessment of the rotator cuff. *Clin Orthop* **254**:87, 1990.
6. Bowyer BL, et al: Sports medicine. Upper extremity injuries. *Arch Phys Med Rehabil* **74**(5):5433–5437, 1993.
7. Breazeale NM, Craig EV: Partial-thickness rotator cuff tears. *Orthop Clin North Am* **28**(2):1997.
8. Burkhart SS: Arthroscopic treatment of massive rotator cuff tears. *Clin Orthop* **267**:15, 1991.
9. Bush LF: The torn shoulder capsule. *J Bone Joint Surg* **57**(2):256, 1975.
10. Cofield RF: Current concepts review: rotator cuff disease of the shoulder. *J Bone Joint Surg* **63B**:198, 1981.
11. Cook DA, Heiner JP: Acromioclavicular injuries. *Orthop Rev* **19**(6):510, 1990.
12. Donatelli RA: Shoulder: Painful arch syndrome. In: *Physical Therapy of the Shoulder*, 2nd ed. New York: Churchill-Livingstone, 1991, pp 86–87.
13. Edeland HG, Stefansson T: Block of the suprascapular nerve in reduction of acute anterior shoulder dislocation. *Acta Anesthesiol Scand.* **17**:46, 1973.
14. Elberger ST, Brody G: Bilateral posterior shoulder dislocations. *Am J Emer Med* **13**(3):1995.
15. Ferry AM, et al: Retrosternal dislocation of the clavicle. J Bone Joint Surg. **39**(4):905, 1957.
16. Frieman G, et al: Rotator cuff disease: A review of diagnosis, pathophysiology and current trends in treatment. *Arch Phys Med Rehabil* **75**(5):604–609, 1994.
17. Glousman RE: Instability versus impingement syndrome in the throwing athlete. *Orthop Clin North Am* **24**(1):1993.
18. Hussein KM: Kocher's method is 3,000 years old. *J Bone Joint Surg* [Br] **50**(3):669, 1968.
19. Iannotti G, et al: Advances in the surgical treatment of disorders of the shoulder. *Surg Ann* **26**:227–250, 1995.
20. Kessel L, Watson M: The painful arch syndrome. *J Bone Joint Surg* [Br] **59**(2):166, 1977.
21. Lacey TH, Crawford HB: Reduction of anterior dislocations of the shoulder by means of Milch abduction technique. *J Bone Joint Surg* **34**(1):108, 1952.
22. Lam SJS: Irreducible anterior dislocation of the shoulder. *J Bone Joint Surg* [Br] **48**(1):132, 1966.
23. Liu SH, Henry MM: Anterior shoulder instability. *Clin Orthop Rel Res* **323**:327–337, 1996.
24. Lynn FS: Erect dislocation if the shoulder. *Surg Gynecol Obstet* **39**:51, 1990.
25. Lyons AR, Tomlinson JE: Clinical diagnosis of tears of the rotator cuff. *J Bone Joint Surg* **74B**(3):414, 1992.
26. Mallon WJ, Bassett FH, Goldner RD: Luxatio erecta: The inferior glenohumeral dislocation. *J Orthop Trauma* **4**(1):19, 1990.
27. Miniaci A, Fowler PJ: Impingement in the athlete. *Clin Sports Med* **12**(1):1993.
28. Miniaci A, Salonen D: Rotator cuff evaluation: Imaging and diagnosis. *Orthop Clin North Am* 28(1):1997.
29. Moseley HF: The basic lesions of recurrent anterior dislocation. *Surg Clin North Am* **43**:1631, 1963.
30. Nicholson GG: Rehabilitation of common shoulder injuries. *Clin Sports Med* **8**(4):633, 1989.
31. Parker AP: Fractures and dislocations of the shoulder girdle. *Surg Clin North Am* **20**:1613, 1940.
32. Pirrallo RG, Bridges TP: Luxatio erecta: A miss diagnosis. *Am J Emerg Med* **8**(4):315, 1990.
33. Pollock RG, Bigliani LU: Recurrent posterior shoulder instability. *Clin Orthop Rel Res* **291**:85–96, 1993.
34. Post M: Complication of rotator cuff tears. *Clin Orthop* **254**:97, 1991.
35. Rames RD, Karzel RP: Injuries to the glenoid labrum, including slap lesions. *Orthop Clin North Am* **24**(1):1993.
36. Rechet MP, Resnick D: Magnetic resonance-imaging studies of the shoulder. *J Bone Joint Surg* **75-A**:8, 1993.
37. Relouis P, Karzel RP: Management of rotator cuff calcifications. *Orthop Clin North Am* 24(1):1993.
38. Riebelg D, McCabe JB: Anterior shoulder dislocation: A review of reduction techniques. *Am J Emerg Med* **9**(2):180, 1991.
39. Roddgers JA, Crosby LA: Rotator cuff disorders. *Am Fam Phys* **54**(1):1996.
40. Rowe CR: Anterior dislocations of the shoulder. *Surg Clin North Am* **43**:1609, 1963.
41. Rowe CR, Zarins B: Recurrent transient subluxation of the shoulder. *J Bone Joint Surg* **63A**:863, 1981.
42. Royle G: Treatment of acute anterior dislocation of the shoulder. *Br J Clin Pract* **27**:11, 1973.
43. Sailer SM, Lewis SB: Rehabilitation and splinting of common upper extremity injuries in athletes. *Clin Sports Med* **14**:2, 1995.
44. Salvatore JE: Steronclavicular joint dislocation. *Clin Orthop* **58**:51, 1968.
45. Sibilia J, et al: Local corticosteroid in the treatment of rotator cuff tendinitis (except for frozen shoulder and calcific tendinitis). *Clin Exper Rheum* **14**:561–566, 1996.
46. Smith DL, Campbell SM: Painful shoulder syndromes: Diagnosis and management. *J Gen Intern Med* **7**(May/June):328, 1992.

47. Smith WS, Klug TJ: Anterior dislocation of the shoulder. A simple and effective method of reduction. *JAMA* **163:**182, 1957.
48. Snyder SJ: Evaluation and treatment of the rotator cuff. *Orthop Clin North Am* **24**(1):1993.
49. Soohoo NF, Rosen P: Diagnosis and treatment of rotator cuff tears in the emergency department. *J Emerg Med* **14**(3):309–317, 1996.
50. Soslowsky LJ, et al: Biomechanics of the rotator cuff. *Orthop Clin North Am* **28**(1):1997.
51. Stimson LA: An easy method of reducing dislocations of the shoulder and hip. *Med Record* March:356–357, 1990.
52. Tibone JE, Bradley JP: The treatment of posterior subluxation in athletes. *Clin Orthop Rel Res* **291:**124–137, 1993.
53. Uhthoff HK, Sano H: Pathology of failure of the rotator cuff tendon. *Orthop Clin North Am* **28:**1, 1997.
54. Uri DS: MR imaging of shoulder impingement and rotator cuff disease. *Radiol Clin North Am* **35:**1, 1997.
55. Weaver JK: Treatment of acromioclavicular injuries, especially complete acromioclavicular separation. *J Bone Joint Surg* **54**(6):1973.
56. Zuckerman JD, Newman D, et al: The painful shoulder. Part II. Intrinsic disorders and impingement syndrome. *Am Fam Phys* **43**(2):497–511, 1991.
57. Zuckerman JD, Mirabello SC, Newman D, et al: The painful shoulder. Part I. Extrinsic disorders. *Am Fam Phys* **43**(1):119, 1991.

BIBLIOGRAPHY

Bacevich BB: Paralytic brachial neuritis. *J Bone Joint Surg* **58**(2):262, 1976.
Cruess RL: Steroid induced avascular necrosis of the head of the humerus. *J Bone Joint Surg* [Br] **58**(3):313, 1976.
Heath RD: The subclavian steal syndrome. *J Bone Joint Surg* **54**(5):1033, 1972.
Imatani RJ, et al: Acute, complete acromioclavicular separation. *J Bone Joint Surg* **57:**328, 1975.
Lunseth PA, et al: Surgical treatment of chronic dislocation of the sterno-clavicular joint. *J Bone Joint Surg* [Br] **57**(2):193, 1975.
McEntire JE, et al: Rupture of the pectoralis major muscle. *J Bone Joint Surg* **54**(5):1040, 1972.
McLaughlin HL, MacLellan DI: Recurrent anterior dislocation of the shoulder. *J Trauma* **7**(2):191, 1967.
Poppen NK, Walker PS: Normal and abnormal motion of the shoulder. *J Bone Joint Surg* **58**(2):195, 1976

SECTION TWO

LOWER EXTREMITIES

18
CHAPTER
FRACTURES OF THE PELVIS

PELVIC FRACTURES

CLASS A: PELVIC FRACTURES

Type I: Avulsion fractures (p. 356)

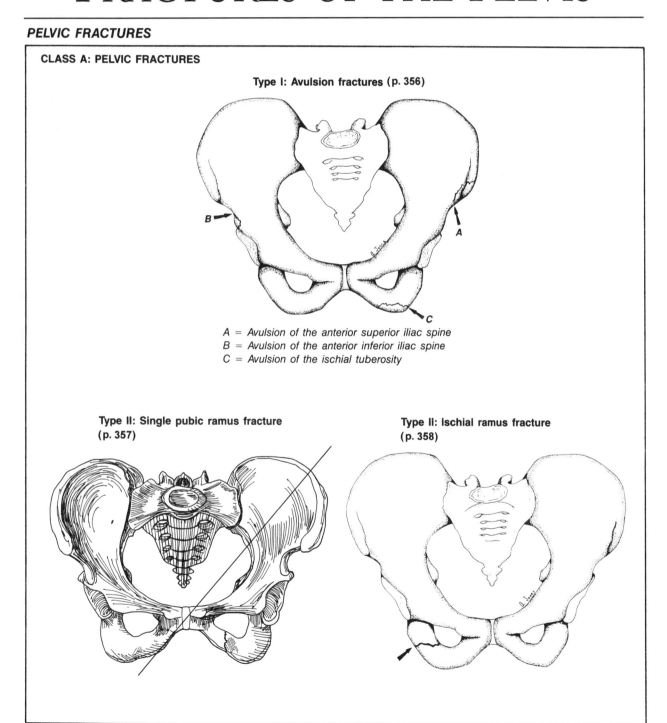

A = Avulsion of the anterior superior iliac spine
B = Avulsion of the anterior inferior iliac spine
C = Avulsion of the ischial tuberosity

Type II: Single pubic ramus fracture (p. 357)

Type II: Ischial ramus fracture (p. 358)

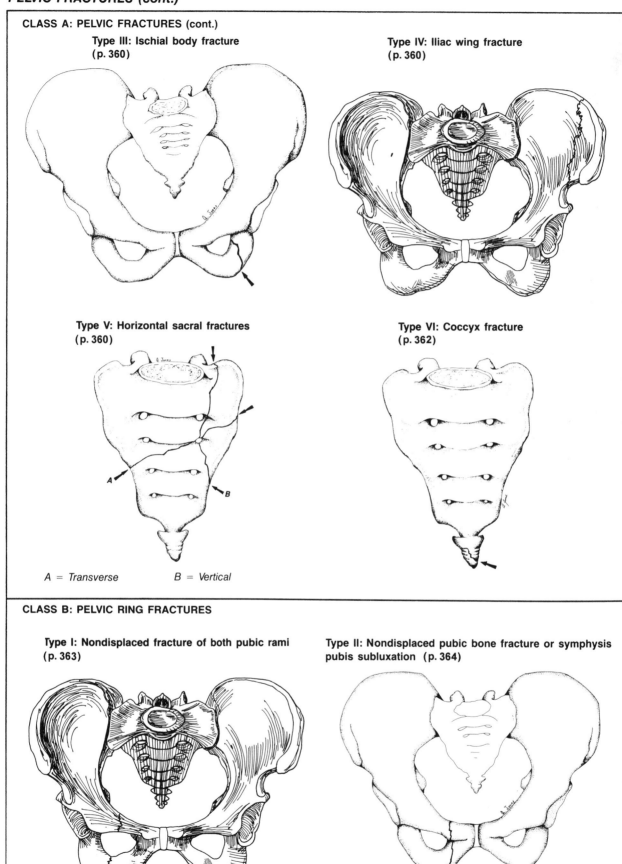

CLASS A: PELVIC FRACTURES (cont.)

Type III: Ischial body fracture
(p. 360)

Type IV: Iliac wing fracture
(p. 360)

Type V: Horizontal sacral fractures
(p. 360)

Type VI: Coccyx fracture
(p. 362)

A = Transverse   B = Vertical

CLASS B: PELVIC RING FRACTURES

Type I: Nondisplaced fracture of both pubic rami
(p. 363)

Type II: Nondisplaced pubic bone fracture or symphysis pubis subluxation (p. 364)

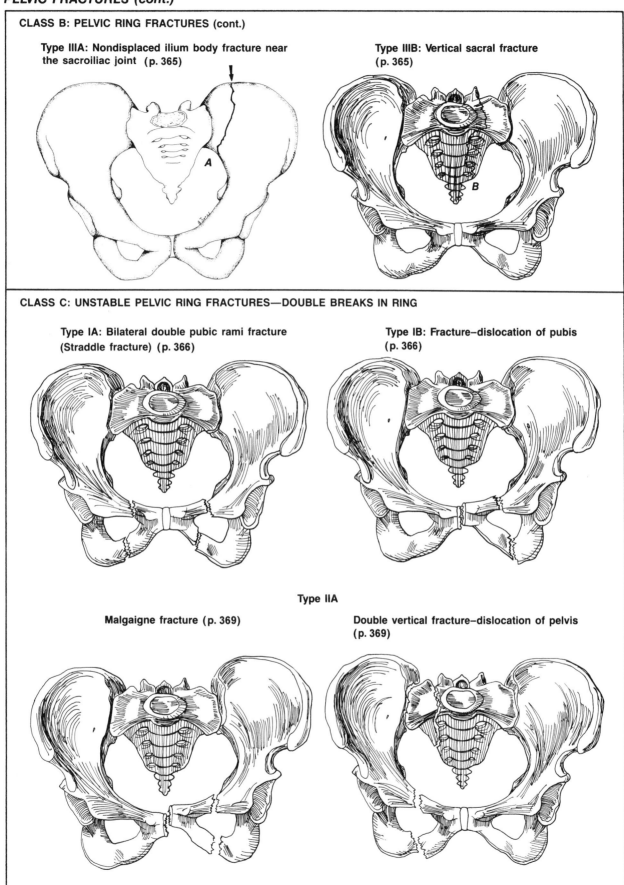

CLASS B: PELVIC RING FRACTURES (cont.)

Type IIIA: Nondisplaced ilium body fracture near the sacroiliac joint (p. 365)

Type IIIB: Vertical sacral fracture (p. 365)

CLASS C: UNSTABLE PELVIC RING FRACTURES—DOUBLE BREAKS IN RING

Type IA: Bilateral double pubic rami fracture (Straddle fracture) (p. 366)

Type IB: Fracture–dislocation of pubis (p. 366)

Type IIA

Malgaigne fracture (p. 369)

Double vertical fracture–dislocation of pelvis (p. 369)

CLASS C: UNSTABLE PELVIC RING FRACTURES

Type IIA (cont.)

Fracture of the symphysis pubis and dislocation of the sacroiliac joint   (p. 369)

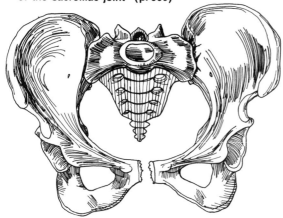

Fracture of the ilium and fracture of the symphysis pubis   (p. 369)

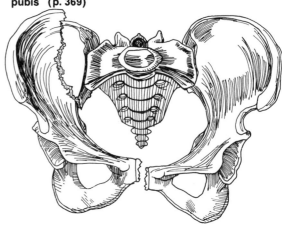

Type IIB: Contralateral double vertical ring fracture (Bucket-handle fracture)   (p. 370)

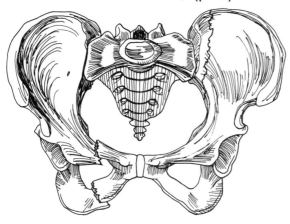

Type IIIA: Pelvic dislocation (Sprung pelvis) (p. 371)

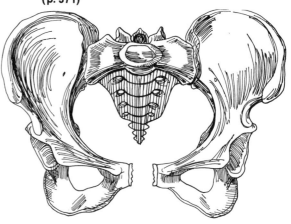

Type IIIB: Multiple displaced pelvic fractures (p. 371)

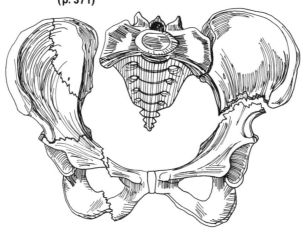

ACETABULAR FRACTURES

CLASS A: NONDISPLACED ACETABULAR FRACTURES
(p. 373)

Type I: Central acetabular fracture

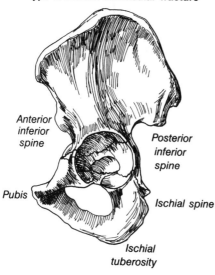

Anterior inferior spine

Posterior inferior spine

Pubis

Ischial spine

Ischial tuberosity

Type II: Posterior rim fracture

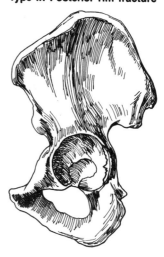

Type III: Anterior column fracture

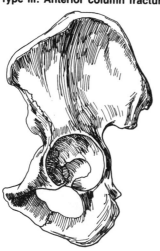

Type IV: Posterior column fracture

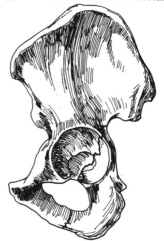

ACETABULAR FRACTURES (cont.)

CLASS B: DISPLACED ACETABULAR FRACTURES
(p. 374)

Type I

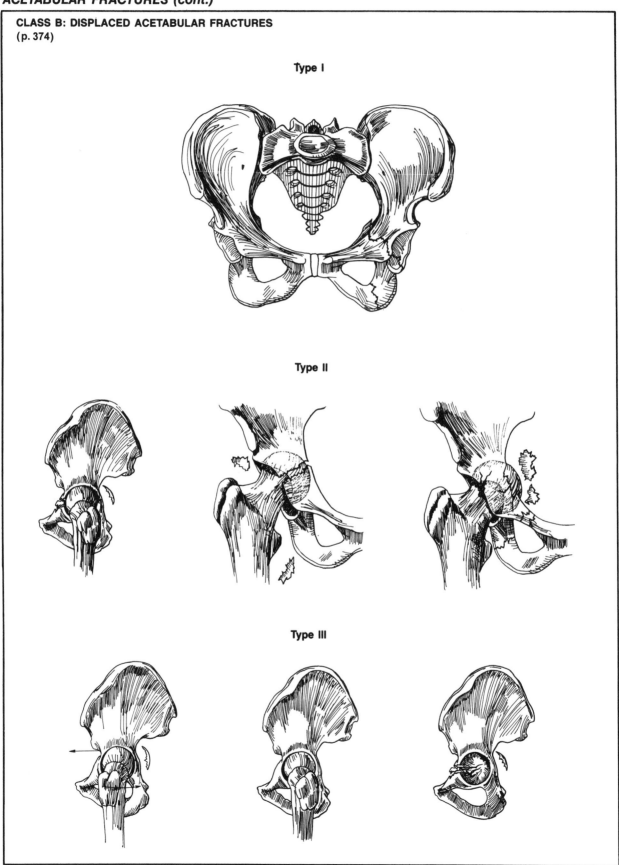

Type II

Type III

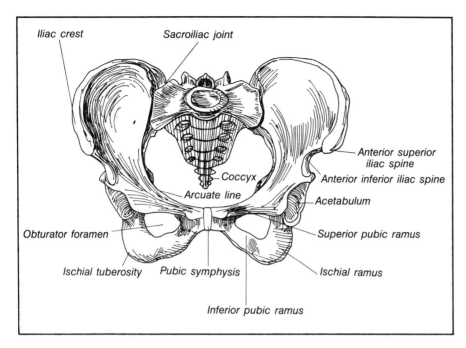

Figure 18-1. The osseous structures of the pelvis.

Pelvic fractures represent 3 percent of all skeletal fractures and are exceeded only by skull fractures in their associated complications and mortality.[1] The mortality rate for pelvic fractures varies from 5 to 20 percent.[1,2] Pelvic fractures secondary to falls are commonly seen in the elderly whereas motor vehicle accidents represent the most common cause in the young.

Pubic rami fractures are the most commonly seen pelvic fractures with the superior ramus more commonly involved than the inferior ramus (Fig. 18-1). The right pubic bone is the second most commonly involved pelvic fracture with superior involvement more common than inferior. Pubic rami and pubic bone fractures account for over 70 percent of all pelvic fractures.[2] The incidence of fractures of the remaining pelvic bones in descending order is right ilium, left ilium, ischium, left acetabular, and right acetabular.[4] Sacroiliac fractures are associated with the most significant bleeding. Patients who have significant bleeding from pelvic fractures may require vascular studies. Vascular occlusive procedures, external fixation or operative intervention may be indicated for severe pelvic hemorrhage.

Essential Anatomy

There are essentially two bones that combine to form the pelvic ring: the innominate bone, composed of the ischium, the ilium, and the pubis, and the sacrum. The coccyx is a third bone, but it is not incorporated into the bony pelvic ring. The two innominate bones and the sacrum are united into a ring by the formation of three joints that are the strongest in the body. Figure 18-2 is a conceptualized drawing of these three joints.

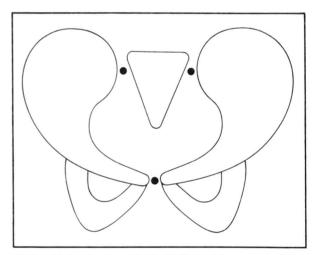

Figure 18-2. The three joints of the pelvis conceptualized. Note the ring structure of the pelvis.

In humans the pelvic ring serves two important functions: weight support and protection of the viscera. Weight support during ambulation and sitting is a combined function of ligaments and bones. Anteriorly, the interpubic ligaments join the two pubic bones forming the symphysis pubis. If these ligaments are disrupted the anterior pelvis opens disrupting its weight support function. Posteriorly, the sacroiliac joint is supported by strong ligaments allowing only a minimal amount of motion. The *posterior sacroiliac ligaments* are much stronger than the *anterior sacroiliac ligaments*. Disruption of the sacroiliac ligaments will alter the normal weight-bearing function of the pelvic ring. The anterior pelvic structures (symphysis and rami) are responsible for only 40% of

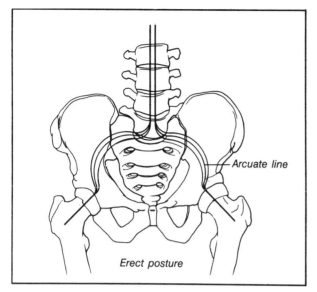

Erect posture

Figure 18–3. In the standing position, the lines of stress due to the weight of the body are transmitted through the lines shown. Patients with a fracture through these lines have much more pain and inability to bear weight as compared with those patients with fractures that do not traverse these lines of stress. For example, a patient with a fracture of the superior pubic ramus may walk into the emergency department whereas a patient with a fracture through the sacrum will not be able to bear weight without significant pain.

pelvic ring stability. The majority of the pelvic ring stability is the result of the posterior sacroiliac integrity (39).

Weight bearing is transmitted through the bony pelvis along two pathways. Figure 18–3 diagrammatically displays the lines of force through the pelvis when standing erect. The weight is transmitted through the spine to the sacrum, the sacroiliac joints, and along the arcuate line to the superior dome of the acetabulum and down the femur. In the sitting position (Fig. 18–4), the force is transmitted down the spine to the sacrum and the sacroiliac joints and to the ischium by way of the inferior ramus. An AP radiograph of the pelvis clearly demonstrates the thick trabecular pattern along these lines of stress. Pelvic fractures that do not interrupt or involve these weight-bearing arches are associated with little discomfort. Fractures involving the erect or sitting weight-bearing arches are associated with much more pain when stressed. Note that 70 percent of all pelvic fractures are through the pubis (a non-weight-supporting area), the most common being a superior ramus fracture.[2]

Axiom: *Pelvic fractures tend to interrupt the ring in areas not involved in weight transmission. A greater force is required to fracture a "weight-bearing" area of the pelvis.*

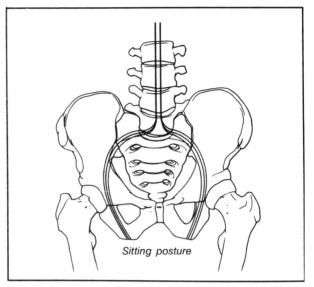

Sitting posture

Figure 18–4. The lines of stress in the sitting position. Note that in this position the lines go through the ischium.

The concept of the pelvis as an anatomic ring has important implications when dealing with displaced fractures. The presence of at least two fractures or one fracture and a dislocation is required to cause a displaced fracture in the ring.

Axiom: *A displaced fracture of the pelvic ring indicates that there is at least a second fracture or a fracture plus a joint dislocation, most commonly the sacroiliac.*

The muscles attached to the pelvis serve to support the body in the erect position and to provide mobility to the lower limbs. For the purpose of this text, the essential muscular anatomy concerns only those muscles responsible for avulsion fractures.

1. The *sartorius* inserts on the *anterior superior iliac spine.*
2. The *rectus femoris* inserts on the *anterior inferior iliac spine.*
3. The *hamstrings* insert on the *ischial tuberosity.*

The spinal nerves leave the protection of the vertebral column by way of the lumbar intervertebral foramina or the sacral foramina and course along the posterior aspect of the pelvis. Pelvic fractures, particularly those involving the posterior half, may be associated with neural damage.[5,6] A thorough neurologic examination of the lower extremities and the sphincters is essential in the assessment of pelvic fractures.

The abdominal aorta descends to the left of the midline and divides at L4 into the two common iliac vessels. At the level of the sacroiliac joints the common iliacs divide forming the external and internal iliacs. The internal iliac artery further divides into anterior and posterior branches. The posterior branch gives rise to the superior gluteal artery, which has an acutely angled base and is exposed to shearing forces with fractures in the area.[6] The anterior branch supplies the viscera of the pelvic cavity. Posterior pelvic (illium and sacroiliac) fractures are associated with more extensive hemorrhage than are anterior pelvic fractures.

The rectum, anus, sigmoid, and descending colon are contained within the bony pelvis. These structures may be damaged with any pelvic fracture but are most commonly injured with fractures associated with penetrating injuries.[7] The genitourinary system is frequently damaged in association with pelvic fractures due to blunt or penetrating trauma. The bladder, lying directly behind the symphysis pubis, is frequently damaged with pelvic fractures involving the pubis. The bladder may rupture in two locations depending on the forces involved and the fullness of the bladder at the time of injury. Most bladder ruptures occur above the urogenital diaphragm and are associated with intrapelvic extra vasation of urine. Bladder dome ruptures result in the intraperitoneal extravasation of urine. Anterior pelvic fractures may be associated with urethral injuries. If the urethra ruptures below the level of the urogenital diaphragm, the extravasation of urine will involve the scrotum, the superficial perineal compartment, and the abdominal wall.[8]

The superior dome of the acetabulum is the chief weight-supporting structure of the region. The superior dome of the acetabulum is formed by the ilium, the posterior rim by the ischium, and the inner rim by the pubis. The posterior rim of the acetabulum serves mainly to stabilize the joint and prevents dislocation during walking. The inner rim is very thin and easily fractured.

Examination

All unconscious patients with multiple injuries must be suspected of having a pelvic fracture until proven otherwise. Pelvic fractures may result in exsanguination and therefore several large intravenous lines must be started, and matched blood made available should the need arise. These patients should be moved or manipulated as little as possible so as not to aggravate the hemorrhaging or induce further complications.

Unlike many other fractures, the treatment of pelvic fractures requires that first priority be given to the diagnosis and the management of associated injuries rather than the fracture per se. The genitourinary system is frequently injured with pelvic fractures and questions relating to urinary urgency, inability to void, last menses, and vaginal bleeding should be asked. The examination of suspected pelvic fractures must include direct palpation of the entire ring with special emphasis on the pubic symphysis, the

sacroiliac joints, and the sacrum. Simultaneous medial or posterior pressure on each iliac wing may elicit or exacerbate the pain of a pelvic ring fracture or ring instability. An examination of each hip and its range of motion should be included to exclude an acetabular injury. In addition, a digital rectal examination assessing the position of the prostate gland is essential when dealing with suspected pelvic fractures. Prostate displacement indicates a likely disruption in the membranous urethra.

Secondary signs of a potential pelvic fracture include the following:

1. *Destot's sign* is a superficial hematoma above the inguinal ligament or in the scrotum.
2. *Roux's sign* occurs when the distance measured from the greater trochanter to the pubic spine is diminished on one side, as compared with the other, as might result from an overlapping anterior ring fracture.
3. *Earle's sign* occurs when a large hematoma, an abnormal palpable bony prominence, or a tender fracture line is detected on a rectal examination.

X ray

All suspected pelvic fractures should be evaluated initially with an AP radiograph of the pelvis. Obvious fracture lines are usually easily diagnosed on this film and suspected fracture areas may be localized and the appropriate oblique studies obtained. Lateral views, inlet projections, or AP views with 35 degrees of cephalic tilt may be necessary to accurately demonstrate suspected fractures. CT is more sensitive in diagnosing fractures of the acetabulum and sacrum.[9,10] CT Scanning is also essential for evaluating the integrity of the posterior pelvic structures which facilitates a more accurate assessment of pelvic injury and stability. CT is also very helpful in the evaluation of hematoma size and location as well as visceral injuries in patients sustaining pelvic fractures. Elderly osteopenic patients with pelvic pain and negative plain films may benefit from a radionucleotide scan. A delay of 3 days from the trauma incident is recommended before scanning.[3,9]

The lower urinary tract should be radiographically examined first by a retrograde urethrogram. If this study is normal, a voiding cystourethrogram using 250 ml of contrast in the adult should be obtained. A post-void film is imperative to exclude the extravasation of dye.

Associated Injuries

The mortality rate for pelvic fractures is high (7.6 to 16%) and is a result of the high incidence of multisystem injury seen with these fractures.[1,2,7,11–13] Hemorrhagic shock is the major cause of death in pelvic fractures.[14] However, a large review established that the majority of patients suffering hemorrhagic fatality after a pelvic fracture did not die as a result of pelvic hemorrhage.[14] 50 percent or more of patients suffering blunt pelvic fractures admitted to the hospital will require blood transfusions (mean volume 7 to 8 units in one study).[4,14,15] Of those patients requiring large transfusion, 30 percent will die.[15] Fractures that involve a displaced double ring break have a twofold increase in the incidence of bleeding requiring transfusion when compared with single ring fractures. As mentioned earlier, posterior pelvic fractures are associated with more bleeding than are anterior fractures. Generally, major vascular injuries are localized to the iliac veins, and arterial injuries and bleeding are not commonly seen.[16,17]

Patients with pelvic fractures require the insertion of short large bore lines and the typing of blood in expectation of serious bleeding. Should hypovolemia become a problem, crystalloids, blood, and use of the mast suit should be employed.[18] Arteriography or venography, or both, have been advocated to localize the source of persistent bleeding in pelvic fractures.[19,20] Problems arise in the interpretation of these studies because of the presence of large overlying and obscuring hematomas.

Surgical control and repair of bleeding vessels associated with pelvic fractures is not routinely indicated. Pelvic fractures are most often treated with bedrest, with or without traction. Unstable fractures may be treated with external fixation or open reduction with internal fixation.[17,21] The type of external fixater and its application should be determined by the orthopedic surgeon based upon the specific fracture pattern. Pelvic fixaters can be inserted in the Emergency Department under local anesthesia with minor skin incisions. Early external fixation of unstable pelvic fractures may be a valuable option in reducing blood loss. Although strict criteria are not available, most surgeons in the past would accept persistent shock after adequate volume replacement or a transfusion requirement of over 20 units as indicative of the need for surgical intervention. Angiography with acute arterial embolization has been successfully utilized in patients suffering from pelvic fractures associated with extensive hemorrhage.[21] The authors recommend this procedure, when available, if bleeding continues beyond 8 units.

Visceral injuries in conjunction with pelvic fractures are associated with a high mortality. The most common visceral injury is to the lower urinary tract consisting of injury to the bladder and the urethra. Urethral injuries are twice as common as bladder injuries.[4]

Axiom: *All pelvic fractures are assumed to have an associated urinary tract injury until proven otherwise.*

Anterior urethral ruptures are more common than are posterior urethral injuries. These injuries generally occur after a straddle fracture or a displaced pubic fracture. Posterior urethral ruptures more commonly involve the membranous rather than the prostatic urethra. Pubic rami fractures are associated with a 10 percent incidence of this injury.[8,22]

There is a 6 percent incidence of bladder injuries associated with pelvic fractures.[8,22] Extraperitoneal rupture of the bladder is usually associated with a full bladder just before the injury. Shock in association with lower abdominal pain, inability to void, or urethral bleeding may be an early sign of a bladder injury.

Patients with pelvic fractures and consequently suspected lower urinary tract injury first should be asked to void spontaneously. Patients with a ruptured bladder will be unable to do so. If urine is obtained it should be examined for the presence of red blood cells. The patient should also be examined for ecchymoses or perineal bleeding along with urethral bleeding and a rectal examination for the localization of the prostate. Only a displaced prostate is considered definitive proof of a urinary tract injury. The remainder of the above mentioned findings including hematuria may be present or absent with a significant lower tract injury. Female patients are also at risk for associated urethral and bladder injuries (4.6% female urethral injury with a pelvic fracture).[23] A meticulous vaginal examination should be considered whenever blood is seen at the introitus. Difficulty with urination should be followed with a urethrogram and a cystogram.

If there is no hematuria and no sign on examination of a urinary tract injury in the presence of an avulsion fracture, or a fracture that does not disrupt the ring (class A fracture), further radiographic evaluation is not warranted. If the patient is unable to void, it is the authors' recommendation that a sterile gentle attempt to pass a urethral catheter should be made. If this attempt is unsuccessful, a urethrogram should be performed.[8,22]

Fractures that disrupt the pelvic ring (class B and C) require a cystourethrogram for evaluation. A urethrogram can be obtained by gently injecting 20 ml of 30 percent pantopaque contrast medium into the urethral meatus followed by an x-ray. Depending on the results of the urethrogram, a catheter, a filliform with followers, or a suprapubic cystostomy may be necessary.

A retrograde cystogram is performed by instilling 250 ml of 30 percent pantopaque contrast medium, by gravity alone, into the bladder. Views in distention and postvoiding should be examined carefully for any evidence of extravasation. Lower tract injuries are generally treated by surgical repair. Small anterior urethral tears are usually not surgically repaired as they heal well over an indwelling Foley catheter. Bladder ruptures and posterior urethral injuries are best treated surgically.

It is essential to determine early on in the management of patients with pelvic fractures if the fracture is open or closed. A thorough visual evaluation of the surrounding skin surfaces is required. Also, a digital rectal evaluation for bone or bone fragments is required when evaluating posterior pelvic or sacral fractures. As mentioned earlier, female patients with a pelvic fracture and blood at the introitus may have a urinary tract injury. These patients may also have an open fracture with bone penetrating the uterus or vaginal mucosa. The source of bleeding in these patients must be determined early in their management. Open pelvic fractures require the early administration of broad spectrum bacteriocidal antibiotics. Those fractures involving the rectum will typically require a diverting colostomy.[24]

Neurologic injuries are frequently associated with sacral fractures. Typically the first and second foramen and their corresponding nerves are damaged due to stretching, small bony fragments, or hematoma formation. This injury is usually detected by a thorough neurologic examination. A lesion impinging on the first or second foramina will typically present with ankle dorsiflexion weakness and weakness of the glutei, hamstrings, and calf muscles. The sciatic nerve may be impaired in association with sacroiliac joint injuries. Again, a neurologic exami-

nation eliciting diminished sensation at the base of the great toe or weakness of the anterior tibial compartment muscles is indicative of this injury.

Gastrointestinal injuries associated with fractures are typically seen only with penetrating trauma. If a lower gastrointestinal injury is suspected, a water-soluble contrast enema should be obtained.

Complications

Pelvic fractures may be associated with many long-term complications.[1]

1. Chronic sacroiliac arthritis presenting as constant low sacral pain may follow sacroiliac joint injury and may require operative intervention.[6,25]
2. Malunion or delayed union may complicate the management of these fractures.
3. Pulmonary and fat emboli may complicate the early management of these fractures.
4. Sepsis may result from a ruptured viscus with bacterial seeding of a hematoma.

PELVIC FRACTURES

☐ Class A: Pelvic fractures [These involve only a portion or a segment of the pelvis without transecting the entire ring.] (Figs. 18–5 to 18–14)
Type I (Avulsion fractures, Fig. 18–5)
Type II (Single pubic or ischial ramus fractures, Figs. 18–6, 18–7)
Type III (Ischial body fractures, Fig. 18–9)
Type IV (Illiac wing fractures, Fig. 18–10)
Type V (Horizontal sacral fractures, Fig. 18–11)
Type VI (Coccyx fractures, Fig. 18–14)

☐ Class B: Pelvic ring fractures [These are nondisplaced and transect the pelvic ring.] (Figs. 18–15 to 18–22)
Type I (Nondisplaced fractures of both pubic rami, Fig. 18–16)
Type II (Nondisplaced pubic bone fractures or symphysis pubis subluxations, Fig. 18–17)
Type IIIA (Nondisplaced ilium body fractures near the sacroiliac joint, Fig. 18–18)
Type IIIB (Vertical sacral fractures, Fig. 18–18)

☐ Class C: Unstable pelvic ring fractures [These involve a double break in the pelvic ring, usually with displacement.] (Figs. 18–19 to 18–30)
Type 1A (Bilateral double pubic rami fractures [Straddle fracture], Fig. 18–19)
Type IB (Fracture, dislocation of the pubis, Fig. 18–20)
Type IIA (Malgaigne fractures, Figs. 18–23 through 18–26)
Type IIB (Contralateral double vertical ring fractures [Bucket-handle fracture], Fig. 18–28)
Type IIA (Pelvic dislocation [Sprung pelvis], Fig. 18–29)
Type IIB (Multiple displaced pelvic fractures, Fig. 18–30)

ACETABULAR FRACTURES

☐ Class A: Nondisplaced acetabular fractures (Fig. 18–32)

☐ Class B: Displaced acetabular fractures [Many authors include class B acetabular injuries under the discussion of hip dislocations. The authors of this book apologize for inconvenience caused by differences in terminology.] (Fig. 18–33)

Classification

The classification system used in this book is a modification of that presented by Key and Conwell[6], Dunn and Morris[26], Furey[27] and Tile and Pennal[39]. The system as presented groups pelvic fractures as to the likelihood of associated injuries and the therapeutic approach recommended by most authors. Fractures of the pelvis are first divided into acetabular and pelvic ring fractures. Pelvic ring fractures are then further subdivided into stable or unstable injuries. Class A and B fractures are considered stable whereas class C fractures are unstable. In general, class A fractures are associated with the lowest incidence of associated injuries and class C the highest. Acetabular fractures are divided into class A nondisplaced and class B displaced fractures.

PELVIC FRACTURES

☐ CLASS A: PELVIC FRACTURES

As mentioned earlier, class A fractures do not transect the pelvic ring and usually are treated symptomatically with good results. These fractures are usually not complicated by serious associated injuries.

☐ Class A: Type I (Avulsion Fractures, Fig. 18–5)

These fractures generally occur in young athletes and are due to a forceful muscular contraction in an area where the apophyseal centers are not yet fused. They typically fuse at the following ages:

- **Type IA:** *Anterior superior iliac spine* (sartorius insertion) fuses at 16 to 20 years.
- **Type IB:** *Anterior inferior iliac spine* (rectus femoris insertion) fuses at 16 to 20 years.
- **Type IC:** *Ischial tuberosity* (hamstrings insertion) fuses at age 25.

In addition to the above, an avulsion at the symphysis pubis by the adductor may be seen in young athletes.

PELVIC FRACTURES

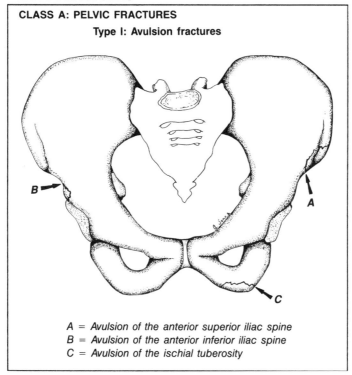

CLASS A: PELVIC FRACTURES

Type I: Avulsion fractures

A = Avulsion of the anterior superior iliac spine
B = Avulsion of the anterior inferior iliac spine
C = Avulsion of the ischial tuberosity

Figure 18–5.

After the fracture, callus formation may be extensive and at times be mistaken for a neoplasm.

Mechanism of Injury

Each type of avulsion fracture is associated with a different mechanism of injury.

☐ *Class A: Type IA*

These fractures are typically seen in young sprinters and are secondary to a forceful contraction of the sartorius. Displacement is usually mild and inhibited by the attachment of the *inguinal ligament* and *fascia lata* to this bone.

☐ *Class A: Type IB*

These fractures are less frequent than type IA injuries and are due to a forceful contraction of the rectus femoris as during a soccer kick.

☐ *Class A: Type IC*

These injuries are typically seen in athletes, such as hurdlers, cheerleaders, and pole vaulters, who vigorously use their hamstrings. The sacrotuberous ligament antagonizes displacement of the ischial tuberosity.

Examination

The examination of each type of avulsion fracture is different and will be discussed separately.

☐ *Class A: Type IA*

There will be pain and tenderness over the anterior superior iliac spine that is exacerbated with use of the sartorius (flexion or abduction of the thigh).

☐ *Class A: Type IB*

The patient will complain of pain and tenderness in the groin. Active hip flexion using the rectus femoris as during walking will be painful.

☐ *Class A: Type IC*

This injury may present with acute or chronic symptoms of pain that worsen with sitting. Tenderness will be elicited with percutaneous and rectal palpation of the ischial tuberosity. Palpation over the sacrotuberous ligament on rectal examination will also greatly exacerbate the pain. In addition, flexion of the thigh with the knee extended is painful although it is painless with the knee flexed.

X ray

An AP view is generally adequate in defining the fracture fragment. Nonossified apophyseal centers may at times confuse the interpretation of these radiographs and the reader is referred to the introduction of this section for further clarification.

Associated Injuries

These fractures are usually not associated with any other significant injuries.

Treatment

The treatment for avulsion pelvic fractures is symptomatic. Referral is indicated if the avulsed fragment is markedly displaced.

☐ *Class A: Type IA*

The patient should rest in bed for 3 to 4 weeks with the hip in flexion and abduction. The patient may sit as tolerated although ambulation and vigorous activity should be restricted. Complete recovery may take as long as 8 weeks or more.

☐ *Class A: Type IB*

The treatment is the same as for type IA injuries except the hip should be in flexion with *no abduction*.

☐ *Class A: Type IC*

The patient should be placed on bed rest with the thigh in extension with external rotation and slight abduction. An inflatable ring cushion for sitting is advised after the period of rest.

Complications

Avulsion fractures may be followed by the persistence of chronic pain for several months or the overzealous growth of callus and new bone requiring surgical excision secondary to chronic pain.

☐ Class A: Type II   (Single Pubic or Ischial Ramus Fractures)   (Figs. 18–6, 18–7)

These fractures do not transect the pelvic ring and are the most commonly seen fractures of the pelvis.[25,28]

PELVIC FRACTURES

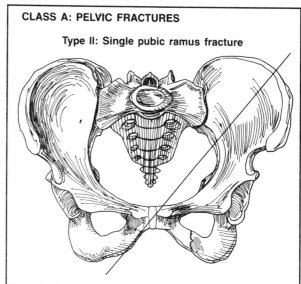

CLASS A: PELVIC FRACTURES

Type II: Single pubic ramus fracture

Figure 18–6.

PELVIC FRACTURES

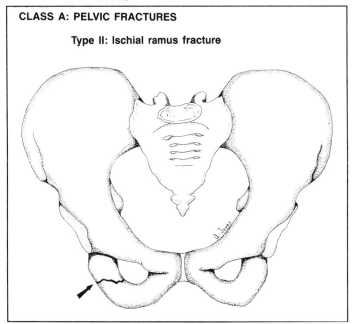

CLASS A: PELVIC FRACTURES

Type II: Ischial ramus fracture

Figure 18–7.

Some authors elect to classify these injuries as stress fractures because they are commonly seen in women during the third trimester of pregnancy or in military recruits after a strenuous march.[29,30] These fractures are also commonly seen in elderly patients. Stress fractures of the pubic rami have recently been described in serious runners.[31] The only way to make a diagnosis is by bone scanning. Most of these patients experience persistent groin discomfort during any activity. All patients recover with an 8- to 12-week rest period and particularly with the avoidance of running.[31]

Mechanism of Injury
In the elderly the mechanism is generally secondary to a fall. In the young, persistent tension on the adductors and the hamstrings may result in a stress fracture of the inferior ramus.

Examination
The patient will complain of a "deep pain" that is exacerbated with deep palpation or walking. Hamstring stressing will elicit or worsen the pain.

X ray (Fig. 18–8)
An AP pelvic view should be obtained first as a general overview of the area. If clinical or radiographic suspicion is high a 35 degree cephalic tilt view should be obtained.

Associated Injuries
These fractures may be accompanied by a hip fracture in elderly patients.

Treatment
Symptomatic treatment is recommended including analgesics and bed rest progressing to crutch walking as tolerated.

Complications
Complications are not commonly seen after these fractures.

☐ Class A: Type III   (Ischial Body Fractures) (Fig. 18–9)
Ischial body fractures are frequently comminuted and are the least frequent of all pelvic fractures.

Mechanism of Injury
These fractures result from a significant fall landing on the buttocks in the seated position.

Examination
There will be pain and tenderness to deep palpation that is exacerbated with tension on the hamstrings.

X ray
An AP view of the pelvis is generally adequate in demonstrating this fracture.

Associated Injuries
These fractures usually follow a significant fall and associated fractures of the lumbar and thoracic spine may accompany these injuries.

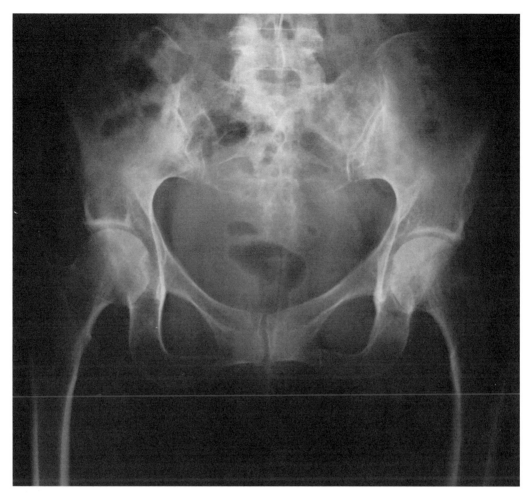

Figure 18–8. Fracture of the inferior pubic ramus.

PELVIC FRACTURES

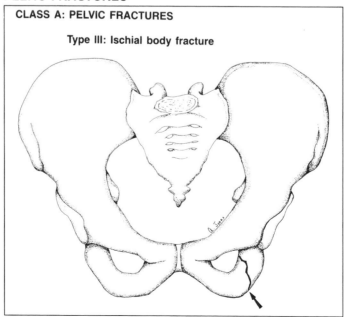

CLASS A: PELVIC FRACTURES

Type III: Ischial body fracture

Figure 18–9.

Treatment

Symptomatic treatment with 4 to 6 weeks of bed rest is usually adequate. Elderly patients typically require active and passive motion exercises along with earlier mobilization. A pneumatic cushion for sitting is helpful during the later stages of healing.

Complications

Ischial body fractures may be complicated by malunion or excessive callus formation resulting in the development of chronic pain exacerbated by sitting or hamstring stress.

□ Class A: Type IV (Iliac Wing Fractures) (Fig. 18–10)

The abductors of the hip insert on the iliac wing.

Mechanism of Injury

These fractures are usually the result of a medially directed force. The iliac wing may at times demonstrate medial displacement.[30]

Examination

The patient will complain of tenderness and swelling over the iliac wing. Pain will be exacerbated with walking or stressing of the hip abductors.

X ray

An AP pelvic view is generally adequate in demonstrating this fracture. Oblique views may be indicated if the fracture is not clearly identified or if displacement is suspected.

Associated Injuries

Iliac wing fractures typically follow severe injuring forces and may be associated with several serious injuries.

1. Acetabular fractures may accompany these injuries.
2. Associated gastrointestinal injuries are uncommon but may be delayed in their presentation. The abdomen should always be evaluated initially for tenderness as well as later for the development of ileus.

Treatment

Symptomatic treatment including bed rest and non-weight bearing until the hip abductors are pain-free is generally adequate. Displaced fractures typically do not require reduction.

Complications

Iliac wing fractures are generally free of long-term complications.

□ Class A: Type V (Horizontal Sacral Fractures) (Fig. 18–11)

Sacrum fractures may be either horizontal or vertical. Vertical fractures are secondary to an indirect mechanism

PELVIC FRACTURES

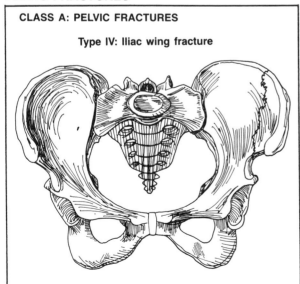

Figure 18–10.

PELVIC FRACTURES

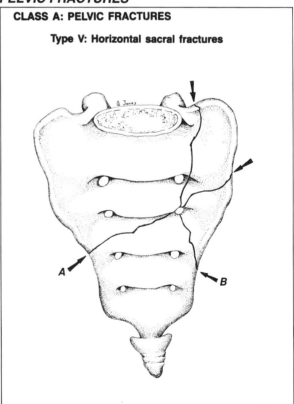

Figure 18–11. Sacrum fractures. A = transverse, B = vertical.

and usually transect the pelvic ring. Vertical sacrum fractures will be discussed under class B injuries, because they usually transect the ring. The following discussion is limited to *horizontal sacrum fractures.*

Mechanism of Injury
A direct blow over the posterior sacrum in an anterior direction is the usual mechanism. These fractures commonly follow a fall with landing in the sitting position or a massive crush injury to the pelvis.

Examination
The patient will complain of tenderness, swelling, and ecchymosis over the sacral prominence. Rectal examination will elicit pain in the sacrum and displacement can be assessed with a bimanual rectal examination. Blood on the examiner's glove following the digital rectal examination suggests an open fracture. Open fractures require emergent broad-spectrum antibiotics and surgical intervention. The neurologic function of the lower sacral nerves including anal sphincter, perineal sensation, and bladder sphincter must be documented early in the patient assessment.

X ray (Fig. 18–12)
Transverse sacral fractures may be difficult to detect on routine pelvic radiographs. Transverse fractures tend to occur distal to the sacroiliac joints. A malalignment or buckling of the sacral foramina may be indicative of a dis-

placed sacral fracture. The lateral view or the AP cephalic view is often better for demonstrating displaced sacral fractures.[32] A CT evaluation or a bone scan is often helpful in delineating these fractures where plain films are not definite.[3]

Associated Injuries
Various series report a 4 to 14 percent incidence of associated pelvic fractures with transverse sacral fractures.[4]

Treatment
☐ *Class A: Type V (Nondisplaced Horizontal Sacral Fracture)*
Symptomatic treatment with bed rest for 4 to 5 weeks along with heat and massage are recommended. An inflated cushion may be used later for sitting.

☐ *Class A: Type V (Displaced Horizontal Sacral Fractures) (Fig. 18–13)*
It is imperative that the examining physician initially perform a thorough neurologic examination of the patient. It is the authors' recommendation that all displaced class A, type V fractures have an emergent orthopedic referral.

Complications
Horizontal sacral fractures may be complicated by the development of chronic pain or nerve dysfunction secondary to overzealous callus formation.

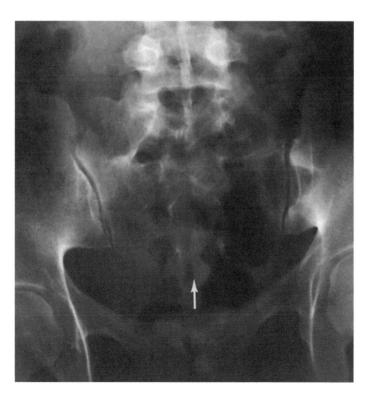

Figure 18–12. A transverse sacral fracture.

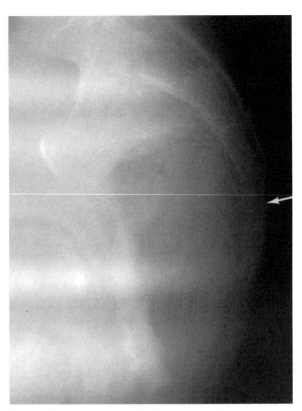

Figure 18–13. A displaced horizontal sacral fracture.

PELVIC FRACTURES

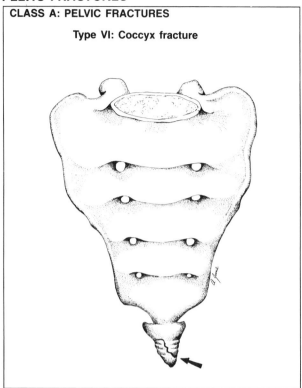

Figure 18–14.

□ Class A: Type VI   (Coccyx Fractures)
(Fig. 18–14)

Coccyx fractures tend to be transverse and because numerous muscle fibers insert here they are impossible to immobilize. Coccyx fractures are among the easiest fractures to treat and yet the most difficult to cure.

Mechanism of Injury

A fall landing in the sitting position is the most common mechanism of injury. In addition, surgical procedures performed in this area may be complicated by the development of a coccyx fracture.

Examination

The patient will complain of tenderness localized to "one spot." Use of the *tensor levator ani* or spasm of the *anococcygeal muscle* as during sitting or defecation will exacerbate the pain. Palpation rectally or externally over the coccyx is usually diagnostic.

X ray (Fig. 18–15)

An AP pelvic view along with a lateral projection with the thighs in flexion is best for demonstrating these fractures. Coccygeal fractures are often not visualized radiographically.

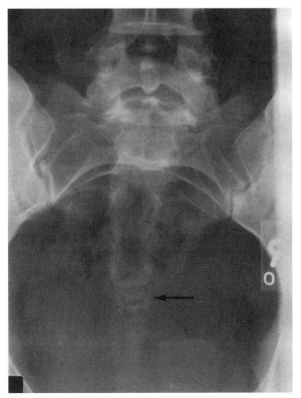

Figure 18–15. A coccyx fracture.

Associated Injuries
Coccygeal fractures are not commonly associated with any other significant injuries.

Treatment
The treatment is symptomatic with bed rest, inflated cushions, sitz baths, and laxatives to avoid straining. Coccygectomy may be indicated if chronic pain persists despite adequate conservative therapy.

Complications
Chronic pain may persist for several years after coccygeal fractures.

☐ CLASS B: PELVIC RING FRACTURES

Class B fractures transect the pelvic ring in one location and are considered stable injuries because there can be no displacement. As mentioned earlier, displaced pelvic fractures require that there be two fractures transecting the ring or one fracture transection with a joint dislocation. Class B fractures are secondary to direct trauma such as a crush injury. These fractures tend to occur near the symphysis pubis or sacroiliac joint as the relative mobility of the pelvis in these areas allows a ring transection without further displacement.

☐ Class B: Type I (Nondisplaced Fractures
of Both Pubic Rami)
(Fig. 18–16)
This fracture is very commonly seen and very stable.

PELVIC FRACTURES

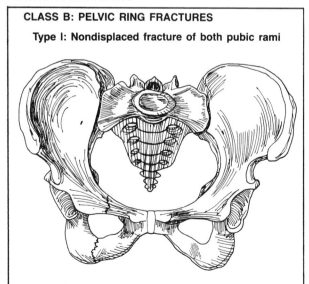

CLASS B: PELVIC RING FRACTURES

Type I: Nondisplaced fracture of both pubic rami

Figure 18–16.

Mechanism of Injury
This fracture usually results from direct trauma to the area.

Examination
The patient will present with tenderness, swelling, and ecchymosis over the fracture site. Lateral compression of the ring or *Patrick's test* will exacerbate the patient's pain.

X ray
A routine AP pelvic view is usually adequate in demonstrating the fracture. The ipsilateral sacroiliac joint must be inspected carefully for any evidence of disruption. CT scanning is recommended if a sacroiliac joint disruption is suspected.

Associated Injuries
As mentioned in the introductory section of this chapter, vascular and visceral injuries frequently accompany pelvic fractures. Class B, type I fractures may be associated with any of these serious injuries. CT scanning is useful in evaluating patients with suspected visceral and/or vascular injuries.

Treatment
Early orthopedic consultation is recommended. These fractures are typically stable and treated symptomatically with bed rest for three weeks. If the fracture is slightly displaced there may be an associated sacroiliac joint injury. With slight displacement, the recommended therapy includes referral for a pelvic sling and bilateral bucks traction for 4 to 6 weeks. After this a pelvic belt with ambulation as tolerated is indicated.

Complications
Class B, type I fractures may be complicated by the persistence of pain secondary to posttraumatic arthritis for prolonged periods.

☐ Class B: Type II (Nondisplaced Pubic
Bone Fractures or
Symphysis Pubis
Subluxations)
(Fig. 18–17)
This is a rare isolated injury and is usually associated with genitourinary injury. The ligaments of the symphysis pubis normally allow for 0.5 to 1 mm of movement. Any separation beyond 1 mm in men and 1.5 mm in women is considered a subluxation or a dislocation. Third trimester and postpartum patients are susceptible to this injury because the hormonally induced ligamentous laxity allows for more mobility.

PELVIC FRACTURES

CLASS B: PELVIC RING FRACTURES

Type II: Nondisplaced pubic bone fracture or symphysis pubis subluxation

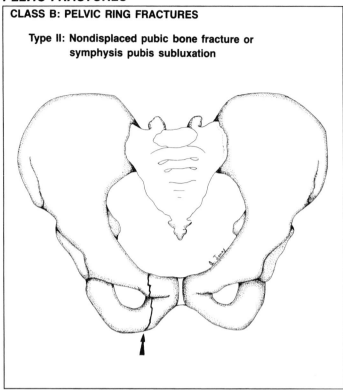

Figure 18–17.

Mechanism of Injury

A direct AP force is the usual mechanism although indirect forces may add to the displacement. There are three common symphysis dislocation patterns seen.

1. Midline overlap
2. Posterior superior displacement
3. Anterior inferior displacement

Examination

The patient will present with tenderness, swelling, or even deformity over the involved area. pregnant patients may complain of an audible click with walking. Pain will be localized and exacerbated with AP or lateral compression of the pelvis. Those injuries with marked displacement may present in a shock state with a sprung pelvis. This will be discussed under class C injuries.

X ray

A routine pelvic view is usually adequate in demonstrating the fracture or subluxation. Urologic imaging studies are indicated for patients with suspected urinary tract disruption.

Associated Injuries

Damage to the urologic system frequently accompanies these injuries.

Treatment

Although these are typically stable injuries, early orthopedic consultation is recommended. The treatment is symptomatic and similar to class B, type 1 fractures except that bed rest in the lateral position is recommended.

Complications

These injuries may be complicated by the development of persistent pain over the involved area.

☐ Class B: Type IIIA (Nondisplaced Ilium Body Fractures Near the Sacroiliac Joint) (Fig. 18–18)
  Type IIIB (Vertical Sacral Fractures) (Fig. 18–18)

Isolated nondisplaced ilium body fractures near the sacroiliac joint are rare injuries. Typically, posterior pelvic fractures are associated with anterior ring fractures. Vertical sacral fractures usually begin at the weakest point that is adjacent to the first and second foramina.

Mechanism of Injury

Type IIIA or ilium body fractures near the sacroiliac joint are usually the result of a direct force pushing the ilium posteriorly and medially. Type IIIB fractures are

PELVIC FRACTURES

CLASS B: PELVIC RING FRACTURES

Type IIIA: Nondisplaced ilium body fracture near the sacroiliac joint

Type IIIB: Vertical sacral fracture

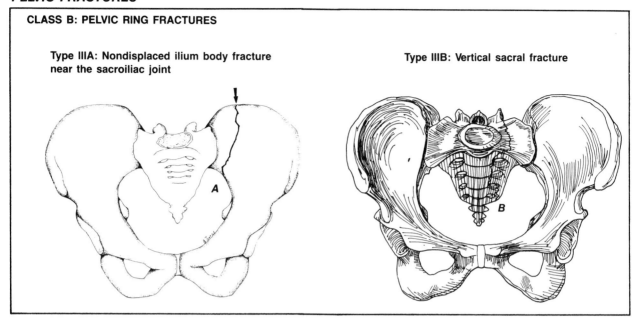

Figure 18–18.

usually the result of indirect trauma as when an anterior force drives the pelvic ring posteriorly resulting in a vertical sacral fracture.[33]

Examination
The patient will present with tenderness over the posterior pelvis that is exacerbated with AP or lateral compression. Straight leg raising is painful for both type IIIA and IIIB fracures. Blood on the examiner's glove following the digital rectal examination suggests an open fracture. Open fractures require open emergent broad-spectrum antibiotics and surgical intervention. Patients with these fractures should have a digital rectal examination.

X ray
An AP pelvic view is usually adequate for both of these injuries. Sacral fractures may be better demonstrated on an AP cephalic tilt view. A CT evaluation or a bone scan is often helpful in delineating these fractures where plain films are not helpful.[3]

Associated Injuries
Class B, type III fractures are frequently associated with anterior pelvic fractures. Sacral fractures may be accompanied by neurologic damage.

Treatment
Although these are typically stable fractures and treated symptomatically, early orthopedic consultation is recommended. Bed rest with a pelvic sling or belt is recommended. Ambulation should progress as tolerated with an expected return to normal function within 3 to 4 months.

Complications
Class B, type III fractures may be complicated by the development of chronic back pain or neurologic compromise.

☐ CLASS C: UNSTABLE PELVIC RING FRACTURES

Class C fractures involve a transection of the pelvic ring in two places with displacement. Class C fractures are seen less often than are class A or B injuries. The mortality rate for displaced pelvic fractures is very high, being second only to skull fractures. In addition, life-threatening associated injuries including hemorrhage and visceral organ damage frequently accompany these injuries. Class C fractures usually are secondary to severe direct forces as those that occur in a high speed car accident. Straddle fractures are the most common type of displaced pelvic fracture seen.

Classification
Class C displaced pelvic fractures have been divided into three types. Type I injuries are bilateral, double vertical fractures of the anterior pelvic ring, or anterior

double vertical fractures with a pubic symphysis dislocation. Type II injuries involve ipsilateral double vertical fractures in any area of the pelvic ring. There are many fracture patterns within this broad group and many of them include sacroiliac dislocations. Type III injuries include the multiply fractured pelvis.

☐ Class C: Type IA   (Bilateral Double Pubic
                        Rami Fractures
                        [Straddle Fracture])
                        (Fig. 18–19)
             Type IB   (Fracture–Dislocation of
                        the Pubis) (Fig. 18–20)

Type I fractures are the most frequent of the class C injuries. Nearly one third of these fractures have an associated lower urinary tract injury.[4]

Mechanism of Injury
The most common mechanism is a fall resulting in the straddling of a hard object. In addition, lateral compression of the pelvis may result is a type I fracture.

Examination
The patient will present with anterior tenderness, swelling, and ecchymosis. It is important to examine and palpate the perineum, rectum and vagina for lacerations, bony deformities and hematomas. It is imperative that patients with type I fractures undergo a radiographic examination of the lower urinary tract.

PELVIC FRACTURES

**CLASS C: UNSTABLE PELVIC RING FRACTURES—
DOUBLE BREAKS IN RING**

**Type IA: Bilateral double pubic rami fracture
(Straddle fracture)**

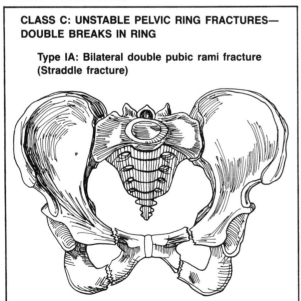

Figure 18–19.

PELVIC FRACTURES

**CLASS C: UNSTABLE PELVIC RING FRACTURES—
DOUBLE BREAKS IN RING**

Type IB: Fracture–dislocation of pubis

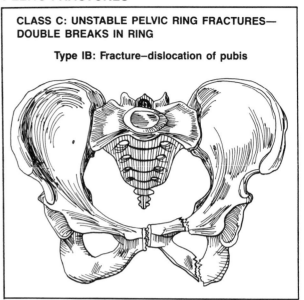

Figure 18–20. A variant of the same injury illustrated in Fig. 18–19.

X ray (Fig. 18–21)
An AP pelvic view is usually adequate in demonstrating the fracture. CT scanning is valuable in determining the extent of the damage to the underlying tissues and organs. Radiographic imaging of the lower urinary tract is recommended with type I fractures.

Associated Injuries
As mentioned earlier, class C injuries are associated with a high incidence of vascular and visceral injuries. Up to 33 percent of type I fractures have an associated lower urinary tract injury, the most common being a urethral rupture[4] (Figure 18–22).

Treatment
Emergent orthopedic consultation is recommended. The emergency management of these fractures includes immobilization of the patient in a recumbent position and stabilization including fluid therapy and the exclusion of serious associated injuries. The physician's priority must be directed at the indentification and stabilization of those life-threatening associated injuries. Once stabilized, the patient should be admitted to an intensive care setting.

Complications
Class C, type I fractures may be complicated by the development of several serious disorders.

1. Posttraumatic arthritis frequeantly follows these injuries.
2. Malunion or nonunion may develop during the recumbency period.

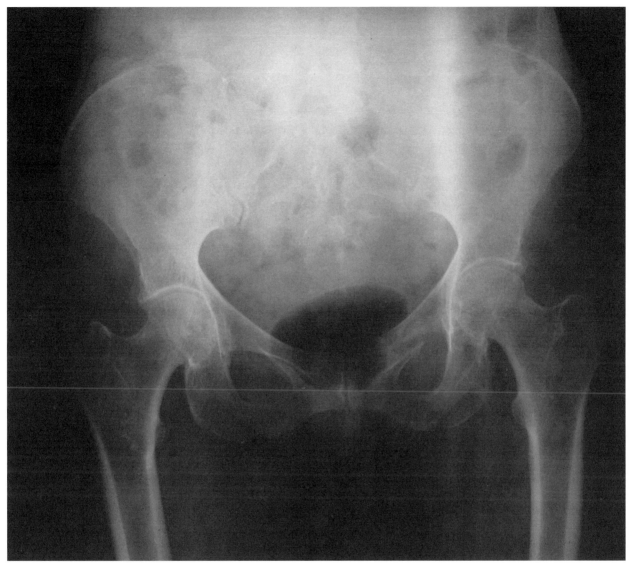

Figure 18–21. Displaced fracture of the superior and inferior pubic rami.

3. Pulmonary or fat emboli may develop during the early stages of healing.
4. A perforated viscus secondary to trauma may later become a source of sepsis.

☐ Class C: Type IIA   (Malgaigne Fractures) (Figs. 18–23 through 18–26)

Type IIB   (Contralateral Double Vertical Ring Fractures [Bucket-handle Fracture] (Fig. 18–28)

Type II injuries involve an anterior symphysis pubis dislocation and/or superior and inferior pubic rami fractures with an ipsilateral sacral fracture and/or sacroiliac dislocation. These fractures may result in posterior and superior displacement of the hemipelvis with secondary leg length changes. These patients should be immobilized as soon as possible as any leg or foot motion will be reflected in the unstable hemipelvis and may further aggravate vascular or visceral injuries.

Mechanism of Injury

There are two mechanisms that may result in class C, type II fractures. A direct blow or anterior compression is the most frequent mechanism of injury. In addition, torsion with the sacrum fixed may result in a type II injury. Axial transmission of force from the femur in abduction and less than 90 degrees of flexion may result in an indirect type II fracture.

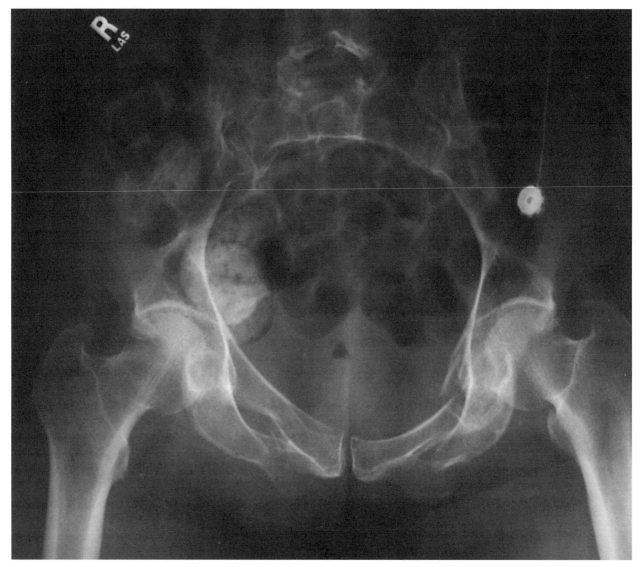

Figure 18–22. A straddle fracture with bilateral breaks of both pubic rami.

Examination

The patient will complain of tenderness and swelling on the involved side. On examination a lower abdominal mass, the hematoma, may be palpable. In addition, the physician will note decreased motion and possibly shortening of the lower extremity on the involved side. Shortening is due to cephalad displacement of the pelvic fragment including the acetabulum. Careful measurements from the umbilicus to the anterior superior iliac spine or the medial malleus will demonstrate shortening on the involved side. Measurements from the anterior superior iliac spine to the malleus will be similar, thus excluding a femoral neck fracture. It is important to palpate and examine the perineum, rectum, and vagina for lacerations, bony deformities, and hematomas. Sacral neurologic deficits may accompany these injuries and must be excluded early on the basis of examination. Visceral injuries frequently accompany these fractures and require a thorough physical and radiographic evaluation.

X ray (Fig. 18–27)

An AP pelvic view is generally adequate for demonstrating these fractures. The physician should closely scrutinize the sacroiliac joints for widening and displacement of the fracture lines. The inferior pubic borders should be examined closely for evidence of asymmetry as an indicator of a displaced pelvic fracture. The symphysis pubis should not exceed 10 mm in the child or 8 mm in the adult; otherwise this raises the suspicion of a dislocation. CT scanning is essential in order to accurately determine the extent of the fracture and ligamentous damage to the pelvis. In addition, CT scanning is essential in evaluating the abdominal and pelvic viscera and vascular structures. Arteriography and/or venography may be valuable diagnostic aids in evaluating patients with significant hemorrhage. Imaging of the lower urinary tract should be strongly considered in these patients.

PELVIC FRACTURES

CLASS C: UNSTABLE PELVIC RING FRACTURES—
DOUBLE BREAKS IN RING

Type IIA: Malgaigne fracture

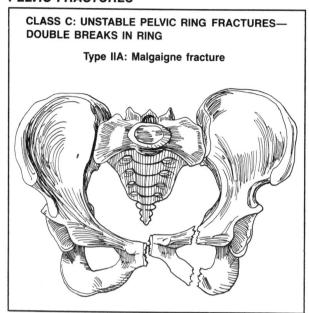

Figure 18–23.

PELVIC FRACTURES

CLASS C: UNSTABLE PELVIC RING FRACTURES

Type IIA: Fracture of the symphysis pubis and
dislocation of the sacroiliac joint.

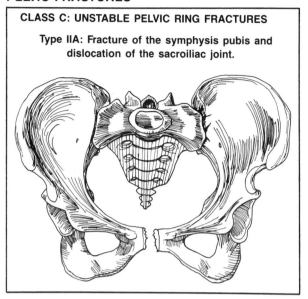

Figure 18–25.

Associated Injuries

All of the vascular, visceral, and neurologic injuries discussed in the introductory section may accompany these fractures.

Treatment

As these injuries are frequently accompanied by other life-threatening injuries, they should be considered within the context of polytrauma management rather than as isolated fractures of the pelvis. Emergent orthopedic consultation is strongly recommended. The emergency management of these fractures includes immobilization along with a rapid and thorough assessment for life-threatening associated injuries. Patients with unstable pelvic fractures with hemodynamic instability despite appropriate fluid therapy should be considered candidates for emergent external fixation (40). External fixation can be done in the emergency department under local anesthesia with only minor skin incisions. The type of external fixater and its application should be determined by the orthopedic surgeon based upon the specific fracture pattern. Early external fixation of unstable pelvic fractures may be a valuable

PELVIC FRACTURES

CLASS C: UNSTABLE PELVIC RING FRACTURES—
DOUBLE BREAKS IN RING

Type IIA: Double vertical fracture–dislocation of pelvis

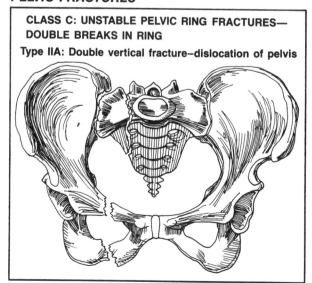

Figure 18–24. Double vertical fracture–dislocation of the pelvis. An unstable injury with a double break in the ring.

PELVIC FRACTURES

CLASS C: UNSTABLE PELVIC RING FRACTURES

Type IIA: Fracture of the ilium and fracture
of the symphysis pubis

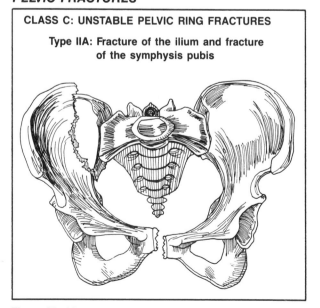

Figure 18–26.

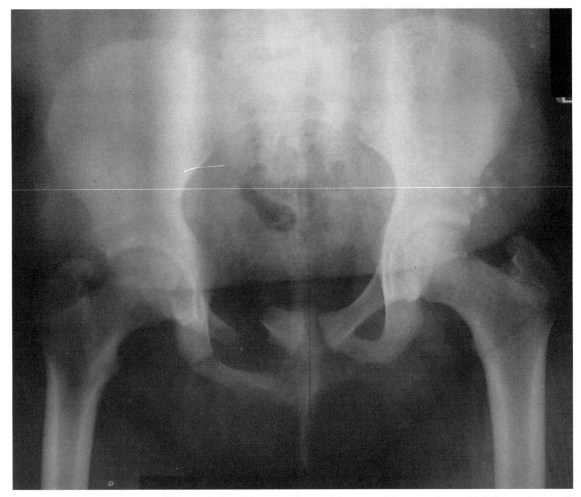

Figure 18–27. Pelvic fracture with symphysis pubic separation and fracture of the superior and inferior rami as well as sacroiliac joint separation.

PELVIC FRACTURES

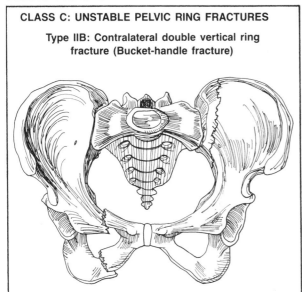

CLASS C: UNSTABLE PELVIC RING FRACTURES

Type IIB: Contralateral double vertical ring fracture (Bucket-handle fracture)

Figure 18–28.

option in reducing blood loss and will reduce the number of patients requiring vascular studies. Stable pelvic fractures with continued bleeding do not benefit from external fixation (34). Continued arterial hemorrhage (4-6 units transfused acutely) may be evaluated with angiography in order to determine the most suitable therapeutic intervention (surgical repair, ligation or embolization) (35, 36).

Complications
Class C, type II fractures may be complicated by the development of sepsis, pulmonary or fat emboli, malunion or nonunion, and posttraumatic arthritis.

☐ Class C: Type IIIA (Pelvic Dislocation [Sprung Pelvis]) (Fig. 18–29)

Type IIIB (Multiple Displaced Pelvic Fractures) (Fig. 18–30)

These fractures are totally unstable as the integrity of the pelvic ring has been abolished. Associated injuries

PELVIC FRACTURES

CLASS C: UNSTABLE PELVIC RING FRACTURES

Type IIIA: Pelvic dislocation (Sprung pelvis)

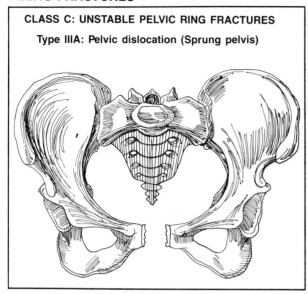

Figure 18–29. This is perhaps the most serious of pelvis dislocations where all the joints are dislocated. The incidence of associated injuries with this fracture is very high (sacroiliac joints).

frequently complicate the management of these fractures resulting in a high morbidity and mortality.

Mechanism of Injury
The most frequent mechanism involves a crush injury to the pelvis.

Examination
The examination of these patients is similar to class C, type II injuries and the reader is referred to that section for further discussion.

X ray (Fig. 18–31)
An AP pelvic view is usually adequate in demonstrating these fractures. Careful scrutiny of the sacroiliac and symphysis pubis joints as discussed under class C, type II fractures is strongly recommended. CT scanning is essential in order to accurately determine the extent of the fracture and ligamentous damage to the pelvis. In addition, CT scanning is essential in evaluating the abdominal and pelvic viscera and vascular structures. Arteriography and/or venography may be valuable diagnostic aids in evaluating patients with significant hemorrhage. Imaging of the lower urinary tract should be strongly considered in these patients.

PELVIC FRACTURES

CLASS C: UNSTABLE PELVIC RING FRACTURES

Type IIIB: Multiple displaced pelvic fractures

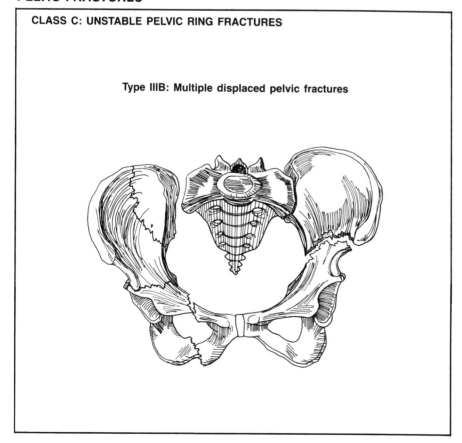

Figure 18–30. Multiple fractures of the pelvis that cannot be classified into any of the other groups.

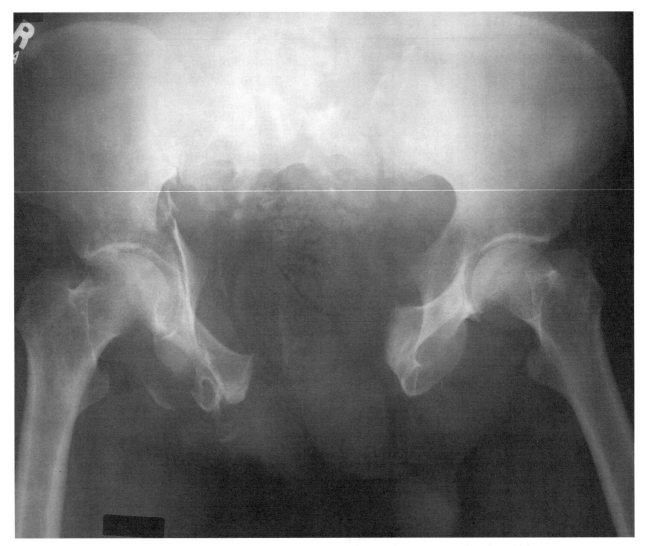

Figure 18–31. Severe pelvic fracture with "Sprung pelvis" involving fracture dislocations in multiple areas.

Associated Injuries

Vascular, visceral, and neurologic injuries frequently accompany these fractures. It is imperative that the emergency physician aggressively evaluate all of these patients for the presence of accompanying life-threatening injuries.

Treatment

As these injuries are frequently accompanied by other life-threatening injuries, they should be considered within the context of polytrauma management rather than as isolated fractures of the pelvis. Emergent orthopedic consultation is strongly recommended. The emergency management of these fractures includes immobilization along with a rapid and thorough assessment for life-threatening associated injuries. Patients with unstable pelvic fractures with hemodynamic instability despite appropriate fluid therapy should be considered candidates for emergent external fixation. (40). External fixation can be done in the emergency department under local anesthesia with only minor skin incisions. The type of external fixater and its application should be determined by the orthopedic surgeon based upon the specific fracture pattern. Early external fixation of unstable pelvic fractures may be a valuable option in reducing blood loss and will reduce the number of patients requiring vascular studies. Stable pelvic fractures with continued bleeding do not benefit from external fixation (34). Continued arterial hemorrhage (4-6 units transfused acutely) may be evaluated with angiography in order to determined the most suitable therapeutic intervention (surgical repair, ligation or embolization) (35, 36).

Complications

Class C, type III fractures may be complicated by the development of pulmonary or fat emboli, sepsis, posttraumatic arthritis, and malunion or nonunion.

ACETABULAR FRACTURES (FIGS. 18–32, 18–33)

Acetabular fractures are classified on the basis of displacement.

- **Class A:** Nondisplaced acetabular fractures
- **Class B:** Displaced acetabular fractures

Displaced acetabular fractures are referred to as *central fracture dislocations* of the hip by several authors. It is the view of the authors of this text that most of these fractures are not true dislocations and therefore they are included under pelvic fractures.

ACETABULAR FRACTURES

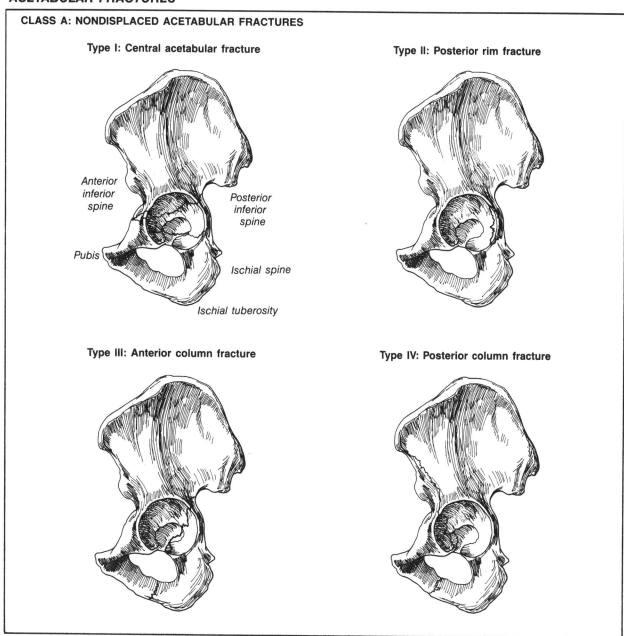

Figure 18–32. Undisplaced acetabular fractures. Many variant types exist.

ACETABULAR FRACTURES

CLASS B: DISPLACED ACETABULAR FRACTURES

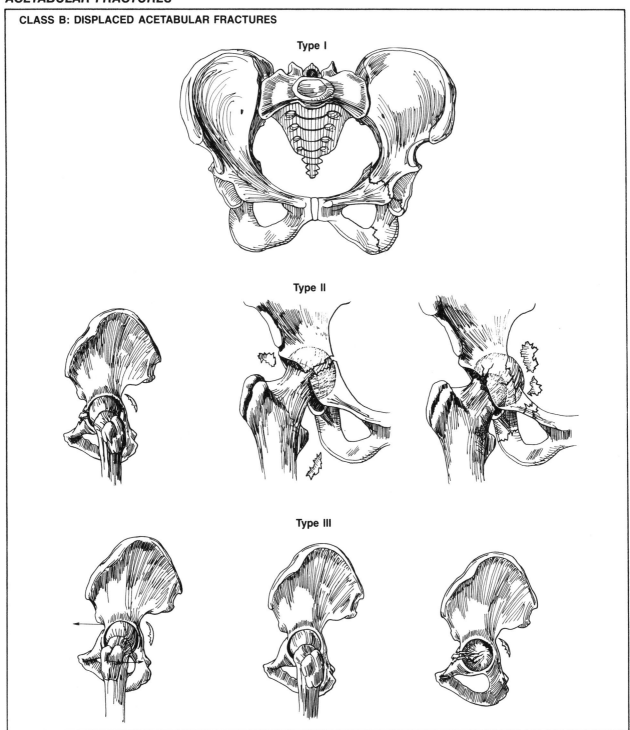

Figure 18–33.

Mechanism of Injury

The most common mechanism of injury is indirect as with a medially directed blow to the greater trochanter. This is commonly seen when a pedestrian is struck by a car, and may result in any type of acetabular fracture except a pos-

terior rim. Another indirect mechanism of injury is by the axial transmission of a force from a blow to the knees transmitted to the femoral head and the acetabulum. This mechanism is encountered frequently in drivers or passengers of cars involved in accidents. This mechanism often results in a central acetabular fracture or less commonly a posterior column fracture. Inner wall injuries comprise the largest group of acetabular fractures and typically are due to a medially directed force against the greater trochanter.

Examination

The patient will present with tenderness, which is increased with attempted weight bearing. Patients with central acetabular fractures may have ipsilateral leg shortening if associated with displacement or dislocation. Patients with acetabular fractures may have accompanying vascular, visceral or neurologic injuries. A thorough examination and evaluation for accompanying injuries is strongly recommended.

X ray (Fig. 18–34 and Fig. 18–35)

Acetabular fractures may be difficult to detect on the initial AP pelvic radiograph. It is essential that the normal anatomic landmarks surrounding the acetabulum, as shown in Fig. 18–36, be carefully scrutinized when these injuries are suspected. If an acetabular fracture is suspected, the following views may be obtained for a complete evaluation.

1. AP of the pelvis
2. AP of the ipsilateral hip
3. 45 degrees external oblique
4. 45 degrees internal oblique

The posterior column and the anterior lip are best visualized on the 45 degree external view whereas the posterior lip and the anterior column are projected best on the 45 degree internal view. In addition, posterior column fractures will distort the *ilioischial line* whereas anterior column fractures will deform the *iliopubic line*. Central acetabular fractures are best visualized on a posterior oblique radiograph. Certain pelvic fractures are

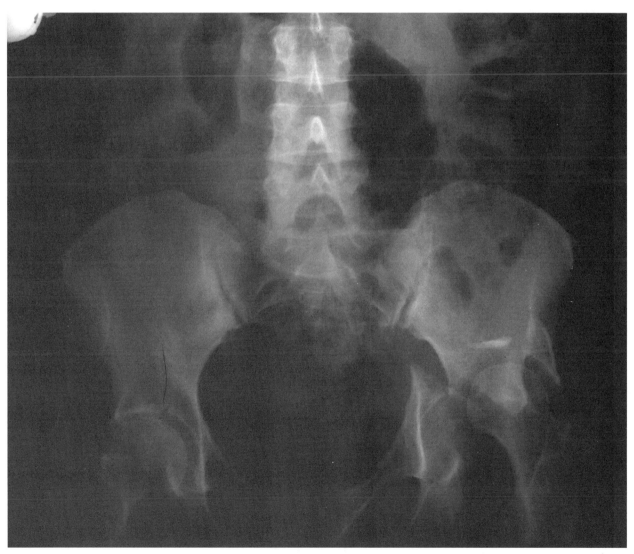

Figure 18–34. Bilateral acetabular fractures. Right side with severe displacement.

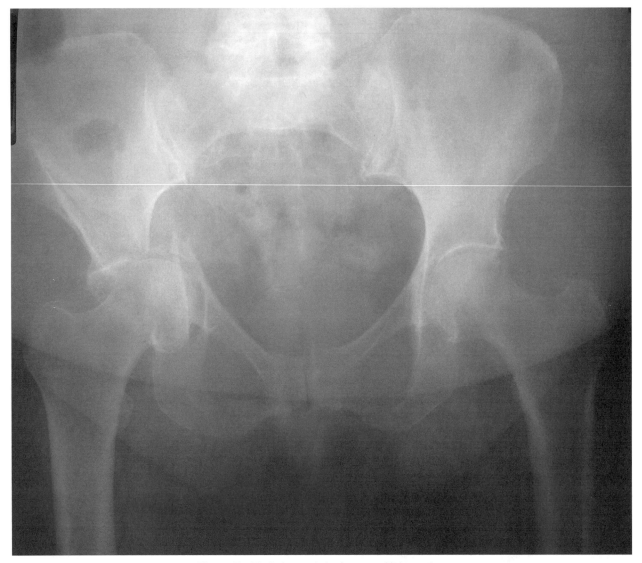

Figure 18–35. Left acetabular fracture with impaction.

frequently associated with acetabular fractures that may not be easily visualized radiographically. Eighty percent of intra-articular fragments in the hip joint are not seen utilizing plain film radiography.[10] CT scanning is recommended in all suspected acetabular injuries.

Axiom: *A fracture of the superior and inferior pubic rami near the ilial junction is frequently associated with an acetabular fracture that may be occult.*

Associated Injuries

Acetabular fractures may be associated with the vascular, visceral, and neurologic complications discussed in the introductory section of this chapter. In ad-

dition, acetabular fractures may be associated with fractures of the femur,[1] the femoral head,[1] pubic rami, and the ipsilateral extremity.[37] Hip dislocations frequently are associated with displaced posterior rim fractures. Associated sciatic nerve injuries occur in 10 to 13 percent of acetabular fractures.[11]

Treatment

Emergent orthopedic referral is recommended. The emergency management of these fractures includes immobilization of the extremity and a thorough evaluation for accompanying vascular, visceral or neurologic injuries. An early normalization of the femoral acetabular relationship is the orthopedic treatment goal. Open reduction with internal fixation is recommended by many orthopedic surgeons (38). Some orthopedic surgeons prefer Russell's traction (Fig. 18–37) for reduction and immobilization.

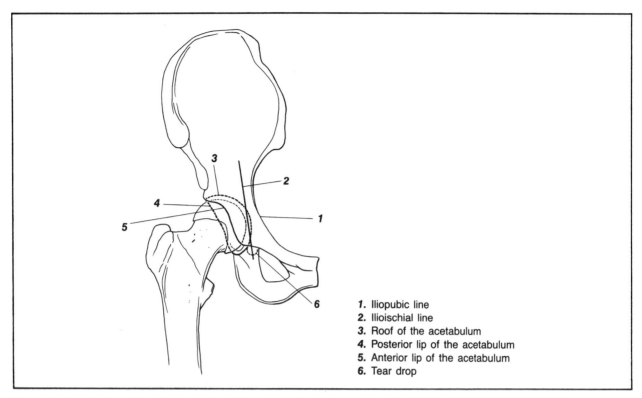

1. Iliopubic line
2. Ilioischial line
3. Roof of the acetabulum
4. Posterior lip of the acetabulum
5. Anterior lip of the acetabulum
6. Tear drop

Figure 18–36. AP view of the hip (acetabulum). These lines should be examined carefully in a patient with suspicion of a fracture. A subtle fracture may displace only one of these lines.

Complications

The management of acetabular fractures may be complicated by the development of several serious disorders.

1. Osteoarthritis commonly follows even the smallest fractures.
2. Traumatic arthritis is commonly noted, especially after displaced central fracture dislocations.
3. Avascular necrosis may occur up to a year after the injury.[11,26] The incidence is dependent on the fracture type and the reduction time. Central acetabular fracture dislocations, which were reduced early, had an aseptic necrosis incidence of 15 percent.[17] If reduction was delayed, there was an incidence of 48 percent.[17] Other authors report no cases of aseptic necrosis after central acetabular fracture dislocations.[2]
4. Sciatic nerve injury may complicate the management of these injuries, especially central displaced fractures.

REFERENCES

1. Peltier LF: Complications associated with fractures of the pelvis. *J Bone Joint Surg* **47:**1060, 1965.
2. Conolly WB, Hedburg EA: Observations on fractures of the pelvis. *J Trauma* **9:**104, 1969.
3. Newhouse KE, EI Khoury Y, Buckwalter A: Occult sacral fractures in osteopenic patients. *J Bone Joint Surg* **74A**(10):1472–1477, 1992.
4. Rockwood CA Jr, Green DP: *Fractures*, Vol. 2. Philadelphia: Lippincott, 1975.
5. Clemente R: *Anatomy*. Philadelphia: Lea & Febiger, 1980.
6. Key JA, Connell HE: Management of Fractures, Dislocations and Sprains. St. Louis: Mosby, 1951.
7. Levine JI, Crampton RS: Major abdominal injuries associated with pelvis fractures. *Surg Gynecol Obstet* **116:**223, 1963.
8. Cass AS: Bladder trauma in the multiple injured patient. *J Urol* **115:**667, 1976.

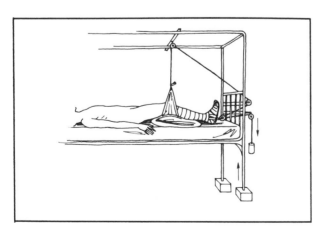

Figure 18–37. Russell's traction. The leg is balanced in a suspension apparatus with minimal flexion; 10 to 15 pounds of weight will provide good traction.

9. Kricun E: Fractures of the pelvis. *Orthop Clin North Am* **21**(3):573–590, 1990.

10. Resnik CS, Stackhouse DJ, Shanmuganathan K, Young JW: Diagnosis of pelvic fractures in patients with acute pelvic trauma: Efficacy of plain radiographs. *AJR* **158**(1):109–112, 1992.

11. Froman C, Stein A: Complicated crushing injuries associated with pelvis fractures. *Surgery* **49**:24, 1967.

12. Fox MA, Mangiante EC, Fabian TC, Voeller GR, Kudsk KA: Pelvic fractures: An analysis of factors affecting prehospital triage and patient outcome. *South Med J* **83**(7): 785–788, 1990.

13. Failinger MS, McGanity PLJ: Current concepts review unstable fractures of the pelvic ring. *J Bone Joint Surg* **74A**(5):781–788, 1992.

14. Poole GV, Ward EF, Muakkassa FF, Hsu HS, Griswold JA, Rhodes RS: Pelvic fractures from major blunt trauma. *Ann Surg* **221**(6):532–538; Discussion 538–539, 1991.

15. Reynolds BM, Balsano NA, Reynolds FS: Pelvic fractures. *J Trauma* **13**:1011, 1973.

16. Braunstein PW, et al: Concealed hemorrhage due to pelvic fracture. *J Trauma* **4**:832, 1964.

17. Gilchrist MR, Peterson DH: Pelvic fracture and associated soft tissue trauma. *Radiology* **88**:278, 1967.

18. Kaplan BH: Pneumatic trousers save accident victims' lives. *JAMA* **225**:686, 1973.

19. Gerlock AJ: Hemorrhage following pelvic fracture controlled by embolization. Case report. *J Trauma* **15**:740, 1975.

20. Margolies MN, et al: Arteriography in the management of hemorrhage from pelvic fractures. *N Engl J Med* **287**:317, 1972.

21. Burgess AR, Eastridge BJ, Young JW, Ellison TS, Ellison PS Jr, Poka A, Bathon GH, Brumback RJ: Pelvic ring disruptions: Effective classification system and treatment protocols. *J Trauma* **30**(7):848–856, 1990.

22. Clasr SS, Prudencia RF: Lower urinary tract injuries associated with pelvic fractures. Diagnosis and management. *Surg Clin North Am* **52**:183, 1972.

23. Perry MO, Husmann DA: Urethral injuries in female subjects following pelvic fractures. *J Urology* **147**(1): 139–143, 1992.

24. Hanson PB, Milne JC, Chapman MW: Open fractures of the pelvis. *J Bone Joint Surg* (Br) **73-B**:325–329, 1991.

25. Trunkey DD, et al: Management of pelvic fractures in blunt trauma injury. *J Trauma* **14**:912, 1974.

26. Dunn AW, Morris HD: Fractures and dislocations of the pelvis. *J Bone Joint Surg* **50**:1639, 1968.

27. Furey WW: Fractures of the pelvis with special reference to associated fractures of the sacrum. *AJR* **47**:89, 1942.

28. Holm CI: Treatment of pelvic fractures and dislocations. Skeletal traction and the dual pelvic fraction sling. *Clin Orthop* **97**:97, 1973.

29. Selakovich W, Love L: Stress fracture of the pubic ramus. *J Bone Joint Surg* **36**:573, 1954.

30. Howard FM, Meany RP: Stress fracture of the pelvis during pregnancy. *J Bone Joint Surg* **43**:538, 1954.

31. Noakes TD, Smith JA, Lindenberg G, Wills CE: Pelvic stress fractures in long distance runners. *Am J Sports Med* **13**:120, 1985.

32. Northrop CH, Eto RT, Loop JW: Vertical fracture of the sacral ala. Significance of noncontinuity of the anterior superior sacral foraminal lines. *AJR* **124**:102, 1975.

33. Waheley CPG: Fractures of the pelvis: An analysis of 100 cases. *Br J Surg* **17**:22, 1930.

34. Trafton PG: Pelvic ring injuries. *Surg Clin North Am* **70**(3):655–669, 1990.

35. Ben-Menachem Y, Coldwell DM, Young JW, Burgess AR: Hemorrhage associated with pelvic fractures: Causes, diagnosis and treatment. *AJR* **157**(5): 1005–1014, 1991.

36. Klein SR, Saroyan RM, Baumgartner F, Bongard FS: Management strategy of vascular injuries associated with pelvic fractures. *J Cardiovasc Surg* **33**(3):349–357, 1992.

37. Holm CI: Pelvic fractures with hemorrhage. *N Engl J Med* **284**:668, 1971.

38. Butler-Manuel PA, James SE, Shepperd JAN: Pelvic underpinning: Eight years' experience. *J Bone Joint Surg* (Br) **74-B**(1):74–77, 1992.

BIBLIOGRAPHY

Ellis R, Green AG: Ischial apophysealysis. *Radiology* **87**:646, 1966.

Hansa WR: Epiphyseal injuries about the hip joint. *Clin Orthop* **10**:19, 1957.

19
CHAPTER

FRACTURES OF THE HIP AND PROXIMAL FEMUR

HIP AND PROXIMAL FEMORAL FRACTURES

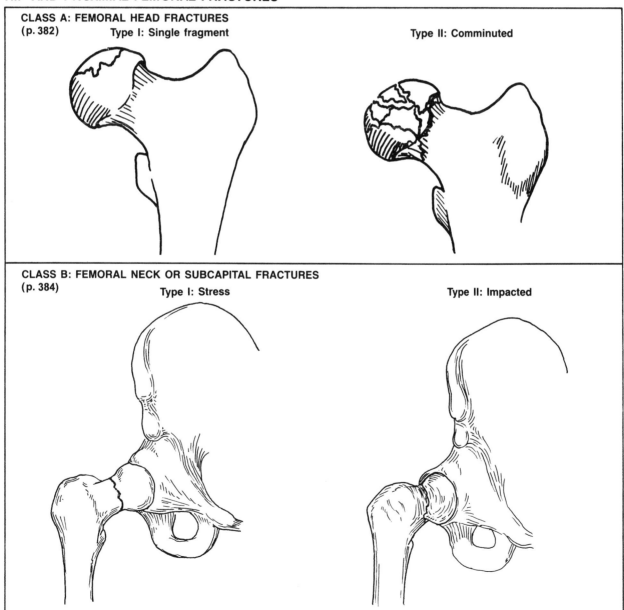

CLASS A: FEMORAL HEAD FRACTURES
(p. 382)

Type I: Single fragment

Type II: Comminuted

CLASS B: FEMORAL NECK OR SUBCAPITAL FRACTURES
(p. 384)

Type I: Stress

Type II: Impacted

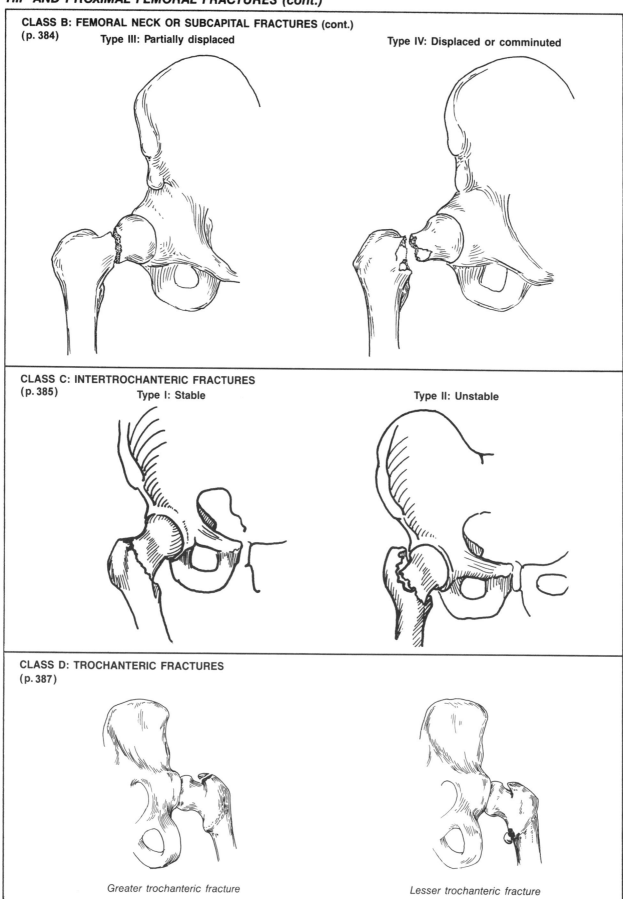

CLASS B: FEMORAL NECK OR SUBCAPITAL FRACTURES (cont.)
(p. 384)

Type III: Partially displaced

Type IV: Displaced or comminuted

CLASS C: INTERTROCHANTERIC FRACTURES
(p. 385)

Type I: Stable

Type II: Unstable

CLASS D: TROCHANTERIC FRACTURES
(p. 387)

Greater trochanteric fracture

Lesser trochanteric fracture

HIP AND PROXIMAL FEMORAL FRACTURES *(cont.)*

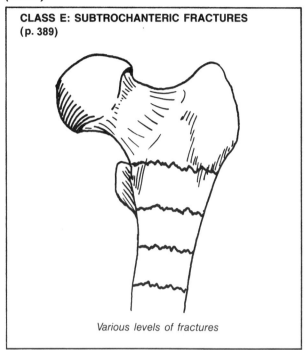

CLASS E: SUBTROCHANTERIC FRACTURES
(p. 389)

Various levels of fractures

Discussed in this section are fractures of the femoral head, neck, trochanters, and shaft up to 5 cm distal to the lesser trochanter. The discussion will focus on the more commonly diagnosed fractures and their management.

Essential Anatomy
The essential bony and vascular anatomy of the proximal femur and hip is demonstrated in Figure 19–1. It is essential that one understand clearly the precarious vascular supply to the proximal femur before assessing these injuries. As shown in Figure 19–1, the vascular supply is by way of three main sources.

1. Vascular ring around the base of the femoral neck
2. Ascending endosteal-metaphyseal blood supply
3. Vessels traversing the joint associated with the ligamentum teres

Any injury that disturbs the normal bony or joint capsular anatomy may compromise this tenuous blood supply.

X Ray
Routine projections including anteroposterior (AP) and internal and external rotation views are usually adequate. Comparison views of the hip are often helpful in diagnosing occult fractures. *Shenton's line* (see Fig. 21–7) must be carefully scrutinized in all patients with a suspected hip injury. In addition, the normal *neck–shaft angle of 120 to 130 degrees* should be evaluated in all suspected fractures. This is obtained by measuring the angle of the intersection of lines drawn down the axis of the femoral shaft and the femoral neck.

Classification
Proximal femoral and hip fractures are classified on the basis of anatomy. The five major classes are listed below.

HIP AND PROXIMAL FEMORAL FRACTURES

☐ Class A: Femoral head   (Figs. 19–2, 19–3)
             fractures
☐ Class B: Femoral neck or   (Fig. 19–4)
             subcapital fractures

☐ Class C: Intertrochanteric   (Fig. 19–6)
             fractures
☐ Class D: Trochanteric fractures (Fig. 19–8)
☐ Class E: Subtrochanteric   (Fig. 19–10)
             fractures

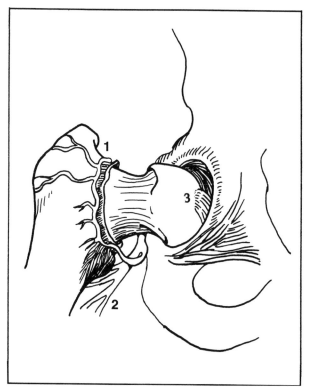

Figure 19-1. The vascular supply of the femoral head is by way of three sources: (1) the endosteal-metaphyseal blood supply; and (2) the vascular ring around the base of the neck, which sends intracapsular vessels; (3) the vessels that traverse through the ligamentum teres.

☐ CLASS A: FEMORAL HEAD FRACTURES (FIGS. 19–2, 19–3)

This is an uncommon fracture that may present with a dislocation or without any significant deformity. The fracture is classified into two types based on the size and number of fragments. Type I fractures present with a single fragment whereas type II injuries are comminuted.

Mechanism of Injury
The mechanism of injury varies depending on the type of fracture.

☐ Class A: Type I (Single Fragment)
These fractures are sheer injuries that usually occur during a dislocation. Anterior dislocations are associated with superior fractures whereas posterior dislocations are associated with inferior fractures.

☐ Class A: Type II (Comminuted)
These fractures are usually the result of direct trauma and may be associated with severe injuries.

Examination
The patient will present with pain on palpation and rotation. There will be a contusion over the lateral aspect of the thigh, although gross bony deformities are uncommon unless there is an associated dislocation.

X Ray
Routine hip views are usually adequate in demonstrating these fractures.

Associated Injuries
Comminuted fractures may be associated with pelvic or ipsilateral upper extremity fractures. Posterior fracture dislocations are associated with sciatic nerve injuries, pelvic fractures, and ipsilateral lower extremity injuries. Anterior fracture dislocations may be associated with arterial injury or venous thrombosis.

Treatment
☐ Class A: Type I (Single Fragment)
The emergency management of these fractures includes immobilization, analgesics, and admission. If associated with a dislocation, reduction followed by immobilization is indicated. Small fragments or superior dome fragments may require operative removal or arthroplasty.

☐ Class A: Type II (Comminuted)
The emergency management of these injuries includes immobilization, analgesics, stabilization of associated

HIP AND PROXIMAL FEMORAL FRACTURES

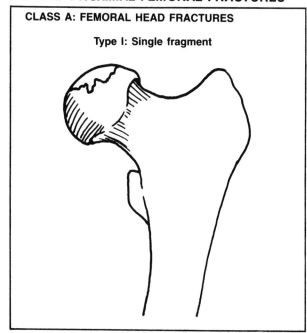

CLASS A: FEMORAL HEAD FRACTURES

Type I: Single fragment

Figure 19–2. The fracture fragment can be large or small.

HIP AND PROXIMAL FEMORAL FRACTURES

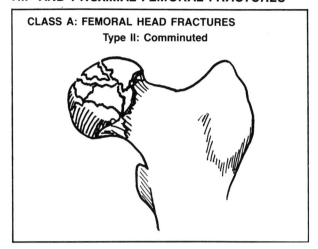

CLASS A: FEMORAL HEAD FRACTURES
Type II: Comminuted

Figure 19–3.

injuries, and admission for arthroplasty as most will undergo aseptic necrosis if treated conservatively.[8]

☐ CLASS B: FEMORAL NECK OR SUBCAPITAL FRACTURES (FIG. 19–4)

These fractures typically occur in the elderly osteoporotic patient with a female to male ratio of 4:1.[1] Femoral neck fractures are rarely seen in young patients. If this injury is diagnosed in a young patient, a pathologic fracture should be suspected. Femoral neck fractures are very serious injuries that may result in long-term disability secondary to the development of femoral head avascular necrosis.

The vascular supply to the femoral head is by way of the ligamentum teres and the epiphyseal ring surrounding the femoral neck (see Fig. 19–1).

In addition, femoral neck fractures are intracapsular and periosteal bone healing is impaired because of the lack of surrounding soft tissues and their potential vascular supply.

Many systems have been used in the classification of femoral neck fractures based on anatomy and therapeutic results. The Protzman et al[11] classification is dependent on the femoral head-to-shaft angle after injury. Under this system 30 degrees or less of angulation is associated with good results whereas 30 to 60 degrees of angulation correlates with a less favorable prognosis. Fractures with over 60 degrees of angulation have a very high incidence of aseptic necrosis. Garden divides femoral neck fractures into incomplete or impacted fractures (stage I), nondisplaced complete fractures (stage II), partially displaced complete fractures (stage III), and displaced complete fractures (stage IV).[1,7] Rockwood and Green classify femoral

neck fractures into four categories: stress, impacted, displaced, and comminuted.[13] The classification system used in this text is a combination of Garden's and that of Rockwood and Green and is shown in Figure 19–4.

- **Class B, type I:** Stress femoral neck fracture
- **Class B, type II:** Impacted femoral neck fracture
- **Class B, type III:** Partially displaced femoral neck fractures
- **Class B, type IV:** Displaced or comminuted femoral neck fractures

Mechanism of Injury

There are two mechanisms that result in femoral neck fractures. Direct minor trauma in the elderly may result in a class B fracture. However, indirect trauma is the more common mechanism in the elderly with osteoporotic bone. Femoral neck stress in combination with a torsion injury may result in a class A, type I, II, or III fracture. The patient then falls, adding displacement or comminution to the injury. Stress fractures are usually initiated along the superior border of the femoral neck.

Examination

Patients with type I and II injuries may present with a complaint of minor groin pain or medial thigh or knee pain that is exacerbated with active or passive motion. There may be no history of trauma and the patient may be ambulatory. There is usually no leg shortening or external rotation, thus making the diagnosis difficult on the basis of examination.

Type III and IV fractures usually present with severe pain along with leg shortening and external rotation.

X Ray

Type I injuries may be very difficult to visualize radiographically during the acute stage. A distortion of the normal trabecular pattern or a cortical defect may be the only clues to an underlying fracture. Clinically, patients with, suspected fractures but normal plain films may benefit from computed tomography (CT), nuclear bone or magnetic resonance imaging (MRI) scans.[10] Displaced fractures are usually well visualized on the AP and lateral views.

Associated Injuries

These fractures are usually not associated with other significant injuries.

Treatment

Horizontal fractures are associated with a more favorable prognosis because reduction is usually better and more easily achieved.

HIP AND PROXIMAL FEMORAL FRACTURES

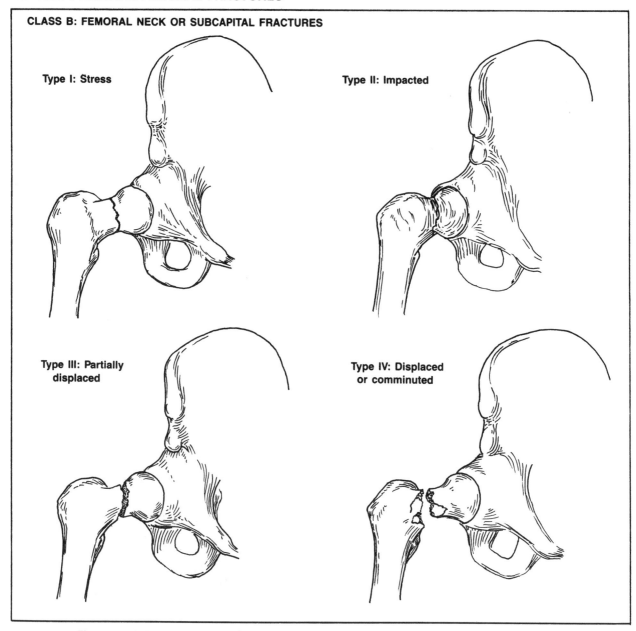

CLASS B: FEMORAL NECK OR SUBCAPITAL FRACTURES

Type I: Stress

Type II: Impacted

Type III: Partially displaced

Type IV: Displaced or comminuted

Figure 19–4. Four types of femoral neck fractures are described. Comminuted fragments are not shown.

☐ Class B: Type I   (Stress)
Elderly patients require internal fixation to protect against increased stress with completion of the fracture. Younger patients can be treated with crutches and nonweight bearing for 6 to 12 weeks, followed by partial weight bearing progressing to full ambulation. Early orthopedic referral for all patients is strongly recommended.

☐ Class B: Type II   (Impacted)
The emergency management of these fractures includes immobilization, analgesics, and emergent orthopedic consultation. The recommended therapy varies from bed rest with protection against external rotation (86 to 90 percent union) to internal fixation (nearly 100 percent union).[13] Conservative treatment in patients over 70 years of age has a 21 percent incidence of instability. In younger patients the incidence of instability with conservative nonsurgical treatment is 5.5 percent.[12]

Emergent orthopedic referral is recommended for all these fractures.

☐ Class B: Type III   (Partially Displaced)
The emergency management of these fractures includes immobilization, analgesics, and admission for reduction

and internal fixation. These fractures should be reduced emergently as within 12 hours 24 percent suffer avascular necrosis and by 48 hours after injury 40 percent will undergo avascular necrosis.[13] Avascular necrosis will occur in 100 percent of those fractures unrepaired at 1 week postinjury.[13]

☐ Class B: Type IV   (Displaced or Comminuted)

The emergency management of these fractures includes immobilization, analgesics, and admission for reduction with internal fixation or prosthetic insertion. Due to the patient's age there is a 10 percent mortality rate for those patients treated with internal fixation and a 60 percent rate for those treated with bed rest.[1] Twenty-one percent of the women and 37 percent of the men over 84 years of age died within 1 month of injury in one study.[1]

Complications

Femoral neck fractures are associated with several significant complications.

1. Avascular necrosis of the femoral head is the most common, occurring in up to 35 percent of patients 3 years after injury.[4]
2. The development of osteoarthritis commonly follows these fractures.
3. Osteomyelitis and nail protrusion are complications of the operative procedure.
4. The overall incidence of nonunion is under 5 percent.[2,8]

☐ CLASS C: INTERTROCHANTERIC FRACTURES (FIG. 19–5)

These fractures are extracapsular and involve the cancellous bone between the greater and lesser trochanters. These fractures are usually seen in elderly patients averaging 66 to 76 years of age with a female to male ratio of 4:1 to 6:1.[13] The vascular supply to this region is very good owing to the large amount of surrounding musculature and the presence of cancellous bone. The internal rotators of the hip remain attached to the proximal fragment whereas the short external rotators remain attached to the distal head and neck.

The Boyd and Griffin classification system[3] is used by most orthopedists; however, the emergency medical specialist need only classify these injuries as stable (type I) or unstable (type II).

- **Class C, type I:** Stable intertrochanteric fractures. A single fracture line transects the cortex between the two trochanters, and there is no displacement between the femoral shaft and neck.

- **Class C, type II:** Unstable intertrochanteric fracture. There are multiple fracture lines or comminution with associated displacement between the femoral shaft and neck.

Mechanism of Injury

The majority of these fractures are secondary to direct trauma such as a fall on the trochanter or transmission of forces along the axis of the femur. With increasing forces, greater or lesser trochanter fractures may be combined with this injury. The muscles inserting on the trochanters act to further displace the fragments.

HIP AND PROXIMAL FEMORAL FRACTURES

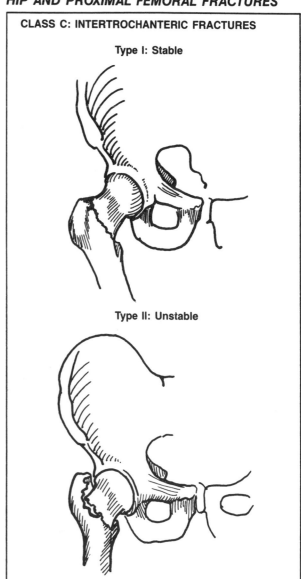

CLASS C: INTERTROCHANTERIC FRACTURES

Type I: Stable

Type II: Unstable

Figure 19–5.

Examination

The patient will present with tenderness, swelling, and ecchymosis over the hip. There is usually leg shortening with external rotation secondary to traction by the iliopsoas.

X Ray (Fig. 19–6)

AP and lateral views are usually adequate in demonstrating the fracture.

Treatment

The emergency management of this fracture includes immobilization and analgesics. Typically, these patients are treated surgically with internal fixation and early mobilization.[9]

Patients who are a very poor surgical risk have been successfully treated with external fixation.[5]

Complications

Intertrochanteric fractures are associated with several significant complications.

1. The mortality rate for these fractures is 10 to 15 percent, which is primarily related to the predominance of elderly patients in the population at risk.[13]
2. Osteomyelitis at a rate of 5 to 8 percent and protrusion of the nail are postoperative complications.[13]
3. Thromboembolism is seen frequently in these patients if prolonged bed rest is not avoided.
4. Avascular necrosis and nonunion are rarely seen after these injuries.

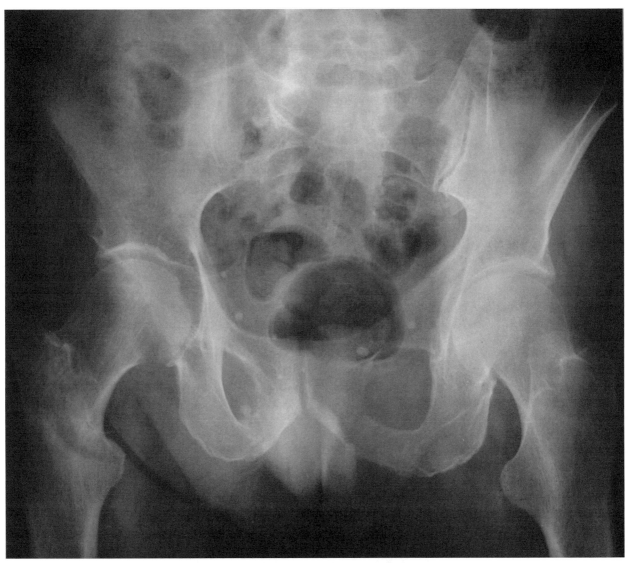

Figure 19–6. Intertrochanteric fracture of the femur.

HIP AND PROXIMAL FEMORAL FRACTURES

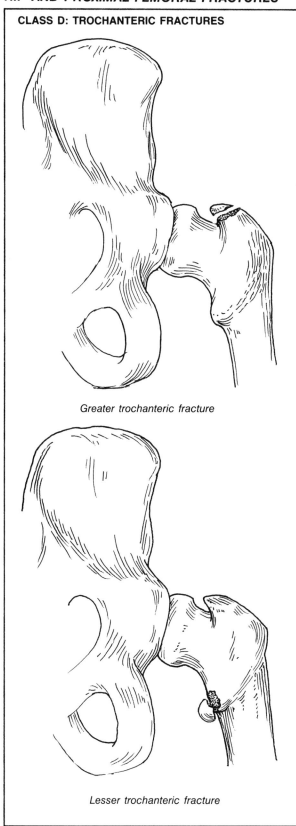

CLASS D: TROCHANTERIC FRACTURES

Greater trochanteric fracture

Lesser trochanteric fracture

Figure 19–7.

☐ CLASS D: TROCHANTERIC FRACTURES (FIG. 19–7)

Trochanteric fractures are uncommon injuries usually seen in young patients. Greater trochanteric fractures may be classified as type I nondisplaced or type II displaced (over 1 cm). Lesser trochanteric fractures may also be classified as type I nondisplaced or type II displaced (over 2 cm).

Mechanism of Injury
Greater trochanteric fractures are usually secondary to direct trauma as, for example, a fall, although a minority may be the result of an avulsion injury. Lesser trochanteric fractures are secondary to an avulsion mechanism.

Examination
Greater trochanteric fractures usually present with tenderness and pain exacerbated with active abduction of the thigh. Lesser trochanteric fractures typically present with tenderness and pain that increase with flexion and rotation of the hip.

X Ray (Fig. 19–8)
AP and lateral views are generally adequate in demonstrating this fracture. Internal and external rotation views may be necessary to accurately determine displacement. There may be significant blood loss at the fracture site.

Associated Injuries
No significant injuries are commonly associated with these fractures.

Treatment
☐ Class D: Type I (Nondisplaced)
This fracture is managed symptomatically with bed rest followed by crutch walking for 3 to 4 weeks. Limited weight bearing should be continued until the patient is pain free. Orthopedic referral for follow-up is recommended.

☐ Class D: Type II (Displaced)
Young patients with greater trochanteric fractures with 1 cm of displacement or lesser trochanteric fractures with 2 cm of displacement require internal fixation. Elderly patients with displaced fractures may be managed symptomatically as described under class D, type I injuries.

Complications
The loss of associated muscle function secondary to atrophy is a long-term complication of these fractures.

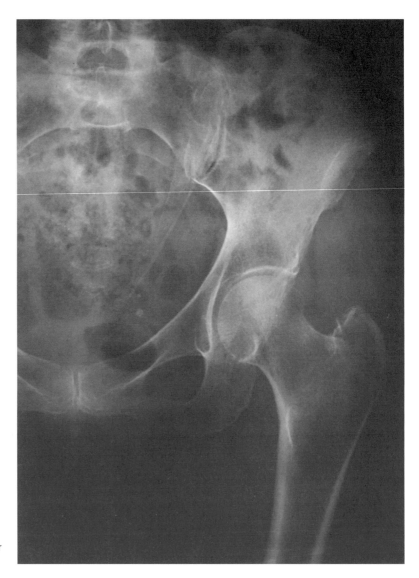

Figure 19–8. Greater trochanter fracture with out displacement.

☐ CLASS E: SUBTROCHANTERIC FRACTURES (FIGS. 19–9, 19–10)

Subtrochanteric fractures include those injuries within 5 cm of the lesser trochanter. These fractures usually occur in younger patients and are often the result of severe injury forces. The fractures may be spiral, comminuted, displaced, or occur as an extension of an itertrochanteric fracture.

The classification system used by most orthopedists is that of Fielding.[6]

- **Class E, type I :** Fracture at the level of the lesser trochanter
- **Class E, type II :** Fracture 1 inch below the lesser trochanter
- **Class E, type III :** Fracture within 1 to 2 inches of the lesser trochanter

The emergency management of all three fracture types is similar.

Mechanism of Injury
The most common mechanism is a fall with a combination of direct and rotational forces.

Examination
The patient will present with pain and swelling in the hip and upper thigh. In addition, ipsilateral knee injuries or lower extremity fractures may be seen due to the large forces necessary to cause these fractures.

HIP AND PROXIMAL FEMORAL FRACTURES

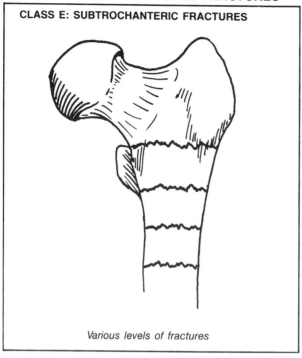

CLASS E: SUBTROCHANTERIC FRACTURES

Various levels of fractures

Figure 19–9.

Treatment

The emergency management of these fractures includes immobilization in a Sager splint (see Fig. 1–7C), ice, analgesics, intravenous fluids to correct volume loss, and admission for open reduction and internal fixation. Severely comminuted fractures are best treated with traction.

Complications

Several significant complications are associated with these fractures.

1. These patients are at risk of developing venous thrombosis with embolism.
2. Osteomyelitis and mechanical failure of the nail or screw are postsurgical complications.
3. Malunion or nonunion may complicate the management of these fractures.

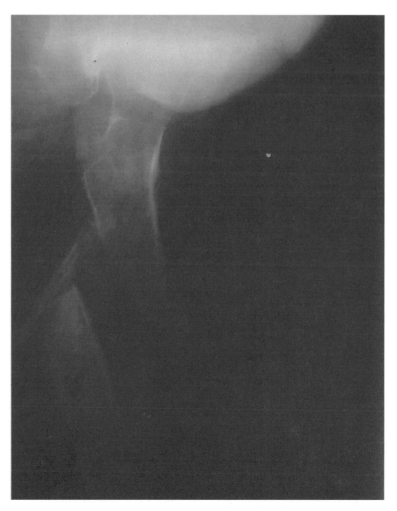

Figure 19–10. Subtrochanteric fracture of the proximal femur.

REFERENCES

1. Barnes R, et al: Subcapital fractures of the femur. *J Bone Joint Surg* [Br] **58**(1):2, 1976.
2. Barr JS: Experience with sliding nail in femoral neck fractures. *Clin Orthop* **92**:63, 1973.
3. Boyd HB, Griffin LL: Classification of intertrochanteric fractures of the femur. *Arch Surg* **58**:853, 1949.
4. Claffey TJ: Avascular necrosis of the femoral head. *J Bone Joint Surg* [Br] **42**:802, 1960.
5. Dhal A, Varghese M, Bhasin VB: External fixation of intertrochanteric fractures of the femur. *J Bone Joint Surg* **11**:955–958, 1991.
6. Fielding JW: Subtrochanteric fractures. *Clin Orthop* **92**:86, 1973.
7. Garden RS: Low angle fixation in fractures of the femoral neck. *J Bone Joint Surg* [Br] **43**:647, 1961.
8. Hunter GAP: Posterior dislocation and fracture-dislocation of the hip. *J Bone Joint Surg* [Br] **51**:38, 1969.
9. Larsson S, Friberg S, Hansson I-I: Trochanteric fractures. *Clin Orthop* [From the department of Orthopedics University Hospital, Umea, Sweden] **11**:232–241, 1990.
10. Norris MA, Desmet AA: Fractures and dislocations of the hip and femur. *Sem Roentgenol* **XXIX**(2):100–112, 1994.
11. Protzman RR, et al: Femoral neck fractures in young adults. *J Bone Joint Surg* **58**(5):689, 1976.
12. Raaymakers ELFB, Marti R: Non-operative treatment of impacted femoral neck fractures. *J Bone Joint Surg* [Br] **11**:950–954, 1990.
13. Rockwood CA, Green DA: *Fractures*. Philadelphia: Lippincott, 1975.

BIBLIOGRAPHY

Bands HH: Factors influencing the results in fractures of the femoral neck. *J Bone Joint Surg* **44**:931, 1962.

Brav EA: Traumatic dislocation of the hip joint. *J Bone Joint Surg* **44**:1115, 1962.

Farrington KD, et al: The management of comminuted unstable intertrochanteric fractures. *J Bone Joint Surg* **55**(7):1367, 1973.

Kelly PJ, et al: Primary Vitallium mold arthroplasty for posterior dislocations of the hip with fracture of the femoral head. *J Bone Joint Surg* **40**:675, 1958.

Mussbrichler H: Arterial supply of the head of the femur. *Acta Radiol Scand* **46**:533, 1956.

20
CHAPTER

FRACTURES OF THE FEMORAL SHAFT

The femoral shaft extends from an area 5 cm distal to the lesser trochanter to a point 6 cm proximal to the adductor tubercle.[4] The femoral shaft is a strong bone with an excellent blood supply and therefore good healing potential. These fractures are more common in children and adolescents. The extensive musculature surrounding the femoral shaft is often the source of displacement. Lateral muscles inserting on the greater trochanter may result in an abduction deformity whereas those inserting on the lesser trochanter (iliopsoas) exert external rotation flexion deformities when associated with proximal femoral shaft fractures. Midshaft fractures undergo a varus deformity because of the pull of the medial adductors, which is resisted by the lateral thigh muscles and fascia lata.

Previously, femoral shaft fractures had a mortality rate as high as 50 percent, primarily because the treatment was prolonged bed rest. Current therapy uses plates or intramedullary rods, thus allowing earlier mobilization. Associated sciatic nerve injuries are rarely encountered with these fractures secondary to the protective surrounding musculature.

Femoral shaft fractures are classified into three types as shown in Figures 20–1 and 20–2.

- **Type I** : Spiral or transverse shaft fractures with or without displacement or angulation
- **Type II** : Comminuted femoral shaft fractures
- **Type III** : Open femoral shaft fractures

Mechanism of Injury

Femoral shaft fractures are usually secondary to severe injuring forces such as a direct blow or an indirect force transmitted through the flexed knee.

FEMORAL SHAFT FRACTURE

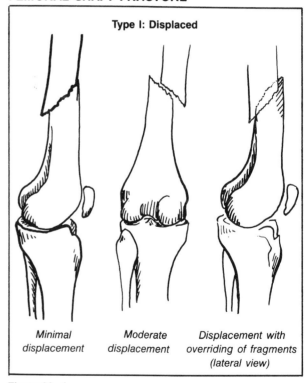

Type I: Displaced

| Minimal displacement | Moderate displacement | Displacement with overriding of fragments (lateral view) |

Figure 20–1.

Examination

The patient will present with severe pain in the involved extremity and usually visible deformities. The extremity may be shortened and there may be crepitation with movement. The thigh may be swollen and tense secondary to hemorrhage and formation of a

FEMORAL SHAFT FRACTURE

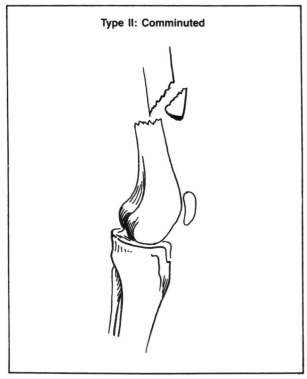

Type II: Comminuted

Figure 20–2.

hematoma. Arterial injuries are rare, but they must be excluded on the initial examination. Arterial injuries associated with a femoral shaft fracture should be suspected when:

1. There is an expanding hematoma
2. There are absent or diminishing pulses
3. There are progressive neurologic signs in the presence of a closed fracture.[5]

X Ray

Routine anteroposterior (AP) and lateral views are usually adequate in demonstrating the fracture. Stress fractures of the femoral shaft may not be visualized on these routine views. Hip and knee views should be included as there is a significant incidence of associated injury.[7]

Associated Injuries

Femoral shaft fractures are usually the result of severe injuring forces. These fractures may be associated with ipsilateral fractures, dislocations, and ligamentous soft tissue injuries to the hip and knee.[6] Muscular contusions and lacerations may accompany these injuries resulting in hematomas acutely and later, myositis ossificans. Because of the severe injuring forces involved, many of these patients have multiple injuries and require a careful systematic initial examination. Femoral shaft fractures have significant bleeding with an average blood loss of 1000 mL.

Treatment

The emergency management of this injury should begin at the time the fracture is first suspected. The extremity should be immobilized in a skin traction splint, Thomas splint, Hare traction splint, or Sager splint as shown in Figure 20–3. These devices provide for sufficient immobilization and also supply a distraction force for initial reduction. Emergent referral and admission are indicated; one must remember to treat the patient for the associated blood loss.

The definitive treatment for type I fractures is closed intramedullary nailing. Immediate nailing of a fracture of the femoral shaft allows for early patient mobilization and reduces the incidence of complications including fat embolisms and acute respiratory distress syndrome (ARDS).[2] The treatment of comminuted fractures can in most instances be successfully accomplished with an intramedullary nailing.[10,11]

Open fractures require emergent operative debridement with delayed intramedullary nailing.

The treatment of femoral shaft fractures in prepubertal patients is more complex. Most children less than 6 years of age can be treated with an immediate hip spica cast or traction followed by a spica cast. Children between 6 and 10 years of age can be treated by an immediate hip spica cast or traction followed by a spica cast or flexible rods or external fixation. Children over 10 can be treated with a locked intramedullary rod, or flexible rods or external fixation.[8] Successful treatment has been reported with the Hoffman external fixator.[9] Patients approaching skeletal maturity or those with injuries precluding prolonged traction may require operative intervention (intramedullary nailing, compression screw plate fixation).[1]

Complications

Femoral shaft fractures are associated with several significant complications.

1. Nonunion or infection is seen in less than 1 percent of these patients. Malunion or delayed union is more common.[2,3]
2. Malrotation of the extremity may lead to a permanent deformity.
3. Knee stiffness secondary to prolonged immobilization is a common problem that is avoided to some extent with the use of an intramedullary nail and early mobilization.
4. Breakage of nails and plates and infection are postsurgical complications.
5. Arterial injury with delayed thrombosis or aneurysm formation is an uncommon complication.
6. Peroneal nerve contusion with loss of function may be the result of compression secondary to traction.

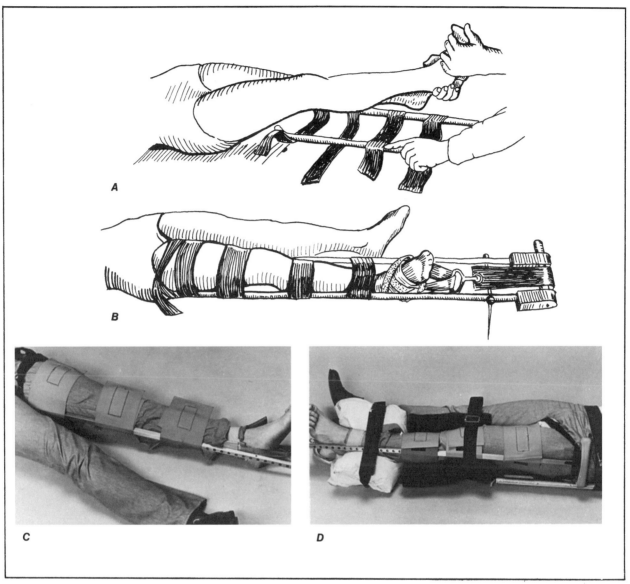

Figure 20–3. **A.** Hare traction applied as shown by applying traction to the lower limb and elevating it with the knee held in extension. **B.** The splint is then inserted under the limb and the foot secured in the traction apparatus. **C.** The Sager traction splint. the gauged meter distally tells the amount of weight being applied to the ankle straps for distraction. **D.** The splint can be applied to the outer side of the leg in patients with groin injuries or pelvic fractures who also have a femoral fracture.

7. Refracture at the initial injury site may occur.
8. The development of a thigh compartment syndrome is a significant although rare complication.[2]
9. Elderly patients over age 60 with closed shaft fractures have a mortality rate of 16 to 20 percent and a complication rate of between 46 and 54 percent.[7]

REFERENCES

1. Bohn WW, Durbin RA: Ipsilateral fractures of the femur and tibia in children and adolescents. *J Bone Joint Surg* **3**:429–439, 1991.
2. Bucholz RW, Jones A: Current concepts review fractures of the shaft of the femur. *J Bone Joint Surg* **73**(10): 1561–1565, 1991.
3. Carr CR, Wingo CH: Fractures of the femoral diaphysis. *J Bone Joint Surg* **55**:690, 1973.
4. Dencker H: Shaft fractures of the femur. *Acta Chir Scand* **130**:173, 1965.
5. Isaacson J, et al: Arterial injury associated with closed femoral shaft fractures. *J Bone Joint Surg* **54**(8):1147, 1975.
6. Karlstorm G, et al: Ipsilateral fracture of the femur and tibia. *J Bone Joint Surg* **59**(2):240, 1977.
7. Mitchell MJ, Ho C, Resnick A, Sartoris D: Diagnostic imaging of the lower extremity trauma. *Radiol Clin North Am* **27**(5):909–928, 1989.

8. Moran CG, Gibson MJ, Cross AT: Intramedullary locking nails for femoral shaft fractures in elderly patients. *J Bone Joint Surg* [Br] **1:**19–22, 1990.

9. Shih H-N, Chen L-M, Lee Z-L, Shih C-H: Treatment of the femoral shaft fractures with the Hoffmann external fixator in pre puberty. *J Trauma* **4:**498–501, 1989.

10. Sojbjerg JO, Eiskjaer S, Moller-Larsen F: Locked nailing of comminuted and unstable fractures of the femur. *J Bone Joint Surg* [Br] **1:**23–25, 1990.

11. Wiss DA, Brien WW, Stetson WB: Interlocked nailing for treatment of segmental fractures of the femur. *J Bone Joint Surg* **6:**724–728, 1990.

21
CHAPTER

SOFT TISSUE INJURIES, DISLOCATIONS, AND DISORDERS OF THE HIP, PELVIS, AND THIGH

The discussion of nontraumatic disorders of the hip includes those that are not entirely in the realm of emergency medicine. The emergency physician must be able to make a diagnosis because he or she often is the only clinician who will see the patient early enough at an opportune time for treatment.

Functional Anatomy of the Hip

The hip joint is a ball and socket joint composed of the head of the femur and the acetabulum. The pelvis that contains this articulation has many palpable bony landmarks. The anterosuperior iliac spine and the greater trochanter are easily palpated laterally, and the pubic symphysis and the tubercle (lying 1 inch lateral to the symphysis) are palpated medially. The hip joint is capable of a very wide range of motion. The joint is enclosed in a capsule that has attachments to the rim of the acetabulum and the femoral neck. Three ligaments are formed by capsular thickenings: the *iliofemoral ligament*, which is located anteriorly and is the thickest and the strongest of the three; the *pubofemoral ligament*, which is located inferiorly; and the *ischiofemoral*, which

is located posteriorly and is the widest of the three ligaments. The iliofemoral ligament is a wide ligament divided into two bands, a lower band that passes obliquely downward and an upper band. This ligament tightens when the hip is extended. Additional support is provided by the *labrum acetabulare*, which is a thick band of cartilage surrounding and extending out from the socket adding depth to the cavity. A flat thin-shaped ligament, the ligament teres, attaches the head of the femur to the acetabulum centrally. There are three sources of blood supply to the femoral head. These are the retinacular arteries, the artery of the ligamentum teres, and the superior branch of the nutrient artery to the femoral shaft. The muscles surrounding the hip joint are massive and powerful and contribute to the force acting on the head of the femur significantly. For the supine patient to merely lift the legs straight places a force acting across the hip joint of one to one-and-one-half times the body weight. Running creates a force of up to five times the patient's weight acting across this joint. A patient with a painful hip will tilt the trunk toward the affected side, displacing the center of gravity laterally toward the femoral head, shortening the lever on the femur, and lessening the force acting across the joint required by the abductor muscles. When walking, such a patient will sway toward the affected side to decrease the pressure on the joint. An alternate method is to carry a cane in the opposite hand. This decreases the force needed by the hip abductors acting across the painful joint.

We will discuss the nontraumatic disorders of the hip in two general categories: Those disorders that affect the hip and are intra-articular (which appear primarily in childhood), and those disorders that are extra-articular. In the intra-articular category are avascular necrosis of the femoral head, Legg-Calvé-Perthes disease, congenital dislocation of the hip, slipped femoral epiphysis, transient synovitis, and suppurative arthritis. In addition, degenerative joint disease is briefly mentioned. In the extra-articular category, bursitis, calcific tendonitis, and snapping hip syndrome are discussed.

Intra-Articular Disorders

☐ AVASCULAR NECROSIS OF THE FEMORAL HEAD

Necrosis of the femoral head is a result of impaired blood supply, a common complication of many affections of the hip from infancy to adult life. This condition occurs most often in males between 40 and 50 years of age and is bilateral in 40 to 80 percent of patients.[59] The chief blood supply to the head comes from branches of the medial and lateral circumflex arteries that enter the capsule distally and pass along the posterior surface of the head. The infarction of the femoral head may be total or incomplete. If incomplete, it is limited to one segment of the femoral head, and the x ray appearance will be spotty.[39]

Pathogenesis
Any condition that disrupts the blood supply to the femoral head can cause this disorder. Trauma to the major blood vessels is perhaps the major cause. Avascular necrosis ensues most commonly after fractures of the neck of the femur, which tear the retinacular vessels causing necrosis in up to 20 to 30 percent of all femoral neck fractures. This condition is more likely to develop with fractures that occur more proximally, such as subcapital fractures and those fractures that are inadequately reduced, thus permitting greater shearing stresses to occur at the fracture site. Tears of the posterior capsule as occur during dislocations of the hip account for a significant number of these cases.

Avascular necrosis is known to be associated with several diseases and disorders. Avascular necrosis can complicate sickle cell disease due to the impaired circulation of the small vessels that supply the femoral head. Metabolic disorders and collagen vascular disorders, such as gout and systemic lupus erythematosus, may also cause avascular necrosis of the femoral head. This condition may occur after prolonged steroid therapy. Other secondary causes for avascular necrosis include alcohol abuse, Caisson disease, Gaucher's disease, and renal osteodystrophy.[59] In some cases, there is no history of trauma or any of the above causes and idiopathic avascular necrosis of the femoral head is then diagnosed.

The articular cartilage covering the necrotic head survives usually because it derives its nutrition from the synovial fluid. If subchondylar bone cortex collapses, the cartilage then undergoes degeneration. The added stress of weight bearing, before bony replacement is complete, can cause collapse and severe degenerative changes (Fig. 21–1).

X Ray
The hip x ray is usually normal in the early stages as the bony architecture is typically normal. When a fracture disrupts the blood supply to the head, the bone distal to the fracture site becomes hyperemic and osteoporotic. Thus, the living bone stands out in contrast to the dead bone. These x ray changes may not be visible for a period of 2 months, by which time union of the fracture may have occurred. The roentgenographic changes classify avascular necrosis of the femoral head into four stages.

Stage	Roentgenogram
1	Normal
2	Density change in femoral head
3	Loss of sphericity, collapse
4	Joint space narrowing, acetabular changes[59]

If this condition is present, the x ray will show an increased density of the head with blotchy shadows of reduced density that will appear just proximal to the fracture site even after union. If the head is protected from weight bearing during the period of reconstitution,

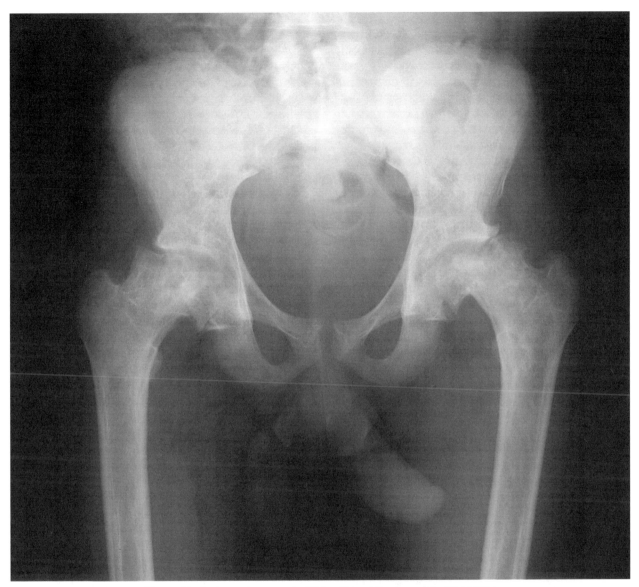

Figure 21–1. Avascular necrosis, bilateral hips. (*Courtesy of Dr. Fitzpatrick.*)

which will take place over several months, then the head will be restored to its normal architecture with no residual deformity. Pressure from weight bearing may cause the necrotic head to collapse, and may be the first thing noted by the physician.

Clinical Presentation

Often there is no history of trauma and the patient complains of slight to moderate pain about the hip, and the examiner notes a limp. Joint motion is decreased, especially *rotation* and *abduction*. The clinical picture will vary, however, depending on the underlying cause and the patient's age. The onset of the symptoms does not correlate well with the appearance on x ray. In a child, spasm about the hip appears to be an early sign. It is not the death of bone cells that causes hip pain, but rather the collapse and fracture of the subchondral bone that heralds the onset of clinical symptoms.[52] In the adult, pain in the groin is usually the first symptom causing complaint. This is often referred to the thigh or to the knee, may be sudden in onset and worse on standing or walking, with relief at rest. Later, the patient experiences atrophy and restriction of *abduction* and *internal rotation*. In the child, a limp or a slight spasm of the hip is often the first clinical manifestation of this disorder. It is followed by pain that is present on weight bearing and often referred to the thigh or to the knee. A high index of suspicion is needed in the absence of x ray findings, as previously noted. This is particularly true in the child who has no history of previous trauma. Nevertheless, it is very important to diagnose this condition early in order to prevent progression to painful osteoarthritis.[42]

Treatment

The treatment for this condition depends on which stage the avascular necrosis has reached. In stage 1 and early stage 2, core decompression is the recommended procedure. This involves removing an 8- to 10-mm core of bone from the anterolateral segment of the femoral head through a lateral trochanteric approach. This procedure is highly effective in relieving pain and prevents further changes in the femoral head. In the later stages of 2 and in stage 3, a trochanteric osteotomy is necessary. Avascular necrosis in stage 4 requires a total hip arthroplasty. It should be noted that core decompression could be used in later stages even after the head shows early collapse in order to relieve the patient of pain.[42]

☐ LEGG-CALVÉ-PERTHES DISEASE (COXA PLANA) (FIG. 21-2)

Legg-Calvé-Perthes disease is an idiopathic form of avascular necrosis of the femoral head occurring in children. This disorder is usually self-limited whereby the femoral head undergoes aseptic necrosis and replacement resulting in some flattening of the femoral head (coxa plana). A variable amount of permanent deformity and restricted motion usually result. This condition, which affects boys 3 to 5 times more often than girls, occurs most often in children between 5 and 7 years of age. It must also be noted that small children with small feet and delayed maturation can be considered to be structurally and biochemically at risk.[29,62] The condition can occur in either hip and is unilateral in 85 percent of cases and bilateral in 15 percent. These children are usually shorter than normal, and the condition seems to be rarer in blacks.

Pathogenesis

The definite cause of the vascular disturbance resulting in Legg-Calvé-Perthes disease is unknown. Repeated episodes of infarction and ensuing abnormalities have been implicated as a cause.[21,33,37] Injury or disease to the blood vessels supplying the head or within the head itself may be responsible but this is not clear. The condition results in necrosis of the head and all or part of the epiphysis that is self-limited. New bone is formed and the necrotic trabecula replaced over a period of 2 to 3 years. The final shape is not normal (coxa plana).

Clinical Presentation

The onset is insidious, and the course is prolonged over a period of several years. An almost constant early sign

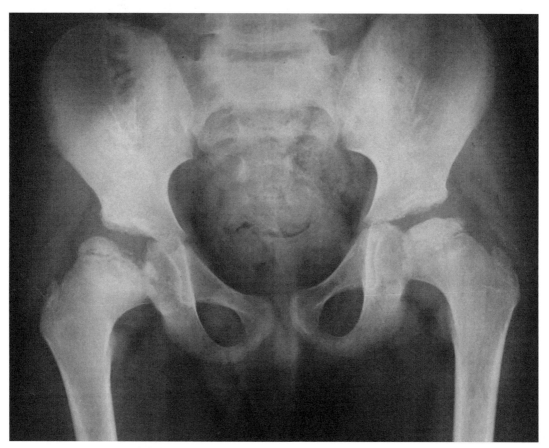

Figure 21-2. Legg-Calvé-Perthes disease is present bilaterally. Osteochondrosis of the femoral head.

is a limp, which is caused by limited abduction of the hip and limited internal rotation in both flexion and extension.[62] The patient complains of a vague ache in the groin that radiates to the medial thigh and inner aspect of the knee. This is aggravated by activity and relieved by rest. The patient may also complain of stiffness in a joint, and tenderness is noted over the anterior aspect of the joint. Muscle spasm is another common complaint in the early stages of the disease. It is not unusual for a patient to present with complaints of muscle spasm and a limp with no pain noted at all. When the disease runs its course, a variable amount of restricted motion with an insignificant limp is the usual result along with slight shortening of the limb. A Trendelenburg-type gait usually develops and can persist for several years even with resolution of the avascular necrosis.[62] The patient is often disabled only for activities that require prolonged standing or running and in some patients, reconstitution of the hip and a complete clinical cure occurs, whereas in others degenerative arthritis ensues years later.[26]

X Ray

The early signs on x ray are of joint space widening, and prominence of the soft tissues over the capsule with a minimal joint effusion.[25] The femoral head may be laterally shifted slightly in the acetabulum. A few weeks later the femoral head will appear more dense than the rest of the bone with later fragmentation. A fragmentation appearance on x ray is evidence of necrosis; ingrowth of new vessels initiates the process of reabsorption. This results in a decreased density of the proximal end of the metaphysis because of the increased vascularity and the osteosclerosis with broadening and shortening of the femoral neck and an increased density of the head. This stage of fragmentation takes place over a period of 1 to 2 years followed by a regenerative phase where new bone is formed in the epiphysis and the final shape of the head varies in size and shape, depending on the degree of collapse that has occurred earlier. As the patient progresses through adult life, changes of secondary osteoarthritis develop.

Treatment

This appears to be a limited disease with a tendency to spontaneous recovery as one progresses through the previously outlined stages. The prognosis appears to be better when involvement of the femoral head is partial rather than complete.[26] The prognosis is much improved when there is no collapse of the femoral head. Children who are less than 5 years of age at the onset of the disease have a higher risk of having poor results after treatment.[62] An important aspect in the treatment is containment of the femoral head in the acetabulum, which is insured by maintaining the hips in abduction and mild internal rotation for a long time.[7,35] This can be accomplished by a Scottish-Rite brace which maintains the hip in fixed abduction. This brace allows the hip to flex to 90 degrees, but it cannot control the rotation of the hip. Patients with Legg-Calvé-Perthes disease are able to run and ride a bicycle while wearing the brace.[62] Early in the disease when pain, spasm, and limited motion are prime features, treatment with traction for 1 to 2 weeks affords relief from spasm, and the patient often regains full range of motion. In one study, operative therapy proved to be better than conservative therapy in these patients. Surgically treated patients were able to lead a more normal life as soon as osteotomy was performed.[18]

☐ CONGENITAL DISLOCATION OF THE HIP

Congenital dislocation of the hip is an intra-articular displacement of the femoral head from its normal position within the acetabulum that leads to an interruption in the normal development of the joint occurring before or shortly after birth.[60] At birth, the acetabular fossa is shallow with the superior portion of the acetabulum, poorly developed, offering little resistance to the upward movement of the head by muscle pull or weight bearing. This can lead to a condition called *congenital subluxation of the femoral head* in which case the femoral head is displaced laterally and proximally and articulates with the outer portion of the acetabulum. In *complete dislocation* of the hip, the femoral head is located completely outside the acetabulum and rests against the lateral wall of the ilium. Later, a false acetabulum forms with a capsule interposed between the femoral head and the ilium.[60]

X Ray

The emergency physician, when seeing this patient for the first time, will see nothing on x ray. So if the clinical picture suggests this disorder, he or she must refer the patient for evaluation by the orthopedist.

Clinical Presentation

In the normal infant, one will see *folds* in the groin, below the buttocks, and several along the thigh, which are symmetrical. In subluxation or dislocation, these folds will be *asymmetrical*. When the examiner places the infant on the table, the pelvis and the limb on the affected side will be pulled proximally by muscle action. This proximal displacement of the limb causes apparent shortening of the limb.

The *Ortolani click test* should be performed as a routine part of every examination on all infants before 1 year of age seen in the emergency department. In the normal infant, when the hip is flexed 90 degrees and the thigh is abducted, the lateral aspect of both thighs will nearly touch the table. In subluxation or dislocation,

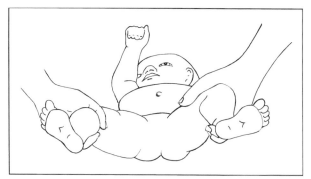

Figure 21–3. The Ortolani click test is shown. See text for discussion.

abduction is restricted and the involved hip is unable to be abducted as far as the opposite one (Fig. 21–3), producing an audible or palpable click as the femoral head slips over the acetabular rim.[26]

Jones and co-workers[34] have demonstrated in a rather large study that repeat examination is mandatory until the child starts walking because the lack of symptoms and subtle physical findings make early diagnosis difficult.[60] Although all the patients have functional disability, only about half have pain. It is for these reasons that the emergency clinician must be aware of this condition and be able to diagnose it early enough so that appropriate therapy can be instituted.

☐ SLIPPED CAPITAL FEMORAL EPIPHYSIS (FIG. 21–4)

This condition occurs in children between the ages of 10 and 16 years. Boys predominate over girls. A seasonal variation in the occurrence of slipped capital femoral epiphysis has been shown. In patients who live north of the 40 degrees latitude, this injury occurs with a peak onset in mid-June.[36] This has been attributed to increased physical activity during these months.[36] In approximately one fourth of the cases both hips are affected. An association between slipped capital femoral epiphysis and hypothyroidism was first reported in 1928.[61] Since then, an increased frequency of this disorder in patients with endocrine disorders, including hypothyroidism, growth hormone deficiency, and hypogonadism, has also been noted.[61] The disorder occurs during the rapid growth period in adolescence. The capital femoral epiphysis is weakened and displaced downward and backward, resulting in a very disabling external rotation deformity of the lower extremity that later goes on to form degenerative arthritis of the hip. This separation occurs between the hypertrophying cells and the calcifying cells of the epiphysis.[54] In many of these patients, there is a history of rapid skeletal growth before

the displacement. The patient may present to the emergency department with a history of minor trauma or strain and symptoms continuing since this trivial episode. Interestingly enough, this condition is found in children who are typically obese with underdeveloped skeletal characteristics, and is less commonly seen in tall, thin children. Weight bearing and muscle contraction cause the displacement to worsen. Therefore, young athletes between the ages of 8 and 12 years with knee discomfort and no effusion must be considered for slipped capital femoral epiphysis.[38,54] The etiology of this condition remains unknown.

X Ray (Figs. 21–5, 21–6)
Antero-posterior (AP) views of both hips should be taken. In addition, a lateral view taken in a frogged position with the hip flexed 90 degrees and abducted 45 degrees will demonstrate the displaced capital femoral epiphysis. In the preslipping stage, one sees a globular swelling in the joint capsule accompanied by a widening of the epiphysis and decalcification of the metaphysis at the epiphyseal border caused by the displacement of the head slipping inferiorly and posteriorly. Other clues to the diagnosis of slipped epiphysis include a wide irregular or mottled epiphyseal plate, metaphyseal rarefaction, and periosteal new bone formation. In addition to this, loss of Shenton's line is commonly seen radiographic finding (Fig. 21–7). Computed tomography (CT) scans have proven very useful in diagnosing diseases of the hip and the shoulder. When the relationship of the femoral head to the acetabulum is uncertain on the plain radiographs, slices taken with a CT scan are often able to diagnose the problem readily.

Clinical Presentation
The onset is insidious and slowly progressive. The early symptoms are fatigue after walking and standing and later slight pain is complained of and stiffness associated with a limp. There may be a history of trivial trauma, several weeks to months before the onset of symptoms. One should suspect this disorder in any adolescent who limps and has complaints of hip or knee pain associated with slight restriction of internal rotation of the hip. On examination, the hip is externally rotated and there is pain and diminished range of motion to internal rotation, abduction, and flexion.[11] When this occurs, the patient's diagnosis is clear and the approach is fairly straightforward. Often, clinical findings are subtle and may be missed.[11] Three stages can be identified with an associated clinical picture.

In the *preslipping stage*, there is first noted a slight discomfort about the groin, which usually occurs after activity and subsides with rest. The patient may complain of stiffness and an occasional limp. Discomfort may radiate along the anterior and medial

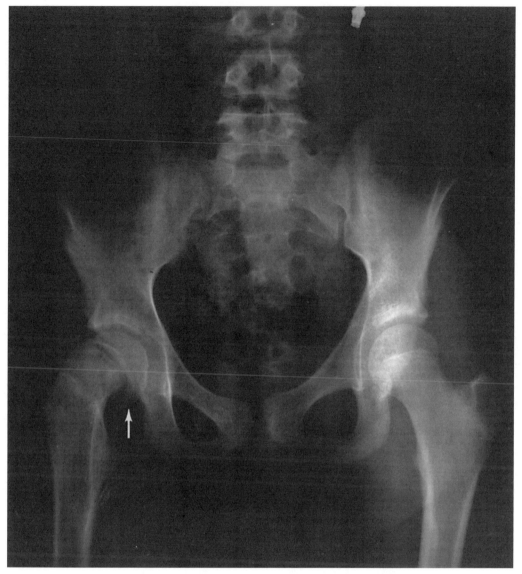

Figure 21–4. Slipped capital femoral epiphysis is demonstrated on the right hip.

aspect of the thigh to the inner aspect of the knee. The symptoms are usually vague, and no objective findings are noted on physical examination. This stage is followed by the *chronic slipping stage* where the epiphysis is separated and gradually shifts backward as is usually noted on x rays taken during that time. In this stage, a patient has tenderness around the hip joint and limitation of motion (particularly abduction and internal rotation). The limb develops an adduction and external rotation deformity. As the hip is flexed and externally rotated, the slipping is accentuated, and the gluteus medius becomes inadequate. The patient develops a positive *Trendelenburg test*. When the condition is bilateral, the patient has a typical gluteus medius or waddling gait. This is followed by a stage of *fixed deformity* in which pain and muscle spasm disap-

pear; however, the limp and external rotation and adduction deformity persist as does the limitation of internal rotation and abduction. These cases must be diagnosed early, and once suspected referred immediately to the orthopedic surgeon for definitive treatment, which involves reduction of the slipped epiphysis and no weight bearing.

Recently, a new classification system based on combination of stability of the physeal area and chronicity has been developed. In an acute slipped capital femoral epiphysis there is an effusion, indicating physeal instability and recent progression. A chronic slipped capital femoral epiphysis is characterized by remodeling of the anterior aspect of the metaphysis, indicating the duration of symptoms for at least 3 weeks. In an acute-on-chronic slipped capital femoral epiphysis, there is an

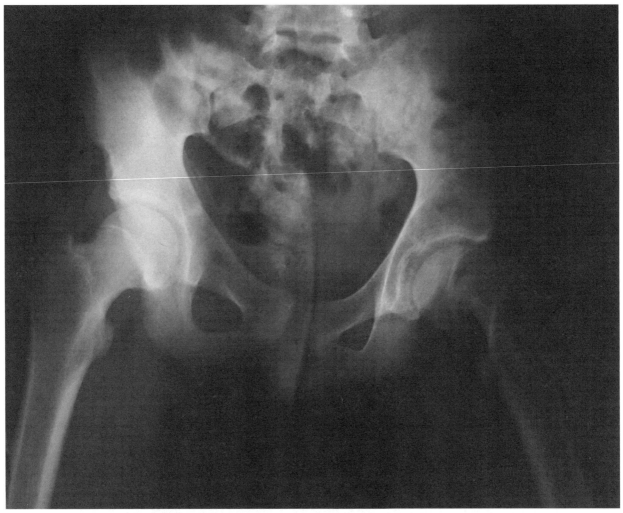

Figure 21–5. Late stage of slipped capital femoral epiphysis is demonstrated.

effusion and remodeling.[3] The importance to this is that treatment is guided by whether the slipped epiphysis is stabile or unstabile. Thus, using this classification system, an acute slipped capital femoral epiphysis has an effusion and no remodeling and is regarded as unstabile. An acute-on-chronic slipped capital femoral epiphysis has an effusion and remodeling and is unstabile. A chronic slipped capital femoral epiphysis has remodeling but no effusion.[3]

Treatment

To reduce the slipped epiphysis, a single cannulated screw must be inserted into the center of the femoral head. The single screw not only preserves the blood supply to the femoral head, but also is easier and has better results than multiple screws. *In situ* pinning is safe and effective to as much as 60 degrees of slipped epiphysis. If the screw is to be removed for total hip replacement, it should be done as soon as there is

radiographic evidence of obliteration of the physeal line.[2]

Slipped capital femoral epiphysis, which is the most common hip disorder in adolescents, has generally been classified according to symptom duration, as previously indicated. An acute slip is one in which there are symptoms for less than 3 weeks; for a chronic slip, there are symptoms for greater than 3 weeks. An acute-on-chronic slip is characterized by a combination of both with a recent exacerbation of symptoms. This classification system is misleading because it does not consider stability. A stable slipped capital femoral epiphysis has a good prognosis, but an unstable slip has a guarded prognosis. The priorities in treating an unstabile (acute) slip are to avoid avascular necrosis, avoid chondrolysis, and prevent further slip as well as correct the deformity.[3] In this new classification system, treatment guidelines have been developed which are beyond the scope of this discussion.[3]

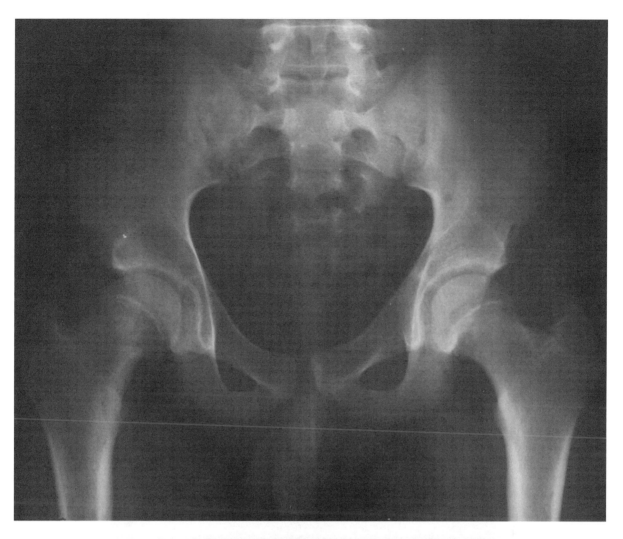

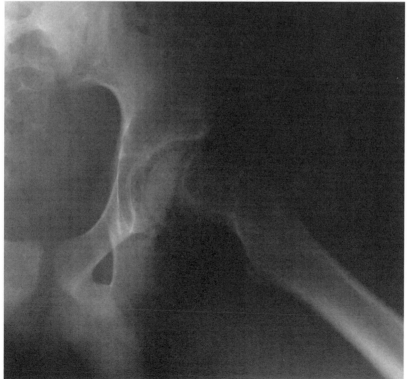

Figure 21–6. Early stages of slipped capital femoral epiphysis are demonstrated.

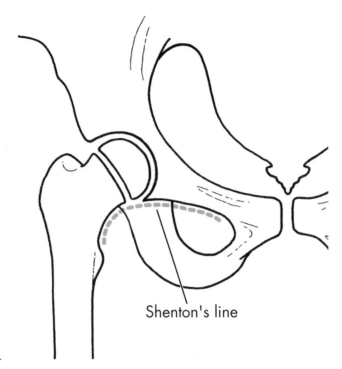

Shenton's line

Figure 21–7. Shenton's line.

☐ TRANSIENT SYNOVITIS OF THE HIP (ACUTE TRANSITORY EPIPHYSITIS)

This is a very common short-lived nonspecific inflammation of the synovium of the hip occurring in children, most often boys, between the ages of 4 and 10 years. The condition is often attributed to a mild traumatic episode or low-grade febrile illness such as occurs in tonsillitis or an acute otitis media. The disorder is usually unilateral although it can be bilateral.

X Ray
The x rays are initially normal; however, in an established case, one does note that the soft tissues that overlay the interpelvic aspect of the acetabulum are swollen and form a very prominent shadow known as the *obturator sign*.

Clinical Presentation
The onset of this condition is usually insidious. The child complains of pain in the hip that radiates down into the thigh and the knee, and the extremity is held in *flexion, adduction,* and *internal rotation* while the child resists all attempts at passive motion resulting from muscle spasm. These children almost always have a limp and the joint is tender to palpation. The temperature is usually normal to slightly elevated and is rarely high.

Differential Diagnosis
One must differentiate this condition from osteomyelitis, pyogenic arthritis, and slipping of the capital femoral epiphysis. This differentiation is aided by the history of a preceding febrile illness and the typical course of transient synovitis that is short lived. If doubt exists, aspiration of the hip joint and culture of the synovial fluid is mandatory.

Treatment
The treatment for this condition is bed rest, and if there is significant pain and muscle spasm, a short period of traction usually leads to a quick recovery. Prolonged follow-up is indicated because some of these patients go on to develop Legg-Calvé-Perthes disease.

☐ SEPTIC ARTHRITIS OF THE HIP JOINT

Septic arthritis is a disease of the young and when the hip joint is affected, the age range is even lower. Seventy percent of cases occur in patients aged 4 years or younger.[27] The younger the child affected by septic arthritis of the hip, the worse is the result.[27] Refusal to walk in children is often attributable to bacterial infections of the hip. In one study in which the authors eliminated all patients who had refused to walk because of definite antecedent pathology, it was found that 21 of 22 patients had bacterial infections.[10] Osteomyelitis and septic arthritis occurred with equal frequency and accounted for 14 of the 22 episodes.[40] Diskitis also accounted for a significant number of cases. Fever was present in 82 percent of patients with bacterial infections but in only 17 percent of those with no infections. The white blood cell count and erythrocyte sedimentation rate were not useful.[10]

Pathogenesis

Staphylococcus aureus is the most prevalent organism causing this condition. The infection usually reaches the hip joint from a focus of osteomyelitis within the joint capsule. The osteomyelitis is usually of hematogenous origin and arises in the metaphysis by way of nutrient vessels. From there it may spread outward and develop as a subperiosteal abscess. As a result, the infection of the hip joint usually arises from a focus of osteomyelitis in the femoral neck that is within the joint capsule.[46] There appears to be a fundamental difference between the disease in children and in infants. In children, the disease is usually secondary to osteomyelitis of the neck of the femur. In infants, it may arise as a result of hematogenous spread from a generalized septicemia.

The articular cartilage is unable to withstand the increased intra-articular pressures resulting from the pus produced by the staphylococcus organism.[31] In addition, the staphylococcus organism produces an activator staphylokinase that aids in the destruction of articular cartilage.[45] The cartilage can withstand these forces for about 4 to 5 days before destructive changes occur.[31,45] Other organisms that can cause septic arthritis of the hip in children include *Streptococcus pyogenes* and *Haemophilus influenzae*. *Streptococcus* infection is usually associated with a much more rapid onset of signs and symptoms. *Haemophilus* infection is generally responsible when septic arthritis occurs during the first 12 months of life but may be seen in the first 2 years. In the young adult, gonococcal arthritis must be suspected.

Clinical Presentation

Characteristically, the child presents to the emergency department with high temperature, irritability, and severe pain in the affected hip, accompanied by grossly restricted motion in all directions and muscle spasm. The child walks with a limp or does not walk at all. The hip is held in the *flexed externally rotated* and *abducted* position.[27] On examination, the patient has tenderness anteriorly in the groin and over the hip joint and appears toxic. The white blood cell count in the synovial fluid averages 57,000 μL, however, it can be as low as 10,000 μL or as high as 250,000 μL.[27] Characteristically, there is a shift to the left and blood cultures are positive in more than 50 percent of the cases.[27,45] The mucin level is decreased in all cases when the joint fluid is examined as is the glucose level when compared with the blood glucose in a majority of patients tested.[27] The sedimentation rate is usually elevated in most cases. Morey and co-workers[40] recommend that the diagnosis be made if any four of the following five are noted: (1) temperature greater than 38.3 C; (2) pain localized to the hip that is worse with gentle passive motion; (3) swelling of the involved joint; (4) systemic symptoms of lethargy, irritability, or toxicity with no other demonstrable pathologic process; or (5) if a satisfactory response is noted to antibiotic therapy.

X Ray

In one study,[27] all patients showed some degree of soft tissue swelling about the hip joint (Fig. 21–8). The younger the child, the more likely one is to see widening of the joint space.[27] In another study[40] many patients had a normal x ray initially. Abnormal subluxation of the hip with widening of the joint space was most common. Osteomyelitis of the proximal femur was noted in some.

Differential Diagnosis

A number of conditions must be differentiated from septic arthritis of the hip. Transient synovitis may present with intense pain, pronounced limp, and restriction of motion of the hip joint. Nuclear scanning helps to differentiate this condition from septic arthritis. If this is not available, skin traction in bed in a hospital is a useful way to differentiate this entity from the septic joint.[46] Significant improvement in the signs and symptoms within 24 hours indicates *transient synovitis*. If one suspects septic arthritis, then the patient should have a joint tap and be begun on antibiotics. Hemophilia may be hard to differentiate; however, the patient is usually a known hemophiliac. When this condition is suspected, urgent decompression is needed to avoid permanent damage to the head of the femur from the increased intra-articular pressures (see discussion in the section on pathogenesis). *Rheumatic fever* can present with severe pain and restriction of motion in the hip joint. Typically this condition shows a migratory type of arthritis and arthralgia, which aids in the differentiation.

Treatment

Perhaps the most important point for the emergency physician to be aware of is that a delay in diagnosis in this condition and thus a delay in treatment is a most important factor affecting the prognosis and poor results in this condition.[40] There was an almost uniformly poor result when treatment was started more than 4 days after the onset of symptoms in one study.[40] The goals of treatment are to clean the joint to avoid articular cartilage destruction and adhesion formation as well as to decompress the joint to avoid vascular embarrassment of the epiphysis.[14] Adequate doses of parenteral antibiotics are a must. The initial agent recommended by Griffin[27] was penicillin; however, other agents are currently used. Arthrotomy and early irrigation form an important part in the treatment protocol.[40,46] One should choose the appropriate antibiotic depending on the most likely organism as determined by age and mode of onset. A Gram stain and cultures are essential in picking the appropriate antibiotic. Staphylococcal arthritis is most common and

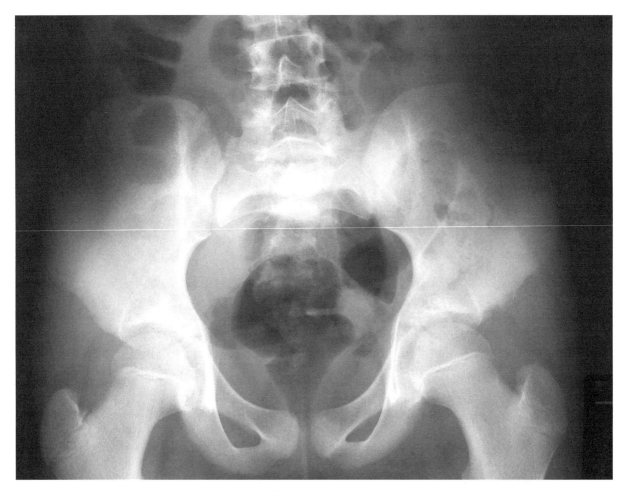

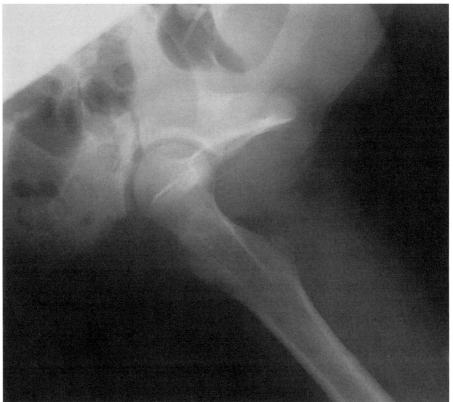

Figure 21–8. Septic left hip is demonstrated.

responds to methicillin or oxacillin. When gonococcal arthritis is suspected, penicillin in a dose of 10 million units IV per day for adults is the recommended initial therapy.

☐ DEGENERATIVE JOINT DISEASE

This condition is discussed briefly here because it is so commonly seen and thus it behooves the emergency physician to be aware of it. Degenerative arthritis of the hip takes place with advancing age. It is accelerated by any incongruity of the articular surface causing abnormal friction such as irregularities of the femoral head, which can result from a number of factors. Although ischemia to the femoral head after fractures of the femoral neck or direct injury to the articular cartilage is implicated in a number of cases, 50 percent of cases are idiopathic.

Clinical Presentation

The patient usually complains of insidious onset of stiffness about the hip which comes on after a rest and is relieved by some activity. At first there are repeated attacks of slight pain lasting only a day or two, made worse by prolonged periods of weight bearing. There is often a protective limp due to muscle spasm accompanied by pain and a sense of stiffness that progressively worsens. The pain may be anterior, lateral, or posterior depending on the site of inflammation. Referral is typically to the anterior and medial aspects of the thigh and the inner aspect of the knee. Characteristically, the pain is worsened with prolonged weight bearing and movement, particularly in the direction of *abduction*, *internal rotation*, and *extension*. Patients often complain of worsening pain in cold and humid weather and relief with heat and salicylates. In an acute exacerbation of osteoarthritis of the hip there is tenderness over the site of capsular inflammation

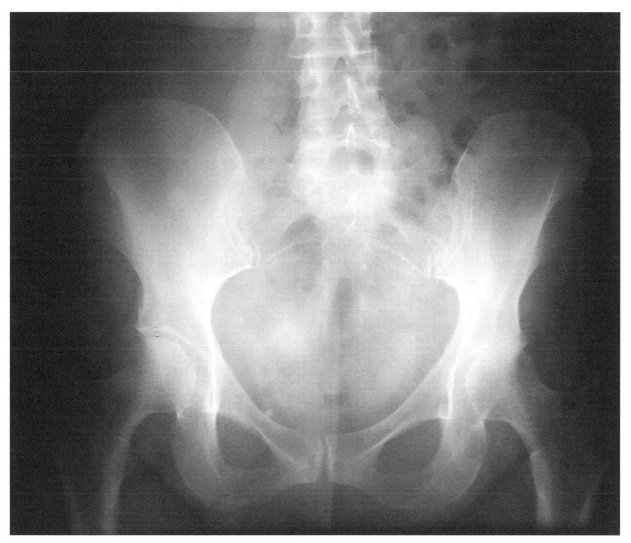

Figure 21–9. Early degenerative joint disease with cartilage narrowing is demonstrated on the left hip. (*Courtesy of G. Shove, MD.*)

accompanied by muscle spasm primarily involving the adductors. The *Fabere test* is usually positive. This test is performed by having the patient place the heel of the affected extremity on the dorsum of the normal foot and "sliding" the heel up the cutaneous portion of the tibia until the knee is reached. This test is not specific for acute exaspirations of degenerative hip disease, but it will be positive in any inflammatory process involving the hip.

X Ray

In the early stages of this disorder, the x rays will be negative (Fig. 21–9). Later, however, one will note an irregular subchondral sclerosis that gradually evolves into joint narrowing. Additional findings will be flattening of the head at the superior pole accompanied by cystic changes in this area.[16,26,32]

Treatment

Conservative treatment is usually indicated for acute exacerbations that present to the emergency department, including abstinence from weight bearing, traction when indicated, heat, and massage. Salicylates are an important adjunct in relieving the inflammatory process.

EXTRA-ARTICULAR DISORDERS

☐ BURSITIS OF THE HIP

Many bursae surround the hip, but only three are clinically important: the trochanteric bursae are divided into both a superficial and deep portion, the iliopectineal bursae, and the ischiogluteal (Fig. 21–10). The deep trochanter bursa is located between tendinous insertion of the gluteus maximus muscle and the posterior lateral prominence of the greater trochanter. A superficial trochanteric bursa is located between the greater trochanter and the skin. The iliopectineal bursa (often called the *iliopsoas bursa*) is the most constant and the largest of all the hip bursae.[9] It lies between the iliopsoas anteriorly and the iliopectoneal eminence posteriorly along the anterior surface of the hip joint capsule. The ischiogluteal bursa is superficial to the tuberosity of the ischium.

The usual causes of bursitis include reactive inflammations secondary to overuse or excessive pressure and trauma-induced inflammations. Other causes of bursitis are infections and metabolic conditions such as gout. Although septic bursitis here is rare, one must understand the microbiology of this condition when it does occur. Approximately 80 percent of the cases of septic bursitis are caused by *Staphylococcus aureus* and other gram-positive organisms. Indications for hospitalization are systemic symptoms and extensive local involve-ment.[64] Patients who fail to respond to intravenous antibiotics and percutaneous aspiration of the bursa may require surgical drainage or bursectomy.[64]

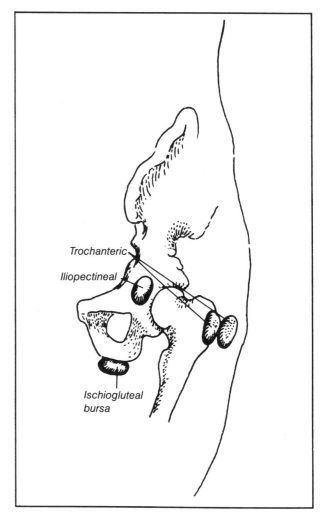

Figure 21–10. The bursae of the hip.

Clinical Presentation

Deep *trochanteric bursitis* characteristically presents with pain and tenderness localized to the posterior aspect of the greater trochanter, which is increased by *flexion of the hip* and *internal rotation*. Abduction and external rotation of the leg relaxes the gluteus maximus and relieves the pressure on the bursa. The pain may radiate down the back of the thigh and any motion of the thigh may cause discomfort. Greater trochanteric bursitis is likely often associated with repetitive microtrauma caused by active use of the muscles inserting on the greater trochanteric that results in degenerative changes of the tendons, muscles, or fibrous tissues.[53] Calcification in the region of the greater trochanteric in association with the bursitis has been observed since initial reports of trochanteric bursitis were first described. Degenerative diseases have been associated with this condition, as well as inflammatory arthritis of the hip, obesity, and iliotibial band syndrome.[53] Calcification around the greater trochanter is evident in 40 percent of the patients with trochanteric bursitis.[53] Sixty percent of the patients with bursitis treated by injection demonstrated total relief of symptoms after a single injection therapy 6 months afterward.[53]

Superficial trochanteric bursitis presents with tenderness and swelling over the inflamed bursa with accentuation on *extreme adduction* of the thigh. In *iliopectineal bursitis*, the patient presents with pain and tenderness over the lateral aspect of Scarpa's triangle. Tenderness is usually localized over the anterior aspect of the hip just inferior to the middle of the inguinal ligament. Irritation of the adjacent femoral nerve causes pain to be referred along the anterior thigh. The patient usually holds the hip in a position of flexion and ab duction with external rotation. Pain is increased by *extension, adduction,* or *internal rotation* of the hip. The examiner often sees a palpable mass or swelling lateral to the femoral vessels, and this must be differentiated from femoral hernia, psoas abscess, synovitis, and infection of the joint.

Patients with occupations requiring prolonged sitting on hard surfaces present with *ischiogluteal bursitis.* Tenderness is elicited over the ischial tuberosity, which radiates down the back of the thigh and along the course of the hamstrings, mimicking a herniated disk.

Treatment

The treatment for all these bursitidies is bed rest, heat application, and anti-inflammatory agents. In ischial gluteal bursitis, a cushion or pillow helps to relieve the discomfort and prevents recurrence. When the bursitis is secondary to an infectious process this presents a true emergency and must be diagnosed early by the emergency physician. When this is suspected, inci-sion and drainage is mandatory and should be done as soon as possible. Parenteral antibiotics are also indicated.

☐ CALCIFIED TENDONITIS OF THE HIP JOINT

This condition is comparable to calcific tendonitis in the shoulder where amorphous calcific deposits occur in the tendons of the gluteus medius lateral to the greater trochanter and the gluteus minimus superior to the capsule.

Clinical Presentation

The patient usually presents with severe pain in the hip. The hip is held in a position of flexion, abduction, and external rotation. Muscle spasm limits motion in all directions. The examiner elicits tenderness over the site of inflammation. The x ray will often reveal a cloudy opacity in the soft tissues overlying the hip joint.

Treatment

Heat application, rest, and anti-inflammatory agents are usually effective. The calcific depositions are more readily absorbed when broken up by a needling of the involved tendons under local anesthesia.[28]

☐ SNAPPING HIP

This is an uncommon condition that affects young adults between the ages of 15 and 40 years and is slightly more common in women. X rays of the hip are usually normal. This syndrome should be differentiated from a painless, deep "pop" that occurs with normal hip motion and that holds no clinical importance.[4] There are different types of snapping hip syndromes. The most common cause is the iliotibial band snapping over the greater trochanteric. This lateral snapping may be associated with development of a bursitis or with increased varus of the hip. It is a common problem causing hip pain in ballet dancers or people with similar exercises. It can also occur as a complication of total hip replacement.

Affected patients often say that they can dislocate their hip. The snapping of the tendon over the greater trochanteric can often be shown voluntarily by patients while standing or lying on their side. Passive internal and external rotation of the abducted limb in the sideline position usually demonstrates the snapping. The snapping can be eliminated by walking with the limb externally rotated. The snapping sensation can also be elicited by flexion of the knee, active internal rotation, and adduction of the hip.[6]

Another cause of snapping hip is the iliopsoas tendon snapping over the iliopectineal eminence of the pelvic brim as it proceeds to its insertion on the lesser tuberosity. In this instance, patients complain of snapping during extension of the flexed hip. It is decreased by internal and increased by external rotation of the hip. The tenderness and pain occur at the anterior superior spine and medial to the sartorius muscle. Fluoroscopy with contrast agents will help demonstrate this problem.

Snapping hip syndrome can also be caused by injuries of the acetabular labrum, a cartilaginous structure

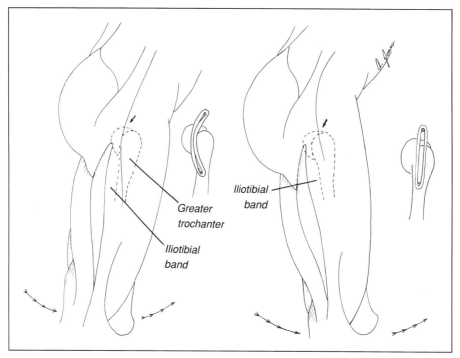

Figure 21–11. In the snapping hip syndrome, the iliotibial band courses over the trochanter.

that encircles the acetabulum. The painful pop or snap is most often anterior but may be posterior and is often accompanied by a sudden weakness of the leg.[4]

Treatment
Most patients with snapping hip could be treated conservatively (Fig. 21–11). If this condition becomes trouble-some, "Z-plasty" could be applied to treat an external snap. "Z-plasty" lengthens the tight iliotibial tract and also brings the thickened band anteriorly so that it no longer flicks over the greater trochanter during hip flexion.[6]

TRAUMATIC CONDITIONS OF THE HIP

The injuries that occur around the hip and the pelvis will be discussed under three general categories: injuries to the hip and trochanter; injuries to the buttocks, sacrum, and coccyx: and finally, injuries near the iliac crest.

☐ INJURIES AROUND THE HIP AND THE TROCHANTER

☐ Strain of the Iliopsoas Tendon
This is an uncommon injury occurring primarily in dancers and gymnasts. Strain of the iliopsoas may occur at its attachment to the lesser trochanter or at the musculotendinus junction. The usual mechanism of injury is excessive stretch placed on the iliopsoas. On examina-tion, the patient characteristically holds the thigh in a flexed adducted and externally rotated position. *Extension* and *internal rotation* of the thigh accentuate pain, as does contraction of the iliopsoas.

Ice packs and bed rest are the mainstay of manage-ment in this injury. The avulsed tendon is usually not repaired surgically even if it is complete or has incorpo-rated a bone fragment with it.

☐ Traumatic Phlebitis of the Femoral Vein
This condition is usually secondary to a direct blow over the femoral vein. Although uncommon, it can be quite serious and should be recognized by the emergency physician, and appropriate therapy instituted.

☐ Strain of the Gluteus Medius

This is more commonly seen in young athletes; however, even in this group it is an uncommon injury. Strain of the gluteus medius usually occurs as a result of overexertion of the gluteus medius. Pain is noted on abduction against resistance and is accentuated by having the patient rotate the thigh medially against resistance.

The treatment of this injury is symptomatic and is the same as for any other muscle strain, including rest, moist heat application, and analgesics.

☐ Tendonitis of the External Rotators

This condition can be acute or chronic and although it can involve the internal rotators of the thigh it more commonly involves the external rotators. The condition is characterized by pain and tenderness on active external rotation and the treatment for the condition is local moist heat application, anti-inflammatory agents, and analgesics.

☐ INJURIES TO THE BUTTOCKS, THE SACRUM, AND THE COCCYX

☐ Contusions

This is a common injury to the buttocks resulting from a direct blow such as during a fall. The buttocks are protected by a large amount of fatty tissue, and contusion of the gluteus maximus requires a significant force. The patient will complain of pain on sitting and on ambulation, and the examiner will note tenderness to palpation. Other conditions resulting from contusions to the buttocks include *periostitis of the ischial tuberosity*, *contusion of the ischial tuberosity*, and *fractures of the tuberosity*. These conditions can be differentiated by appropriate x rays and clinical evaluation. In the patient with periostitis of the ischial tuberosity, the examiner will note exquisite pain over the tuberosity with very little discomfort elsewhere.

The treatment of contusions to the buttocks is symptomatic, with ice packs and rest in a prone position. A pillow or a cushion affords relief from the discomfort until the condition improves. In the patient with periostitis of the ischial tuberosity, injection of the tuberosity, after adequate preparation, with 2 percent lidocaine affords good relief. In addition to this, the patient should be discharged with instructions to use a cushion until the condition clears, as well as appropriate analgesics and ice packs during the first 24 to 48 hours.

☐ *Contusions of the Sacrum and the Coccyx*

This is a common injury and is due to a direct blow over the subcutaneous portion of the sacrum or the coccyx. Owing to the subcutaneous nature of these bones, contusions maybe extremely painful, and the patient usually complains of a sharp localized area of pain that may be quite disabling. On examination, one finds a *well-localized* area of tenderness over the sacrum or the coccyx with little discomfort elsewhere. Appropriate x rays should be ordered to exclude fractures of the sacrum or the coccyx.

Although other authors have stated that this condition is not disabling, we have found it tends to be extremely disabling to the patient. Contusions of the coccyx can lead to a condition called *coccydynia*, which has a poor prognosis and for which there is little in the way of adequate treatment. The emergency treatment of contusions of the sacrum and the coccyx includes the early application of cold compresses and the dispensing of a "doughnut" and appropriate analgesics, along with referral for follow-up care. Because of the guarded prognosis in contusions of the coccyx, the authors believe that all contusions of this bone should be referred for follow-up care.

☐ *Contusion of the Perineum*

Contusions of the perineum are uncommon and result from direct blows such as during a fall on a hard object. On examination, the patient will have a painful ecchymotic and swollen perineum and may have a painful hematoma. The treatment is cold compresses for the first 48 hours followed by warm sitz baths. A patient with a hematoma should be referred for follow-up because x rays taken at a later date may show consolidation in this region. One must be certain that urethral injury has not occurred.

☐ Sprain of the Iliosacral Ligament

This is an uncommon injury; however, missing its diagnosis in the emergency department can lead to inappropriate treatment for a herniated disk. The sacroiliac articulation is a strong unyielding joint, which is rarely injured. When injury does occur, the patient complains of pain localized to the region of the sacroiliac joint and referral to the groin and the posterior aspect of the thigh. The mechanism of injury involves wide abduction of the thighs or extremes of hyperextension or hyperflexion. The best maneuvers to diagnose this condition are to have the patient lie on the side, with the examiner placing his or her hands over the iliac crest and compressing downward, thereby compressing this articulation and eliciting pain. Alternately, wide abduction of the supine patient's elevated extended legs will elicit pain over the injured iliosacral or lumbosacral ligaments.

Localized injection of the joint with 2 percent lidocaine often affords relief, and the dispension of analgesics, hot packs, and bed rest is usually all that is needed. A constricting strap has been advised by some; however, the authors have not found this to be a useful treatment. If symptoms persist, referral is indicated.

☐ Strain of the Ischial Attachment of the Biceps Femoris and Semitendinosis

This condition results from forcible flexion of the hip while the knee is extended. In the adolescent, when the epiphysis is not closed, avulsion of the tuberosity with wide separation of the epiphysis can occur. On examination, the patient will present with tenderness over the attachment to the bone with little swelling. A history compatible with the afore-mentioned mechanism accompanied by pain increased with passive flexion of the hip with the knee extended or active extension of the hip against resistance will help make the diagnosis. X rays should always be taken in these cases.

With incomplete avulsion, treatment consists of splinting the knee in a flexed position to relieve the pressure on the ischial attachment of the tendons and avoidance of active flexion of the thigh. In cases where complete avulsion is suspected, the patient should be referred for evaluation of the need for surgical repair.

☐ Compression of Sciatic Nerve

There are several causes of this condition which include sitting in an awkward position for a prolonged period of time, hematoma following a fracture of the hip, or fibrosis following an injection to the buttock. This condition is also seen in patients who undergo anesthesia and are recumbent for a prolonged period of time or bedridden.

Compression of the sciatic nerve will elicit classical symptoms of sciatica. In patients with the *piriformis syndrome*, an atypical fibrose band develops and constricts a group of small vessels. There is functional loss of the piriformis which is minimal because three stronger, short external rotators of the hip exist. Sectioning of the piriformis muscle at its tendinous origin releases the fibrous band and compressed vessels. The diagnosis of sciatic nerve compression at the level of the piriformis can be confirmed by neurophysiologic tests which can be done prior to operative treatment.[30]

☐ Pudendal Nerve Palsy

Pudendal nerve palsy is caused by a compression neuropathy due to the forces applied to the perineal region. This is usually a condition that occurs postoperatively following an intramedullary nailing of the femur; however, it can be seen posttraumatically.[8] Numbness of the penis and scrotum along with erectile dysfunction is present. The sensory terminal branches of the pudendal nerve are more susceptible to this palsy postoperatively than the motor branches.

☐ Gluteal Compartment Syndrome[43]

Gluteal compartment syndrome is an extremely rare condition; however, it is one the emergency physician

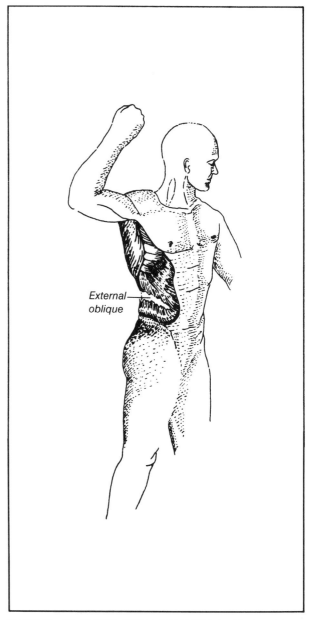

External oblique

Figure 21–12. Rupture of the external oblique aponeurosis.

must be aware of because its consequences may be quite serious. The gluteal muscles behave as if they were divided into three separate compartments: the *tensor compartment*, enclosing the tensor fascia lata muscle and the fascia lata; the *medius-minimus compartment*, enclosing the gluteus medius and minimus; and the *maximus compartment*, enclosing the gluteus maximus. After severe contusions to the buttocks as would occur during a fall from a height, the patient may present to the emergency department with tensely swollen buttocks and increasing pain and pressures that, over the ensuing 4 to 6 hours, may result in necrosis of the muscles.[43] In addition, because of the inverse relationship between peripheral nerve conduction block and intracompartmental pressure,[49] the high pressures may cause sciatic neuropathy that may lead to further problems.[5,11,43]

Patients who have a history and examination compatible with this syndrome should be admitted and consulted by the orthopedic surgeons. A fasciotomy could be performed if the pressure within the compartment is 30 mm Hg or more for a duration of 6 to 8 hours.[51]

☐ INJURIES NEAR THE ILIAC CREST

☐ Contusions

The most common injury to occur at the iliac crest is a contusion. Contusions of the iliac crest have been called "hip pointers."[19,44] This diagnosis should not be made without ruling out an intra-abdominal injury. *Periostitis of the iliac crest* results from a contusion of the bone and usually poses no problem in diagnosis and treatment. On examination, the patient presents with tenderness localized to any region along the iliac crest from the anterior superior spine to the posterior superior spine. Treatment of the condition is symptomatic.

☐ Rupture of the External Oblique Aponeurosis on the Iliac Crest

This uncommon condition results from forceful contraction of the abdominal muscles while the trunk is rapidly pushed to the contralateral side. The patient presents with very severe pain over the iliac crest and characteristically walks into the emergency department in a stooped-over posture from which he or she cannot straighten out due to pain. Examination discloses exquisite tenderness along the entire iliac crest, and in the early stages one may feel a palpable defect if a large rupture has occurred (Fig. 21–12). In mild cases, only tenderness is noted to palpation. Contraction of the involved muscle elicits significant pain that aids in clinching the diagnosis and separating it from contusion of the iliac crest. The patient will also complain of pain at the involved iliac crest on *flexion* to the *opposite side*.

Treatment for incomplete avulsions of the muscle includes ice for the first 24 to 48 hours followed by heat, analgesics, and rest. Strapping and taping have been used by some physicians; however, this has not proved to be entirely beneficial and is not used in the acute stage of this injury. When extensive tears of the aponeurosis exist and a hematoma is present, consultation should be obtained from the orthopedic surgeon.

Injuries to the Thigh

☐ QUADRICEPS CONTUSIONS

The term *charley-horse* is listed as synonymous with a quadriceps contusion in the standard nomenclature of athletic injuries of the American Medical Association.[31] Contusions of the quadriceps are quite common, usually not disabling at the time of the injury and are variable in their degree of discomfort. Quadriceps contusions are usually due to a direct blow and can be differentiated from rupture because there is usually residual function with contusion. Contusions are often not disabling at the time of the injury. The vastus lateralis and intermedius are the most frequently involved muscles in quadriceps contusions. The rectus femoris is less commonly injured.

Examination

The patient complains of a dull aching pain over the anterior lateral aspect of the thigh. Tenderness is noted to palpation and variable swelling will be noted. If the swelling is extreme and rapidly follows the injury, the physician should suspect an injury to major vessels. The pain is increased by flexion of the knee and is accompanied by muscle spasm. There is often a diffuse hematoma that may or may not be palpable initially. In a large study by Jackson,[31] a clinically and prognostically useful classification system was presented. Grading of quadriceps contusions was divided into mild, moderate, and severe. In a mild contusion, the patient has localized tenderness over the quadriceps with no alteration of gait and knee motion without pain up to at least 90 degrees or more. In a moderate contusion, the patient displays swelling and a tender muscle mass with knee motion restricted to less than 90 degrees and an antalgic gait. The patient is unable to climb stairs or arise from a chair without considerable discomfort. In patients with severe contusions, the diagnosis was made when a markedly tender and swollen thigh was noted in which the contour of the muscle was unable to be palpated and not well defined. In these cases, knee motion was less than 45 degrees, and there was a severe limp. These patients usually present with inability to walk unaided and frequently had an effusion in the ipsilateral knee. The patients were started on a treatment program that included bed rest, ice packs, and elevation for the first 24 to 48 hours and a compressive dressing when indicated, followed by a rehabilitation program. In this series, myositis ossificans occurred in over 70 percent of the patients classified as having moderate or severe contusions.

Treatment

One should not be complacent in the treatment of the contusions of the quadriceps. Early recognition and classification as to the severity of the initial quadriceps contusion will lead to appropriate restrictions of activity and follow-up care. The patient with moderate to severe contusion should be initially placed at bed rest with ice packs and elevation and a firm compressive dressing should be applied extending from the toes to the groin. The patient should then be referred for appropriate follow-up care. During the ensuing 48 hours, immobilization is important and massage should be strongly discouraged in the initial stages as well as early vigorous activity.

In treating this condition, the goal is to limit swelling and hemorrhage, and minimize the amount of scar formation while preserving contractility and strength of the muscle.[49] In *Phase 1* the goal is to limit hemorrhage by using rest, ice, elevation, and compressive dressings for 24 hours for mild contusions and 48 hours for severe contusions.

In *Phase 2* the goal is to restore motion to the muscle. In this phase, ice or cold whirlpool is continued and gravity-assisted movement is used. Active flexion and extension exercises as well as weight bearing as tolerated are used only when this does not cause significant pain.

In *Phase 3* the goal is functional rehabilitation. This is begun when there is 120 degrees of pain-free motion in the knee. If there is a return of pain or loss of motion during this phase of rehabilitation, then return to the prior phase is indicated. During the functional rehabilitative phase, weight bearing is increased and active flexion and extension exercises are performed using weights.

□ MYOSITIS OSSIFICANS (TRAUMATIC)

Myositis ossificans is a common condition in which traskeletal ossification occurs within a muscle or a group of muscles (Fig. 21–13). The condition is most often seen in the thigh after a moderate or severe contusion. The patient is usually a young athletically inclined person who has returned to active use of the quadriceps too early after a contusion. This can occur, however, even with adequate treatment in severe contusions of the quadriceps.[31] In most cases of myositis ossificans, the involvement is limited to the middle one third of the thigh; however, in some it extends into the proximal one

third. The lesion may be attached to the femur by a stalk or have a very broad periosteal base. Myositis ossificans can usually be diagnosed 2 to 4 weeks after injury to the thigh.

Examination

After a severe contusion to the thigh, the patient experiences a swelling that persists and becomes increasingly tender and warm. X rays taken 2 to 4 weeks after an injury usually show the heterotopic bone. The sedimentation rate is usually elevated early and remains elevated during the myositis stage of this lesion.

X Ray

As previously mentioned, the x ray usually shows evidence of the heterotopic bone within 2 to 4 weeks after an injury. Three forms of myositis ossificans have been discussed:[31] a type with a stalked connection to the adjacent femur; a periosteal type with continuity between the heterotopic bone and the adjacent femur, in which case the continuity is almost total; and a third, broad-base type with a portion of the ectopic bone projecting into the quadriceps muscle.

Treatment

The emergency physician should be aware of the *preventive measures* relating to myositis ossificans. The patient with a quadricep contusion should be cautioned against early active use of the quadriceps, and forceful passive flexion of the knee. The condition is usually not severely disabling and generally requires no surgical removal of the mass. Once the diagnosis is established, appropriate referral and follow-up are indicated.

□ ADDUCTOR MUSCLE STRAINS

This injury is usually caused by a straddling injury secondary to forceful abduction of the thigh and is commonly seen in cheerleaders and others undergoing similar activities.

Examination

The patient complains of pain that is localized to the pubic region. With incomplete rupture, the pain is made worse by *passive abduction* of the thigh and is accentuated by *active adduction against resistance*. If complete rupture has occurred, the examiner will often see bunching of the muscle along the medial aspect of the thigh near the groin.

Treatment

The treatment for incomplete rupture is ice, crutches, and rest for at least 3 to 6 weeks. X rays should always be taken in these patients to determine if avulsion has

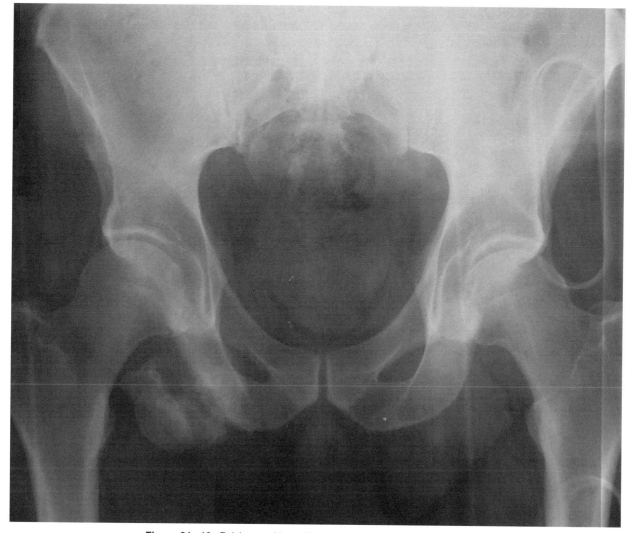

Figure 21–13. Pelvic myositis ossificans. (*Courtesy of D. Wrensch, PA-C.*)

occurred at the origin of the adductor longus that is most commonly involved in this injury. If the examiner suspects a complete rupture, referral is indicated for evaluation to determine if surgical repair is warranted.

☐ Strains of the Hamstrings

The hamstring is a commonly strained muscle, particularly in runners and in patients participating in basketball. The patient complains of pain and often presents to the emergency department with spasm that restricts motion of the hamstrings. On questioning, the patient will often give the history that he or she continued to run after the initial episode.

Treatment

It is important to emphasize to the patient that he or she must avoid early return to sports until pain has subsided. The patient should use pain as a guide, and gradual re-

turn to running is emphasized. The treatment is similar to strains in other muscles of the thigh.

Because inflammation follows muscle strain, nonsteroidal anti-inflammatory drugs are the first step. Ice provides the most efficient clinical method to limit inflammation.[63] The ice should be left on for 20–45 minutes, 2 to 4 times a day. If the athlete continues to experience pain with activity, daily ice applications should continue until symptoms resolve, usually within 7 to 14 days after injury. Limiting ice treatment to the first 24 to 36 hours is probably too short a time.[63] During the acute phase of rehabilitation for a moderate strain, a single clutch on the opposite side of the injury may be advised.

In the subacute phase, symptoms start to resolve. Resistance exercises can begin, in addition to range of motion exercises. Swimming pool activities, in particular, will facilitate motion and strength without pain.

In the remodeling phase, the hamstrings are at 100 percent strength. Recent evidence demonstrates that hamstring-injured athletes showed less hamstring flexibility than a controlled group.[63] Thus, hamstring muscle strains are complex, multifactorial injuries. The rehabilitation for these injuries requires follow-up with an appropriate clinician.[63]

☐ RUPTURES OF MUSCLES OF THE THIGH

The rectus femoris and adductor longus as well as the hamstrings can rupture anywhere from their origin to their insertion. The patient is often misdiagnosed as having a contusion, only to appear several days later with a definite mass that is the contracted bunched-up muscle. The diagnosis is often difficult to make and emphasizes the need for appropriate follow-up for all strains and contusions involving the muscles of the thigh.

Treatment
A minimum of 6 weeks is needed for healing when partial rupture occurs involving the muscles of the thigh. Activity can be permitted to the tolerance of pain; however, no sports or vigorous activity can be allowed. Ambulation with crutches and a gradual return to activity is advised. Patients with complete ruptures should be splinted and referred.

☐ Fascial Hernia
The muscles of the thigh are invested in fascial sheaths. The fascial sheaths along the anterior and lateral aspect of the thigh are thinner just anterior to the iliotibial band.

The patient may present to the emergency department with a complaint of a small palpable mass that appears when the quadriceps is contracted and *disappears* when the *muscle is relaxed*. Treatment is usually not necessary; however, if the symptoms warrant, surgical repair may be indicated.

☐ Compartment Syndrome of the Anterior Thigh
Compartment syndrome of the anterior thigh is uncommon but may result from fractures of the femur, crush injuries of the quadriceps, or following blunt trauma to the muscle with a resulting hematoma. Postischemic edema following the revascularization can also be a cause of anterior compartment syndrome of the thigh.

The symptoms of compartment syndrome in this area are similar to other compartment syndromes with pain experienced when the muscles in the compartment are passively stretched. Pain is excessive and cannot be relieved by medication, and the compartment is firm on palpation. Neurologic changes as well as vascular changes are late to develop.

Conservative therapy in this syndrome is superior to surgical therapy when this condition occurs as an isolated injury in a young athlete without any accompanying wound or fracture. The subcutaneous semiopen fasciotomy can cause severe stretching of the skin and skin necrosis may develop which limits knee flexion. An emergency fasciotomy should be performed only when neurologic dysfunction develops.[48,57]

HIP DISLOCATIONS

Hip dislocations (Figs. 21–14, 21–15) require large forces such as occur in automobile accidents where the knee strikes the dashboard or as with pedestrian automobile accidents. Hip dislocations are frequently associated with acetabular fractures or ipsilateral extremity injuries.[13,20] Approximately 25 percent of hip dislocations are associated with knee injuries and 4 percent with ipsilateral femoral fractures.[13,24] Also, avascular necrosis of the femoral head is seen in about 10 percent of the uncomplicated dislocations.[15] All hip dislocations must be regarded as true emergencies and reduced promptly in order to minimize the incidence of avascular necrosis of the femoral head.[47]

The classification of posterior hip dislocations is based on the system developed by Stewart and

Milford.[24,55] Posterior dislocations are the most common type of hip dislocation and may be classified as follows:

1. Simple dislocation (no fracture)
2. Dislocation with large acetabular rim fragments stabilized after reduction
3. Dislocations with unstable or comminuted fractures
4. Dislocation with femoral head or neck fractures[55]

Anterior dislocations account for 5 to 10 percent of all traumatic hip dislocations[15] and are classified as follows:[1]

1. Obturator dislocation
2. Iliac dislocation

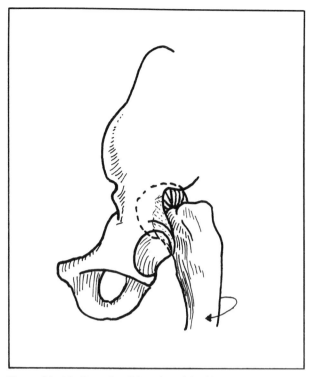

Figure 21–14. Posterior dislocation of the hip.

3. Pubic dislocation
4. Anterior dislocation with a femoral head fracture

Acetabular fractures may be associated with a central dislocation of the femoral head. This injury is discussed under *pelvic and acetabular fractures*.

Mechanism of Injury

Anterior dislocations are the result of forced abduction resulting in impingement of the femoral neck or trochanter against the superior dome of the acetabulum and a levering of the femoral head out through a tear in the anterior capsule. If the hip was in flexion, an obturator dislocation results and the limb becomes fixed in up to 60 degrees of abduction, full external rotation, and some flexion. Injuries to an extended hip results in a pubic or iliac dislocation. The limb in the pubic type reveals a marked external rotation in full extension and some abduction.[15] A pubic dislocation can also be the result of severe hyperextension with external rotation, thus forcing the head of the femur anteriorly. Obturator dislocations are more common than are pubic and iliac dislocations. Dislocation may be associated with a shear fracture of the femoral head.[12,22]

Posterior dislocations are more common than are anterior dislocations.[12] These injuries often occur after a blow to the knee with the hip and knee in flexion. This injury is commonly seen after automobile accidents where the knee has struck the dashboard (Fig. 21–16).

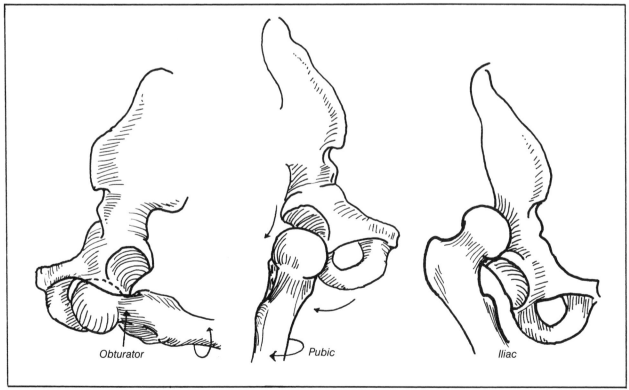

Figure 21–15. Anterior dislocations of the hip. Three types are demonstrated: obturator, pubic, and iliac.

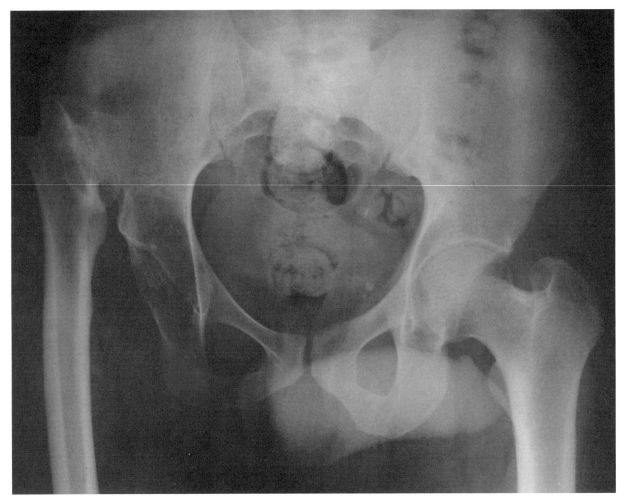

Figure 21–16. Posterior dislocation of the hip is shown on the right side.

X Ray

Routine hip and pelvic views are usually adequate in demonstrating these injuries. Shenton's line, as shown in Figure 21–7, should be evaluated whenever a hip injury is suspected. Additional radiographs of the ipsilateral extremity may be indicated on the basis of the physical examination.

Examination

Anterior obturator dislocations usually present with abduction, external rotation, and flexion of the involved extremity. Anterior iliac or pubic dislocations present with extension and slight abduction with external rotation. The femoral head is palpable near the anterior superior iliac spine with iliac dislocations and near the pubis after a pubic dislocation. The neurovascular status of the extremity must be documented in all patients with hip dislocations.

Posterior dislocations present with limb shortening and adduction with internal rotation of the involved extremity as shown in Figure 21–17. The femoral head

may be palpable within the muscle of the buttock. The patient should be carefully evaluated for associated femoral head or shaft fractures along with sciatic nerve injuries.

Associated Injuries

Hip dislocations may be associated with several significant injuries.

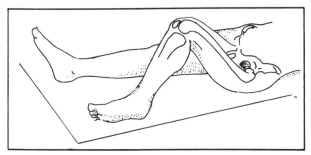

Figure 21–17. The typical position of posterior dislocation of the hip.

1. Femoral head fractures occur in up to 16 percent of posterior hip dislocations.[41] Femoral shaft fractures may also occur in association with hip dislocation. More recently, many causes have been identified for this condition.[52] With the advent of magnetic resonance imaging (MRI), the diagnosis can be made prior to the development of radiographic changes. An 18-fold increase in the prevalence of this condition has been found in patients who have a high consumption of alcohol compared to nondrinkers.[52] Steroid-associated cases have been reported to be high as well. This condition is seen in association with renal failure, rheumatic diseases, inflammatory bowel disease, and leukemia.[52] Rotation of the shaft after fracture may alter the position of the extremity and confuse the diagnosis.[13]
2. Injury to the sciatic nerve occurs in 10 to 13 percent of posterior hip dislocations.[23]
3. Posterior dislocations may be associated with ipsilateral knee injuries (25 percent in one series).[24] These injuries vary from ligamentous damage to the cruciates, medial, or lateral collateral ligaments, to fractures of the patella, femoral, or tibial condyles.
4. Anterior dislocations may be associated with arterial injuries or venous thrombosis.

Treatment

Anterior dislocations of the hip are best managed with early closed reduction under spinal or general anesthesia. Open reduction is applied if attempts at closed reduction fail. Emergent referral for reduction is strongly recommended.

Posterior hip dislocations are best managed with immobilization and emergent referral for reduction within 24 hours.[17] If emergent referral is not available, closed reduction using the following method may be attempted (Fig. 21–18):

1. The patient should be placed on a backboard and given intravenous diazepam (Valium) and intramuscular meperidine (Demerol) for analgesia and skeletal muscle relaxation.
2. The patient should be lowered to the floor while on the backboard where an assistant immobilizes the pelvis as demonstrated in Figure 21–18A by holding the iliac crests down.
3. The physician then applies traction in line with the deformity along with gently flexing the hip to 90 degrees (Fig. 21–18B).
4. At this point gentle but firm pulling of the hip forward will result in reduction. If unsuccessful, reduction should be performed under general anesthesia.
5. The patient should be admitted for traction, strict non-weight bearing and observation (Fig. 21–19).

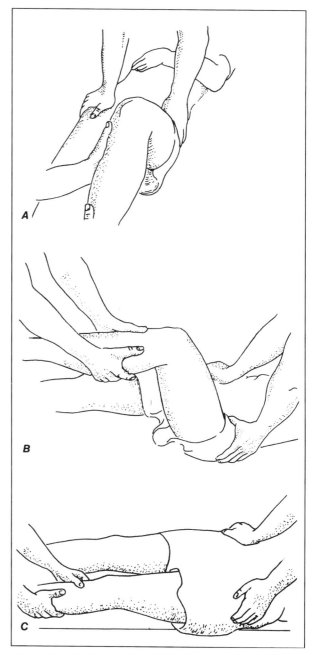

Figure 21–18. Technique for reducing a posterior hip dislocation.

Stimson's method of reducing posterior hip dislocations is shown in Figure 21–20. This method is also safe and effective, providing of course there is good skeletal muscle relaxation and analgesia. In those dislocations complicated by an acetabular fracture, an attempt at closed reduction is indicated. If the reduction is unstable, operative fixation is indicated. Some authors believe that operative reduction and fixation provide better results with posterior hip fracture–dislocations; therefore early consultation is recommended. Whichever

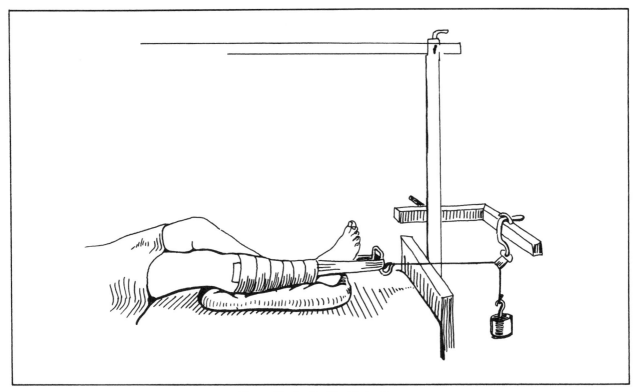

Figure 21–19. Buck's skin traction.

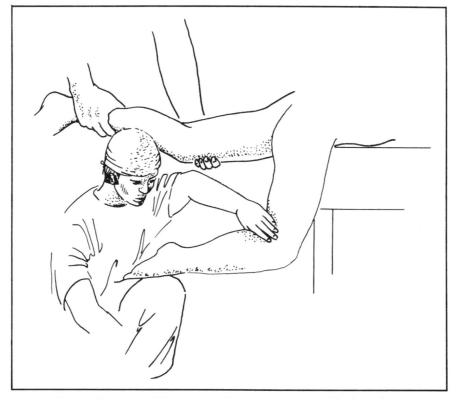

Figure 21–20. The Stimson method for reducing posterior hip dislocation.

technique is applied for anterior or posterior dislocations, it is mandatory to evaluate the femoral arterial pulse before and after the reduction.

Complications

Hip dislocations are associated with several significant complications. In one study in which follow-up of traumatic posterior dislocations of the hip for an average of 12 $\frac{1}{2}$ years was undertaken, it was found that even with simple dislocations, 24 percent of the patients had poor results and up to 70 percent of the patients had fair to poor results. It is clear that even with simple posterior dislocations of the hip treated properly, late osteoarthritis may develop in as many as 20 percent of cases. Thus, posterior dislocations of the hip have a very guarded prognosis.

1. Avascular necrosis of the femoral head occurs in 15 percent of patients 17 months to 2 years after injury.[27] The incidence increases to 48 percent if reduction is delayed.[20]
2. Sciatic nerve contusion, laceration, or traction injuries may complicate the management of posterior dislocations.[24] Early diagnosis and management often result in a reduction in the morbidity associated with this complication.
3. Traumatic arthritis may complicate the management of these fractures years after the initial injury.[50]

REFERENCES

1. Adams JC: *Outline of Fractures Including Joint Injuries.* Baltimore: Williams and Wilkkins, 1972.
2. Aronsson DD, Carlson WE: Slipped capital femoral epiphysis. *J Bone Joint Surg* **74A**(6):810, 1992.
3. Aronsson DD, Loder RT: Treatment of the unstable acute slipped capital femoral epiphysis. *Clin Orthop Rel Res* **322**:99–110, 1996.
4. Beals RK: Epitomes: Important advances in clinical medicine. *Orthopedics* **81**:481–482, 1996.
5. Bleicher RJ, et al: Bilateral gluteal compartment syndrome. *J Trauma Injury, Infec Crit Care* **42**:1, 1997.
6. Brignall CG, Stainsby GD: The snapping hip: *J Bone Joint Surg* **73B**(2):253, 1991.
7. Brotherton BJ: Perthes disease treated by prolong recumbency and femoral head containment. *J Bone Joint Surg* **57**(8):620, 1975.
8. Brumback RJ, Ellison S, Molligan H, et al: Pudendal nerve palsy complicating intramedullary nailing of the femur. *J Bone Joint Surg* **74A**(10):1450, 1992.
9. Butcher JD, et al: Lower extremity bursitis. *Am Fam Phys* **53**:7, 1996.
10. Callahan DL: Causes of refusal to walk in childhood. *South Med J* **75**:20, 1982.
11. Causey AL, et al: Missed slipped capital femoral epiphysis: Illustrative cases and review. *J Emerg Med* **13**:175–189, 1995.
12. Clark SS, et al: Lower urinary tract injuries associated with pelvic fractures. *Surg Clin North Am* **52**:183, 1972.
13. Conolly WB, et al: Observations on fractures of the pelvis. *J Trauma* **9**:104, 1969.
14. Curtiss PH, et al: Destruction of articular cartilage in septic arthritis of the hip. *J Bone Joint Surg* **47**:1595, 1965.
15. Dawson I, Van Rijn ABB: Traumatic anterior dislocation of the hip. *Arch Orthop Trauma Surg* **108**(1):55, 1989.
16. Day WH: Contact pressures in the loaded human cadaver hip. *J Bone Joint Surg* **52**(3):210, 1970.
17. Divoenney JG: *Traite des maladies des Os*, vol I. Paris: De Biore L'Auire, 1751.
18. Edvardsen P, Siordahl J, Svennigsen S: Operative vs conservative treatment of Legg-Calvé-Perthes disease. *Acta Orthop Scand* **52**:553, 1981.
19. Fanciullo JJ, Bell Carolyn L: Stress fractures of the sacrum and lower extremity. *Curr Opinion Rheum* **8**:158–162, 1996.
20. Fina CP, et al: Dislocations of the hip with fractures of the proximal femur. *J Trauma* **10**:104, 1969.
21. Freeman MAR: The pathogenesis of Perthes disease. *J Bone Joint Surg* [Br] **58**(4):453, 1976.
22. Friedenberg ZB: Fracture of the hip. *J Trauma* **10**(1):51, 1974.
23. Gander RS: Reduction and fixation of subcapital fractures of the femur. *Orthop Clin North Am* **5**:683, 1974.
24. Gillespie WJ: The incidence and pattern of knee injury associated with dislocation of the hip. *J Bone Joint Surg* [Br] **57**(3):376, 1975.
25. Gopalakrishnan KC, Lewis J: Traumatic haemarthrosis causing femoral head subluxation. *J Bone Joint Surg* **72B**(4):554, 1990.
26. Gower WE, et al: Legg-Calvé-Perthes disease. *J Bone Joint Surg* **53**(4):759, 1971.
27. Griffin PP: Hip joint infections in infants and children. *J Bone Joint Surg* [Br] **9**(1):123, 1978.
28. Holt PD, Keats TE: Calcific tendinitis: A review of the usual and unusual. *Skeletal Radiol* **22**:1–9, 1993.
29. Hubbard AM, Dormans JP: Evaluation of developmental dysplasia, Perthes disease, and neuromuscular dysplasia of the hip in children before and after surgery: An imaging update. *AJR* **164**:1067–1073, 1995.
30. Hughes SS, Goldstein MN, Hicks DG, et al: Extrapelvic compression of the sciatic nerve. *J Bone Joint Surg* **74A**(10):1553, 1991.
31. Jackson DW: Quadriceps contusions in the young athlete. *J Bone Joint Surg* **55**(1):95, 1973.
32. Jeffreys A: Osteophytes and osteoarthritic femoral head. *J Bone Joint Surg* [Br] **52**(2):172, 1969.
33. Jensen OM, et al: Legg-Calvé-Perthes disease. *J Bone Joint Surg* [Br] **58**(3):332, 1976.
34. Jones D, et al: An assessment of the value of examination of the hip in the newborn. *J Bone Joint Surg* **53**(2):514, 1971.
35. Kamhi E: Treatment of Legg-Calvé-Perthes disease. *J Bone Joint Surg* **57**(5):651, 1975.
36. Loder RT: A worldwide study on the seasonal variation of slipped capital femoral epiphysis. *Clin Orthop Rel Res* **322**:28–36, 1996.

37. Martinez AG, Weinstein SL: Recurrent Legg-Calvé-Perthes disease *J Bone Joint Surg* **73A**(7):1081, 1991.
38. Meier MC, Meyer LC, Ferguson RL: Treatment of slipped capital femoral epiphysis with special cast. *J Bone Joint Surg* **74A**(10):1522, 1992.
39. Moran MC: Osteonecrosis of the hip in sickle cell hemoglobinopathy. *Am J Orthop* **24**(1):18–24, 1995.
40. Morey BF, et al: Suppurative arthritis of the hip in children. *J Bone Joint Surg* **58**(3):388, 1976.
41. Norris MA. De Smet A: Fractures and dislocations of the hip and femur. *Sem Roentgenol* **29**(2):100–112, 1994.
42. Ohzono K, Saito M, Takaoka K, et al: Natural history of non-traumatic avascular necrosis of the femoral head. *J Bone Joint Surg* **73B**(1):68, 1991.
43. Owen CA, et al: Gluteal compartment syndromes. *Clin Orthop* **132**:57, 1978.
44. Paletta GWA, Andrish JT: Injuries about the hip and pelvis in the young athlete. *Clin Sports Med* **14**:3, 1995.
45. Paterson DC: Acute suppurative arthritis in infancy and childhood. *J Bone Joint Surg* [Br] **52**:474, 1970.
46. Patterson D: Septic arthritis of the hip joint. *Orthop Clin North Am* **9**(1):135, 1978.
47. Rath E, et al: Bilateral dislocation of the hip during convultion: A case report. *J Bone Joint Surg* **79B**:2, 1997.
48. Robinson D, On E, Halperin N: Anterior compartment syndrome of the thigh in athletes: Indications for conservative treatment. *J Trauma* **32**(2):183, 1992.
49. Ryan JB, Wheeler JH, Hopkinson WJ, et al: Quadriceps contusions (West Point update). *Am J Sports Med* **19**(3):299, 1991.
50. Schlickewei W, et al: Hip dislocation without fracture: Traction or mobilization after reduction? *Injury* **24**(1):27–31, 1993.
51. Schmalzried TP, Neal WC, Eckardt JJ: Gluteal compartment and crush syndromes. *Clin Orthop* **277**:161, 1992.
52. Schroer WC: Current concepts on the pathogenesis of osteonecrosis of the femoral head. *Orthop Rev* **23**(6):487–497, 1994.
53. Shbeeb MI, Matteson EL: Trochanteric bursitis (greater trochanter pain syndrome). *Mayo Clin Proc* **71**:565–569, 1996.
54. Sports injury assessment and rehabilitation. Slipped capital femoral epiphysis (adolescent coxa vera). *Orthop Clin North Am* **24**:644, 1993.
55. Stewart JM, et al: Fracture dislocation of the hip. *J Bone Joint Surg* **36**:315, 1954.
56. Teitz CC, et al: Tendon problems in athletic individuals. *Sport Medicine* Chapter 55, (46):569–582, 1997.
57. Tischenko GJ, Goodman SB: Compartment syndrome after intramedullary nailing of tibia. *J Bone Joint Surg* **41**, 1990.
58. Umans H, Pavlov H: Stress of the lower extremities *Sem Roentgenol* **29**(2):176–193, 1994.
59. Ware HE, Brooks AP, Toye R, et al: Sikle cell disease and silent avascular necrosis of the hip. *J Bone Joint Surg* **73B**(6):947, 1991.
60. Wedge JH: The natural history of dislocation of the hip. *Clin Orthop* **137**:154, 1978.
61. Wells D, et al: Review of slipped capital femoral epiphysis associated with endocrine disease. *J Pediatr Orthop* **13**(5):610–614, 1993.
62. Wenger DR, Ward WT, Herring JA: Current concepts review Legg-Calvé-Perthes disease. *J Bone Joint Surg* **73A**(5):778, 1991.
63. Worrell TW: Factors associated with hamstring injuries. An approach to treatment and preventative measures. *Sports Med* **17**(5):338–345, 1994.
64. Zimmermann AM III, et al: Septic bursitis. *Sem Art Rheumatism* **24**(6):391–410, 1995.

BIBLIOGRAPHY

Baimes ST, et al: Pseudotumor of the ischimus. *J Bone Joint Surg* **58**:24, 1976.
Coley WB: Myositis ossificans traumatic. *Ann Surg* **57**:305, 1913.
Cruess RL: Cortisone-induced avascular necrosis of the femoral head. *J Bone Joint Surg* **52**(3):113, 1969.
Eisenberg KS, et al: Posterior dislocations of the hip producing lumbosacral nerve root avulsion. *J Bone Joint Surg* **54**:1083, 1972.
Epstein H: Traumatic dislocations of the hip. *Clin Orthop* **92**:116, 1973.
Epstein H: Posterior fracture dislocation of the hip. *J Bone Joint Surg* **56**(6):1103, 1974.
Hunter GA: Posterior dislocation and fracture dislocations of the hip. *J Bone Joint Surg* [Br] **51**:1, 1969.
Iversen LD, Clawson DK: *Manual of Acute Orthopedic Therapeutics*. Boston: Little, Brown, 1977.
Juclet R, et al: Fractures of the acetabulum. *J Bone Joint Surg* **46**:1615, 1964.
Kaufman G, et al: Ischemic necrosis of muscles of the buttocks. *J Bone Joint Surg* **54**(5):1079, 1973.
Rockwood CA, Green DP: *Fractures*, vol 2. Philadelphia: Lippincott, 1975.
Rowe CR, et al: Prognosis of fractures of the acetabulum. *J Bone Joint Surg* **43**:30, 1961.
Thompson VP, et al: Traumatic dislocations of the hip. *J Bone Joint Surg* **33**:746, 1951.
Tipton WW, et al: Non-operative management of central & fracture dislocations of the hip. *J Bone Joint Surg* **57**(7):888, 1975.

22
CHAPTER

FRACTURES OF THE DISTAL FEMUR

Distal femoral fractures are uncommon injuries.[1] These fractures may be divided into four types on the basis of anatomy (Fig. 22–1). Type I supracondylar fractures involve the area between the femoral condyles and the junction of the metaphysis with the femoral shaft. These fractures are extra-articular and therefore not associated with knee joint distention. The remaining fracture types are intra-articular and include condylar, intercondylar, and epiphyseal injuries.

The musculature surrounding the distal femur is often responsible for fragment displacement after a distal femoral fracture. The quadriceps extends along the anterior surface of the femur and inserts on the anterior–superior tibia (Fig. 22–2). After a distal femoral fracture this muscle tends to pull the tibia and the attached distal fragment in an anterior–superior direction. The hamstrings extend along the posterior surface of the tibia and insert on the posterior–superior tibia. This muscle tends to displace the tibia and the distal fragment in a posterior–superior direction. The gastrocnemius and the soleus insert on the posterior distal femur and provide for inferior displacement after a fracture. The typical combined effect of these muscles is posterior–superior displacement as shown in Figure 22–2.

It is important to recall the close proximity to the distal femur of the popliteal artery and vein along with the tibial and common peroneal nerves.

Distal femoral epiphyseal fractures are uncommon but serious injuries, which occur typically in children older than 10 years of age.[1,2] In children, 65 percent of the longitudinal growth of the lower extremity occurs around the knee and primarily the distal femoral epiphysis.[2] Leg shortening despite the maintenance of an anatomic reduction is common after these injuries occurring in 25 percent of Salter type II injuries.[11] A Salter

type II injury is the most common type of distal femoral epiphyseal fracture and the poor prognosis is in contradistinction to the generally favorable prognosis associated with Salter type I and II injuries in most other joints which have a good prognosis.[3,6,11]

The classification system divides femoral fractures into four types.[1,8]

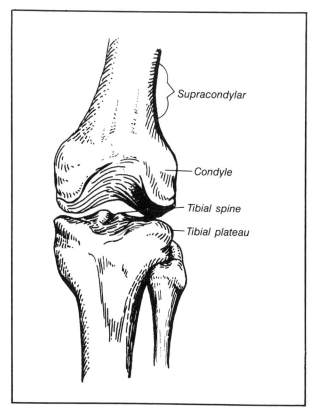

Figure 22–1. The anterior view of the knee. Note the supracondylar and condylar regions.

□ Class A:	Supracondylar fractures	(Fig. 22−3)		□ Class D:	Distal femoral epiphyseal	(Fig. 22−6)
□ Class B:	Intercondylar fractures	(Fig. 22−4)			fractures	
□ Class C:	Condylar fractures	(Fig. 22−5)				

Mechanism of Injury

Most of these fractures are secondary to direct trauma or have a component of direct force. Typical mechanisms include automobile accidents and falls. Condylar fractures are typically secondary to a combination of hyperabduction or adduction with direct trauma. Distal femoral epiphyseal fractures are usually secondary to a medial or lateral blow resulting in fracture of the weaker epiphysis rather than the metaphysis.[3] Another common mechanism involves hyperextension and torsion of the knee.

Examination

The patient with a distal femoral fracture will present with pain, swelling, and deformity of the involved extremity. There may be palpable crepitus or bone fragments within the popliteal space.[3] Displaced supracondylar fractures typically present with leg shortening and external rotation of the femoral shaft. It is essential that the neurovascular status of the involved extremity

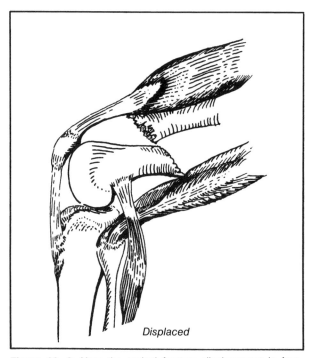

Figure 22−2. Note the typical fracture displacement in fractures of the supracondylar region of the distal femur. This displacement is caused by the traction of the hamstrings and quadriceps muscles in one direction and the traction of the gastrocnemius muscle on the distal fragment, producing posterior angulation and displacement.

DISTAL FEMORAL FRACTURES

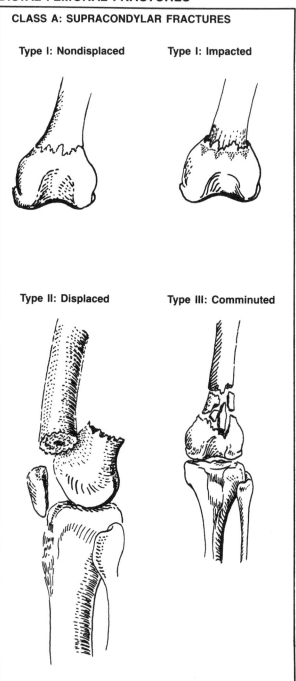

Figure 22−3.

be documented early in the patient assessment. Neurovascular injuries are uncommon but they may be devastating if uncorrected. The web space between the

DISTAL FEMORAL FRACTURES

CLASS B: INTERCONDYLAR FRACTURES

Type I: Nondisplaced (T or Y fractures)

Type II: Displaced

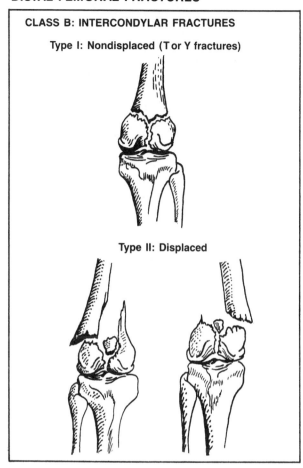

Figure 22-4.

DISTAL FEMORAL FRACTURES

CLASS C: CONDYLAR FRACTURES
Type I: Nondisplaced (AP view)   Type II: Displaced (AP view)

Type II: Coronal (lateral view)   Type III: Both condyles (AP view)

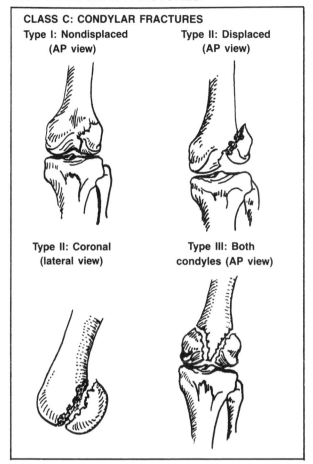

Figure 22-5.

first and second toe innervated by the deep peroneal nerve should be examined. Distal pulses should be examined and their absence documented. Distal capillary filling may persist despite an arterial injury secondary to an abundant collateral supply.[3] Examine the popliteal space carefully for a pulsatile hematoma indicating an arterial injury.

X Ray (Fig. 22-7)
Antero-posterior (AP) and lateral views are usually adequate in demonstrating the fracture. Radiographs of the entire femur and hip should be obtained. Oblique, tangential, and comparison views may be necessary for accurately diagnosing a small condylar fracture. Comparison views should be obtained in all children less than 10 years of age.[2] Distal femoral epiphyseal injuries may require valgus and varus stress views to differentiate a ligamentous injury from an epiphyseal fracture.

Associated Injuries
Distal femoral fractures may be associated with the following:

DISTAL FEMORAL FRACTURES

CLASS D: DISTAL FEMORAL EPIPHYSEAL FRACTURES

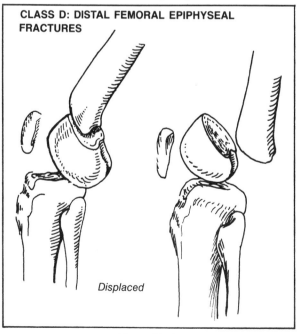

Displaced

Figure 22-6.

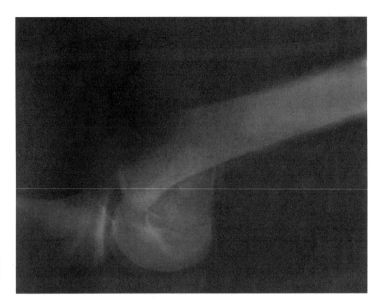

Figure 22–7. Displaced type II supracondylar fracture of the distal femur.

1. Ipsilateral hip fracture or dislocation
2. Vascular injury[1–3]
3. Peroneal nerve injury
4. Damage to the quadriceps apparatus

Treatment

The emergency department management of these fractures includes immobilization, analgesics, and emergent referral. The definitive treatment of these fractures varies from open reduction with internal fixation to cast immobilization depending on the type of fracture, the amount of displacement, and the success of reduction. Displaced fractures may be reduced surgically or by using skeletal traction as shown in Figures 22–8 and 22–9. After skeletal traction reduction, many authors prefer to use a cast-brace for immobilization as this permits early ambulation and knee motion.[7,10]

A relatively recent development in the treatment of fractures around the knee is the hinged cast-brace. This provides safe and reliable means of treating distal femoral fractures. It combines the advantages of nonoperative management with early mobilization.[12]

☐ CLASS A: SUPRACONDYLAR FRACTURES

☐ Class A: Type I (Nondisplaced or Impacted)

Nondisplaced fractures can be managed utilizing traction (Figs. 22–8 and 22–9), casting, or a cast-brace. Early stable joint mobilization is imperative in order to prevent cartilage deterioration, adhesions, and subsequent joint stiffness. The nonsurgical management of these fractures frequently does not allow for early mobilization. For this reason, many surgeons prefer early surgical management of these fractures.[5,9]

☐ Class A: Type II (Displaced)

These fractures are typically treated with operative reduction and internal fixation.

☐ Class A: Type III (Comminuted)

The treatment varies from open reduction and internal fixation to skeletal traction depending on the degree of comminution.

☐ CLASS B: INTERCONDYLAR FRACTURES

☐ Class B: Type I (Nondisplaced)

These intra-articular fractures require that all rotation and angulation be corrected early.

☐ Class B: Type II (Displaced)

This intra-articular fracture requires accurate reduction.

☐ CLASS C: CONDYLAR FRACTURES

☐ Class C: Type I (Nondisplaced)

These injuries may be managed with a cast, cast brace, spica, skeletal traction, or internal fixation depending on the size of the fragment and the preference of the surgeon.

☐ Class C: Type II (Displaced)

Most surgeons prefer operative management with internal fixation of these fractures.[5]

☐ Class C: Type III (Both Condyles)

The recommended therapy is open reduction with internal fixation. If the fragments are small, closed treatment may be preferred.[5]

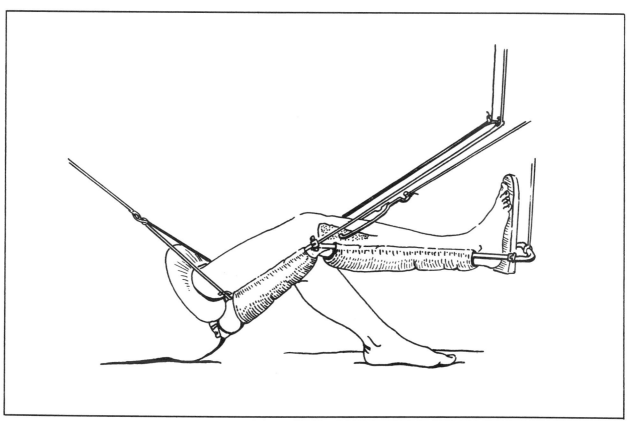

Figure 22-8. Skeletal traction is shown through the proximal tibia.

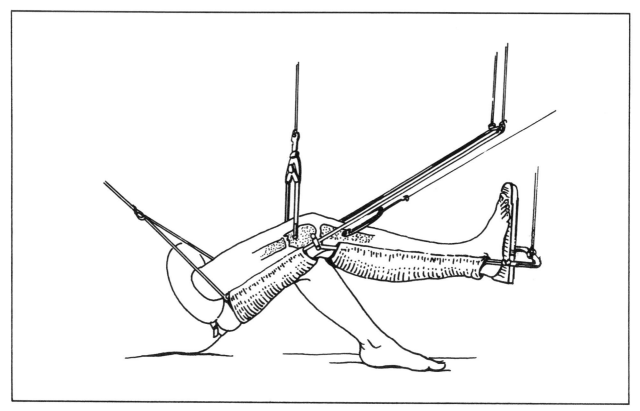

Figure 22-9. Two-pin traction is shown with one pin through the proximal tibia and another pin distal to the fracture site through the distal femur.

☐ CLASS D: DISTAL FEMORAL EPIPHYSEAL FRACTURES

Thirty-six percent of these fractures present with a valgus or varus deformity of 5 degrees or more. Medial or lateral displacement is a more difficult management problem than is anterior or posterior displacement. Displaced fractures are usually managed with manipulation under general anesthesia followed by traction. Maintaining an anatomic reduction is very important. Associated physeal fractures (Salter-Harris type II) may be managed with the judicious use of internal fixation screws in order to maintain an anatomic reduction.[4]

Complications

Distal femoral fractures are associated with several significant complications.

1. The development of thrombophlebitis or fat embolism may complicate the management of these fractures.
2. Delayed union or malunion may occur if reduction is incomplete or not maintained.
3. Intra-articular fractures may develop intra-articular or quadriceps adhesions or valgus/varus angulation deformities.
4. Intra-articular fractures may be complicated by the development of arthritis.
5. Femoral epiphyseal fractures are often followed by a growth disturbance in the involved extremity.

REFERENCES

1. Brown RB: Fractures about the knee. *Surg Clin North Am* **20:**1763, 1940.
2. Crawford AH: Fractures about the knee in children. *Orthop Clin North Am* **7**(3):639, 1976.
3. Ehrlich MG, et al: Epiphyseal injuries about the knee. *Orthop Clin North Am* **10**(1):91, 1979.
4. Graham JM, Gross RH: Distal femoral physeal problem fractures. *Clin Orthop* **6:**51–53, 1990.
5. Leung KS, Shen WY, So WS, Mui LT, Gross A: Interlocking intramedullary nailing for supracondylar and intercondylar fractures of the distal part of the femur. *J Bone Joint Surg* **3:**332–340, 1991.
6. Lombargo SJ, et al: Fractures of the distal femoral epiphysis. *J Bone Joint Surg* **59A**(6):742, 1977.
7. Moll J: The cast brace walking treatment of open and closed femur fractures. *South Med J* **66:**345, 1973.
8. Neer CS, et al: Supracondylar fractures of the femur in adults. *J Bone Joint Surg* **49:**591, 1973.
9. Newman JH: Supracondylar fractures of the femur. *Injury* **21**(9):280–282, 1990.
10. Rockford CA, et al: Experience with quadrilateral cast brace. *J Bone Joint Surg* **55:**421, 1973.
11. Stephens DC, et al: Traumatic separation of the distal femoral epiphyseal cartilage plate. *J Bone Joint Surg* **56**(7): 1383, 1974.
12. Thomas TL, Meggitt BF: A comparative study of methods for treating fractures of the distal half of the femur. *J Bone Joint Surg* **63B:**3, 1981.

BIBLIOGRAPHY

Criswell AR, et al: Abduction injuries of the distal femoral epiphysis. *Clin Orthop* **115:**184, 1976.

Elliot RB: Fractures of the femoral condyles. *South Med J* **52:**80, 1959.

Holt EP: Blade-plate internal fixation of supracondylar fractures of the femur. *South Med J* **52:**1331, 1959.

Hoover NW: Injuries of the popliteal artery associated with fractures and dislocations. *Surg Clin North Am* **41:**1099, 1961.

Klingensmith WOP, et al: Arterial injuries associated with dislocation of the knee or fracture of the lower femur. *Surg Gynecol Obstet* **120:**961, 1965.

Neer CS, et al: Supracondylar fractures of the femur. *J Bone Joint Surg* **49:**591, 1973.

Stewart MN, et al: Fractures of the distal third of the femur. *J Bone Joint Surg* **48:**784, 1966.

White EH, et al: Supracondylar fractures of the femur treated by internal fixation with immediate knee motion. *Am Surg* **22:**801, 1956.

Zimmerman AJ: Intraarticular fractures of the distal femur. *Orthop Clin North Am* **10**(1):75, 1979.

23
CHAPTER

FRACTURES OF THE PROXIMAL TIBIA AND FIBULA

PROXIMAL TIBIAL FRACTURES

CLASS A: CONDYLAR FRACTURES
(p. 434)

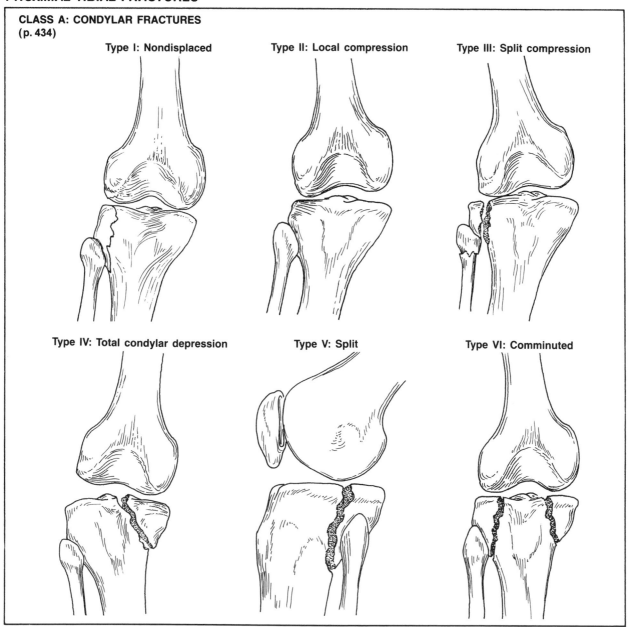

Type I: Nondisplaced　　Type II: Local compression　　Type III: Split compression

Type IV: Total condylar depression　　Type V: Split　　Type VI: Comminuted

CLASS B: SPINE FRACTURES
(p. 437)

Type I: Incomplete avulsion without displacement

Type II: Displaced incomplete avulsion

Type III: Complete

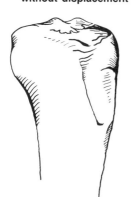
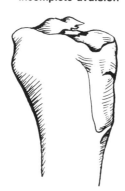
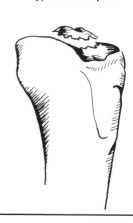

CLASS C: TUBEROSITY FRACTURES
(p. 438)

Type I: Incomplete avulsion

Type II: Complete avulsion extra-articular

Type III: Complete avulsion intra-articular

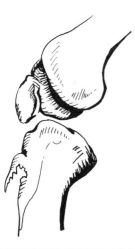
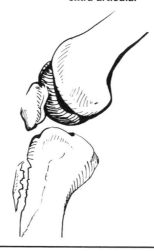
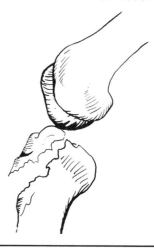

CLASS D: SUBCONDYLAR FRACTURES
(p. 439)

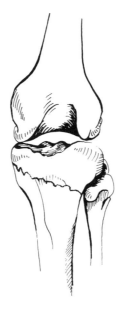

(p. 440)

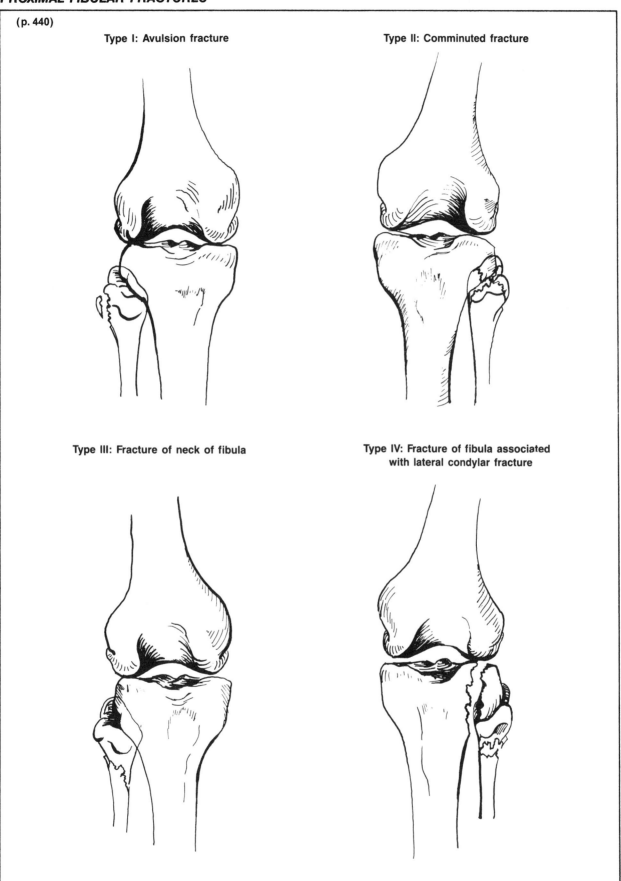

Type I: Avulsion fracture

Type II: Comminuted fracture

Type III: Fracture of neck of fibula

Type IV: Fracture of fibula associated with lateral condylar fracture

Proximal tibial fractures include those fractures above the tibial tuberosity. These fractures can be divided into extra-articular or articular injuries. Articular fractures include the condylar injuries whereas extra-articular injuries include tibial spine, tubercle, and subcondylar fractures. Tibial epiphyseal fractures are considered intra-articular. Proximal fibular fractures are relatively unimportant as no weight is supported by the fibula. Fibular fractures are discussed at the end of this section.

Essential Anatomy
The medial and lateral tibial condyles form a plateau that transmits the weight of the body from the femoral condyles to the tibial shafts. Condylar fractures typically are associated with some degree of depression secondary to the axillary transmission of the body's weight. Condylar depression will then result in a valgus or varus strain on the knee.

As shown in Figure 23–1 the intercondylar eminence includes the tibial spines, which provide the attachment site for the cruciates and the semilunar cartilages.

Classification
Proximal tibial fractures may be divided into five categories on the basis of anatomy.

PROXIMAL TIBIAL FRACTURES

☐ Class A: Condylar fractures   (Fig. 23–2)
☐ Class B: Spine fractures   (Fig. 23–7)
☐ Class C: Tuberosity fractures   (Fig. 23–8)
☐ Class D: Subcondylar fractures   (Fig. 23–9)
☐ Class E: Epiphyseal fractures   (Not shown)

PROXIMAL FIBULAR FRACTURES   (Fig. 23–10)

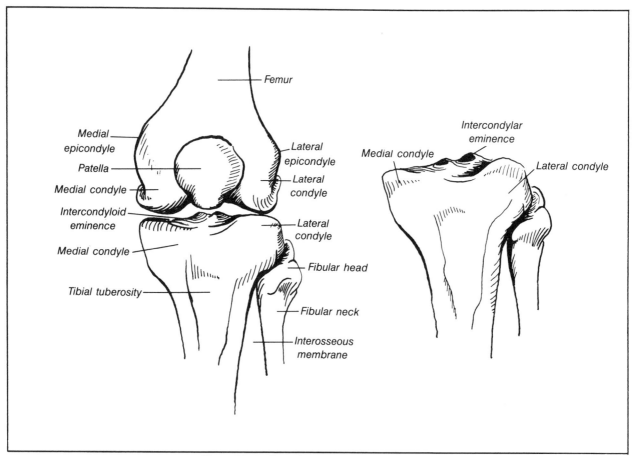

Figure 23–1. Essential bony anatomy of the knee.

PROXIMAL TIBIAL FRACTURES

☐ CLASS A: CONDYLAR FRACTURES (FIG. 23–2)

These fractures are commonly seen and were classified by Hohl on the basis of anatomy and therapy.[6] In discussing tibial condylar fractures, depression indicates more than 4 mm of inferior displacement.

Serious knock-knee deformity may result from innocent appearing fractures of the proximal tibia in children. The cause is obscure. It occurs in children less than 4 years of age and presents genu valgum deformity between 6 and 15 months later. This deformity seems to occur primarily because of bowing of the tibial shaft below the fracture site. Thus, the emergency physician should refer all proximal tibial fractures to an orthopedic specialist for follow-up.

Insufficiency fractures of the tibial condyles occur in elderly people. The initial x rays are normal; however, the patient continues to have pain, particularly in the medial condyle. These are fatigue fractures, and when one suspects them a scan should be ordered.

Mechanism of Injury

The forces that normally act on the tibial plateau include axial compression and rotation. Fractures result when these forces exceed the strength of the bone.

A direct mechanism, such as a fall from a height, is responsible for approximately 20 percent of condylar fractures.[1] Automobile-pedestrian accidents where the car bumper strikes the patient over the proximal tibia are responsible for approximately 50 percent of these fractures.[1] The remainder of the fractures result from a combination of axial compression and rotational strain. Fractures of the lateral tibial plateau usually result from an abduction force on the leg. Medial plateau fractures typically result from adduction forces on the distal leg. If the knee is extended at the time of injury, the fracture tends to be anterior. Posterior condylar fractures usually follow injuries where the knee was flexed at the time of impact.

Examination

The patient will usually present with a chief complaint of pain and swelling with the knee slightly flexed. On examination, there frequently is an abrasion indicating the point of impact along with an effusion and reduced range of motion secondary to pain. A valgus or varus deformity usually indicates a depressed fracture. Stress radiographs may be necessary following plain views to diagnose occult ligamentous or meniscal injuries.

X Ray

Antero-posterior (AP), lateral, and oblique views are usually adequate for demonstrating these fractures. In addition, a *tibial plateau view*, as shown in Figure 23–3, is very helpful in assessing the amount of depression.[9] Anatomically, the tibial plateau slopes from anterior superiorly to posterior inferiorly. Routine AP views do not detect this slope and may mask some depression fractures. The tibial plateau view compensates for this slope and allows a more accurate estimation of depressed tibial plateau fractures. Oblique views of the knee are always helpful in determining the extent of the fracture.

All knee radiographs should be examined closely for bony avulsion fragments from the fibular head, femoral condyles, and intercondylar eminence indicating ligamentous injury. Widened joint spaces associated with a fracture of the opposite condyle may indicate a ligamentous injury.[7] Tomograms may be necessary for the detection of occult compression fractures. Computed tomography (CT) scanning or magnetic resonance imaging (MRI), or both, are frequently utilized to determine the full extent of the injury.[13]

Associated Injuries

Tibial condylar fractures are associated frequently with several significant knee injuries.

1. Ligamentous or meniscal injuries or both frequently accompany these fractures.[2] With a lateral condylar fracture, tibial collateral ligament, anterior cruciate, and lateral meniscal injuries should be suspected. With a medial condylar fracture, fibular collateral ligament, cruciate, and medial meniscal injuries should be suspected.
2. Vascular injuries either acute or delayed in presentation may be seen after these fractures.

Treatment

The four most common treatment modalities include compressive dressing, closed reduction and casting, skeletal traction, and open reduction with internal fixation.[1] Regardless of which therapy is selected the therapeutic goals are:

1. To restore the articular surface to normal
2. To begin early knee motion to prevent stiffness
3. To delay weight bearing until healing is complete.

The therapeutic modality selected is dependent on the type of fracture, the past experiences and training of

PROXIMAL TIBIAL FRACTURES

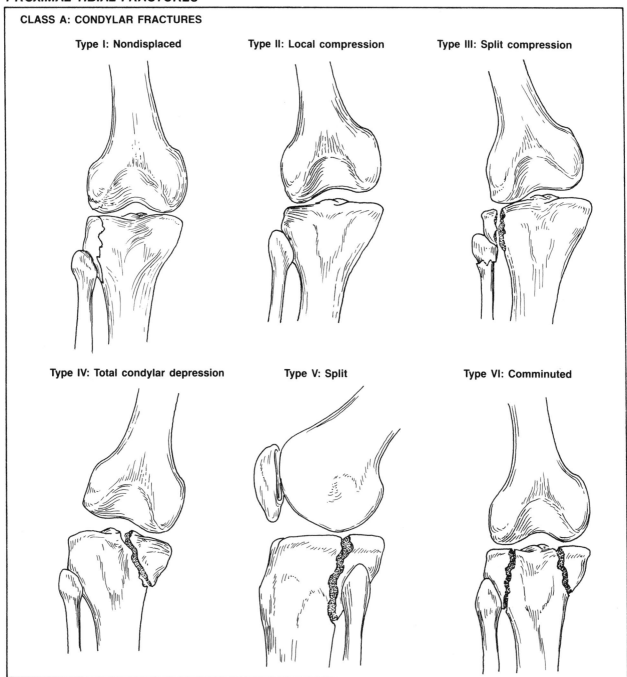

Figure 23–2.

the orthopedic surgeon, and the age and reliability of the patient. Early consultation with an orthopedic surgeon is recommended strongly.

☐ Class A: Type I   (Nondisplaced)

In the reliable, otherwise ambulatory, patient with no associated ligamentous injuries, this fracture can be managed with aspiration of the hemarthrosis followed by the application of a compressive dressing with ice and eleva-

tion for a minimum of 48 hours.[1,11] If after 48 hours the radiographs remain unchanged, knee motion and quadriceps exercises can be started. The patient should not bear weight until healing is complete. At this point partial weight bearing with crutch ambulation or the use of a cast-brace device may be used.[1] Casting at the time of injury for 4 to 8 weeks is not advocated in the reliable patient because of the high incidence of knee stiffness.[1,11] If the patient is otherwise ambulatory and has no liga-

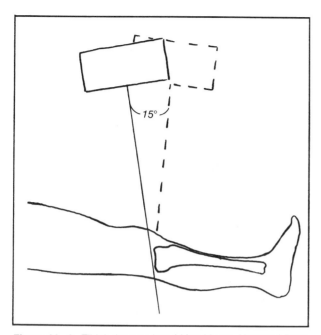

Figure 23-3. Tibial plateau view. (*After Moore, Harvey:* J Bone Joint Surg *56:155, 1974.*)

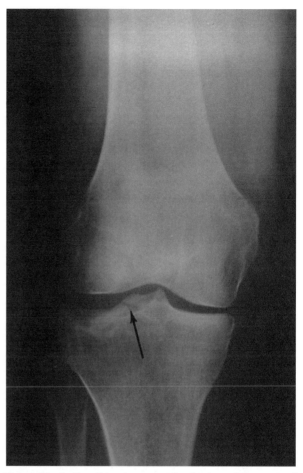

Figure 23-4. Type II local compression fracture of the proximal tibia involving the lateral plateau.

mentous injuries but is unreliable, casting is the recommended mode of therapy. Active quadriceps exercises (isometric) should be initiated early and the cast should remain in place until healing is complete. Nonambulatory patients without ligamentous injuries are usually treated with traction and early motion exercises.[11]

□ Class A: Type II (Local Compression) (Fig. 23-4)

The emergency management of these fractures is dependent on the following points:

1. A depression of 3 mm or more with greater than 20 percent of the articular surface requires immediate referral for consideration of surgical repair[3,14]
2. The location of the depression, as anterior or middle injuries are more ominous than are posterior fractures
3. The presence of associated ligamentous injuries

The assessment of these fractures requires a tibial plateau view and stress tests of the ligaments surrounding the knee. If the ligaments are damaged, operative repair is indicated. Conservative therapy for nondisplaced fractures without ligamentous injuries includes:

1. Aspiration of the hemarthrosis
2. A compression dressing or posterior splint for several days to 3 weeks with non-weight bearing
3. Early consultation

If the patient is nonambulatory, Buck's traction with active motion exercises are recommended.

□ Class A: Type III (Split Compression) (Fig. 23-5)

The emergency management of these fractures includes ice, immobilization in a posterior splint, and accurate radiographic assessment with emergent referral. The therapy frequently involves operative fragment elevation and stabilization.[3] Cast immobilization with non-weight bearing may be utilized in selected poor risk patients.[1,11]

□ Class A: Type IV (Total Condylar Depression)

The emergency management of these fractures includes ice, immobilization, and accurate radiographic assessment with early referral. Fractures depressed 3 mm or more are considered significantly displaced and require emergent orthopedic referral.[3]

□ Class A: Type V (Split)

These fractures usually involve the medial condyle and may be anterior or posterior. Open reduction with internal fixation is the recommended therapy.

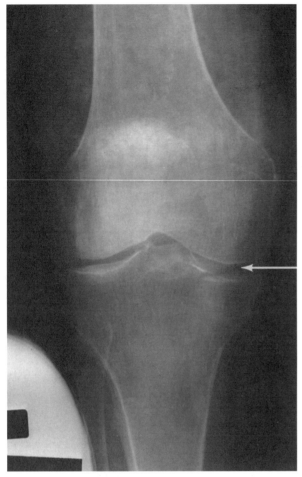

Figure 23–5. Type III split compression fracture of the proximal tibia involving the medial plateau.

☐ Class A: Type VI (Comminuted) (Fig. 23–6)

The emergency management of these fractures includes ice, elevation, immobilization in a posterior splint, and emergent referral for operative repair.[3]

Complications

Tibial condylar fractures may be followed by the development of several significant complications.

1. Loss of full knee motion may follow prolonged immobilization.[1]
2. Degenerative arthritis may develop despite optimum therapy.[2]
3. Angular deformity of the knee may develop in the first several weeks even with initially nondisplaced fractures.
4. Knee instability or persistent subluxation secondary to ligamentous damage may complicate these injuries.
5. Infection may complicate the course of open fractures or those treated surgically.

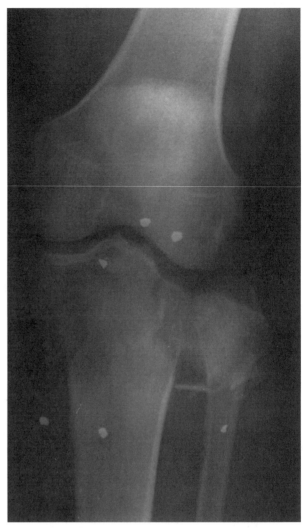

Figure 23–6. Comminuted fracture of the proximal tibia and fibula.

6. Neurovascular injuries are usually the result of compartment syndromes and may complicate the management of these fractures.

☐ CLASS B: SPINE FRACTURES (FIG. 23–7)

Isolated tibial spine fractures are uncommon injuries. Typically these fractures result in damage to the cruciate ligaments. The classification of these fractures is based on the system developed by Meyers and McKeever.[8]

- **Type I:** Incomplete avulsions of the tibial spine without displacement
- **Type II:** Displaced incomplete avulsions of the tibial spine
- **Type III:** Complete fractures of the tibial spine

PROXIMAL TIBIAL FRACTURES

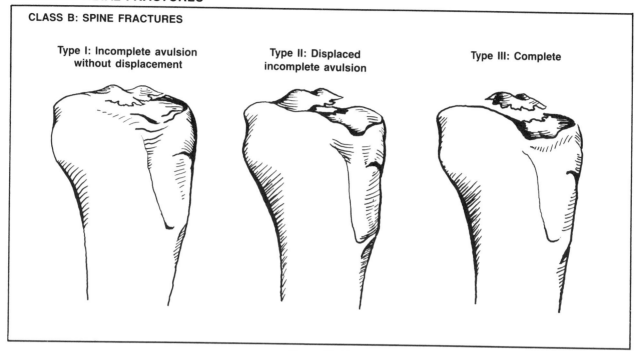

CLASS B: SPINE FRACTURES

Type I: Incomplete avulsion without displacement

Type II: Displaced incomplete avulsion

Type III: Complete

Figure 23–7.

Mechanisms of Injury

Tibial spine fractures are the result of indirect trauma such as with an anterior or posterior force directed against the flexed proximal tibia resulting in cruciate tension and avulsion of the spine. Hyperextension or violent abduction, adduction, or rotational forces may also result in fractures.

Examination

The patient will usually present with a suggestive history and a painful swollen knee. On examination there will be an effusion, a block to full extension, and a positive drawer sign in most patients. Surrounding muscle spasm may prevent an accurate assessment of the drawer sign. The remaining ligaments surrounding the knee should be examined carefully to exclude associated injuries.

X Ray

Routine radiographs including a tunnel view are usually adequate in defining the fracture. CT scanning or MRI, or both often used to determine the full extent of the injury.

Associated Injuries

Collateral and cruciate ligamentous injuries are commonly associated with these fractures.

Treatment

The therapeutic objectives include joint stability and the early restoration of motion. Early orthopedic consultation is recommended.

☐ Class B: Type I   (Incomplete Avulsion without Displacement)
            Type II   (Displaced Incomplete Avulsion)

These fractures can be reduced with closed manipulation, which should then be followed by cast immobilization in full extension for 4 to 6 weeks. Closed treatment is not indicated when there are associated ligamentous injuries.

☐ Class B: Type III   (Complete)

Operative therapy for these fractures is indicated.[15] In addition, type I and II fractures that are inadequately reduced with closed manipulation or are associated with ligamentous damage should be treated operatively.

Complications

The most frequent complication after this fracture is persistent pain and instability in the AP plane of the knee.

☐ CLASS C: TUBEROSITY FRACTURES (FIG. 23–8)

These are uncommon fractures most often seen in young patients.[5] The tibial tubercle is the insertion point of the quadriceps mechanism and accurate reduction with healing is essential. These fractures may be classified into three types.[5]

PROXIMAL TIBIAL FRACTURES

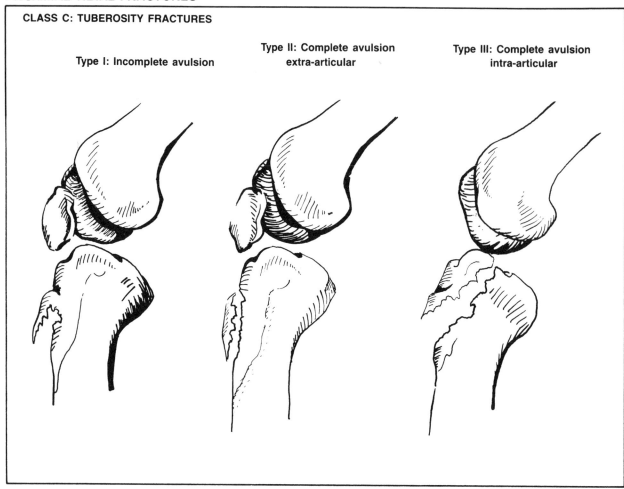

CLASS C: TUBEROSITY FRACTURES

Type I: Incomplete avulsion   Type II: Complete avulsion extra-articular   Type III: Complete avulsion intra-articular

Figure 23–8.

- **Type I:** Incomplete avulsion of the tibial tubercle
- **Type II:** Complete avulsion extra-articular of the tibial tubercle
- **Type III:** Complete avulsion with intra-articular extension of the tubercle fragment

Mechanism of Injury

The mechanism of injury is indirect as described by Hand et al.[5] With the knee in flexion and the quadriceps tightly contracted, a sudden flexion force is applied to the joint. The tightly contracted quadriceps resists this force and avulses the tibial tubercle.

Examination

The patient will present with pain that is exacerbated with attempted extension. Patients with incomplete or complete fractures may retain some degree of active extension as the patellar retinaculum usually remains intact.

X Ray

Routine radiographs are usually adequate in demonstrating the fracture. In young patients, comparison views may be necessary when a type I injury is suspected. CT scanning or MRI, or both are frequently utilized to determine the full extent of the injury.

Associated Injuries

A tear of the patellar retinaculum including avulsion of the patellar ligament may be associated with these fractures.[4]

Treatment

The emergency management of these fractures includes ice, immobilization, and emergent orthopedic consultation as operative repair is often necessary.

Complications

Most of these fractures heal without complications. Secondary postoperative displacement may follow inadequate immobilization or surgical fixation.

☐ CLASS D: SUBCONDYLAR FRACTURES (FIG. 23–9)

This fracture involves the proximal tibial metaphysis and typically is transverse or oblique. The fracture line may extend into the knee joint.

Mechanism of Injury
The fracture mechanism involves a rotational or angular stress accompanied by vertical compression.

Examination
The patient will present with tenderness and swelling over the involved area. A hemarthrosis may indicate extension of the fracture line into the joint.

X Ray
Routine views are usually adequate in demonstrating this fracture. CT scanning or MRI, or both, are often used to determine the full extent of the injury.

Associated Injuries
Tibial condylar fractures are frequently associated with these injuries.

Treatment
The emergency management of these fractures includes ice, immobilization in a posterior splint, and early consultation. Stable extra-articular nondisplaced transverse fractures are usually treated with a long leg cast for 8 weeks. Comminuted fractures or those associated with a condylar component require open reduction and internal fixation or are treated with traction.

Complications
Subcondylar fractures are frequently associated with condylar injuries and are thus subject to similar complications. The reader is referred to the section on condylar fractures for a review of these complications.

☐ CLASS E: EPIPHYSEAL FRACTURES

These are uncommon injuries and are seen less frequently than are distal femoral or tibial tubercle epiphyseal fractures.

Mechanism of Injury
These injuries usually result from a severe valgus or varus strain on the knee.

Examination
The patient will present with pain and deformity of the knee. On examination, angulation is usually evident. Knee effusions are usually not seen with this fracture.

X Ray
Most of these fractures are Salter-Harris type II injuries and require comparison views for an accurate diagnosis. CT scanning or MRI, or both, are frequently utilized to determine the full extent of the injury.

Associated Injuries
These fractures are only infrequently associated with ligamentous or meniscal injuries.

Treatment
The emergency management of these fractures includes ice, immobilization in a posterior splint, and early orthopedic consultation for reduction. After reduction most patients are immobilized in a long leg cast for 6 weeks.

Complications
Growth abnormalities may follow proximal tibial epiphyseal fractures.

PROXIMAL TIBIAL FRACTURES

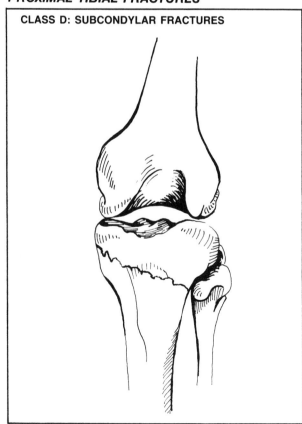

CLASS D: SUBCONDYLAR FRACTURES

Figure 23–9.

PROXIMAL FIBULAR FRACTURES

PROXIMAL FIBULAR FRACTURES

Type I: Avulsion fracture

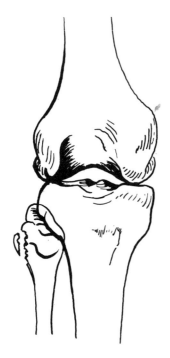

Type II: Comminuted fracture

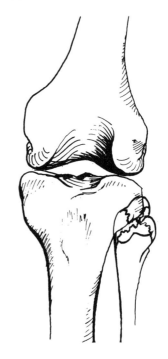

Type III: Fracture of neck of fibula

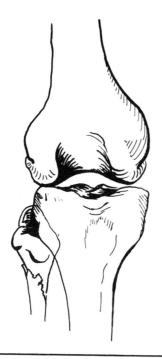

Type IV: Fracture of fibula associated with lateral condylar fracture

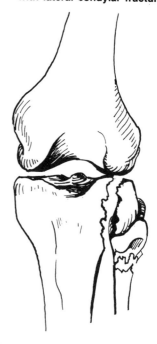

Figure 23–10.

Isolated proximal fibular fractures are relatively unimportant as no weight is supported by the fibula. These fractures are significant in that they are frequently associated with other more serious knee injuries.

Axiom: *Proximal fibular fractures should be considered indicative of a significant knee injury until proven otherwise.*

Figure 23–10 categorizes several of the types of fibular fractures.

Mechanism of Injury
There are two mechanisms that result in fractures of the proximal fibula. A direct blow over the fibular head may result in a comminuted fracture. An indirect varus stress to the knee may result in an avulsion fracture of the fibular head. A valgus strain on the knee may result in a tibial condylar fracture associated with a proximal fibular fracture.

Examination
The patient will present with pain and tenderness over the fracture site. It is essential that the knee and distal leg and foot be thoroughly examined to exclude associated serious neurovascular or ligamentous injuries.

Associated Injuries
As mentioned earlier, proximal fibular fractures may be associated with several serious neurovascular or ligamentous injuries.

1. The common peroneal nerve may be contused or lacerated at the time of injury. Most orthopedic surgeons will follow these injuries and repair them later if function does not return.[10,12]
2. The lateral collateral ligament may be ruptured or strained at the time of injury.
3. Anterior tibial arterial injury with thrombosis may be associated with these fractures.

Treatment
The emergency management of these fractures includes ice, analgesics, and thorough evaluation and exclusion of serious occult associated injuries. Isolated fibular fractures are treated symptomatically.

Complications
Injuries associated with proximal fibular fractures are responsible for the majority of complications seen with this fracture.

REFERENCES

1. Apley GA: Fractures of the tibial plateau. *Orthop Clin North Am* **10**(1):61, 1979.
2. Brodetti A: An experimental study on the use if the nails and bolt screws in the fixation of fractures of the femoral neck. *Acta Orthop Scand* **31**:247, 1961.
3. Dirschl DR, Dahners LE: Current treatment of the tibial plateau fractures. *J South Orthop Assoc* **6**(1):54–61, 1997.
4. Frankl U, Wasilewsky SA, Healy WL: Avulsion fracture of the tibial tubercle with avulsion of the patellar ligament. *J Bone Joint Surg* **10**:1411–1413, 1990.
5. Hand WL, et al: Avulsion fractures of the tibial tubercle. *J Bone Joint Surg* **53**:1579, 1971.
6. Hohl MLJ: Tibial condylar fractures. *J Bone Joint Surg* **49**:1456, 1967.
7. Martin AF: The pathomechanics of the knee joint. The medial collateral ligament and lateral tibial plateau fractures. *J Bone Joint Surg* **42**:13, 1960.
8. Meyers MH, Mckeever FMB: Tibial condylar fractures with delayed diagnosis. *J Bone Joint Surg* **52**:1677, 1970.
9. Moore TM, et al: Roentgenographic measurement of the tibial-plateau depression due to fracture. *J Bone Joint Surg* **56**(1):155, 1974.
10. Novich MM: Abduction injury of the knee with rupture of the common peroneal nerve. *J Bone Joint Surg* **42**:1372, 1960.
11. Salter RB, et al: The effect of continuous passive motion on the healing of articular cartilage defects: An experimental investigation in rabbits. *J Bone Joint Surg* **57**:570, 1975.
12. Smille IW: *Injuries of the Knee Joint*, 4th ed. Baltimore: Williams and Wilkins, 1971.
13. Walker CW, Moore TE: Imaging of skeletal and soft tissue injuries in and around the knee. *Radiol Clin North Am* **35**(3):631–653, 1997.
14. Watson JT: High-energy fractures of the tibial plateau. *Orthop Clin* **25**(4):723–752, 1994.
15. Wiley JJ, Baxter MP: Tibial spine fractures in children. *Clin Orthop* **6**:54–60, 1990.

BIBLIOGRAPHY

Banks HH: Factors influencing the result in fractures of the femoral neck. *J Bone Joint Surg* **44**:931, 1962.

Chiron HS, et al: Fractures of the distal third of the femur treated by internal fixation. *Clin Orthop* **100**:160, 1974.

Hohl M, et al: Fractures of the tibial condyles. *J Bone Joint Surg* **38**:1001, 1956.

Hymbert R: Contribution à l'étude du traitement des fractures du plateau tibial par l'extension au fil de Dirschner. *Rev Med Suisse Romande* **59**:641, 1939.

24
CHAPTER

FRACTURES OF THE PATELLA

Patellar fractures represent only a small percentage of skeletal body injuries and generally occur in patients 40 to 50 years old. Patellar fractures are of three general types; the most common being a transverse fracture. Stellate fractures (comminuted) are the second most common type representing about one third of patellar fractures. Longitudinal or vertical fractures represent 10 to 20 percent of patellar fractures and are the least common.[1,3]

The blood supply to the patella enters by way of central and distal polar vessels. Fractures may interrupt the blood supply resulting in the development of avascular necrosis.

Classification
Patellar fractures are classified on the basis of mechanism of injury as either *direct fractures* secondary to direct trauma or *indirect fractures*, which are avulsion injuries due to the pull of the quadriceps against resistance.

PATELLAR FRACTURES

☐ Class A: Fractures secondary   (Fig. 24–1)
            to a direct blow
            Type I (Nondisplaced)
            Type II (Comminuted)
            Type III (Vertical)
            Type IV (Osteochondral)

☐ Class B: Fractures secondary to   (Fig. 24–2)
            quadriceps avulsion
            Type I (Transverse
            [displaced])
            Type II (Upper or lower
            pole fracture)
            Type III (Vertical or
            longitudinal fracture)

Mechanism of Injury
There are two mechanisms that result in fractures of the patella. A direct blow or fall on the patella may result in a nondisplaced fracture. Secondary quadriceps pull may result in distraction of the fragments. Indirectly, an intense quadriceps contraction as occurs during a fall may result in an avulsion fracture.

Examination
The patient will present with tenderness and swelling of the knee. The undersurface of the patella must be pal-

pated if an osteochondral fracture is suspected. The knee should be examined for active extension. If this is absent, the quadriceps mechanism may be disrupted requiring surgery. Occasionally, a palpable defect along the inferior pole of the patella may indicate a disruption of the distal extensor mechanism.[5]

X Ray (Fig. 24–3)
Anteroposterior (AP), lateral, and axial (skyline) views are usually adequate in defining these fractures. A bipartite patella may at times be difficult to differentiate from

PATELLAR FRACTURES

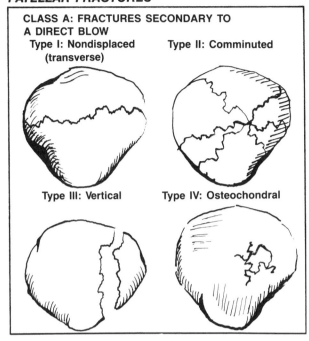

CLASS A: FRACTURES SECONDARY TO
A DIRECT BLOW
Type I: Nondisplaced   Type II: Comminuted
(transverse)

Type III: Vertical   Type IV: Osteochondral

Figure 24–1.

PATELLAR FRACTURES

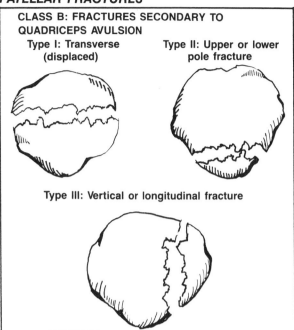

CLASS B: FRACTURES SECONDARY TO
QUADRICEPS AVULSION
Type I: Transverse   Type II: Upper or lower
(displaced)   pole fracture

Type III: Vertical or longitudinal fracture

Figure 24–2.

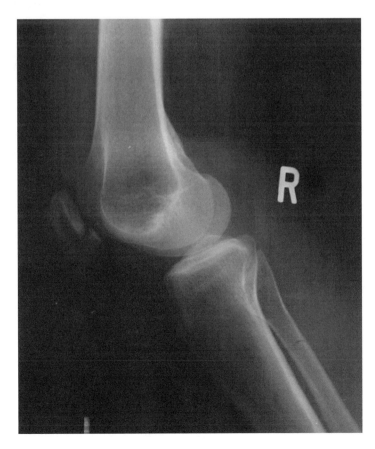

Figure 24–3. Transverse fracture of the patella with minimal displacement.

a fracture. Comparison views and recognition that a bipartite patella is typically in the superior lateral position are helpful in distinguishing these two entities. Osteochondral fractures are usually not detected on plain radiographs although at times a small defect on the undersurface of the patella may be seen. Disruption of the distal extensor mechanism may allow the patella to "ride high" in the patella alta position best visualized on the lateral and AP views. Magnetic resonance imaging (MRI) may be useful in delineating the full extent of the osseous and soft tissue injuries.[6]

Associated Injuries
Direct patellar fractures are often associated with traumatic chondromalacia.

□ CLASS A: FRACTURES SECONDARY TO A DIRECT BLOW

□ CLASS B: FRACTURES SECONDARY TO A QUADRICEPS AVULSION

Treatment
□ Class A: Type I   (Nondisplaced [Transverse])

The emergency management of these fractures includes aspiration of the hemarthrosis when present and the application of a long leg cylinder cast extending from the groin to the malleoli. The cast should be well molded around the patella, and the knee must be in full extension. Alternatively, nondisplaced patellar fractures can be treated with a long leg posterior splint in full extension. The patient should then be referred for follow-up and the institution of quadriceps exercises within the first several days.

□ Class A: Type II   (Comminuted)
             Type III   (Vertical)
             Type IV   (Osteochondral)

□ Class B: Type I   (Transverse [Displaced])
             Type II   (Upper or Lower Pole Fracture)
             Type III   (Vertical or Longitudinal Fracture)

The emergency management of these fractures includes ice, immobilization in extension, analgesics, and admission for operative treatment if the displacement exceeds 4 mm. Severely comminuted fractures are usually treated with patellectomy and are associated with a high incidence of degenerative arthritis (39 percent in one series[4]). Partial patellectomy in comminuted fractures of the patella have given satisfactory results if at least three fifths of the patella could be preserved. Total excision of the patella is sometimes unavoidable; however, one should try to preserve as much of the patella as possible for optimal results.[2]

Complications
Patellar fractures may be followed by the development of several significant complications.

1. Degenerative arthritis is common, especially after osteochondral or comminuted fractures.
2. Postoperative displacement of the fragments secondary to inadequate fixation or immobilization may be seen after surgical repair.
3. Focal avascular necrosis may be seen after transverse or polar fractures.

REFERENCES

1. Bostmam O, Kiviluoto O, Nirhamo J: Comminuted displaced fractures of the patella. *Injury* **13**:196, 1981.
2. Bostrom A: Fractures of the patella. *Acta Orthop Scand* **143**(suppl):1, 1972.
3. Campbell WC: Fractures of the patella. *South Med J* **28**:401, 1935.
4. Crenshaw AH, Wilson FD: The surgical treatment of fractures of the patella. *South Med J* **47**:716, 1954.
5. Ray JM, Hendrix J: Incidence, mechanism of injury, and treatment of fractures of the patella in children. *J Trauma* **32**(4):464–467, 1992.
6. Walker CW, Moore TE: Imaging of skeletal and soft tissue injuries in and around the knee. *Radiol Clin North Am* **35**(3):631–653, 1997.

BIBLIOGRAPHY

Black JK Jr, Conners JJ: Vertical fractures of the patella. *South Med J* **62**:76, 1969.
Blodgett WE, et al: Fractures of the patella. Results of total and partial exclusion of the patella for acute fractures. *JAMA* **106**:2121, 1936.

25
CHAPTER

SOFT TISSUE INJURIES AND DISORDERS OF THE KNEE

The knee is a complex joint that is commonly injured and frequently misdiagnosed, often resulting in an unnecessary delay in the institution of therapy. The accurate diagnosis of knee injuries requires a rather detailed knowledge of anatomy. In this chapter, the discussion centers around a review of knee anatomy followed by a discussion of the soft tissue injuries about the knee. These disorders are organized anatomically into *superficial disorders*, *muscular injuries*, *ligamentous injuries*, and *meniscal injuries*.

Essential Anatomy

The knee is a complex joint composed of three articulations: the medial and lateral condylar joints and the patellofemoral joint. The knee is capable of a wide range of motion including flexion, extension, internal and external rotation, abduction, and adduction. In full extension, no rotary motion is permitted as the ligamentous structures are taut. This tightening with extension is referred to as "the screwing home mechanism." Beyond 20 degrees of flexion, the supporting ligaments are relaxed and axial rotation is permitted.[62] At 90 degrees of flexion, there is a maximum of laxity allowing up to 40 degrees of rotation.

The surface anatomy including the major muscles surrounding the knee can be easily visualized and palpated. With the knee extended, the large dominant vastus medialis and the smaller vastus lateralis can be visualized and palpated. The larger medialis pulls the patella medially during extension, thus preventing lateral subluxation or dislocation. The sartorius, the gracilis, and the semitendinosus are palpable medially along their common insertion on the tibia referred to as the pes anserinus. Laterally, the iliotibial tract and the tendon of the biceps femoris can be palpated.

The bony anatomy of the knee can also be palpated. The patella and patellar tendon are palpated along the anterior surface of the knee. Medially, the medial tibial plateau and medial femoral condyle are noted. The adductor tubercle extends posteriorly from the medial femoral condyle and can be palpated. The joint line can be readily located by noting the natural depression just medial and lateral to the patellar tendon with the knee in flexion. These indentations overlie the articular surfaces.

The patellar ligament inserts on the anterior tibial tubercle, which is easily palpable. The lateral tibial plateau is located just lateral to the tubercle. Posterior and lateral to the plateau is the fibular head palpable just inferior to the lateral femoral condyle.

The medial meniscus is palpable along the medial joint line (at the depression indicated above) as the knee is internally rotated and gently extended. The lateral meniscus is not palpable although injury to this structure reliably produces joint line tenderness. The lateral collateral ligament and occasionally the common peroneal nerve can be palpated laterally with the patient sitting cross-legged and the knee in 90 degrees of flexion. The menisci of the knee migrate anteriorly with extension. The medial meniscus is less mobile because of its attachment to the medial collateral ligament. With flexion there is posterior migration of both menisci, secondary to the pull of the (medial) semimembranosus and the (lateral) popliteus.

The supporting structures surrounding the knee can be divided into two groups, *static* (ligaments) and *dynamic* (muscles) *stabilizers*. The static stabilizers can be further divided into medial, lateral, and posterior compartments.

The medial compartment static stabilizer is the tibial collateral ligament (Fig. 25–1). This capsular structure also known as the superficial tibial collateral ligament is the primary medial stabilizer against a valgus or rotary stress.[1,113] This superficial ligament inserts on the medial femoral and tibial condyles. A deep portion of the ligament referred to as the medial capsular ligament inserts on the medial meniscus and thus the division into meniscotibial and meniscofemoral components. The tibial collateral ligament can also be divided into anterior, middle, and posterior components. The posterior component merges with the oblique popliteal ligament.[29,47] The semimembranosus tendon inserts on the oblique popliteal ligament adding stability and posterior mobility to the ligament as well as the medial meniscus during flexion (Fig. 25–2).

The tibial collateral ligament is the most commonly injured ligament of the knee. This ligament normally glides anteriorly during extension and posteriorly during flexion and is taut only in extension.[29,113] The ligament's normal function is to limit forward glide of the tibia on the femur and to limit rotation and abduction. Wang and co-workers have demonstrated that the collaterals are twice as effective at inhibiting rotational laxity when compared with the cruciates.[111]

The lateral compartment static stabilizer is the *lateral collateral ligament* as shown in Figure 25–3. This band-shaped ligament extends from the lateral femoral epicondyle to the fibular head. The ligament is *extracapsular*

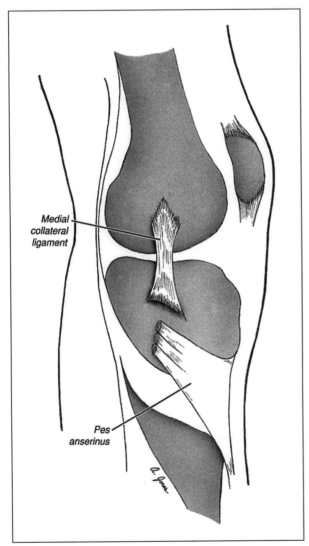

Figure 25–1. Medial aspect of the knee. Note the complex inter-digitations of the semimembranosus.

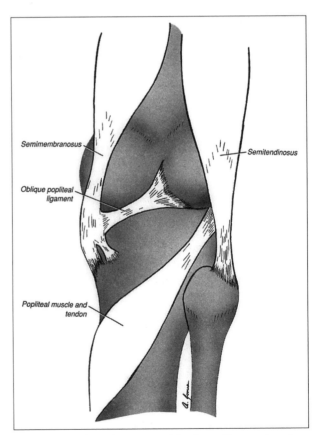

Figure 25–2. Posterior aspect of the knee. The semimembranosus tendon sends extensions to the medial meniscus and to the posterior aspect of the capsule.

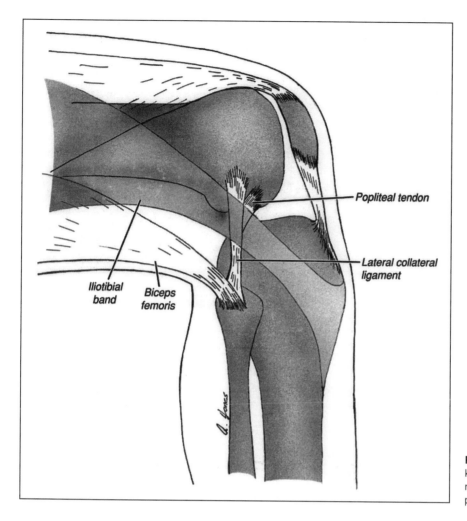

Iliotibial band

Biceps femoris

Popliteal tendon

Lateral collateral ligament

Figure 25–3. Lateral aspect of the knee. Note the lateral collateral ligament and its close relationship to the popliteal tendon.

and does not insert on the lateral meniscus. This ligament offers little stability and is uncommonly injured.

The posterior compartment static stabilizer is the *posterior capsule*, which in reality is a continuation of the medial capsular ligament.[28] The posterior capsular ligament is taut in extension and is the first line of defense against anteromedial or anterolateral rotary instability.[47]

There are two noncapsular static stabilizers of the knee: the anterior and posterior cruciates. The cruciates extend from the area of the intercondylar fossa of the femur to the tibial intercondylar eminence. The ligaments cross over each other forming the letter "X" on lateral inspection. The ligaments are named on the basis of their tibial attachment.

The anterior cruciate prevents anterior displacement of the tibia, excessve lateral mobility in flexion and extension, and controls tibial rotation. Some authors believe the ligament serves to prevent hyperextension and acts as a rotational guide in the screwing home (extension) mechanism.[47] Anterior cruciate injuries are rarely isolated and typically are associated with medial collateral tears. The anterior cruciate has a plentiful vascular supply and with appropriate treatment usually heals well

after an injury. When it ruptures, a hemarthrosis is almost always present.

The posterior cruciate is regarded as the primary static knee stabilizer in preventing rotation. If ruptured, true anteroposterior and mediolateral instability can occur. Posterior cruciate injuries are rarely isolated and typically are associated with severe knee injuries.

The *quadriceps tendon*, a *dynamic stabilizer*, is a combination of the tendons of the vastus medialis, lateralis, and intermedius, along with the rectus femoris. The tendon encircles the patella and continues distally as the patellar tendon inserting on the tibial tubercle. The quadriceps tendon is considered the primary dynamic stabilizer of the knee.

The *pes anserinus*, a *dynamic stabilizer*, is a medial structure formed from the conjoined tendons of the graciles, sartorius, and the semitendinosus (see Fig. 25–1). This tendon stabilizes the knee against excessive rotary and valgus motion.

The *semimembranosus*, a *dynamic stabilizer*, has three extensions that aid in stabilizing the knee (see Fig. 25–2). The oblique popliteal ligament extends from the tendon of the semimembranosus to the posterior capsule (posterior oblique ligament) and tightens the capsule when stressed. This tendon also inserts on the posterior horn of the medial meniscus, pulling it posteriorly during flexion. A final extension of the tendon inserts on the medial tibial condyle serving to flex and internally rotate the knee.

On the lateral surface of the knee there are *three dynamic stabilizing structures:* the *iliotibial tract*, the *biceps femoris*, and the *popliteus muscle* (see Fig. 25–3). The iliotibial tract inserts on the lateral tibial condyle and moves anteriorly with extension and posteriorly with flexion. The biceps tendon inserts on the fibular head, lateral to the insertion of the lateral collateral ligament. The biceps affords lateral stability as well as assisting the knee in flexion and external rotation. The popliteus is a posterior muscle inserting with a Y- shaped tendon called the *arcuate ligament*. One limb of the ligament inserts on the lateral femoral condyle and the other on the fibular head. At the junction of these two portions another limb inserts on the posterior portion of the lateral meniscus providing for posterior mobility of the meniscus during flexion (see Fig. 25–2).

SUPERFICIAL DISORDERS

□ TRAUMATIC PREPATELLAR NEURALGIA

The patient typically presents with a chief complaint of a persistent, dull ache over the patella that may be exacerbated with the slightest pressure as from overlying clothing. The disorder usually follows direct trauma to the area with a resultant contusion of the superficial prepatellar neurovascular bundle. The neurovascular bundle may at times undergo secondary fibrosis after repeated trauma. On examination, the patient will complain of *focal tenderness* over the middle and outer borders of the patella with no discomfort over the remainder of the patella. Most patients respond to an injection of a lidocaine-hydrocortisone mixture. Symptoms of chondromalacia patella are often present bilaterally, and a family history of similar problems may be noted.[38] Patients often complain of pain behind the knee on one or both sides.[38]

□ FAT PAD SYNDROME

The fat pad, located beneath the patellar tendon, may become swollen, resulting in pain on forced extension, catching, and discomfort when sitting for long periods. This condition, which is usually found in football, soccer, and volleyball players, is characterized by point tenderness over the anteromedial or anterolateral joint line. During examination, the knee appears tender, puffy, and the fat pad bulges out on either side of the patellar tendon. The physician must not confuse these symptoms with patellar tendinitis or superficial or deep infrapatellar bursitis. Fat pad syndrome is thought to be caused by secondary effects of premenstrual fluid retention or by irritations in arthroscopy.

The treatment of this condition consists of ice, ultrasound, or inferential currents. Also, aspirin or nonsteroidal anti-inflammatory drugs (NSAIDs) could be used as well as a steroid injection into the fat pad. Fat pad syndromes rarely require an operative resection.[27]

□ JUMPER'S KNEE

Commonly called *patellar tendinitis*, jumper's knee is an overuse syndrome caused by rapid repetitive actions of acceleration, deceleration, jumping, and landing. These actions result in microtears of the tendon matrix at three distinct locations: (1) the bone–tendon junction at the superior aspect of the patella, (2) the bone–tendon junction at the inferior aspect of the patella, and (3) the patellar tendon insertion into the tibial tubercle. According to Colosimo and Bassett,[13] jumper's knee could be classified into four stages:

- **Stage 1:** Pain after practice or after a game
- **Stage 2:** Pain at the beginning of activity, disappearing after warming up and reappearing after completion of activity
- **Stage 3:** Pain remains during and after activity and the patient is unable to participate in sports
- **Stage 4:** A complete rupture of the tendon

X Ray

Radiographic changes are rare before 6 months of symptoms. After this quiescent period, a sonogram can reveal an enlarged and hypoechoic tendon. Furthermore, a bone scan may show an increased blood pooling and localization tracer activity in the region of inflammation.

Examination

During examination, the knee should be held at full extension. Tenderness will be felt during palpation over the insertion of either the quadriceps tendon or the upper pole of the patella. The patellar tendon at the lower pole or at the tibial tuberosity could also become tender upon palpation.

Treatment

Treatment of jumper's knee includes avoiding the inciting activity and resting the affected extremity. The extent of treatment depends on the developmental stage of the knee:

- **Stage 1:** Adequate warming up. Ice packs or ice massage after the activity. Local anti-inflammatory treatment and anti-inflammatory drugs during 10 to 14 days. Physiotherapy. Elastic knee support. No injections.
- **Stage 2:** Same as in stage 1. Some form of heat before activity. Injection of steroids is questionable and the patient should be made aware of the potential hazards.
- **Stage 3:** Same as in stage 2. Prolonged period of rest. The patient should either give up sports or consider surgery.
- **Stage 4:** Surgery.

It must be noted that the use of a steroid injection could lead to further damage and eventual rupture since it allows the athlete to continue to overload the weak tendon.[13]

MUSCLE INJURIES

☐ EXTENSOR MECHANISM INJURIES

The quadriceps mechanism may be disrupted at four locations: rupture of the quadriceps tendon, patellar fracture, patellar tendon rupture, and avulsion of the tibial tubercle (Fig. 25–4). Factors predisposing to this injury include tendon calcifications, arthritis, collagen disorders, fatty tendon degeneration, and metabolic disorders. Rupture of the quadriceps tendon is often seen in elderly patients whereas patellar tendon ruptures, although rare, are typically seen in young athletes with a closed tibial tubercle epiphysis.

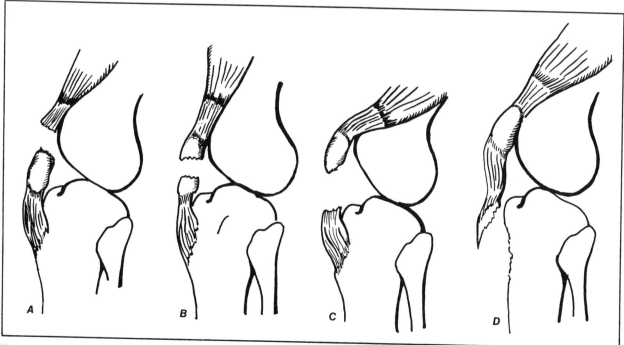

Figure 25–4. **A.** Rupture of quadriceps tendon. **B.** Fracture of the patella. **C.** Rupture of the patella tendon. **D.** Avulsion of the tibial tuberosity.

The *mechanism of injury* may be either direct or indirect. The direct mechanism is less common and is the result of a violent impact against a taut quadriceps tendon. The more common indirect mechanism results from forced flexion when the quadriceps is contracted. This mechanism is commonly seen in patients who stumble while descending a staircase or stepping down from a curb.[66]

The *clinical picture* of an extensor mechanism disruption typically includes a history of a sudden buckling of the knee with extreme pain. After the acute injury the pain is reduced. On examination, the position of the patella should be assessed. Inferior displacement of the patella with proximal ecchymosis and swelling indicate a quadriceps rupture. Proximal displacement of the patella along with inferior pole tenderness and swelling indicate a patellar tendon rupture.[96] In both instances, the patient may have intact, "active" extension but it will be very weak when compared with the uninjured extremity. A quadriceps tendon rupture results in swelling superior to the patella (Fig. 25–5). The most significant finding on clinical examination with extensor mechanism rupture is that the patient has loss of active extension of the knee or inability to maintain the passively extended knee against gravity.[98] With partial ruptures, the patient may have active extension as indicated above; however, it will be markedly weakened. Thirty-eight percent of these patients are misdiagnosed by the initial examiner.[98] When treatment is initiated early, approximation with suture and cast immobilization give good results.[98] Old disruptions typically present with complaints of knee buckling and the inability to climb stairs without support.

The x-ray examination of these injuries may be highly suggestive. Inferior patellar displacement along with a superior pole bony avulsion fragment suggests a quadriceps tendon rupture.[70] Superior displacement with an inferior bony avulsion fragment indicates a patellar tendon rupture. Comparison views may be helpful in diagnosing subtle patellar displacements.

The treatment of a partial quadriceps tendon rupture includes early referral for the placement of a long leg cylinder cast with the knee in extension for 6 weeks. Partial or complete patellar tendon ruptures, avulsion fractures of the patella, and complete quadriceps tendon tears are best treated with early surgical repair, although there are advocates of conservative treatment.

☐ BICEPS AND MEDIAL FLEXOR INJURIES

The medial knee flexors including the gracilis, the sartorius, and the semitendinosus insert on the tibia via the pesanserinus. In addition, the semimembranosus inserts both medially and posteriorly along the knee. The biceps tendon inserts on the fibular head and the lateral collateral ligament. Sudden contraction against resistance as in running or jumping may strain or rupture these tendons or the muscles.

The treatment of these injuries requires rest to prevent muscle or tendon ossification. Moderate strains consist of partial fiber tears with pain and bleeding. These injuries require 3 to 4 weeks of rest, possibly with posterior splinting along with analgesics and heat (after 48 hours). Complete ruptures are rare injuries that are best treated surgically.

☐ ILIOTIBIAL BAND FRICTION SYNDROME

With the knee in extension, the iliotibial band lies anterior to the lateral femoral epicondyle. With flexion, the band slides posteriorly over the epicondyle (Fig. 25–6). Repetitive flexion and extension may result in irritation of the iliotibial band as it slides over the epicondyle.[29]

The *clinical picture* of this syndrome typically includes runners[3] between the ages of 21 and 25 years.[29] The presenting complaint is usually a painful limp that is exacerbated with walking or running. Most patients in one study (Renne) had a history of walking 10 miles or running 2 miles or more just before the onset of pain.[29]

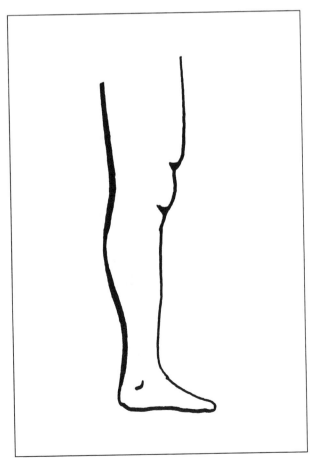

Figure 25–5. With a rupture of quadriceps tendon a swollen area is noted just superior to the upper border of the patella.

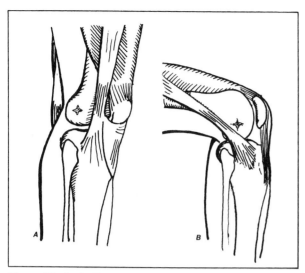

Figure 25–6. A. The iliotibial band lies anterior to the lateral femoral epicondyle when the knee is in extension and passes posterior to it with flexion. **B.** The coursing back and forth over this bony prominence is the cause of a symptom complex referred to as the iliotibial band syndrome.

Climbing stairs or walking up an incline will exacerbate the pain whereas straight leg walking typically relieves the pain.[29] On examination there will be a focal area of tenderness over the lateral femoral epicondyle approximately 3 cm proximal to the joint. There typically is full range of motion, and the pain will be exacerbated with weight bearing on the flexed knee.

The recommended treatment includes the reduction of activities, such as the weekly mileage of running, and changing to a new pair of shoes. Iliotibial band stretching, local modalities (heat or ice), local steroid injections, and oral anti-inflammatory medication are also applied. If conservative treatment is inadequate, the physician could recommend a surgical approach. This includes splitting the posterior 2 cm of the iliotibial band transversely at the area of the lateral condyle so that the portion of the band is not taut at 30 degrees of flexion.[3]

□ FABELLA SYNDROME

The fabella is a sesamoid bone embedded in the tendon of the gastrocnemius muscle that articulates with the posterior portion of the lateral femoral condyle. The fabella is present in 11.5 to 13 percent of normal knees and bilaterally in 50 percent of these patients.[103,115]

The fabella may undergo a degenerative or inflammatory process secondary to irritation resulting in the fabella syndrome.[103] The *clinical picture* typically includes intermittent posterolateral knee pain exacerbated with extension.[115] Tenderness to palpation is localized

over the fabella and is exacerbated with compression against the condylar surface. The recommended treatment includes analgesics and referral as surgical resection may be necessary for lasting relief of pain.

□ BURSITIS

The normal function of a bursa is to permit friction-free movement between two structures. There are several bursae surrounding the knee that can undergo an inflammatory reaction (Fig. 25–7). Typically, acute trauma or chronic occupational stress is the etiologic agent for bursitis surrounding the knee. Other less common etiologies include infection or metabolic disorders such as gout or bursitis associated with chronic arthritis. The treatment of bursitis surrounding the knee is similar and will be discussed at the end of this section.

□ Acute Prepatellar Bursitis
This bursa is located superficial to the patella and usually becomes inflamed 1 to 2 weeks after a direct traumatic injury, such as a fall on the knee (patella).

The *clinical presentation* typically is one of pain with erythema, swelling, and increased warmth of the skin overlying the bursa. With palpation, crepitation of the walls of the bursa may be noted. Limited knee motion is painless up to the point of skin tension at which time pain is noted. Repeated trauma as with an occupational stress results in less pronounced symptoms and a palpably thickened bursal wall. Many cases of prepatellar bursitis are infectious (see olecranon bursitis, p. 253–254).

□ Superficial Infrapatellar Bursitis
This bursa is located just beneath the skin and superficial to the tibial tubercle. When inflamed there will be tenderness over the tubercle that may be difficult to differentiate from Osgood-Schlatter's disease.

□ Deep Infrapatellar Bursitis
This bursa is located beneath the patellar tendon separating it from the underlying fat pad and tibia. The *clinical picture* includes pain-free, passive extension and flexion. *Pain* will be elicited with active complete flexion and extension. *Pain* is also elicited with palpation of the margins of the patellar tendon. It may be difficult to differentiate fat pad inflammation from the disorder although complete passive extension is usually painful with a fat pad disorder.

Infrapatellar fat pad syndrome, often called Hoffa's disease, is caused by hypertrophy and inflammation of the infrapatellar fat pad. This syndrome is characterized

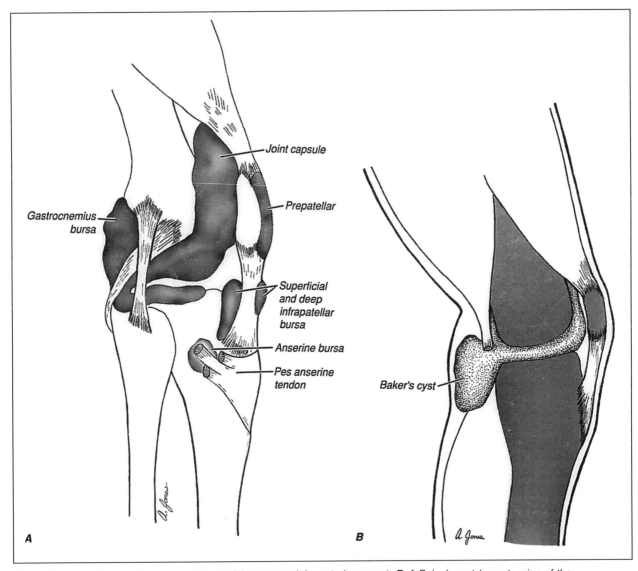

Figure 25-7. A. Bursa of the knee on the medial aspect and the anterior aspect. **B.** A Baker's cyst (an extension of the semimembranosus bursa).

by the appearance of pain during hyperextension of the knee, anterior pain with passive hyperextension of the knee, such as with the bounce test, and in normal radiographs of the knee.[93] The treatment is nonoperative. Treatment involves rest, ice, and NSAIDs. Occasionally, an injection of corticosteroid is useful.[93]

☐ Anserine Bursitis

The anserine bursa lies under the pes anserine tendon. This is a conjoined tendon composed of the sartorius, gracilis, and semitendinosus muscles. Symptoms include knee pain, often nocturnal, particularly on walking up stairs or rising from a sitting position. Morning stiffness may last up to 1 hour, and giving way of the leg occurs. The findings on physical examination are marked ten-

derness over the pes anserine, which is 2 inches below the medial joint line.[82] Often, coexisting osteoarthritis is frequently present. An ultrasound may show an enlarged anserine bursa. Bursal fluid is difficult to obtain; however, if obtained one would find mononuclear cells. Physical stress occurs at this site in obese patients and when walking up stairs. In women, the broad pelvis with resulting angulation of the knee may also add to this stress, which is why the condition is more common in women.[82]

Treatment consists of local injection of an anesthetic and a steroid, which gives immediate relief. The response is quite good and repeated injections are rarely needed. Alternately, ultrasonic treatment is said to have caused dramatic treatment results.[82]

☐ Baker's Cyst

A Baker's cyst is an inflammation of the semimembranosus or medial gastrocnemius bursa and is produced by a herniation of the synovial membrane through the posterior part of the knee's capsule.[90] The bursa of the semimembranosus may communicate with the synovial cavity of the knee. This communication may be congenital in origin or secondary to chronic trauma with damage to the medial portion of the joint capsule. The development of synovitis, arthritis, or any internal derangement of the knee may result in the flow of excess synovial fluid into this bursa. The bursa can then expand posteriorly as there is no limiting obstruction.

The *clinical picture* usually includes a history of intermittent swelling behind the knee. On examination, a tense and sometimes painful fluid-filled sac may be palpated within the popliteal fossa. Additional complaints include chronic pain or a giving way of the knee. In addition to the fluctuant swelling in the popliteal space, the most common presentation is diffuse swelling in one or both legs. There is evidence of posterior tibial nerve compression, such as foot drop, and symptoms of intermittent claudication from arterial compression and local knee discomfort on extension of the knee in some cases.[105] Ruptured Baker's cysts with subsequent inferior dissection of the synovial fluid may be clinically indistinguishable from thrombophlebitis of the calf. Nonruptured cysts must be differentiated from popliteal artery aneurysms, neoplasms, and true synovial hernias.

The change in pressure in a popliteal or Baker's cyst with extension and flexion of the knee (Foucher's sign) suggest the diagnosis of Baker's cyst. This diagnosis is commonly made by ultrasonography, computed tomography (CT) or magnetic resonance imaging (MRI).[105]

Axiom: *A patient with arthritis of the knee who presents with what appears to be thrombophlebitis of the calf must have a ruptured Baker's cyst ruled out by arthrogram.*

☐ Popliteal Bursitis

The popliteal bursa lies proximal to the joint line between the fibular collateral ligament and the popliteus tendon. The patient presents with lateral joint line tenderness and swelling.

☐ Gastrocnemius and Fibular Head Bursitis

The gastrocnemius bursa lies deep to the biceps tendon and may become inflamed secondary to chronic friction or a direct blow. The fibular head is surrounded by several bursae, including the large bicipital bursa lying between the biceps tendon and the fibular collateral ligament.

The *clinical picture* includes pain and tenderness around the fibular head, the fibular collateral ligament, and the head of the biceps. It may at times be difficult to differentiate this from injuries to the fibular collateral ligament, the bicipital tendon, or the lateral meniscus.

☐ Treatment

The treatment of acute traumatic or chronic occupational bursitis includes local heat, rest, and anti-inflammatory agents with protection from recurrent irritation. Chronically inflamed bursae may require aspiration and the application of a pressure dressing. Some patients respond to the injection of a lidocaine-hydrocortisone mixture. Those cases resistant to treatment may require surgical excision of the bursa. The treatment of a Baker's cyst must be directed at the etiology, and early referral is recommended for diagnostic tests and possible closure of the synovial defect.

LIGAMENTOUS INJURIES

The stability of the knee is dependent on its surrounding ligaments and muscles. The knee is most stable in extension and yet the predominance of everyday activities are performed in some degree of flexion. The knee is thus predisposed to injury. The ligaments surrounding the knee function to guide knee motion, and protect the knee from nonphysiologic movement.

The ligaments surrounding the knee are innervated by myelin-free nerve fibers. It is characteristic of ligamentous injuries that a partial tear is typically more painful than a complete rupture. It is imperative that the physician examining a patient with a knee injury obtain a thorough history including the mechanism of injury.

Mechanism of Injury

The following discussion will center around the five common mechanisms resulting in ligamentous injuries. It is imperative to determine if the knee was *weight bearing* at the time of injury as this will increase the likelihood of an associated meniscal injury. In addition,

TABLE 25–1. VALGUS STRAIN

Flexion with external rotation	Extension
↓	↓
Medial collateral ligament injury	Medial collateral ligament injury
↓	↓
Anterior cruciate injury	Anterior cruciate and medial portion posterior capsule injury
↓	↓
Medial meniscus and/or posterior cruciate injury	Deep medial capsular ligament injury
	↓
	Posterior cruciate injury

When a valgus stress is applied to the knee in flexion and extension, a different sequence of events is initiated. Serious flexion injuries are often referred to as the *unhappy triad.*

TABLE 25–2. VARUS STRAIN

Extension with internal rotation	Extension or flexion	Flexion with internal rotation
↓	↓	↓
Anterior cruciate and/or lateral collateral and/or popliteus injury	Lateral collateral injury	Lateral collateral injury
↓	↓	↓
Posterior cruciate and lateral posterior capsule injury	Iliotibial band and/or biceps femoris injury	Lateral posterior capsule and/or lateral meniscus injury
		↓
		Posterior cruciate injury

When a varus stress is applied to the knee in flexion or extension with or without internal rotation, a different sequence of events is initiated.[49,80,112]

a *rotational* force at the time of injury will further increase the possibility of a meniscal injury.[80] Tables 25–1 through 25–5 should serve as a general guide to the types of injuries that are frequently the result of a particular mechanism. This is a controversial area and the following tables include what the authors believe are the predominant theories.[63,71,80,84,88,89]

The most common mechanism of injury resulting in ligamentous damage is a *valgus stress* with an external rotary component on the flexed knee.[47,53,80,112] This is a common skiing or football injury where the patient typically complains of being clipped from the blind side or of catching a ski tip. On examination there will be medial joint line tenderness and anteromedial rotary instability along with a positive valgus stress test in flexion. (Refer to the examination section for a discussion of the valgus stress test.) Table 25–1 lists the sequence of events as an increasing valgus force is applied to the knee in flexion and extension.[80,81,112]

Varus stress is thought to be the second most common mechanism resulting in ligamentous knee injuries.[112] As shown in Table 25–2, a varus stress may or may not be accompanied by an internal rotary force.[40,49,80]

A *hyperextension stress* usually results in injury to the cruciate ligaments. The cruciates may rupture at their

midpoint or at their femoral attachment.[41,64,74,75,79,80] An additional rotational stress may result in damage to the collateral ligaments. Table 25–3 illustrates the sequence of injuries with hyperextension.

There are two types of *rotational injuries:* internal and external. Meniscal injuries may accompany external rotary injuries, especially if there is weight bearing at the time of injury. Table 25–4 illustrates the sequence of injuries accompanying a rotational strain.

Anterior and *posterior* forces of the tibia on the femur may result in injuries to the cruciate ligaments as shown in Table 25–5.

These injuries typically occur with the knee in flexion.

X Ray

A radiographic examination of the knee should precede an in-depth physical examination. Diagnostic manipulation and stress testing should *follow* a normal x ray examination.

Examination

Before the examination the physician should obtain a thorough history. Pertinent questions in subacute and

TABLE 25–3. HYPEREXTENSION STRAIN

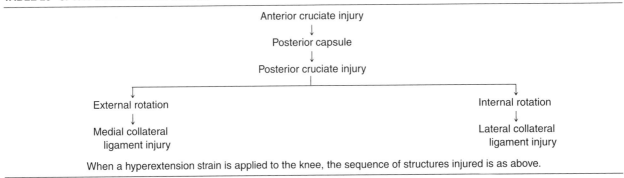

When a hyperextension strain is applied to the knee, the sequence of structures injured is as above.

TABLE 25–4. ROTATIONAL STRAIN

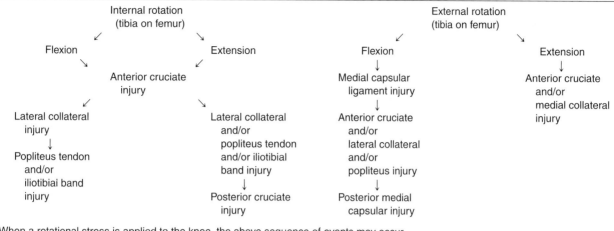

When a rotational stress is applied to the knee, the above sequence of events may occur.

chronic cases include the *location of the swelling* and also what activities reliably *induce* swelling. The usual *duration* of symptoms as well as the response to rest should be assessed.

The exact *location* of the pain after an injury and those factors that *exacerbate* the symptoms give important clues in the specific localization of a ligamentous injury. Partial ligament ruptures typically produce more pain than do complete tears.[41,47] In one study, 76 percent of patients with a complete rupture of a ligament in the knee walked without assistance.[47]

Several studies have indicated that during an injury an audible pop or snap is a reliable indicator of an anterior cruciate rupture.[36,44,80,112] Some authors have stated that patients with this history have a 90 percent incidence of anterior cruciate rupture at surgery.[72,80,92] Sixty-five percent of patients with a torn anterior cruciate, however, did not hear a pop or snap at the time of injury. Rupture of the anterior cruciate is usually followed by the rapid onset of a bloody effusion.[36] The most common etiology for a traumatic hemarthrosis within 2 hours of injury is a rupture of the anterior cruciate.[72,80]

TABLE 25–5. ANTERIOR OR POSTERIOR STRAIN

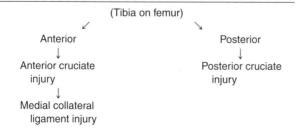

An anterior or posterior force applied to the tibia on the femur typically results in the above sequence of events.

Axiom: *A history that includes a pop or snap at the time of injury suggests a rupture of the anterior cruciate ligament until proven otherwise, especially when associated with the rapid development of a knee effusion.*

Patellar and quadriceps disorders frequently become symptomatic, resulting in a giving way when the patient steps down as, for example, from a curb.[45] Patients with anterior cruciate injuries frequently complain of a painless sensation of one bone going forward on the other along with giving way.[61]

There is controversy surrounding the use and interpretation of various tests often employed in examining the acutely injured knee.[36,47,80] The following discussion is based on published data and personal experience.[7,34,36,73] It is imperative to recall that a patient with complete disruption of the medial compartment may present acutely with little pain, swelling, or instability when walking.[47] The *time* between the injury and the examination is important in determining the physical findings. Immediately after an injury there will be no effusion or spasm and ligamentous injuries will be easily demonstrated. Hours later these same injuries will be difficult to detect secondary to the surrounding ligamentous tension and muscular spasm.[36] If spasm is present, ligamentous laxity may not be demonstrable. This patient must be reexamined after 24 hours when the spasm has been relieved.[36,47] Between the examinations, the patient's knee should be immobilized in a posterior splint, elevated, and iced. If the spasm persists, systemic analgesics or a lidocaine joint injection is recommended. An examination under general anesthesia may be necessary if the spasm is unrelieved.

The acutely injured knee should be examined methodically noting first any *swelling*. Houghton notes that up to 64 percent of patients have localized edema at the site corresponding to the acute ligamentous tear when seen early.[47] *Complete* ligamentous ruptures or capsule disruption may have *no swelling* as the fluid extravasates through the torn capsule. Tense effusions may present with pseudolocking, which is relieved with aspiration of the effusion. Effusions seen within 2 hours of an injury are suggestive of torn tissues whereas those presenting 12 to 24 hours postinjury are typically reactive synovial effusions. A hemarthrosis associated with a negative x ray indicates one of the following:

1. Anterior cruciate tear
2. Osteochondral fracture
3. Peripheral meniscal tear
4. Ligamentous tear

The initial inspection of an acutely injured knee should emphasize the detection of any deformity suggesting a dislocation. Next, the physician should gently palpate the knee in an attempt to localize *tenderness.* In one series 76 percent of patients had

their surgically confirmed injury localized initially on the basis of focal tenderness.[47] At this point a gentle examination to document the range of motion is indicated.

Stress testing for ligamentous injuries often yields valuable information but should be employed only after radiographs have ruled out the possibility of a fracture. It is important to document the feel of the joint at maximum stress (firm or "mushy") along with the amount of joint opening. An objective classification (of limited use) of joint opening is as follows:

1. 1+ = 5 mm or less of joint opening
2. 2+ = 5 to 10 mm joint opening
3. 3+ = 10 mm or more of joint opening

Valgus and varus stress examinations should be performed with the joint in 20 degrees of flexion (Figs. 25–8 and 25–9). It is essential that the stress examination of the injured extremity be compared with that of the uninjured extremity. Ligamentous injuries of the knee or "knee sprains" may be classified into three types on the basis of severity (Table 25–6).

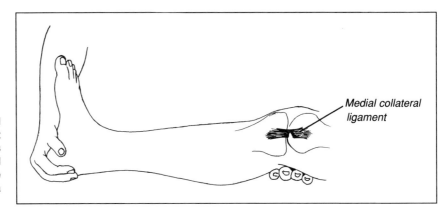

Figure 25–8. Stress test of the medial collateral ligament is shown. One must flex the knee approximately 20 degrees and cup the heel so as to have control over internal and external rotation. The stress test is performed by applying a valgus stress.

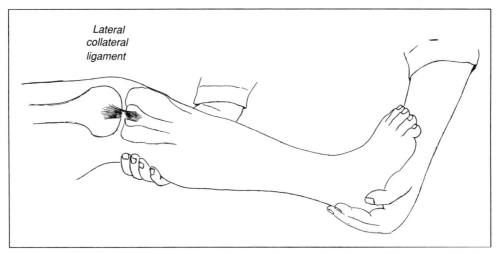

Figure 25–9. Stress test for the lateral collateral ligament is shown. In performing this stress test flex the knee approximately 20 degrees and apply a varus stress.

TABLE 25-6. CLASSIFICATION OF LIGAMENT INJURY

Grade 1 (small incomplete tear)
1. Local tenderness
2. Minimal swelling
3. No stress test instability with firm end point
4. Little pain with stress testing

Grade 2 (moderate incomplete tear)
1. Local tenderness
2. Moderate swelling
3. 1+ stress instability with firm end point when compared with normal knee
4. Moderately disabling

Grade 3 (complete rupture)
1. Local tenderness but pain not proportional to degree of injury
2. Swelling may be minimal or marked
3. 2 to 3+ stress instability with mushy end point
4. Severe disability may be present

The *valgus stress test in flexion* should be performed on the normal knee first. The hip should be in slight extension to relax the hamstrings. This can be accomplished by hanging the thigh and the leg over the side of the table with the knee in 20 degrees of flexion and the patient supine. The examiner should place one hand on the lateral aspect of the knee and grasp the foot and the ankle with the other hand. A gentle abduction stress, with external rotation of the foot and the ankle, should then be applied. The slight external rotary stress tightens the medial capsular ligaments. The test should be performed repeatedly to detect the maximum amount of laxity. This test is a reliable indicator of injury to the tibial collateral ligament (superficial medial collateral ligament).[47] There is controversy surrounding the effect of a torn anterior cruciate on the valgus stress test.[29,47] In the experience of the authors and others, a torn anterior cruciate will result in a greater degree of valgus instability. The grading system for the valgus stress test in flexion is as follows (must be compared with normal knee):

1. 1+ opening indicates a complete medial collateral rupture, or severe partial tear
2. 2+ opening indicates a complete medial collateral and anterior cruciate rupture
3. 3+ opening indicates a complete medial collateral anterior cruciate tear and possibly a posterior cruciate rupture.[24,26]

The *valgus stress test in extension* is performed after the flexion examination using the same technique, but with the knee extended. The interpretation of this test is controversial. Joint opening indicates a rupture of the medial collateral ligament. Some authors also feel that this is indicative of an anterior cruciate and a posterior capsular rupture.[80] Hyperex-

tension or a markedly positive test is indicative of a posterior cruciate injury.[47]

The *varus stress test in flexion* is applied with the knee in 20 degrees of flexion with the foot and the leg internally rotated.[3,31,47,49] Joint opening is indicative of a rupture of the lateral collateral ligament. The varus stress test in flexion with wide opening also indicates anterior cruciate rupture. If the patient experiences 3+ opening, usually the capsule is torn and there may be extension into the iliotibial band.

The *varus stress test in extension* with internal rotation of the leg is effective in examining the lateral compartment ligaments and tendons. Joint opening indicates, in addition to rupture of the lateral collateral ligament, a possible rupture of the lateral capsule (which is separate), the iliotibial band, or the popliteus tendon. Wide opening may indicate a posterior cruciate rupture.[57]

The *anterior and posterior drawer tests have received much attention in the literature.*[36,43,47–49,60,80] There is controversy regarding the interpretation of these tests. The predominant opinion favors the importance of assessing for rotary instability when performing these tests. There are then six types of instability assessed in this examination: anterior, posterior, anteromedial, anterolateral, posterolateral, and posteromedial.[6]

When performing this examination the patient must be in a supine, relaxed position. The hip should be in 45 degrees of flexion with the knee in 80 degrees to 90 degrees of flexion, and the foot immobilized. The examiner should then place the hands on the upper tibia with the fingers in the popliteal fossa and ensure that the hamstring muscles are relaxed (Fig. 25–10). At this point laxity should be assessed by attempting to push and pull the tibia in an anterior posterior direction. This test should then be performed with leg in internal and external rotation. It is important to perform the test on both the injured and uninjured knee.

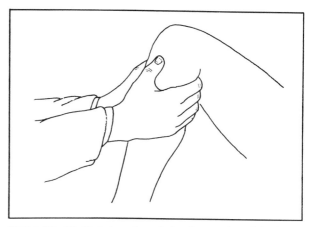

Figure 25-10. Technique for anterior drawer sign of the knee.

Anterior displacement in the *neutral* position is indicative of an anterior cruciate rupture.[17,60] Medial condylar displacement alone is indicative of anteromedial rotary instability and a tear of the meniscotibial portion of the medial capsular ligament.[47] Lateral condylar displacement is indicative of anterolateral rotary instability. Posterior displacement in the neutral position indicates a rupture of the posterior cruciate. With the advent of MRI, the delineation of soft tissue injuries has been revolutionized. The accuracy in diagnosing posterior cruciate ligament injuries and other ligamentous injuries based on confirmation by arthroscopic findings, may be as high as 99 percent.[2] With the leg externally rotated, anteromedial rotary instability can be assessed. The combination of a negative neutral and a positive external rotation drawer test is indicative of a rupture of the deep portion of the medial capsule and possibly a rupture of the posterior oblique ligament. An anterior cruciate rupture will augment the findings of anteromedial instability. In addition, a previous medial meniscectomy will enhance the findings of anteromedial instability.[47] If the test is markedly positive the anterior cruciate is usually ruptured.[36] With the leg in internal rotation an intact posterior cruciate will prevent posterior medial displacement of the tibia on the femur. The reader is referred to Table 25–7 for a further discussion of the significance of rotary laxity when performing the drawer test.

The anterior drawer test may be positive in up to 77 percent of patients with an anterior cruciate rupture.[35,37,47] An anterior cruciate tear will result in anteromedial rotary instability. A positive posterior drawer test indicates a rupture of the posterior cruciate ligament. A negative test, however, does not exclude this injury.[80]

The Lachman test is more sensitive for acute rupture of the anterior or posterior cruciate.[102] Begin with the knee in full extension. Cup the distal femur in one hand and elevate it allowing the knee to flex proximally (Fig. 25–11).[87] Place the other hand on the proximal tibia at approximately the level of the tibial tuberosity and attempt to displace the tibia anteriorly on the femur. Anterior displacement as compared with the opposite side indicates a positive test. In one study, the Lachman test was positive in 99 percent of patients with rupture of

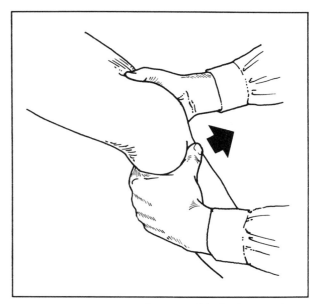

Figure 25–11. The performance of the Lachman test.

the anterior cruciate ligament.[21] This test is more easily performed than the anterior drawer sign in the patient who has a markedly swollen knee.

The Lachman and the pivot shift test (described below) are important adjuncts in the diagnosis of anterior cruciate ligament injuries. In addition, sports medicine physicians use the KT–1,000, an arthrometer, in their assessment of these injuries. This has become routine; however, it is not useful in the emergency department. If the KT–1,000 shows laxity, there is a greater need for surgical intervention in treating the injury.[51,58]

Palpable hamstring spasm should be carefully looked for when performing the Lachman maneuver or the anterior drawer. It has been shown that hamstring spasm will interfere with the interpretation of this test in the awake patient.[32] A predominance of lateral meniscal tears has been demonstrated to occur in association with acute anterior crucsiate rupture, whereas the incidence of medial meniscus tears increases significantly with chronic anterior cruciate ligament insufficiency.[4]

The jerk test is an excellent mechanism for assessing anteromedial rotary instability. To perform the test

TABLE 25–7. ROTARY INSTABILITY ON THE DRAWER TEST

Injury	Positive Test	Injured Structures
Anteromedial instability	1. Valgus stress test in flexion 2. External rotation anterior drawer	Medial compartment and/or posterior oblique and/or anterior cruciate
Anterolateral instability	1. Neutral anterior drawer 2. Jerk test	Lateral capsular (middle 1/3) and/or anterior cruciate[25,34,36,47,49]
Posterolateral instability	Varus stress test in flexion internal rotation posterior drawer	Arcuate complex,* including popliteus tendon[47,49]

*Arcuate complex includes the oblique popliteal ligament and the arcuate ligament.

the patient should be supine with the hip and knee in 45 and 90 degrees of flexion, respectively. When examining the right knee, the internally rotated foot should be held in the examiner's right hand while the left hand applies a valgus stress to the knee. As the knee is extended, subluxation of the lateral femoral tibial articulation will occur at approximately 30 degrees of flexion in the positive test. With further extension a spontaneous relocation will occur.[47] A false-positive jerk test may be seen with an interposed torn meniscus.[49]

The pivot shift test has also been described for the diagnosis of capsular tears. In this test the examiner cups the heel of the tibia and internally rotates the leg while the other hand rests laterally at approximately the level of the fibular head while a mild stress is applied. The knee is gradually flexed. With a positive test, reduction of the subluxated lateral femoral tibial articulation is felt at approximately 30 degrees of flexion.

After a negative examination for ligamentous instability the *muscle power* of the involved extremity should be assessed and compared with the normal extremity. Loss of muscular strength may be seen after rupture of a musculotendon unit.[14]

Ligamentous injuries should be classified on the basis of involved ligaments as well as the degree of involvement. *Grade 1* sprains imply a stretching of the fibers without a tear. On stress testing, grade 1 injuries have a firm end point. *Grade 2* sprains imply a tear in the ligament fibers without a complete rupture. On stress testing there will be a firm end point. *Grade 3* sprains indicate a complete rupture of the ligament. Clinically, a mush end point on stress testing is found with a grade 3 injury.[11]

The posterior cruciate ligament is the primary stabilizer of the knee. Posterior cruciate ligament injuries are more common than was once believed and may represent up to 20 percent of all new ligament injuries.[77] There are three common events that can result in posterior cruciate ligament injury:

1. Hyperflexion, with or without anterior tibial force
2. Hyperflexion with a downward force applied to the thigh
3. Hyperflexion, often with an associated varus/valgus force[77]

Most injuries occur in young males involved in motor vehicle–related accidents and contact sports.[77]

The most characteristic diagnostic finding of posterior cruciate ligament tears is the "sag sign." This is an apparent disappearance of the tibial tubercle on lateral inspection when the knee is flexed to 90 degrees. Gravity-assisted posterior displacement of the tibia accentuates this. This may be misinterpreted as a positive anterior drawer sign.[59]

Treatment

The literature supports a wide spectrum of treatment modalities in managing acute ligamentous injuries of the knee. Treatment modalities varying from immobilization (conservative) to operative intervention are recommended for ligamentous injuries.[1,7,29] The one exception to this is in treating severe disruption of the medial ligaments and capsule. For this injury, surgical repair is generally recommended.[36,83]

The initial management of ligamentous injuries of the knee should include ice, elevation, and soft tissue compressive dressing extending from the midcalf to the midthigh (Jones' dressing; see Appendix). Alternately, a posterior splint may be used. If there is mild instability and little ligamentous distraction conservative treatment is indicated.[9,12,15,19,23,29,36] Nonoperative therapy for complete tears of the medial collateral ligament with only mild to moderate instability has been advocated.[53,54] The treatment has been divided into three phases. In *phase A* the leg is placed in an orthosis in approximately 30 degrees of flexion with partial weight bearing with crutches allowed. Isometric quadriceps exercises and hip strengthening exercises are started in the second week. In *phase B*, which lasts for an additional 4 weeks, the orthosis is adjusted to allow 30 to 90 degrees of motion and isotonic as well as isokinetic exercises are performed.[10] In *phase C*, which occurs 6 weeks after diagnosis, the orthosis is removed and exercises are continued with a mild running program begun. In using conservative therapy there should not be any associated anterior cruciate ligament or meniscus injury. Surgery is indicated when there are injuries involving multiple ligaments or when moderate instability is present.[29,80] It is, of course, imperative that the initial assessment of the injury be accurate. Frequently, an accurate initial examination will be impossible secondary to swelling and muscular spasm. In addition, a negative initial examination cannot entirely exclude the presence of a significant injury. In the presence of significant spasm and a negative initial examination, the injured extremity should be reexamined 24 hours later for confirmation of the previous findings.[47,118] Table 25–8 is a management scheme developed on the basis of the authors' personal experiences, and supported by existing literature.[47,85] The protocol implemented in a particular patient is of course dependent on consultation with the orthopedic surgeon.

Stable knee injuries refer to single ligament involvement of grade 1 or 2 severity. The involvement of multiple ligaments or a single ligament with a grade 3 injury is an unstable injury requiring immobilization and orthopedic referral. If the initial examination is inconclusive or negative, the patient should be reexamined 24 hours later for confirmation of the initial findings. This also applies if any of the criteria listed in

TABLE 25–8. MANAGEMENT SCHEME FOR LIGAMENTOUS INJURIES OF THE KNEE

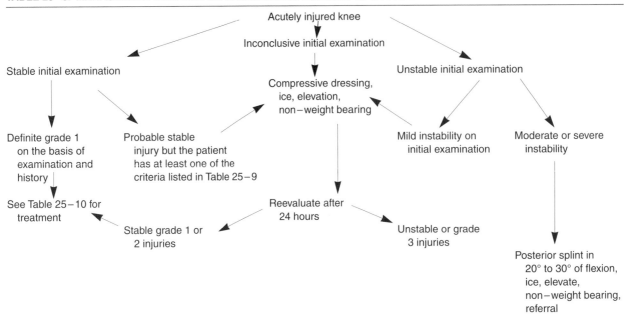

Table 25–9 are present. If a stable grade 1 or 2 injury is diagnosed after reevaluating a patient who has undergone 24 hours of ice and immobilization, the treatment protocol outlined in Table 25–10 can be implemented. There remains controversy surrounding the definitive treatment of complete ruptures of the collateral ligaments. Some orthopedic surgeons believe that complete ruptures of only one ligament as an isolated injury can be treated conservatively whereas others believe that operative intervention is the preferred approach. The authors recommend that after a diagnosis is made of a third-degree rupture of either the cruciates or the collateral ligaments, the patient should be referred. If after 24 hours there is uncertainty as to the extent of damage, immobilization and referral for arthrogram or arthroscopy is indicated.[95]

A small percentage of sprains become more painful during the healing phase. As the pain becomes severe, flexion may be limited. After 3 to 4 weeks, the x ray will show calcification in the area of the injured ligament. This condition is commonly referred to as *posttraumatic periarticular ossification* or *Pellegrini-Streida disease*. Pathologically, calcium is deposited in the hematoma surrounding the partially torn ligament. This calcified mass may be connected to the underlying bone by way of a pedicle. In the early stages of development, massage or manipulation may worsen the symptoms. The recommended treatment includes a compressive dressing and multiple punctures to enhance resorption of the calcium.

Posterior cruciate ligament injuries, as an isolated injury, are usually treated nonoperatively.[77] Surgical

TABLE 25–9. CRITERIA FOR REEVALUATING A STABLE KNEE

1. The mechanism of injury suggests a more severe injury than found on the initial examination.
2. History of an audible snap or pop at the time of injury.
3. The presence of a hemarthrosis on the initial examination.
4. The presence of muscular spasm on the initial examination.
5. Any patient with severe symptoms and a stable initial examination.
6. Any grade 2 injury on initial examination to be certain it is not a "masked" grade 3 injury.

TABLE 25–10. TREATMENT OF GRADE 1 AND 2 LIGAMENTOUS INJURIES OF THE KNEE

Grade 1
1. Soft tissue compression dressing from midthigh to midcalf
2. Ice
3. Elevation
4. Ambulation with quadriceps exercises as soon as comfortable

Grade 2
1. Initial management same as numbers 1, 2, and 3 above followed by reexamination at 24 hours.
2. Posterior splint, immobilizer, or compression dressing for 3 days with ice and elevation.
3. A knee immobilizer should be applied for 2 to 4 weeks. Graduated weight bearing with protection of the injured knee should be instituted as comfort permits.
4. Early isometric quadriceps exercise: In the reliable patient a compressive dressing with non–weight bearing until pain-free may be implemented in place of casting. Orthopedic consultation and follow-up are strongly recommended.

reconstruction is reserved for symptomatic chronic posterior cruciate ligament injuries and acute combined injuries.[22,77] Isolated acute posterior cruciate ligament injuries should be managed by splinting the knee in extension until the pain subsides, then allow-ing early motion. It is essential that the rehabilitation of this ligament emphasize quadriceps strengthening. In patients where posterior cruciate ligament injury is accompanied by a bony avulsion, operative treatment is recommended.[77]

MENISCAL INJURIES

The medial meniscus is a "C"-shaped structure attached on each end to the intercondylar eminence and at its midpoint to the deep medial capsular ligament; the lateral meniscus is "O"-shaped and attached medially to the intercondylar eminence (Fig. 25–12). The lateral meniscus has no attachment laterally. The medial meniscus is injured more frequently owing to its relative immobility. The menisci are relatively avascular with a capillary supply limited to the peripheral one quarter. There are several factors that increase the propensity for meniscal injuries, which include congenital discoid meniscus, weakness of the surrounding musculature, and ligamentous laxity. In addition, meniscal injuries frequently accompany ligamentous knee injuries and particularly injuries to the deep medial collateral ligament. Meniscal degenerative changes, which are rare before the age of 10,[5] typically begin in the second decade and progress more rapidly under conditions of undue stress. One half to two thirds of meniscal tears are longitudinal, extending from the anterior portion to an area posterior to the attachment of the medial collateral ligament. Typically, these injuries result in migration of the torn meniscus (Fig. 25–13A and B). Transverse tears are uncommon and are usually seen in the lateral meniscus. Transverse tears or a spontaneous detachment are usually seen after a degenerative process with repeated exposure to minor stress (Fig. 25–13E). Acute traumatic tears are usually longitudinal and peripheral in location. Ligamentous injuries frequently accompany and may mask these injuries.

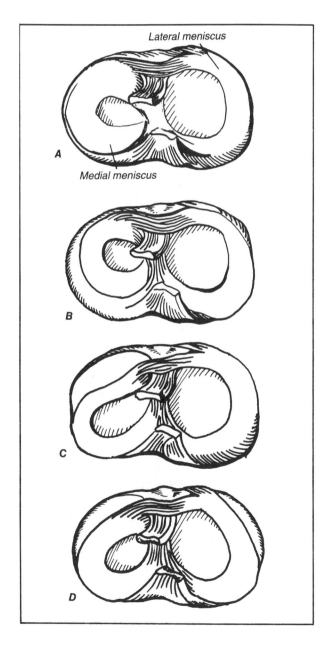

Figure 25–12. A. Articular surface of the tibia is shown with the menisci (as seen above). Note the "O" shape of the lateral meniscus and the "C" shape of the medial meniscus. **B.** The position of the menisci with the knee in extension. **C.** Note the position of the menisci when the knee is flexed and in external rotation. The lateral meniscus is displaced posteriorly and the anterior border of the medial meniscus protrudes forward. **D.** The position of the menisci with the knee in flexion and internal rotation of the tibia. Note that the medial meniscus retracts posteriorly.

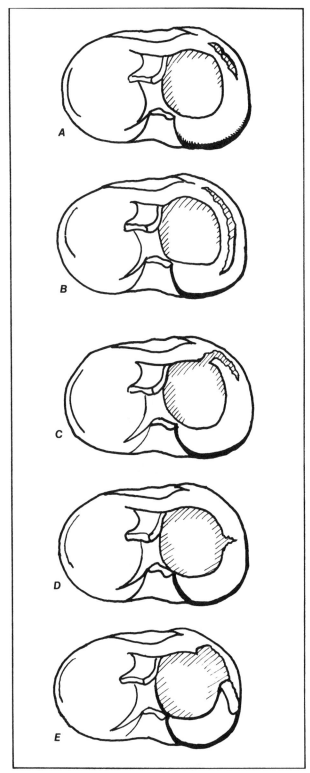

Figure 25-13. Typical meniscal tears. **A.** A partial longitudinal tear of the medial meniscus is shown. **B.** The tear is shown extending across the length of the meniscus in what is called a "bucket handle tear." The inner fragment can displace into the interior of the knee joint. **C.** A tear of the anterior horn is shown. **D.** The fragment is shown uplifted, which can produce locking of the knee. **E.** A transverse tear of the meniscus is shown. This type of tear is more common in the lateral meniscus.

Mechanism of Injury

The menisci move posteriorly with flexion and in an anterior direction with extension. Because of its single medial attachment, the lateral meniscus is more mobile than the medial meniscus. Meniscal tears are usually the result of violent stretching or a crushing force between the femoral and tibial condyles. With knee flexion the femur rotates internally on the fixed tibia, thus displacing the medial meniscus toward the center of the joint. With a rapid forceful extension the meniscus may be trapped centrally, resulting in peripheral segment stretching or tearing. Extension of the tear results in a free segment that may become displaced into the joint, resulting in joint locking (Fig. 25-13C and D). With knee flexion the lateral meniscus is also displaced centrally and a sudden forceful extension often results in a transverse tear at the junction of the anterior and middle thirds (see Fig. 25-12C).

Examination

Meniscal injuries occur frequently in patients with sudden rotary or extension flexion injuries. In older patients with degenerative disease of the menisci, a simple twist or squatting motion may result in a tear. The menisci have no sensory nerve fibers, and the pain results from irritation of the ligaments near the joint line. Meniscal tears often present with a triad of symptoms including *joint line pain*, *swelling*, and *locking*. In addition, giving way of the injured knee is a frequent complaint.

Traumatic ruptures of the meniscus are rare before the age of 10. The diagnosis may require arthroscopy in that the accuracy of clinical examination is below 60 percent.[5] Arthroscopy has an accuracy of 60 to 97 percent depending on the skill and the experience of the arthroscopist.[5] The medial patellofemoral ligament, a component ligament of the medial retinacular complex, is often torn. Without repair, redislocation occurs in up to 44 percent of patients.[100] Consequently, surgical correction is often advocated to reduce the rate of dislocation when this is a problem.

MRI has been reported by some authors to have an accuracy of 90 percent to 98 percent in diagnosing meniscal tears.[18] This has never been the authors' experience and recent studies correlate with our findings. The overall accuracy of clinical diagnosis of meniscal tear is approximately 80.7 percent, with the corresponding accuracy of MRI being 73.7 percent in a recent study.[76] Surgical pathology was found in all knees at arthroscopy. Relying blindly on MRI to determine surgical intervention would have resulted in inappropriate treatment in 35 percent of the knees.[76]

Ligamentous injuries are frequently associated with meniscus injuries and cause "knee locking." Knee locking may be of two types, true or pseudo. Pseudo locking typically follows an episode of increasing pain and swelling. The locking is usually secondary to an effusion which causes pain and muscle spasm. True locking, which occurs spontaneously and only with some degree of flexion to the knee is caused by the following:

- Torn meniscus
- A loose body
- Rupture of the cruciate ligament
- Osteochondral fracture

Childhood locking is rare; however it may indicate congenital discoid meniscus.[46]

Frequently patients present with a history of *giving way*.[101] In addition to ascertaining the frequency of exacerbation of this, the physician must determine if there has been any previous injury to the knee. The most common causes of giving way are the following:

- Meniscal tears
- True locking
- Quadriceps weakness or patellar disorders
- Anterior cruciate injuries

Joint pain or tenderness on palpation of the *joint line* is seen frequently after a meniscal injury. *Bragard's sign* (indicating medial meniscus injury) refers to point tenderness along the anterior medial joint line that is increased with internal rotation and extension of the tibia. With internal rotation and extension the torn medial meniscus is forced against the palpating finger of the examiner.

A joint effusion *immediately* after an injury suggests a ligamentous injury or an osteochondral fracture. Effusions developing 6 to 12 hours after an injury typically follow minor ligamentous sprains or meniscal tears. An acute tear in a degenerated meniscus may produce no effusion.

Only 30 percent of patients with meniscal injuries have *true locking*. Classically, the patient will complain of a sudden inability to fully extend the knee. Extension can be completed by rotating and passively extending the knee. True locking due to a meniscal tear is never complete, as some extension against a rubbery resistance will be present. In addition, meniscal injuries rarely lock in full extension. An inability to fully extend the knee after trauma is usually secondary to muscular splinting, a loose body, or an effusion. Loose bodies are typically seen in patients with osteoarthritis, osteochondritis dissecans, synovial chondromatosis, or a cruciate avulsion with an attached bony fragment.

There are several clinical signs that suggest the presence of a meniscal tear or help to differentiate it from a ligamentous tear.

1. Payr's sign (Fig. 25–14)
2. First Steinmann's sign (Fig. 25–15)
3. Second Steinmann's sign (Fig. 25–16)
4. McMurray's test (Fig. 25–17)
5. Apley's test (Fig. 25–18)

Treatment

Manipulation of the acutely locked knee may further damage the involved meniscus. These injuries should be reduced, however, within 24 hours after the injury. The knee can be reduced by positioning the patient with the extremity hanging off the edge of the table and the knee in 90 degrees of flexion.[65] Gravity will distract the tibia from the femur. Mild rotation of the tibia performed after a period of rest in the aforementioned position, with careful

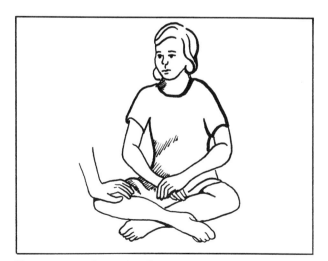

Figure 25–14. Payr's sign. This produces pain with a lesion of the posterior horn of the medial meniscus.

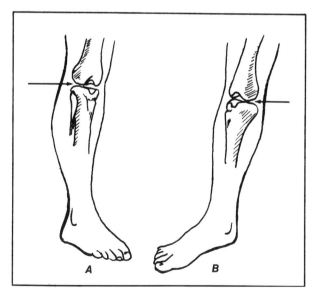

Figure 25–15. First Steinmann's sign. **A.** Pain in the anterolateral joint space is noted with internal rotation of the flexed knee and indicates a lesion of the lateral meniscus. **B.** Pain in the anteromedial joint space occurs with external rotation of the flexed knee. This indicates a lesion of the medial meniscus.

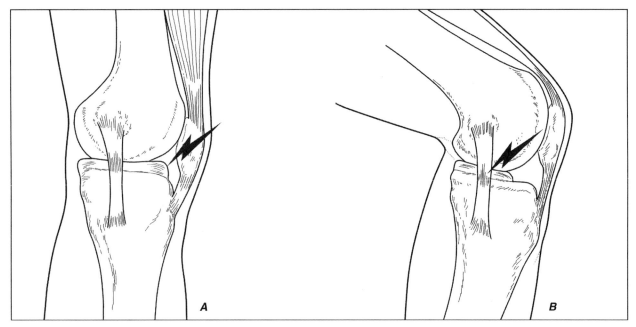

Figure 25–16. Secondary Steinmann's sign. **A.** When the knee joint is extended, the meniscus lies anteriorly. **B.** Flexion of the knee displaces the point of tenderness from the anterior joint line back toward the collateral ligament. This indicates a meniscal problem rather than a ligamentous problem, as the latter does not displace the point of maximal tenderness.

traction along the axis of the leg, will usually result in reduction. If unsuccessful after a gentle attempt, a posterior splint should be applied. Consultation before further attempts at reduction is strongly recommended.

Patients presenting with an acute meniscal tear without ligamentous injuries should have their effusion aspirated and a bulky compression dressing or a splint applied (see Appendix). Twenty-four hours after the initial injury and treatment the patient should be reexamined to exclude an occult ligamentous injury.[86] Those patients with stable ligamentous injuries should be referred for casting and follow-up. For those patients with meniscal tears without associated ligamentous injuries non–weight bearing and active quadriceps exercises are recommended. Recurrent or persistent symptoms are considered operative indications. In some patients, meniscal suture, rather than removal of the meniscus, has been performed.[102] Meniscal tears that are definitely suitable for repair have the following characteristics in common: (1) a tear is located no more than 3 mm from the meniscosynovial junction; (2) minimal damage has occurred to the body of the meniscus; (3) the length of the tear is such that with probing of the meniscus, it sublaxes into

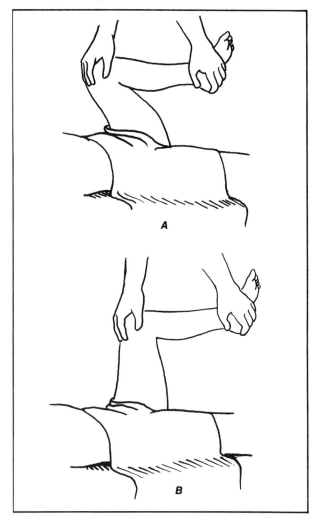

Figure 25–17. McMurray's test. This test is used for evaluation of the medial meniscus. The patient's knee joint is markedly flexed and the foot externally rotated. **A.** The externally rotated leg is gradually extended beyond a right angle. **B.** This produces pain and elicits a crepitation when the test is positive. Evaluation of the lateral meniscus is carried out in a similar manner with the leg in internal rotation.

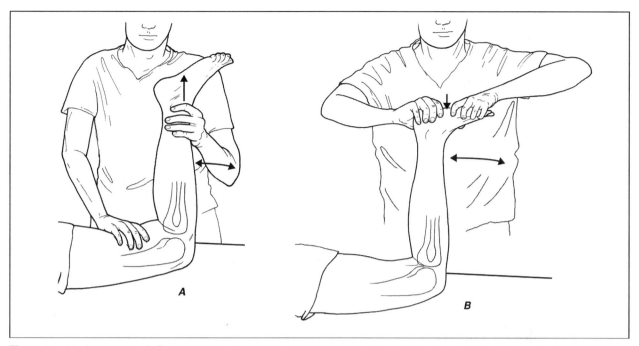

Figure 25–18. Apley's test. **A.** Distraction test. Knee pain on rotation of the foot under traction indicates damage to the capsule and ligamentous structures. **B.** Compression test. Knee pain on rotation of the foot under compression indicates a meniscal injury. While performing the maneuvers, flex and extend the knee.

the joint and is obviously unstable.[20,55,91] Arthroscopy and arthrography are procedures often used in confirming the diagnosis of a suspected meniscal injury. Arthroscopic surgery is now used to resect a segment of the torn meniscus.[80,104] Casts, if employed, should extend from the groin to just above the malleoli.

☐ OSTEOCHONDRITIS DISSECANS

The knee joint, particularly the lateral portion of the medial femoral condyle, frequently develops osteochondritis dissecans (Fig. 25–19). Other areas frequently involved include the lateral femoral condyle and the patella. There are several proposed theories as to the etiology, including localized ischemia and repeated trauma. Whatever the etiology, a fragment of cartilage separates from the underlying bony matrix and the cavity fills with granulation tissue and is followed by the development of fibrocartilage (Fig. 25–20). The surface of the joint becomes irregular, predisposing toward the development of osteoarthritis. In some instances, a sequestrum of bone or cartilage may become free in the joint, and true locking may occur.

Clinical Presentation
Frequently, this diagnosis is made in an asymptomatic patient on the basis of x ray findings alone. Symptoms can include a persistent ache at rest, which is exacer-

bated with exercise. Some patients complain of a stiff sensation that is relieved by kicking. Recurrent knee effusions may be associated with this disorder. Percussion of the patella with the knee in flexion typically exacerbates the pain. The x ray will be negative in recent lesions or when the cavity is filled with fibrocartilage. A cavity surrounded by dense aseptic bone may be seen in older lesions.[94]

Osteochrondritic lesions may occasionally be radiographically occult. Anderson reported that 57 percent of 30 patients with chronic pain after trauma had an occult osteochrondritis dissecans. These lesions were found by using radionuclide bone scans, CT, and MRI.[106] Recent reports on the imaging of osteochrondritis dissecans have stressed the value of MRI.[106]

Treatment
In children under 12, immobilization in a cast with non–weight bearing for 6 to 12 months may result in resolution of a newly acquired lesion. In older children and adults, surgery is recommended to prevent the development of premature degenerative arthritis.

☐ OSTEOCHONDRAL AND CHONDRAL FRACTURES

These injuries typically present with persistent pain after an injury without radiographic abnormalities. Chondral

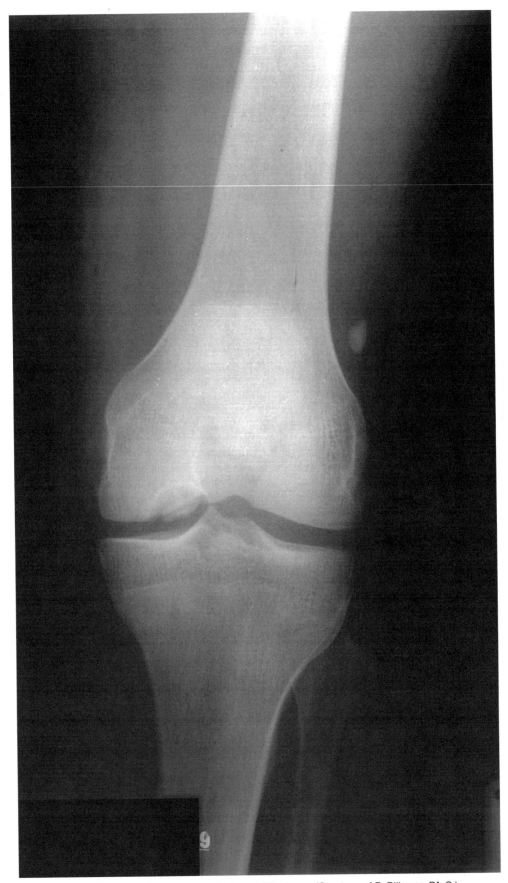

Figure 25–19. Osteochondritis dissicans of the knee. *(Courtesy of D. Billmyer, PA-C.)*

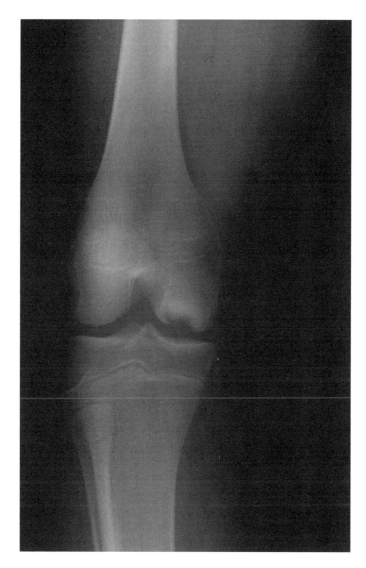

Figure 25–20. Osteochondritis dissicans. Note development of fibrous tissue. *(Courtesy of Dr. Fitzpatrick.)*

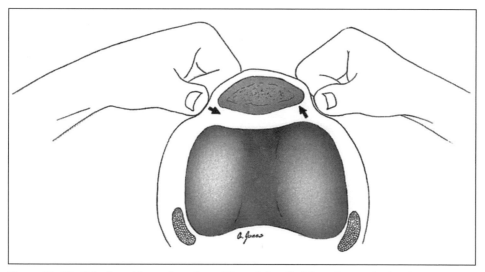

Figure 25–21. Palpation of the undersurface of the patella will elicit tenderness in chondromalacia of the patella.

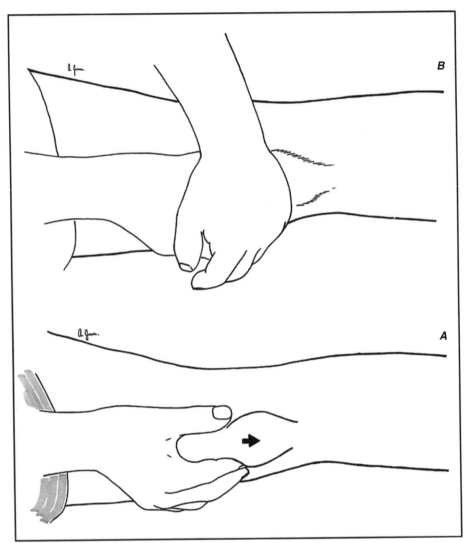

Figure 25–22. The patellar inhibition test is shown. **A.** With the quadriceps muscle relaxed push the patella interiorly. **B.** Compress the patella into the femoral groove and ask the patient to tighten the quadriceps muscle. This will elicit pain and tenderness as the patella courses proximally.

fractures involve only cartilage whereas osteochondral fractures involve the cartilage as well as the subchondral bone. The most common mechanism is a direct impact over the involved area.

Examination

These injuries should be suspected if the patient's complaints are significant in the absence of physical findings. Acutely localized tenderness, joint locking, and hemarthrosis are frequently associated with this injury. These injuries are often confused with a meniscal tear although arthroscopy or arthrography or both will definitely exclude this problem.

Treatment

In children, immobilization with non–weight bearing is recommended. Adults or those with locking or a loose body in the joint require operative intervention. Chondromalacia or osteochrondritis dissecans with chronic pain, locking, and effusions develop if these "fractur remain" untreated.

☐ CHONDROMALACIA PATELLAE (PATELLAR MALALIGNMENT SYNDROME)

Chondromalacia patellae is the premature erosion and degeneration of the patellar cartilage.[30] This disorder is seen commonly in young adults, particularly women. Recently, several authors have noted that this disorder occurs in patients without the characteristic morphologic cartilagenous changes and have renamed the disorder *patellar malalignment syndrome*.[55,56,118] A combined injury of the anterior cruciate ligament and the posterior cruciate ligament strongly suggest the possibility of an acute knee dislocation with spontaneous reduction.[8] Thus, serious consideration should be given to neurovascular injuries. The incidence of popliteal artery injury with knee dislocations ranges from 16 percent to 64 percent.[8,57] Normally, the patellar cartilage is approximately 7 mm thick whereas that of the femoral condyles is only 3 mm thick. Friction is greatest at the patellofemoral interval where compression as well as quadriceps tension forces act.[87] Degeneration of the patellar cartilage begins by the age of 30 and in most cases remains asymptomatic.[55]

Pathogenesis

Patellar pain and the syndrome of chondromalacia patellae may be the result of one or more of the following:

1. Patellar malalignment
2. Direct blow
3. Congenital abnormal shape to patella or femoral groove
4. Recurrent patellar subluxation or dislocation
5. Excessive knee strain (as in athletes)

Clinical Presentation

Typically, symptoms begin in the adolescent age group or the young adult with a complaint of a deep aching in the knees without a history of recent trauma. Some authors differentiate between chondromalacia patella, which occurs commonly in older patients, and patella from a pain syndrome. In emergency medicine, they are regarded as the same condition.[16,67] Strenuous athletic activities or prolonged sitting may exacerbate the pain hours later. Eventually, as the disorder progresses, slight exertion, as with climbing steps, will exacerbate the pain.[39,55] The pain is usually localized to the knee cap or surrounding the medial portion of the knee.[55] Acute trauma to the knee as during a fall may result in retropatellar pain and, in some instances, the development of chondromalacia patellae over a period of several weeks.[39]

During the physical examination, the knee should be in slight flexion, thus drawing the patella into the femoral groove.[69,78] Palpation and compression in this position will avoid synovial entrapment. Firm compression of the patella into the medial femoral groove will elicit pain, which is virtually pathognomonic of chondromalacia patellae. In addition, palpation of the undersurface of the medially displaced patella will typically yield tenderness on the ridge between the medial and odd facet. (Fig. 25–21). Frequently, the examiner will note palpable crepitus with medial patellar displacement and lateral palpation.

In addition to "patellar cartilage tenderness," knee extension against resistance is often painful through the terminal 30 to 40 degrees.[87] The *patellar inhibition test* is performed by asking the patient to contract the quadri-

ceps while the patella is held firmly against the femoral condyles with the knee extended (Fig. 25–22). Pain, tenderness, and crepitus may be diagnostic of patellar dysfunction if synovial entrapment can be excluded. This can be avoided during direct palpation and the inhibition test by placing the knee in slight flexion, thereby drawing the patella into the femoral groove.

As discussed earlier, malalignment of the patella may predispose a person to experience chondromalacia patellae. Patellar malalignment may be determined by measuring the *Q angle* (Fig. 25–23). The Q angle is determined by measuring the angle formed by two lines intersecting through the center of the patella. The first line is drawn from the anterior inferior iliac spine or middle of the femur through the center of the patella. The second line is drawn from the center of the patella through the tibial tubercle. The intersection of these lines forms the Q angle that is normally 15 degrees. Q angles of 20 degrees or more are considered abnormal.[39,55] Clinically, in the standing patient the knee caps will face inward toward each other when the Q angle is increased. This is often referred to as *squinting of the knee caps*.[55]

In addition to the Q angle, the examiner should note the course of the patella through flexion and extension of the knee. Normally with extension the patella moves vertically with a slight medial shift as full extension is approached. Hypermobile or wandering patellae (patellar

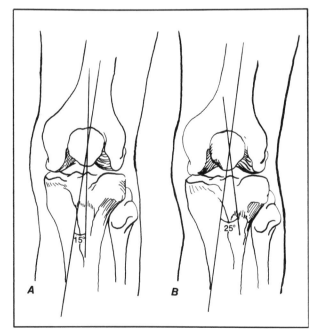

Figure 25–23. The Q angle is formed by a line drawn from the midpoint of the patella through the midpoint of the femoral shaft and a second line, drawn from the midpoint of the patella through the tibial tuberosity. **A.** The normal Q angle as shown above is approximately 15 degrees. **B.** A Q angle of greater than 20 degrees is considered to be abnormal.

malalignment) with knee extension may predispose toward the development of chondromalacia patellae. A high-riding patella is often referred to as *patella alta* and may be diagnosed by measuring the vertical length of the patella and the length of the patellar ligament on a lateral x ray of the knee. If the length of the ligament is greater than 1 cm more than the vertical length of the patella, a high-riding patella should be suspected. These patients frequently have lateral displacement of their patella resulting in a reduced or normal Q angle.

X Ray

Radiographs are typically of little diagnostic value in a patient with chondromalacia patella. Chronic changes including sclerosis or osteophyte development, however, may occasionally be seen in these patients. Surgical treatment in a number of patients by excision of the subcutaneous tissue in the tender area and the prepatellar bursa cured virtually all cases.[52]

Differential Diagnosis

Patients with osteoarthritis may present with symptoms similar to those of chondromalacia patellae. Typically, these patients are older and demonstrate x ray changes including the presence of osteophytes, sclerosis, and joint space narrowing. In addition, patients with chondromalacia patellae typically have medial ridge involvement whereas those with osteoarthritis usually have a predominance of lateral facet involvement. Other conditions that may be confused with chondromalacia patellae include:

1. Torn medial meniscus
2. Prepatellar bursitis
3. Pes anserinus bursitis
4. Fat pad syndrome
5. Osteochondritis dissecans

Treatment

Conservative treatment including rest, salicylates, and *isometric* quadriceps strengthening exercises are recommended. Therapeutic salicylate levels for 3 to 4 months are essential and have, in some cases, resulted in healing of the chondromalacia lesion. Steroid use is not recommended as it may increase the rate of cartilage degradation. The avoid-ance of squatting, running, kneeling, and climbing of steps is strongly recommended during the initial management phase. Casting is contraindicated as it leads to quadriceps atrophy that may exaggerate patellar malalignment.

□ LARSEN-JOHANSSON DISEASE OF THE PATELLA

Larsen-Johansson disease is similar to chondromalacia except that it is limited to the poles of the patella. This condition is also called *inferior pole patellar chondropathy* and is nine times more prevalent in boys, aged 10 to 14 years, than girls. Patients present a lower pole pain exacerbated by running or kneeling.[68] On examination pain is noted with extension against resistance along with localized tenderness. With protracted symptoms, there is an elongation of the involved pole which may develop a stress fracture and eventually an avulsion fracture if not diagnosed.[68] Radiographs are usually normal although blurring of the poles may be seen in chronic cases.[97] Salicylates and rest are recommended and cases of spontaneous healing have been reported. Casting may also expedite healing.

□ OSGOOD-SCHLATTER DISEASE

Osgood-Schlatter disease represents a disturbance in the development of the tibial tuberosity caused by repeated and rapid application of tensile forces by the quadriceps muscles at its tendonis insertion on to the tuberosity. The most widely accepted cause of Osgood-Schlatter disease is chronic repetitive trauma to the anterior portion of the maturing proximal tibial growth plate.[99]

This disease is typically seen in girls who are 8 to 13 years of age and in boys between the ages of 10 and 15 years. The disorder has been associated with inflexibility of the quadriceps muscle. It is bilateral in 20 to 30 percent of cases. It may be associated with a hereditary component.[99] In addition, males are affected three times more often than females.[85] The symptoms of pain and swelling over the tibial tuberosity are bilateral in 25 to 33 percent of the cases[85] and usually remit by the age of 18, when the apophysis fuses to the main bone. The symptoms are secondary to incomplete separation of the cartilagenous link between the patellar tendon and the tibia. The separation interrupts the blood supply, resulting in aseptic necrosis fragmentation, and eventually new bone formation. Fusion of the tubercle to the tibia occurs by 18 years of age, thus eliminating any further symptoms.

On examination there is typically pain, swelling, and tenderness localized over the tibial tubercle. Quadriceps use against resistance aggravates the pain as during climbing of steps or kneeling. The treatment includes a reduction of activity (ie, sprinting, jumping, and kicking), anti-inflammatory modalities and medications, and a short course of NSAIDs. In severe cases, place the affected leg in a cast or brace at 0 to 30 degrees for 6 to

8 weeks. Surgery may be required if the conservative treatment fails, but it cannot be implemented until the epiphysis is closed, at which time the problem is usually resolved.[85] Nevertheless, salicylates and rest are the mainstay of treatment.

REFERENCES

1. Abbott LC, et al: Injuries to the ligaments of the knee joint. *J Bone Joint Surg* [Br] **26:**503, 1944.
2. Andrews JR, et al: Isolated posterior cruciate ligament injuries. *Clin Sports Med* **13:**3, 1994.
3. Barber FA, Sutker AN: Iliotibial band syndrome. *Sports Med* **14:**2, 1992.
4. Bellabarba C, et al: Patterns of meniscal injuries in the anterior cruciate-deficient knee: A review of the literature. *Am J Orthop* **26**(1):18–23, 1997.
5. Bessette GC: The meniscus. *Orthopedics* **15**(1):35, 1992.
6. Boynton MD, Fadale PD: The basic science of anterior cruciate ligament surgery. *Orthop Rev* **22**(6):673–679, 1993.
7. Brantigan OC, Voshell AP: The mechanics of the ligaments and menisci of the knee joint. *J Bone Joint Surg* **23:**44, 1941.
8. Bratt HD, Newsman AP: Complete dislocation of the knee without disruption of both cruciate ligaments. *J Trauma* **34:**3, 1993.
9. Bristow WR: Internal derangement of the knee joint. *Am J Surg* **43:**458, 1949.
10. Cameron JC, Saha S: Management of medial collateral ligament laxity. *Orthop Clin North Am* **25,** 1994.
11. Clancy W Jr, Sutherland TB: Combined posterior ligament injuries. *Clin Sports Med* **13:**3, 1994.
12. Clayton MI: Experimental investigations of ligamentous healing. *Am J Surg* **98:**373, 1959.
13. Colosimo AJ, Bassett FH: Jumper's knee. *Ortho Rev* **XIX**(2):139, 1990.
14. Covoy DC, Sapega AA: Anatomy and function of the posterior cruciate ligament. *Clin Sports Med* **13:**3, 1994.
15. Cubbins W: Cruciate ligaments. *Am J Surg* **43:**481, 1939.
16. Davidson K: Patellofemoral pain syndrome. *Fam Phy* **48:**7, 1993.
17. Dehaven KE, et al: Diagnosis of internal derangement of the knee. The role of arthroscopy. *J Bone Joint Surg* **57:**802, 1975.
18. Dehaven KE, Bronstein RD: Arthroscopic medal meniscal repair in the athlete. *Clin Sports Med* **16:**1, 1997.
19. Delorme TL: Restoration of muscle power by heavy resistive exercise. *J Bone Joint Surg* [Br] **27:**645, 1945.
20. Diment MT, et al: Current concepts in meniscal repair. *Orthopedics* **6:**9, 1993.
21. Donaldson WF, Warren RF, Wickiewicz T: A comparison of acute anterior cruciate ligament examinations. Initial vs. examination under anesthesia. *Am J Sports Med* **13:**5, 1985.
22. Dye SF: The future of anterior cruciate ligament restoration. *Clin Orthop Rel Res* **325:**130–139, 1996.
23. Ellasser JC, et al: The non-operative treatment of collateral ligament injuries of the knee in professional football players. *J Bone Joint Surg* **56**(6):1186, 1974.
24. Emerson J: Basketball knee injuries and the anterior cruciate ligament. *Clin Sports Med* **12:**2, 1993.
25. Eriksson E: Reconstruction of the anterior cruciate ligament. *Orthop Clin North Am* **7:**167, 1976.
26. Fanelli C, et al: The posterior cruciate ligament arthroscopic evaluation and treatment. *J Arthro Rel Surg* **10**(6):673–688, 1994.
27. Fat pad syndromes. Sports injury assessment and rehabilitation. *J Bone Joint Surg* **32:**433–434, 1991.
28. Ferguson AB, et al: The isolated medial capsular lesion of the knee. *Clin Orthop* **97:**119, 1973.
29. Fetto JF, et al: Medial collateral ligament injuries of the knee. *Clin Orthop* **132:**206, 1978.
30. Flandry F, Hughston JC: Complications of extensor mechanism surgury for patellar malalinment. *Am J Orthop* **12:**534–543, 1995.
31. Fowler PJ: Bone injuries associated with anterior cruciate ligament disruption. *Arthroscopy* **10**(4):453–460, 1994.
32. Frank CB, Gravet JC: Hamstring in anterior ligament injuries. *Arthroscopy* **11**(4):444–448, 1995.
33. Furman W, et al: The anterior cruciate ligament. *J Bone Joint Surg* **58:**179, 1976.
34. Galway RD: Pivot-shift syndrome. *J Bone Joint Surg* **54:**558, 1972.
35. Gibbs N: Common rugby league injuries. Recommendations for treatment and preventative measures. *Sports Med* **18**(6):438–450, 1994.
36. Ginsburg JH, et al: Problem areas in the diagnosis and treatment of ligament injuries of the knee. *Clin Orthop* **132:**201, 1978.
37. Girgis FC, et al: The cruciate ligaments of the knee joint. *Clin Orthop* **106:**216, 1975.
38. Goldberg B: Patellofemoral malalignment. *Pediatr Ann* **26**(1):32–35, 1997.
39. Gruber MA: The conservative treatment of chondromalacia patellae. *Orthop Clin North Am* **10**(1):106, 1979.
40. Hartlepool MF, et al: Local excision of cyst of the lateral meniscus without recurrence. *J Bone Joint Surg* [Br] **58**(2):88, 1976.
41. Hawkins RJ, Kennedy JC: Tension studies of knee ligaments. Presented at American Orthopaedic Society for Sports Medicine, Dallas, January 22, 1974.
42. Hayes CW: MRI of the patellofemoral Joint. *Semin Ultrasound CT MRI* **15**(5):383–395, 1994.
43. Hefet AF: Function of the cruciate ligaments of the knee joint. *Lancet* **2:**665, 1948.
44. Hey A, Groves EW: The cruciate ligaments of the knee joint. *J Surg* **7:**505, 1920.
45. Hoppenfeld S: Physical examination of the knee joint by complaint. *Orthop Clin North Am* **10**(1):3, 1979.
46. Hough AJ, Webber RJ: Pathology of the meniscus. *Clin Orthop* **252:**32, 1990.
47. Houghton JC, et al: Classification of knee ligament instabilies. I. The medial compartment and cruciate ligaments. *J Bone Joint Surg* **58**(2):159, 1976.
48. Hughston JC: Acute knee injuries in athletes. *Clin Orthop* **23:**114, 1962.
49. Hughston JC, et al: Classification of knee ligament instabilities. II. The lateral compartment. *J Bone Joint Surg* **58**(2):174, 1976.

50. Hughston JC, Eilers AF: The role of the posterior oblique ligament in repairs of acute medial ligament tears of the knee. *J Bone Joint Surg* **55:**923, 1973.

51. Hutchinson MR, Ireland ML: Knee injuries in female athletes. *Sports Med* **19**(4):288–302, 1995.

52. Ikpeme JO, Gray C: Traumatic prepatellar neuralgia. *Injury* **26:**225–229, 1995.

53. Indelicato PA: Nonoperative management of complete tears of the medial collateral ligament. *Orthop Rev* **XVIII**(9):974, 1989.

54. Indelicato PA, Hermansdorfer J, Huegel M: Nonoperative management of complete tears of the medial collateral ligament of the knee in intercollegiate football players. *Clin Orthop* **256:**174, 1990.

55. Install J: Chondromalacia patella: Patella malalignment syndrome. *J Bone Joint Surg* **10**(1):117, 1979.

56. Install J: Chondromalacia patellae. *J Bone Joint Surg* **58**(1):1, 1976.

57. Irrgang JJ: Modern trends in anterior cruciate ligament rehabilitation: Nonoperative and postoperative management. *Clin Sports Med* **12:**4, 1993.

58. Johnson DL, Warner JP: Diagnosis for anterior cruciate ligament surgery. *Clin Sports Med* **12:**4, 1993.

59. Kannus P, Bergfeld J, Jarvinenn M, et al: Injuries to the posterior cruciate ligament of the knee. *Sports Med* **12**(2):110, 1991.

60. Kaplan EB: Factor responsible for the stability of the knee joint. *Bull Hosp Joint Dis* **18:**51, 1957.

61. Kaplan EB: The iliotibial tract. Clinical and morphological significance. *J Bone Joint Surg* **40:**817, 1958.

62. Kennedy JC, et al: Medial and anterior instability of the knee. *J Bone Joint Surg* **53**(7):1257, 1971.

63. Kennedy JC, Fowler PJ: Medial and anterior instability of the knee. An anatomical and clinical study using stress machines. *J Bone Joint Surg* **53:**1257, 1971.

64. Kennedy JC, et al: The anatomy and function of the anterior cruciate ligament. *J Bone Joint Surg* **56**(2):223, 1974.

65. Kollias SL, Fox JM: Meniscal repair. *Clin Sports Med* **15:**3, 1996.

66. Kuo RS, Sonnabend DH: Simultaneous rupture of the patellar tendons bilaterally: Case report and review of the literature. *J Trauma* **34:**3, 1993.

67. Labrier K, O'Neill DB: Patellofemoral stress syndromes. Current concepts. *Sports Med* **16**(6):449–459, 1993.

68. Larsen J: Disease of the patella. Sports injury assessment and rehabilitation. *J Bone Joint Surg* **73A:**406–408, 1991.

69. Liu S, Mirzayan R: Section III: Regular and special features. Current review. *Clin Orthop Rel Res* **317,** 1995.

70. Manaster BJ, Andrews CL: Factures and dislocations of the knee and proximal tibia and fibula. *Sem Roentgenogr* **29**(2):113–133, 1994.

71. Markolf KL, et al: Stiffness and laxity of the knee. The contributions of the supporting structuress. *J Bone Joint Surg* [Br] **58:**583, 1976.

72. Marshall JL, et al: Ligamentous injuries of the knee in skiing. *Clin Orthop* **115:**196, 1975.

73. Marshall JL, et al: The anterior drawer sign. What is it? *J Sports Med* **3:**152, 1975.

74. McCaroll JR, et al: Anterior cruciate ligament injuries in young athletes. Recommendations for treatment and rehabililtation. *Sports Med* **20**(2):117–127, 1995.

75. Merrill KD: Knee dislocations with vascular injuries. *Orthop Clin North Am* **25:**4, 1994.

76. Miller KG: A prospective study comparing the accuracy of the clinical diagnosis of meniscus tear with magnetic resonance imaging and its effect on clinical outcome. *J Arthro Rel Surg* **12:**406–413, 1996.

77. Miller MD, et al: Posterior cruciate ligament injuries. *Orthop Rev* **22**(11):1201–1210, 1993.

78. Molnar TJ, Fox JM: Overuse injuries of the knee in basketball. *Clin Sports Med* **12:**2, 1993.

79. Moyer R, Marchetto PA: Injuries of the posterior cruciate ligament. *Clin Sports Med* **12:**2, 1993.

80. Nicholas JA: Injuries in sports: Recent developments. *Orthop Clin North Am* **8**(3):523, 1977.

81. Nicholas JA: Injuries to knee ligaments. Relationship to loosness and tightness in football players. *JAMA* **212:** 2236, 1970.

82. Obedian RS, Grelsamer RP: Osteochondritis dissecans of the distal femer and patella. *Clin Sports Med* **16:**1, 1997.

83. O'Donoghue DH: Surgical treatment of fresh injuries to the major ligaments of the knee. *J Bone Joint Surg* **32:**721, 1950.

84. O'Donoghue DH: Treatment of acute ligamentous injuries of the knee. *Orthop Clin North Am* **4:**617, 1973.

85. Osgood-Schlatter Disease: Sports injury assessment and rehabilitation. *J Bone Joint Surg* **73A:**409–412, 1991.

86. Ott JW, Clancy WG: Review: Functional knee braces. *Orthopaedics* **16:**2, 1993.

87. Outridge RE, et al: The problem of chondromalacia patellae. *Clin Orthop* **110:**177, 1975.

88. Palmer I: On the injuries to the ligaments of the knee. *Acta Chir Scand* (supp) **81:**53, 1938.

89. Pickett JC, et al: Injuries of the ligaments of the knee. *Clin Orthop* **76:**27, 1971.

90. Polly H, Hayden G: *Physical Examination of the Joints.* Philadelphia Saunders, 1988.

91. Poulsen KA, et al: Thromboembolic complications after arthroscopy of the knee. *Arthroscopy* **9**(5):570–573, 1993.

92. Reider B: Medial collateral ligament injuries in athletes. *Sports Med* **21**(2):147–156, 1996.

93. Safran MR, Fu FH: Uncommon causes of knee pain in the athlete. *Orthop Clin North Am* **26:**3, 1995.

94. Schenck RC, Goodnight JM: Current concepts review. Osteochondritis dissecans. *J Bone Joint Surg* **78A:**3, 1996.

95. Schulte KR, et al: Arthroscopic posterior cruciate ligament reconstruction. *Clin Sports Med* **16:**1, 1997.

96. Schwartzber G, Csencsitz TA: Bilateral spontaneous patellar tendon rupture. *Am J Orthop* **25**(5):369–372, 1996.

97. Semonian RH, et al: Proximal tibiofibular subluxation relationship to lateral knee pain: A review of proximal tibiofibular joint pathologies. *J Orthop Sports Phys Ther* **21:**5, 1995.

98. Siwek CW, Rao JP: Ruptures of the extensor mechanism of the knee joint. *J Bone Joint Surg* **63A:**932, 1981.

99. Smith AD, Tao SS: Knee injuries in young athletes. *Clin Sports Med* **14**:3, 1995.

100. Spritzer CE, et al: Medial retinacular complex injury in acute patellar dislocation: MR findings and surgical implications. *AJR* **168**(1):117–122, 1997.

101. Steadman JR, Sterett WI: The surgical treatment of knee injuries in skiers. *Med Sci Sports Exerc* **27**(3):328–333, 1995.

102. Strand T, Engesaeter LB, Molster AO: Meniscus repair in knee ligament injuries. *Acta Orthop Scand* **56**:130, 1985.

103. Sutro CJ, et al: Fabella. *Arch Surg* **30**:777, 1935.

104. Swenson TM, Harner CD: Knee ligament and meniscal injuries. Current concepts. *Orthop Clin North Am* **26**: 1995.

105. Treadwell EL: Synovial cysts and ganglia: The value of magnetic resonance imaging. *Semin Arthritis Rheum* **24**(1):61–70, 1994.

106. Tuite MJ, Desmet AA: MRI of selected sports injuries: Muscle tears, groin pain, and osteochondritis dissecans. *Semin Ultrasound CT MRI* **15**(5):318–340, 1994.

107. Vailas JC, Pink M: Biomechanical effect of functional knee bracing. Practical implications. *Sports Med* **15**(3):210–218, 1993.

108. Veltri DM: Arthroscopic anterior cruciate ligament reconstruction. *Clin Sports Med* **16**:1, 1997.

109. Veltri DM, Warren RF: Anatomy, biomechanics, and physical findings in posterolateral knee instability. *Clin Sports Med* **13**(3):599–614, 1994.

110. Walker CW, Moore TE: Imaging of skeletal and soft tissue injuries in and around the knee. *Radiol Clin North Am* **35**:3, 1997.

111. Wang C, et al: Rotary laxity of the human knee joint. *J Bone Joint Surg* **56**(1):161, 1974.

112. Warren LF, et al: Injuries of the anterior cruciate ligaments of the knee. *Clin Orthop* **136**:191, 1978.

113. Warren LF, et al: The prime static stabilizer of the medial side of the knee. *Clin Orthop* **123**:206, 1978.

114. Wasilewski SA, Koth J: Effect of surgical timing on return to sports activity after significant knee injuries. *Sports Med* **18**(3):156–161, 1994.

115. Weiner D, et al: The fabella syndrome. *Clin Orthop* **116**:213, 1975.

116. Westrich GH, et al: Occupational knee injuries. *Orthop Clin North Am* **27**(4):805–814, 1996.

117. Woo SLY, et al: Biomechanics of knee ligament healing, repair and reconstruction. *J Biomechanics* **30**(5):431–439, 1997.

118. Goodfellow J: Patello-femoral joint, mechanics and pathology. *J Bone Joint Surg* [Br] **58**(3):291, 1976.

BIBLIOGRAPHY

Abbott LC, et al: Injuries to the ligaments of the knee joint. *J Bone Joint Surg* **26**:503, 1944.

American Medical Association: *Standard Nomenclature of Athletic Injuries*. Chicago: American Medical Association, 1966.

Ashby ME: Low velocity gunshot wounds involving the knee joint. *J Bone Joint Surg* **56**(5):1047, 1974.

Ballard A, et al: The functional treatment of pyogenic arthritis of the adult knee. *J Bone Joint Surg* **57**(8):1119, 1975.

Bartel DL, et al: Surgical repositioning of the medial collateral ligament. An anatomical and mechanical analysis. *J Bone Joint Surg* **59**(5):107, 1977.

Blackburne JS: A new method of measuring patellar height. *J Bone Joint Surg* **59**(2):241, 1977.

Campbell WC: Reconstruction of the ligaments of the knee. *Am J Surg* **43**:473, 1939.

Casscells SW: Arthroscopy of the knee joint. *J Bone Joint Surg* **52**:287, 1971.

Casscells SW: The torn or degenerated meniscus and its relationship to degeneration of the weight bearing areas of the femur and tibia. *Clin Orthop* **132**:196, 1978.

Chrisman OD, et al: Cartilage degeneration and salicylates. *J Bone Joint Surg* **50**:1258, 1968.

Dehaven KE, et al: Diagnosis of internal derangement of the knee. *J Bone Joint Surg* **57**(6):802, 1975.

Edward DH: Osteochondritis dissecans patellae. *J Bone Joint Surg* **59**(1):58, 1977.

Ellsasser JC, et al: The nonoperative treatment of collateral ligament injuries of the knee in professional football players. *J Bone Joint Surg* **56**:1185, 1974.

Furman W, et al: The anterior cruciate ligament. A functional analysis based on postmortem studies. *J Bone Joint Surg* **58**:179, 1976.

Gurgis FG, et al: The cruciate ligaments of the knee joint. Anatomical functional and experimental analysis. *Clin Orthop* **106**:216, 1975.

Hallen LG, Lindahl D: Rotation in the knee-joint in experimental injury to the ligaments. *Acta Orthop Scand* **36**:400, 1965.

Handelsman JE: The knee joint in hemophilia. *Orthop Clin North Am* **10**(1):139, 1979.

Houghton JC: Subluxation of the patella. *J Bone Joint Surg* [Br] **50**:1003, 1968.

Insall J, et al: Chondromalacia patellae. A prospective study. *J Bone Joint Surg* **58**:1, 1976.

Insall J, Salvati F: Patella position in the normal knee joint. *Radiology* **101**:101, 1971.

Karlson S: Chondromalacia patellae. *Acta Chir Scand* **83**:347, 1939.

Krause WR: Mechanical changes in the knee after meniscectomy. *J Bone Joint Surg* **58**(5):599, 1976.

Lancourt JE, et al: Patella alta and patella infera. *J Bone Joint Surg* **57**(8):1112, 1975.

Liljedahl SL, et al: Early diagnosis and treatment of acute ruptures of the anterior cruciate ligament. *J Bone Joint Surg* [Br] **47**:1503, 1965.

Maquet PG, et al: Femorotibial weight bearing areas. *J Bone Joint Surg* **57**(6):766, 1975.

Marshall JL: Knee ligament injuries. *Clin Orthop* **123**:115, 1977.

Nicholas JA, et al: Double-contrast arthrography of the knee. *J Bone Joint Surg* [Br] **52**(2):203, 1979.

Noble J: Lesions of the menisci. *J Bone Joint Surg* **59**(4):480, 1977.

O'Donoghue DH, et al: Repair and reconstruction of the anterior cruciate ligament in dogs. Factors influencing long-term results. *J Bone Joint Surg* **53**:710, 1971.

Roach JE, et al: Comparison of the effects of steroid, aspirin and sodium salicylate on articular cartilage. *Clin Orthop* **106:**350, 1975.

Schlonsky J, et al: Lateral meniscus tears in young children. *Clin Orthop* **117:**222, 1977.

Slocum DB, Larson RL: Rotary instability of the knee. *J Bone Joint Surg* **50:**211, 1968.

Wang JB, et al: Acute ligamentous injuries of the knee. Single contrast arthrography. A diagnostic aid. *J Trauma* **15:**431, 1975.

26
CHAPTER

DISLOCATIONS OF THE KNEE, FIBULA, AND PATELLA

☐ KNEE DISLOCATIONS (FIGS. 26–1 THROUGH 26–5)

Dislocations of the knee are caused most often by motor-vehicle accidents and vehicle-pedestrian accidents[9] and should be considered orthopedic emergencies. Patients infrequently present with a dislocation as most are reduced by the time they arrive in the emergency department. The diagnosis can only be made if the examining physician retains a high index of suspicion. Neurovascular injuries are commonly seen after a knee dislocation. For example, the popliteal artery is injured in 30 to 40 percent of all knee dislocations.[7,8,15,16] Also, traction injuries to the peroneal and tibial nerves are frequently seen after these dislocations.[8,15,16]

Dislocations are classified on the basis of the direction of tibial movement in relation to the femur. Anterior dislocations are the most common, representing nearly 60 percent of all knee dislocations in one series.[8] In the authors' experience, however, the posterior dislocation is more common. Knee dislocations may be classified as anterior, posterior, medial, lateral, or rotary, which include anterolateral, posteromedial, and posterolateral. Knee dislocations may be further categorized into open or closed injuries and into fracture–dislocations or simple dislocations.

Mechanism of Injury

Each type of knee dislocation has a distinct mechanism and also characteristic associated injuries. Both the

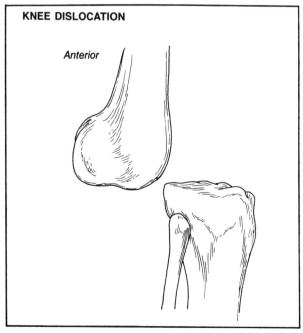

KNEE DISLOCATION

Anterior

Figure 26–1.

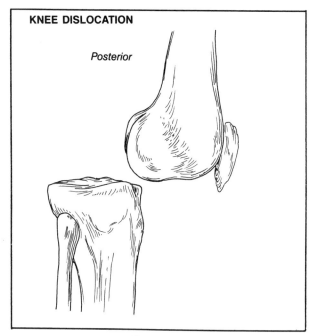

Figure 26–2.

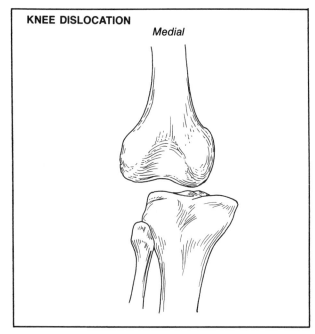

Figure 26–4.

mechanism of injury and the associated injuries will be discussed in this section.

☐ Anterior
This is the most common type of knee dislocation and typically results from hyperextension.[8] A common history is one of walking briskly and then stepping in a hole, resulting in hyperextension and dislocation. Hyperextension results in a tear of the *posterior capsule* fol-

lowed by a rupture of the *anterior cruciate* and a partial tear of the *posterior cruciate*. The *collateral ligaments* of the knee usually remain intact; however, there is a high incidence of *popliteal arterial injuries* secondary to traction or laceration.[8]

☐ Posterior
These dislocations usually result from a direct posterior force applied to the anterior tibia with the knee flexed

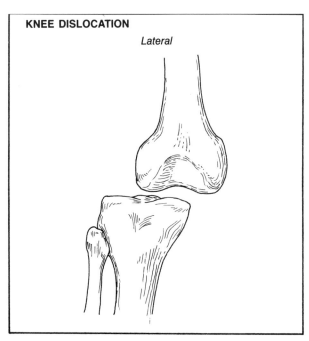

Figure 26–3.

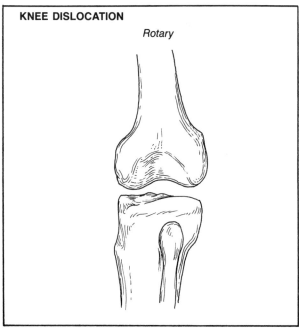

Figure 26–5.

slightly. There is posterior displacement of the tibia with rupture of the *posterior capsule* and *cruciates*. Arterial injuries are not commonly seen after a posterior dislocation.

☐ Lateral

A violent abduction force on the tibia against the femur may result in a lateral dislocation. The *medial collateral*, *both cruciates*, and the *medial posterior capsule* are damaged after a lateral dislocation. Arterial injuries are uncommon after true lateral dislocations.

☐ Medial

A violent adduction force on the tibia against the femur may result in a medial dislocation. The lateral collateral, both cruciates, and the posterior capsule are damaged after a medial dislocation. Peroneal nerve injuries are common with this dislocation. Popliteal arterial damage, however, is not commonly seen after this injury.

☐ Rotary

Posterolateral dislocations are seen when an anteromedial force acts on the anterior tibia, resulting in a posterior dislocation with rotation. There are usually ruptures of the *posterior* and *medial capsules* with partial *avulsion of the gastrocnemii* along with *meniscal damage* and a *chondral fracture*. The *peroneal nerve* is frequently damaged after these injuries. A posteromedial dislocation is the result of an anterolateral force acting on the anterior tibia, resulting in a posterior dislocation with rotation. There is usually rupture of the *medial collateral*, both *cruciates*, the *medial posterior capsule* with a partial *avulsion of the gastrocnemii* along with *meniscal damage* and *chondral fractures*.

Associated Injuries

As mentioned earlier, each type of knee dislocation is associated with several significant injuries. The reader is referred to the previous section on mechanism of injury for a complete discussion.

Under mechanism of injury, we have listed each dislocation of the common arterial injury associated with that dislocation. However, a general discussion is warranted. Popliteal artery injury is the most devastating complication of traumatic knee dislocations. Various authors have reported amputation rates ranging from less than 10 percent up to 90 percent. The critical period for arterial repairs is 6 to 8 hours after injury. When the time interval has approached 6 hours or when marked swelling or increased compartment pressures are evident, fasciotomy is recommended to avoid compartment syndromes and subsequent contracture. The incidence of associated popliteal artery injury within the dislocation has been reported to be approximately 33 percent, with a range anywhere from 16 percent to 64 percent. Routine use of arteriography in patients with knee dislocation

has been a subject of much debate. One must rely on clinical judgment and resource availability to make the decision.

Nerve injuries associated with knee dislocations are less frequent than vascular injuries. The tibial and common peroneal nerves are not anchored as securely as the popliteal artery and, therefore, are injured less often. Reported incidents of nerve injury ranges from 10 percent to 37 percent. These injuries range from simple neuropiraxia to complete disruption of the neural elements, which is rare. The mechanism of neural damage is usually a traction injury. The treatment of these injuries is controversial and left to the consultant.

Examination

An accurate diagnosis of a knee dislocation is imperative and is based on a high index of suspicion.

Axiom: *A grossly unstable knee after a traumatic injury is a reduced dislocation until proven otherwise.*

The oversight of an undiagnosed reduced knee dislocation may have disastrous consequences. In one large series of 245 knee dislocations, 32 percent suffered injury to the popliteal artery.[7] Popliteal arterial injuries must be repaired within 8 hours of injury or up to 86 percent of these injuries will result in amputation.[7] Sixty-six percent of those not requiring amputation had permanent ischemic changes of the leg and the foot.[7]

Axiom: *An acutely traumatized unstable knee with absent distal pulses requires emergent surgical exploration.*

Spasm of the popliteal artery is not a likely cause of distal ischemia and the obtaining of angiograms should not delay operative exploration. The distal leg and foot should always be examined for warmth, pulses, and Doppler pressures. Any obvious temperature difference between feet suggests arterial occlusion in the cooler extremity. Nevertheless, a serious arterial injury may be present despite a warm noncyanotic foot or the presence of a distal pulse.[8,15]

The initial assessment of an acutely traumatized knee in which one suspects dislocation should be limited to inspection, palpation, and a distal neurovascular examination. The patient will present with a history of trauma and a chief complaint of pain. There may or may not be an effusion because a tear in the joint capsule will allow the blood to dissect into the surrounding tissues. If the compartment pressure increases, fasciotomy is

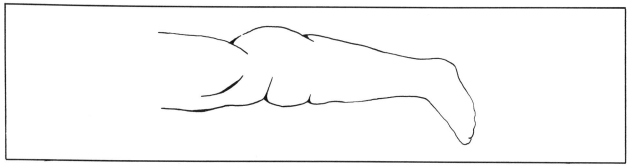

Figure 26–6. Swelling in the popliteal space associated with injury to the popliteal artery after a dislocation.

recommended to avoid compartment syndrome and foot drop.[9] As shown in Figure 26–6, a full popliteal fossa may indicate a popliteal arterial injury.[8,15] The distal neurovascular status must be assessed early and completely in all patients. The ligamentous structures should also be examined carefully at this time. Hyperextension should be avoided because it places unnecessary traction on the peroneal nerve. If there is hypoesthesia in the first web space or loss of dorsiflexion of the foot, with equal temperatures bilaterally, one can suspect peroneal nerve injury.[1] A valgus tilt with the knee in extension acts to protect the peroneal nerve from traction.

X Ray

Anteroposterior (AP) and lateral views are usually adequate in demonstrating any associated fractures. In those patients with diminished distal circulation, arteriography should not delay operative exploration. For those patients who have had anterior or posterior dislocations and whose distal pulses are normal, arteriography should be performed to exclude arterial damage. Those patients with medial or lateral dislocations and normal distal pulses should be observed closely for signs of ischemia.

Treatment

The emergency management of these injuries includes reduction, immobilization, the assessment of vascular injuries, and emergent referral. Spinal anesthesia for reduction is recommended but may be difficult to administer. Parenteral analgesics and muscle relaxants can also be used before reduction.

Anterior. The knee may be reduced by having an assistant place longitudinal traction on the leg while the femur is lifted anteriorly into a reduced position.[8] Pressure over the popliteal space should be avoided. After reduction, the knee should be immobilized in 15 degrees of flexion to avoid tension on the popliteal artery.

Posterior. The knee may be reduced by having an assistant exert longitudinal traction while the proximal tibia

is lifted anteriorly and reduced (Fig. 26–7). The knee should be immobilized in 15 degrees of flexion.

Lateral, Medial, and Rotary. Longitudinal traction along with lifting of the tibia into position will result in reduction. However, a posterolateral dislocation is irreducible because of the evangination of the medial femoral condyle through the medial capsule. These cases require an operative reduction.[9] After reduction the knee should be immobilized in 15 degrees of flexion.

Eighteen percent of patients who were pulseless before reduction will have a return of the pulse after reduction.[7,8]

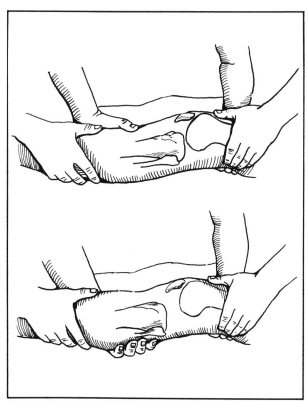

Figure 26–7. Reduction of a posterior dislocation. Note that distraction is a critical maneuver.

Although initially it seemed that magnetic resonance imaging (MRI) would be a gold standard in the evaluation of cartilage, the technique has not yet fulfilled this promise. Arthroscopy is still regarded as the most reliable means of the diagnosis of chondromalacia. Some accurate anatomical details can be obtained by MRI.

Because vascular injury concominent with knee dislocation occurs in about 40 percent of dislocations, it is critical to identify this injury and treat it early. The window of opportunity, as previously indicated, is short. In approximately 10 percent of cases, normal pulses are restored after reduction of the knee. However, in approximately 90 percent of cases, pulses are not restored to normal with reduction. Expeditious treatment of the vascular injury is critical to a good outcome. A one-shot arteriogram can be obtained in the operating room, but proceeding directly with popliteal artery exploration is reasonable if the pulses have not returned to normal.

Complications

Knee dislocations are often complicated by the development of significant problems.

1. Progressive distal ischemia may develop, resulting in amputation.
2. Degenerative joint disease with arthritis is common after knee dislocations.
3. Persistent joint instability secondary to extensive ligamentous injuries is common after these injuries.

☐ PROXIMAL TIBIOFIBULAR DISLOCATIONS AND SUBLUXATIONS (FIG. 26–8)

These are uncommon injuries usually limited to skydivers, hang-gliding enthusiasts, or patients who have suffered a significant fall. It is important to recall that the peroneal nerve passes inferior to the fibular head and encircles the neck of the fibula. The following classification system was developed by Lyle.[10]

Anterior dislocation:	Most common[2,4]
Posterior dislocation:	Sometimes referred to as posteromedial
Superior dislocation:	Always accompanied by superior displacement of the lateral malleolus

Proximal tibiofibular subluxation (Fig. 26–9) is a symptomatic hypermobility of the proximal tibiofibular joint. Pain along the lateral aspect of the knee must be carefully evaluated as the anatomy and the biomechanics of this region are very complex. Anatomic variance of the proximal tibiofibular joint may be key to understand-

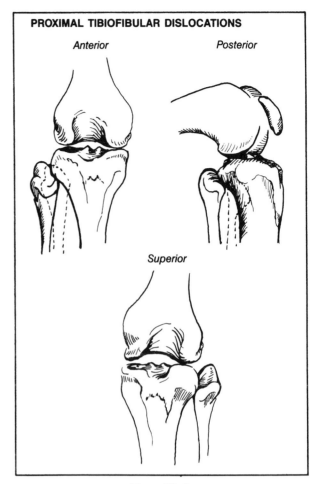

PROXIMAL TIBIOFIBULAR DISLOCATIONS

Anterior   Posterior

Superior

Figure 26–8.

ing the proper mechanics and, thus, treatment of this joint. Treatment of proximal tibiofibular subluxation will involve modifying the patient's activities and the utilization of a supportive strap along with lower leg strengthening exercises.

The location of the pain is generally along the lateral aspect of the knee. It radiates proximally into the region of the iliotibial band and medially into the patellofemoral joint. The patient specifically grabs around the lateral head of the gastroinemius, noting pain along the posterior lateral joint line of the knee. The patient also complains of swelling which disappears and reports clicks somewhere in the front of the knee. Usually there is no specific mechanism described by the patient. Inspection of the knee will reveal a prominent fibular head in the anterior lateral subluxation or dislocation. Movement of the fibula is from side to side (Fig. 25–9).

Mechanism of Injury

Anterior dislocations typically result from a fall where the leg is flexed and adducted. A secondary mechanism involves a violent twisting motion.[12] Posterior

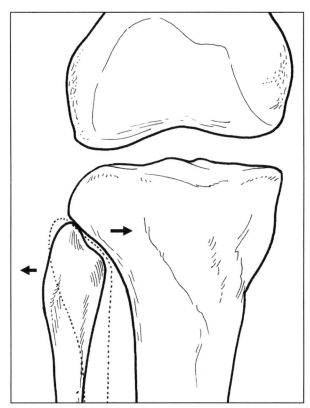

Figure 26–9. Proximal tibiofibular joint subluxation.

dislocations are usually secondary to direct trauma to the flexed knee.[11] In addition, violent twisting may rupture the ligaments and result in dislocation.[12]

Examination

The patient may present with only minimal symptoms and a suggestive history. On examination there will be a localized exacerbation of pain with inversion or eversion of the ankle. The pain will increase with palpation over the fibular head. With an anterior dislocation the fibular head will be more prominent when the knee is flexed. In addition, dorsiflexion and eversion will exacerbate the pain.[11] Superior dislocations present with a proximal displacement of the lateral malleolus.[12]

X Ray

If this injury is suspected, comparison views are recommended. AP and lateral views are usually adequate in defining this injury.

Associated Injuries

Posterior dislocations are associated frequently with peroneal nerve injuries. Superior dislocations are always associated with interosseous membrane damage.[12]

Treatment

These dislocations should be reduced by direct manipulation with the knee in flexion. An audible click is often

heard as the fibula snaps back into position.[11,12] Posterior dislocations with interposed soft tissues require an operative reduction.[12] After reduction the patient should be on crutches with non–weight bearing for 2 weeks followed by progressive weight bearing over the next 6 weeks.[12]

Complications

Peroneal nerve injury occurs in 5 percent of these dislocations and may present as a complication during the recuperation period.[12] Posterior dislocations have a tendency to remain unstable and to develop recurrent subluxation.[12] Degenerative joint disease with arthritis may develop after any of these dislocations.[13]

☐ PATELLAR DISLOCATIONS (FIG. 26–10)

Patellar dislocations are typically seen in patients with chronic patellofemoral anatomic abnormalities. Severe trauma is necessary for a dislocation to occur with a normal patellofemoral relationship.

Anatomically, the patella is an oval-shaped bone with two facets divided by a vertical ridge. The patella normally articulates in the groove between the femoral condyles. The vastus medialis, medial retinaculum along with the medial and lateral patellofemoral and the patellotibial ligaments keep the patella from dislocating. Patellar dislocations tend to occur in patients with the following:

1. Genu valgum
2. Genu recurvatum
3. Excessive femoral neck anteversion or internal femoral torsion
4. External tibial torsion
5. Lateral insertion of patellar ligament on the tibia
6. Contracture of the lateral patellar retinaculum
7. Relaxation or attenuation of medial patellar retinaculum
8. Hypoplasia or dysplasia of the patella
9. Hypoplasia or flattening of the trochlear groove
10. Patella alta or high riding patella
11. Atrophy of the vastus medialis muscle
12. Pes planus
13. Generalized joint laxity

Mechanism of Injury

There are two mechanisms that result in patellar dislocations. Direct trauma to the patella with the knee in flexion may result in a dislocation although this is uncommon. Horizontal dislocations are secondary to a direct blow on the superior pole of the patella followed by rotation.[5,6]

A powerful contraction of the quadriceps in combination with sudden flexion and external rotation of the tibia on the femur frequently results in a lateral patellar dislocation.

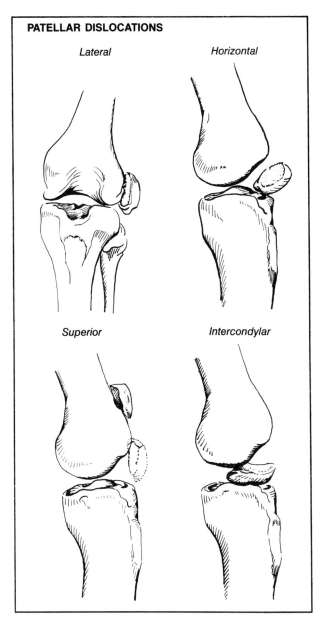

PATELLAR DISLOCATIONS

Lateral

Horizontal

Superior

Intercondylar

Figure 26–10.

Dislocations and subluxations tend to be recurrent as the supporting structures tend to become lax and the femoral condyles erode and thin out.

The classification of patellar dislocations is diagramed in Figure 26–10. Lateral dislocations are by far the most common type.

Examination

If this is the patient's first patellar dislocation, he or she typically will relate a history of feeling the knee go out and noting a deformity followed by swelling.[13] On examination there may be a hemarthrosis if the dislocation is not a chronic problem. There is generally tenderness along the undersurface of the patella and the *Fairbands* or *patellar apprehension test* is positive. This test is performed by simply attempting to push the patella laterally. If positive, the patient will grab for the knee as this reproduces the sensation of impending dislocation.

The examining physician should always search for predisposing factors for dislocation as well as accompanying bony or cartilagenous injuries.

X Ray

AP and lateral views are usually adequate in assessing this injury. Radiographs should always be obtained even if the patella is reduced to exclude a fracture. The presence of a fat-fluid level is indicative of a bony or osteochondral fracture. Note that an abnormal patellofemoral angle is not a reliable radiologic sign of patellar instability in acute dislocation.[17]

Associated Injuries

Osteochondral fractures of the patella or lateral femoral condyle occur in 5 percent of all patellar dislocations.[14]

Treatment

Lateral dislocations can be reduced by flexing the hip and applying a gentle medially directed pressure while extending the knee. Intra-articular and horizontal dislocations are sometimes reduced by closed manipulation although most require open reduction. Superior dislocations usually require operative reduction.

After reduction, radiographs documenting the position of the patella should be obtained. Consultation with an orthopedic surgeon at this point is recommended. Many orthopedic surgeons will elect a conservative approach with long leg casting for 6 weeks in full extension.[3] Some orthopedic surgeons believe that all first-time dislocations should be surgically repaired initially.[13,14] Most surgeons would agree that those dislocations associated with an osteochondral fracture are best treated surgically.

Complications

Patellar dislocations are subject to the following complications: degenerative arthritis, osteochondral fractures not diagnosed initially, and recurrent dislocations and subluxations.[1]

□ PATELLAR SUBLUXATION

Patellar subluxation is a common condition and is seen quite frequently. The diagnosis can be made by palpating tenderness over the superior-medial border of the patella. A subluxation of the patella usually occurs laterally and is associated with a tear of the retinaculum along the vastus medialis.

The initial therapy is nonoperative and includes rest and the administration of nonsteroidal anti-inflammatory agents. Isometric exercises to strengthen the quadriceps are included. Stretch exercises for the hamstrings are also advocated. In cases where tenderness is severe and one notices substantial laxity, the use of a patellar restraining brace is used. Operative therapy is not recommended unless there is no success with nonoperative therapy for 6 to 12 months.

REFERENCES

1. Arnbjornsson A, Negund N, Rydling O, et al: The natural history of recurrent dislocation of the patella. *J Bone Joint Surg* **74B**(1):140, 1992.
2. Christensen S: Dislocations of the upper end of the fibula. *Can Med Assoc J* **98:**169, 1968.
3. Cofield RH, et al: Acute dislocation of the patella. *J Trauma* **17**(7):526, 1977.
4. Dennis JB, et al: Bilateral recurrent dislocations of the superior tibiofibular joint with peronal-nerve palsy. *J Bone Joint Surg* **40:**1146, 1958.
5. Frangakis EK: Intra-articular dislocation of the patella. *J Bone Joint Surg* **56**(2):423, 1974.
6. Gore DR: Horizontal dislocation of the patella. *JAMA* **214**(6):1119, 1970.
7. Green NE, et al: Vascular injury associated with dislocation of the knee. *J Bone Joint Surg* [Br] **59**(2):236, 1977.
8. Kennedy JC: Complete dislocation of the knee joint. *J Bone Joint Surg* **45**(5):889, 1963.
9. Kremcheck TE, Welling RE, Kremcheck EJ: Traumatic dislocation of the knee. *Orthop Rev* **XVIII**(10):1501, 1989.
10. Lyle HHM: Tramatic luxation of the head of the fibula. *Ann Surg* **82:**635, 1925.
11. Ogden JA: Dislocations of the proximal tibiofibular joint. *J Bone Joint Surg* **56**(1):147, 1974.
12. Parkes JC, et al: Isolated acute dislocation of the proximal tibiofibular joint. *J Bone Joint Surg* **55**(1):177, 1973.
13. Percy EC: Acute dislocation of the patella. *Can Med Assoc J* **105:**1176, 1971.
14. Rorabeck CH: Acute dislocation of the patella with osteochondral fracture. *J Bone Joint Surg* [Br] **50**(2):237, 1976.
15. Shields L, et al: Complete dislocation of the knee. *J Trauma* **9**(3):192, 1969.
16. Taylor AR, et al: Traumatic dislocation of the knee. *J Bone Joint Surg* [Br] **54**(1):96, 1972.
17. Vainionpaa S, Laasonen E, Silvennoinen T, et al: Acute dislocation of the patella. *J Bone Joint Surg* **72B**(3):366, 1990.

27
CHAPTER

FRACTURES OF THE TIBIAL AND FIBULAR SHAFT

The tibia and the fibula run parallel to each other and are tightly bound together by ligaments. Typically, a displaced fracture of one bone is associated with an obligatory fracture or ligamentous injury of the other bone.[4] Tibial fractures are not only the most common of the long bone fractures, they are the most common open fracture seen. Fibular shaft fractures are uncommon injuries alone and are usually associated with a tibial fracture. The fibula is a non–weight-bearing bone that can be resected proximally without any loss of function. Distally, of course, the fibula is essential for ankle stability. Fibular shaft fractures alone are usually treated only symptomatically, and they usually heal without complications (Figs. 27–1 and 27–2).

Tibial fractures are classified on the basis of principles established by Nicoll and used by Rockwood and Green.[8,9] Nicoll established that three factors determine the outcome of tibial fractures:

1. Initial displacement
2. Comminution
3. Soft tissue injury (open)

A type I fracture is only slightly displaced (0 to 50 percent) and noncomminuted. Type II fractures have greater than 50 percent displacement but continued bony contact and may be slightly comminuted. Type III fractures have complete displacement with comminution. Type II or III fractures may be open or closed. Type I

TIBIAL AND FIBULAR SHAFT FRACTURES

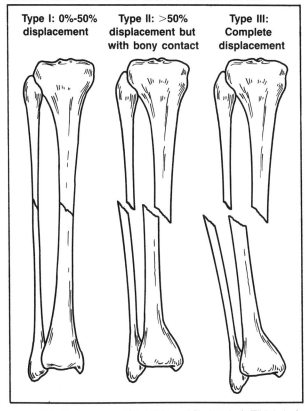

Type I: 0%-50% displacement

Type II: >50% displacement but with bony contact

Type III: Complete displacement

Figure 27–1. Fractures of the tibia and fibular shaft. Tibial shaft fractures can occur alone but are treated similarly to the above.

483

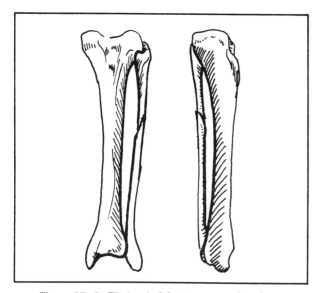

Figure 27–2. Fibular shaft fractures occurring alone.

fractures have a 90 percent chance of union whereas those classified as type III have only a 70 percent chance of union.

Essential Anatomy

There are three compartments in the leg containing the muscles, nerves, and vessels:

1. The *anterior* compartment contains the tibialis anterior, extensor hallucis longus, peroneus tertius, extensor digitorum longus, anterior tibial artery, and the deep peroneal nerve.
2. The lateral compartment includes the peroneus longus and brevis and the superficial peroneal nerve.
3. The posterior compartment contains the soleus, gastrocnemius, tibialis posterior, flexor hallucis longus, and the flexor digitorum longus.

Mechanism of Injury

There are two mechanisms that result in fractures of the tibial and fibular shafts. Direct trauma, as with automobile accidents, or certain types of skiing injuries (boot-top fractures) are responsible for the majority of tibial and fibular shaft fractures. Direct trauma typically results in transverse or comminuted fractures.

Indirect trauma is associated with rotary and compressive forces as from skiing or a fall, and usually results in a spiral or oblique fracture. A tibial plafond fracture is typically secondary to a fall from a height that drives the talus up into the tibia.

Examination

Fibular shaft fractures present with pain that is exacerbated with walking. Tibial shaft fractures usually present with pain, swelling, and deformity. Although neurovascular damage is not commonly seen after these injuries documentation of pulses as well as the function of the peroneal nerve (dorsiflexion and plantar flexion of the toes) is imperative.

X Rays (Figs. 27–3, 27–4)

Anteroposterior (AP) and lateral views are generally adequate in defining the position of the fracture fragments. When describing these fractures it is important to assess the following:

1. Position: upper middle or lower third
2. Type: transverse, oblique, spiral, or comminuted
3. Displacement: percentage of fracture surface contact
4. Angulation: valgus or varus of the distal fragment

Associated Injuries

As mentioned earlier, neurovascular damage at the time of injury is not common although severe injuries may have incomplete or complete disruption of the neurovascular structures.[6] Anterior compartment syndromes may follow tibial fractures and usually present within the first 24 to 48 hours. If suspected, the anterior compartment muscles should be palpated for tenderness or rigidity. The dorsalis pedis pulse should be palpated and compared with the uninjured extremity as well as the sensation between the first and second toes as an indicator of peroneal nerve function. If a compartment syndrome is suspected, emergent orthopedic consultation is recommended. The determination of anterior and/or posterior compartment pressures in addition to a thorough clinical examination will determine the subsequent management plan.[11]

Treatment

The emergency center management of tibial shaft fractures includes initial examination, immobilization in a long leg splint, and emergent referral. Open fractures may be gently cleaned and dressed. Tetanus prophylaxis (when indicated) and parenteral cephalosporins should be initiated. Emergency operative debridement with external or internal fixation is recommended.[1,7,10,12] An emergent reduction of a closed fracture before x rays may be indicated when there is a limb threatening vascular compromise. After the radiographic examination, emergent orthopedic consultation is advised because of the high incidence of complications. Patients with tibial shaft fractures may have an associated compartment syndrome which will evolve later. For this reason, most patients with significant tibial shaft fractures should have an emergent orthopedic consultation and be hospitalized with elevation of the extremity and close observation for the development of a compart-

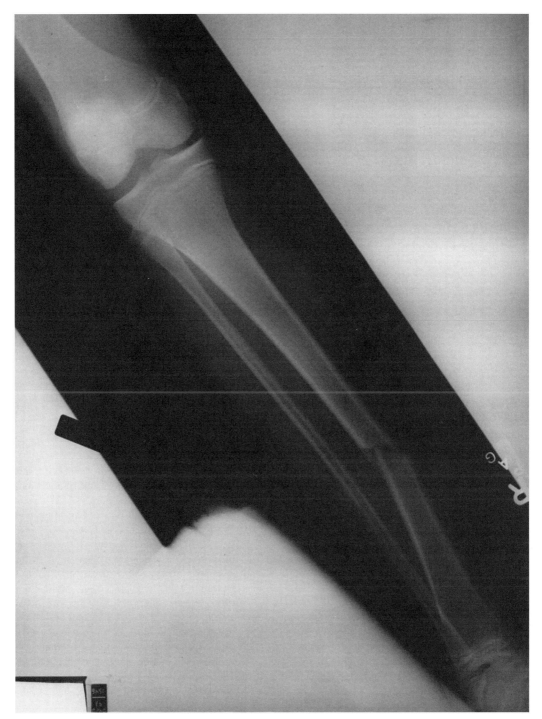

Figure 27–3. Midshaft of the tibia fracture with minimal bowing of the fibula. (*Courtesy of G.A. Peyer, Racine, WI.*)

ment syndrome. A nondisplaced type I tibial shaft fracture can be treated with a long leg non–weight-bearing cast. There is some controversy in the literature concerning the advantages of conservative closed reduction with casting versus open reduction with internal fixation of closed displaced tibial shaft fractures.[3,5]

Emergent orthopedic consultation is strongly recommended in the management of these fractures.

The average healing time for uncomplicated nondisplaced fractures is 10 to 13 weeks. For displaced, open, or comminuted fractures the average healing time is 16 to 26 weeks.

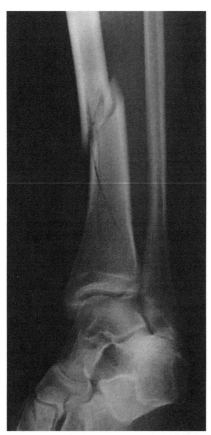

Figure 27–4. Comminuted fracture of the distal tibia with minimal displacement.

In patients with an ununited fracture of the tibia a small portion of the fibula has been removed by some investigators, and this has been found to increase the compressive force on the two ends of the tibia. This has resulted in an increased incidence of union in patients with complicated tibial fractures.[2,12]

Ununited tibial diaphyseal fractures have posed a difficult problem. Pulsing electromagnetic fields have been used to improve the incidence of union in these fractures. Successful results have occurred in approximately 87 percent of cases without any further surgery needed.

Isolated fibular shaft fractures are treated symptomatically and may be casted for relief of pain. Initially, a long leg cast is most comfortable, and this may be reduced to a short leg cast after 2 weeks and removed after 4 weeks. Some patients have little pain and tolerate initial crutch walking without casting very well.

Complications
Shaft fractures of the tibia and fibula have several significant complications.

1. Nonunion or delayed union are common especially when there is:
   a. severe displacement
   b. comminution
   c. open fracture or severe soft tissue damage
   d. infection
2. Neurovascular compromise may develop after treatment secondary to swelling.
3. Chronic joint pain or stiffness are uncommon except in those fractures involving the tibial plafond.

Axiom: *Any patient with a tibial fracture and increasing pain 24 to 48 hours after casting should be suspected of having a compartment syndrome. The cast should be bivalved and the leg thoroughly examined.*

REFERENCES

1. Blachut PA, Meek N, O'Brian P: External fixation and delayed intramedullary nailing of open fractures of the tibial shaft. *J Bone Joint Surg* [Br] **6:**729–735, 1990.
2. DeLee JC, Heckman JD, Lewis AG: Partial fibulectomy for united fractures of the tibia. *J Bone Joint Surg* **63A:**1390, 1981.
3. Den Outer AJ, Meeuwis J, Zwaveling A: Conservative versus operative treatment of displaced noncomminuted tibial shaft fractures. *Clin Orthop* **3:**231–237, 1990.
4. Goldsmith R: Fractures of the shaft of the tibia and fibula. *Surg Clin North Am* **3:**1781, 1940.
5. Hooper GJ, Keddell RG, Penny ID: Conservative management or closed nailing for tibial shaft fractures. *J Bone Joint Surg* **73B**(1):83–85, 1991.
6. Howard PW, Making GS: Lower limb fractures with associated vascular injury. *J Bone Joint Surg* **72B**(1):116–120, 1990.
7. Korovessis PN, Milis Z, Christodoulou G, et al: Open tibial shaft fractures: A comparative analysis of different methods of fixation in southwestern Greece. *J Trauma* **1:**77–81, 1992.
8. Nicoll EA: Fractures of the tibial shaft. *J Bone Joint Surg* [Br] **46:**373, 1964.
9. Rockwood CA, Green DP: *Fractures*, vol 2. Philadelphia: Lippincott, 1975.
10. Thakur J, Patankar J: Open tibial fractures. *J Bone Joint Surg* **73B:**448–451, 1991.
11. Triffitt PD, Konig D, Harper WM, et al: Compartment pressures after closed tibial shaft fracture. *J Bone Joint Surg* **74B**(3):195–198, 1992.
12. Whittle A, Russell A, Taylor J, Lavelle G: Treatment of open fractures of the tibial shaft with the use of interlocking nailing without reaming. *J Bone Joint Surg* **10:**1162–1171, 1992.

BIBLIOGRAPHY

Brown PW, Urban JG: Early weight bearing treatment of open fractures of the tibia. *J Bone Joint Surg* **51:**59, 1969.

Burwell HN: Plate fixation of tibial shaft fractures. *J Bone Joint Surg* [Br] **53:**258, 1971.

Campanacci M, Zanoli S: Double tibiofibular synostosis for nonunion and delayed union of the tibia. *J Bone Joint Surg* **48:**44, 1966.

Dehne E: Treatment of fractures of the tibial shaft. *Clin Orthop* **66:**159, 1969.

Hamza KN, et al: Fractures of the tibia. *J Bone Joint Surg* [Br] **53:**696, 1971.

Johnson RJ, et al: Boot top fractures of the fibula. *Clin Orthop Relat Res* **101:**198, 1974.

Linden W, et al: Fractures of the tibial shaft after skiing and other accidents. *J Bone Joint Surg* **57:**321, 1975.

Olerud S, Karlstrom G: Secondary intramedullary nailing of tibial fractures. *J Bone Joint Surg* **54:**1419, 1972.

Pantazopoulos T, et al: Treatment of double tibial fractures of blind intramedullary nailing. *Clin Orthop* **84:**137, 1972.

Rorabeck CH, Macnab I: Anterior tibial-compartment syndrome complicating fractures of the shaft of the tibia. *J Bone Joint Surg* **58:**549, 1976.

Sakellarides HT, et al: Delayed union and nonunion of tibial shaft fractures. *J Bone Joint Surg* **46:**557, 1964.

Sarmiento A: A functional below the knee cast for tibial fractures. *J Bone Joint Surg* **49:**855, 1967.

Sarmiento A: A functional below the knee brace for tibial fractures. *J Bone Joint Surg* **52:**295, 1970.

Souter WA: Autogenous cancellous strip grafts in the treatment of delayed union of long bone fractures. *J Bone Joint Surg* [Br] **51:**63, 1969.

28
CHAPTER

SOFT TISSUE INJURIES, DISLOCATIONS, AND DISORDERS OF THE LEG

The leg contains the tibia and the fibula, but the tibia is the only weight-bearing bone. Also, the thigh muscles attach to the upper portion of the tibia. The fibula is bound to the tibia by the interosseous membrane, which divides into a "Y" both above and below to surround the talofibular joint. One arm of the "Y" is called the *antero-superior tibiofibular ligament* and the other the *postero-superior tibiofibular ligament*. A similar division occurs below with an anterior and posterior inferior tibiofibular ligament. The fibula is of little importance in its upper portion, which can be excised with little consequence. The lower portion cannot because of its importance in forming the ankle mortise.

The muscles of the leg are enclosed in fascial compartments of which there are four: anterior, peroneal, deep posterior, and superficial posterior compartments. The anterior compartment houses the dorsiflexors of the ankle and foot and the posterior compartment contains the plantar flexors. The peroneal compartment houses the everters of the foot.

□ CONTUSIONS

Contusions are extremely common in the lower extremity because direct blows are frequent there. Four types of contusions are seen: (1) of the anterior compartment musculature producing severe pain caused by pressure

on this closed compartment; (2) of the subcutaneous portion of the tibia, which, because of the superficial location of the tibia, often results in a *traumatic periostitis;* (3) over the posterior compartment, which is less common and not nearly as painful as contusions of the anterior compartment; and (4) over the peroneal nerve where it winds around the upper fibula, producing a painful neuritis or even transient paralysis of the peroneal nerve with a secondary foot drop.

A hematoma may form at the site of the contusion, and if this occurs in the anterior compartment, the patient may present as a surgical emergency requiring fasciotomy to prevent ischemia and subsequent muscle necrosis.

The treatment of these injuries is contingent on the extent of damage and the structures involved. If there is a fresh, palpable hematoma one may aspirate it by using an aseptic technique followed by a pressure bandage and cold compresses for the next 12 hours. If the contusion is limited to diffuse muscle involvement, the initial treatment should include ice packs and rest of the extremity with elevation for the first 48 hours. When the periosteum is involved, a protective padding is all that is necessary, supplemented with analgesics for pain. In contusions involving the nerve, the patient will have local swelling and pain with paresthesias noted. The patient will complain of a shocklike sensation, with pain shooting throughout the distribution of the nerve to the lateral side of the leg and extending into the foot. A sharp tingling and numbness will remain after the pain is gone. In patients with severe contusions to the common peroneal nerve these initial symptoms will be followed by an asymptomatic period where symptoms subside, and the patient complains only of pressure sensation over the nerve and functional loss, with sensory hyperthesia and weakness of the dorsiflexors. This period of functional loss is followed by a period when there is return of nerve function, the first to return being sensation. The return of nerve function may be complete or partial. The treatment for a nerve contusion is initially nonspecific with ice packs followed in 48 hours by heat applications. If paresis is noted, the muscles must be protected by supporting the ankle and the foot in a brace holding the foot in a neutral position. In patients in whom the contusion is followed by a quiescent period and then rapid paralysis, exploration is justified. When paralysis is immediate a more conservative approach is usually taken. Referral is indicated in all patients with nerve involvement.

MUSCLE STRAINS

Muscle strains are common in the calf due to chronic overuse or forcible contraction. The treatment is symptomatic with a period of rest, local heat, and gradual return to activity.

A common question relates to the use of stretching, a commonly used method to prevent muscle strains. Clinical studies have clearly demonstrated that cyclic stretching appears to be beneficial. Stretching that leads to forces in excess of 70 percent of the contractile force of that muscle may make the muscle *more rather than less* likely for injury. Thus, when using stretching to running or other activities, one should use minimal force. Viscoelasticity is known to be temperature dependent and warm-up is considered to protect against muscle strain. Remember to remind the athlete that early return to activity before complete healing entails a risk for further and more major injury of that muscle.

Recent studies clearly demonstrate that nonsteroidal anti-inflammatory agents may be of some benefit early during treatment for pain control and functional improvement; however, long-term use of these agents beyond 2 to 3 days is detrimental to the repair process.

☐ SHIN SPLINTS

The term *shin splints* refers to the syndrome of transient pain in the leg from running or hiking and should exclude stress fractures or ischemic disorders.[1] They usually occur early in the training period of athletes when running on hard surfaces. Many causes have been implicated, including periostitis of the tibia and strain at the attachment of the posterior tibial muscle. The most common site of pain is the anteromedial surface of the distal two thirds of the leg.

Many forms of treatment of shin splints have been advocated,[4] but Andrish[1] has shown that they all seem to be about the same and that the pain did not subside until the patient stopped running. The basic treatment is rest, local heat when it affords comfort, and analgesics.

☐ COMPARTMENT SYNDROMES

This condition occurs after exercise when the intramuscular pressure increases. Also 30 to 60 percent of chronic compartment syndromes have muscular herniations. These herniations occur mostly in the lower one third of the leg overlying the anterior intermuscular septum between the anterior and lateral compartment.[2,3]

There are a number of compartments enclosing various muscle groups throughout the body; however, the most widely recognized syndromes in which these muscle groups are "squeezed" and subject to compression within their compartments are those in the leg, the most common being the anterior compartment. Other compartment syndromes, which have been described in the leg, include the deep posterior compartment and the fascial compartment enclosing the peroneal muscles and the soleus.[5,6] A closed tibial fracture is one of the conditions most frequently associated with the development of compartment syndrome. This occurs in both closed and open tibial fractures.

Compartment syndromes are among the most potentially devastating problems presenting to emergency departments. Early diagnosis and understanding of the pathophysiology and the early signs of this process are crucial to the emergency physician (Table 28–1).

Pathophysiology

Compartment syndromes are caused by increased pressure within a closed-tissue space that compromises the flow of blood through the capillaries in the muscles and nerves. A complex relationship between systemic and venous pressures is not completely understood. The detailed explanation of how capillary blood flow is compromised depends on a number of clinical variables. Compartment syndromes can be caused by a number of conditions, including the following:

Decreased compartment size

- Constrictive dressings and casts
- Thermal injuries and frost bite
- Application of excessive traction to a fractured limb
- Localized external pressure

TABLE 28–1. RELATED ANATOMY OF TISSUE COMPARTMENTS OF LEG

Compartment	Muscles	Vessels	Nerves	Weakness	Paresthesia	Pain	Tenseness
Anterior	Ant. tibialis Extensor hallucis longus Extensor digitorum longus Peroneus tertus	Anterior tibial artery & vein	Deep peroneal	Ankle dorsiflexion Toe extension	1st interspace between great and 2nd toes	Ankle plantar flexion Toe flexion	Anterior leg
Lateral	Peroneus longus Peroneus brevis	None	Superficial peroneal	Ankle dorsiflexion Foot eversion	Dorsum of foot	Ankle plantar flexion Foot eversion	Lateral leg
Deep posterior	Post. tibialis Flexor digitorum longus Flexor hallucis longus	Peroneal artery & vein Posterior tibial artery & vein	Posterior tibial	Ankle plantar flexion Foot inversion Toe flexion	Bottom of the foot	Ankle dorsiflexion Foot eversion Toe flexion	Medial leg

Adapted from: Bouche, R.T. (1990). Chronic compartment syndrome of the leg. *Journal of the American Pediatric Medical Association, 80*(12). 633–648.

Increased compartment contents

- Fractures
- Soft tissue injury
- Popliteal cyst
- Bleeding secondary to vascular injury
- Increased capillary permeability ability secondary to postischemic swelling
- Intensive use of muscles such as exercise and seizures
- Severe contusions
- Reduction and fixation of fractures
- Snakebites
- Vessel laceration
- Prolonged immobilization with limb compression
- Edema accumulation due to arterial injury

Thus, an increase in compartmental pressure can be caused by (1) compression of the compartment, for example by a burn, a circumferential cast, or pneumatic pressure garment; and (2) by a volume increase within the compartment due to hematoma and edema.

The normal tissue pressure is approximately zero and always less than 10 mmHg of mercury. Capillary blood flow within the compartment is compromised at pressures greater than 20 mmHg of mercury, and muscle and nerves are at risk for ischemic necrosis at pressures greater than 30 to 40 mmHg of mercury. Of the tissues within the compartments, muscle is most sensitive followed by nerve tissue. Blood flow through the arteries, arterials, and collaterals is not compromised significantly at these pressures. Tissues within the compartment become ischemic and then necrotic if the compartment pressure is not reduced promptly. By the time that distal pulses are reduced, muscle necrosis has already occurred. Ischemic muscles are painful and this pain is exacerbated by both active muscle contraction and passive stretching of the muscle.

Virtually any muscle mass invested in fascia is at risk given the right conditions. The compartments clinically relevant to the emergency physician are the upper-extremity and lower-extremity compartments. In the upper-extremity within the *arm* are an anterior and posterior compartment. The anterior compartment contains the biceps-brachialis muscle and the ulnar, median, and radial nerves. The posterior compartment contains the triceps muscle. In the *forearm* there are a volar and a dorsal compartment (Fig. 28–1). These are subdivided into smaller compartments by the investing fascia at the midforearm. The volar compartment contains the wrist and finger flexors, and the dorsal compartment contains the wrist and finger extenders. The interosseous muscles of the hand are contained in their own compartments.

In the lower extremity there are three *gluteal* compartments in the buttock. One contains the tensor muscle of the fascia lata, another the gluteus medius and minimus, and a third the gluteus maximus. The *thigh* has an anterior compartment containing the quadriceps group and a posterior compartment containing the hamstring group of muscles as well as the sciatic nerve. In the *leg* there are four compartments (Fig. 28–2). The anterior compartment, the compartment most frequently

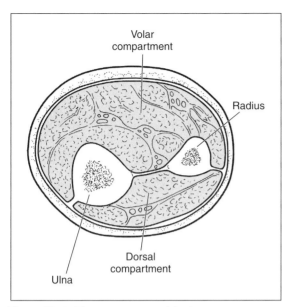

Figure 28–1. The compartment of the forearm.

involved by this syndrome, contains the tibialis anterior muscle and the extensor muscles of the toes. The peroneal compartment contains the evertors of the foot, the peroneus longus, and the peroneus brevis as well as the peroneal nerve. The deep posterior compartment contains the tibialis posterior and the flexors of the toes. The superficial posterior compartment contains the gastrocnemius and the soleus muscles as well as the sural nerve.

Chronic compartment syndrome has been described.[4]

Extract: *"In a consecutive series of 100 patients with chronic compartment syndrome involving 233 compartments, most of these patients were found to be runners. Exercise-induced recurrent tightness, aching, and sharp pains were noted. The main length of symptoms before operation was 22 months. Bilaterality occurred in 82 patients. The majority of these patients had compartment syndrome in either the anterior or posterior compartment. Fasciotomy was performed with a good outcome."[4]*

A conservative treatment for compartment syndromes has also been indicated. This procedure includes prolonged rest, modifying the offending activity, altering the training program, stretching exercises, orthosis, shoe modifications, anti-inflammatory medications, and physical therapy.[2]

☐ Anterior Compartment Syndromes
The anterior compartment of the leg encloses the anterior tibial muscle, the extensor hallucis longus, and the extensor digitorum longus muscles. These muscles are tightly bound to one another and are roofed by the fascia of the anterior part of the leg. Most of the anterior compartment syndromes are secondary to tibial and fibular

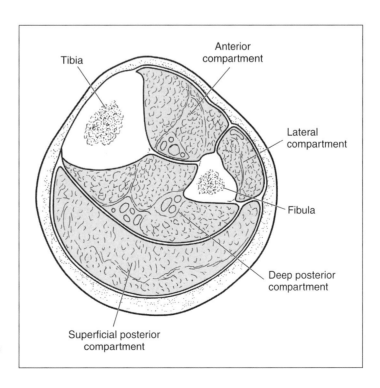

Figure 28–2. The compartments of the leg.

fractures, usually the simple type. Other causes include thrombotic occlusion of the femoral artery, exercise, blunt trauma, and ischemia.[10] In other words, anything that causes swelling in the compartment can cause the syndrome. Experimental studies demonstrate that regardless of the etiology, the common pathway resulting in a compartment syndrome is increased intracompartmental pressure that compromises the blood flow to the compartmental musculature.

Clinical Presentation

The syndrome is characterized by anterior tibial pain, weakness of dorsiflexion of the ankle and the toes, and variable degree of sensory loss over the distribution of the deep peroneal nerve.[9] Clinical evaluation begins with a high degree of suspicion. The earliest and most reliable sign of a compartment syndrome is *severe pain*. This is the first and most important symptom. The pain is not well localized and is out of proportion to the severity of the injury. In addition, intercompartmental pressure is elevated, causing a *palpably tense compartment* as an early sign. *Pain with passive stretch* may be present and can be confused when there is a contusion. One must remember that pareses and paresthesias are not reliable and occur late, as do reduction in pulses.

The emergency physician must not wait for the development of foot drop or paresthesias over the distribution of the deep peroneal nerve as this most assuredly will have disastrous consequences. With the onset of severe pain over the anterior compartment, there is loss of function so that it becomes almost impossible to contract the muscles within the compartment. This will result in foot drop as well as pain caused by passive stretching of the muscles. The skin over the compartment becomes erythematous and shiny and is warm and tender to palpation with what is described as a "woody" feeling. The muscles go on to develop ischemic necrosis and will be replaced by scar tissue.

The examiner must suspect the syndrome in any patient with a cramping pain over the anterior compartment. The pain is typically described as a constant bo-ring pain worsened by walking and relieved somewhat although not completely with rest. Also, when examining the patient, the physician must realize that patients with very low diastolic blood pressures are more susceptible to compartment syndromes.[3] Anterior compartment syndrome may be misdiagnosed as muscle spasms, shin splints, or contusions. However, if the examiner is aware that the previously mentioned conditions can result in a compartment syndrome, he or she will not miss the diagnosis.

Four signs of an anterior compartment syndrome are

1. Pain on passive plantar flexion of the foot
2. Pain increased by dorsiflexion of the foot against resistance
3. Paresthesias in the space between the first and second toes
4. Tenderness over the anterior compartment

Axiom: *Any time a patient complains of intractable pain in the front of the leg with some loss of dorsiflexion of the toes and the foot, an anterior compartment syndrome should be suspected.*

Treatment

One must remember in treating this condition to be alert to the diagnosis. Active contraction of the involved muscle will increase pain as well as passive stretch of the involved muscle. Hypesthesia resulting from compromise of nerves traversing the involved compartment appears later than muscle weakness and pain. If one suspects this diagnosis, the compartment pressures must be measured in the emergency department. Compartment pressure can be quickly and easily measured using a commercially available battery-powered monitor (Stryker STIC monitor). Pressures can also be measured by using a device made up of items in the emergency department after careful aseptic preparation and insertion of an 18-gauge needle into the compartment.

Early ice packs and elevation without any pressure dressings are essential once the diagnosis is suspected. If there is no response, fasciotomy as an emergency surgical procedure is indicated. When a wick catheter is not readily available, a simple technique for measuring compartment pressures, which has proven reliable and accurate, has been described. Figure 28–3 shows a technique of measuring compartment pressures using items that are readily available in any emergency department.

In using the method shown in Figure 28–3, the following supplies are needed:

- A 20-mL syringe
- Two IV extension tubes
- A four-way stop-cock
- A small bottle of sterile saline
- A blood pressure manometer
- An 18-gauge needle

These should be assembled as shown in Figure 28–3. The 18-gauge needle is attached to an IV extension tube and then to the stop-cock. First insert the needle into the sterile saline and aspirate to approximately half the distance of the IV extension tubing. It is important to avoid getting any air into the tubing (one must close one of the ports of the four-way stop-cock with a finger or syringe). This can be facilitated by placing a

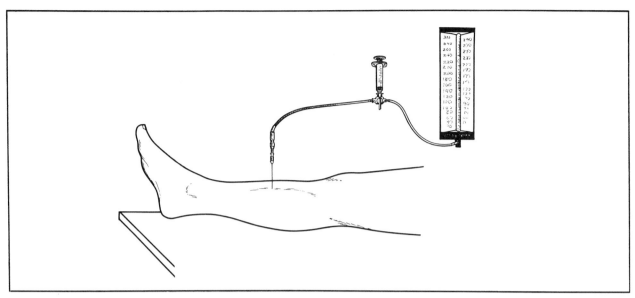

Figure 28–3. Technique for measuring compartment pressure.

small needle into the bottle of saline to allow air entry. The second IV extension tube is then attached to the four-way stop-cock with the opposite end attached to the manometer having removed the black hose from the manometer. The needle is then placed in the compartment and the apparatus kept at the level of the needle. The stop-cock is then turned so that it is open in all three directions: IV tubing on either side and the syringe. Slowly compress the syringe when it is filled with air. The plunger causes air to move into both IV extension tubes. *Watch* the meniscus created by the saline in the extension tube attached to the 18-gauge needle for any movement. As soon as movement occurs in the fluid column, look at the blood pressure manometer. The pressure noted on the manometer *is the compartment pressure.*

Compartment pressures between 15 and 20 are problematic. If the pressure is elevated slightly, the patient can be observed. A pressure of 20 mmHg of mercury can be damaging if it persists for several hours; therefore, admission is required. Pressures greater than 20 mmHg of mercury demand admission and surgical consultation. A pressure of 30 to 40 mmHg of mercury is generally considered grounds for an emergent fasciotomy in the operating room. The fasciotomy is accomplished by making a longitudinal skin incision over the compartment. The underlying fascia is split the length of the compartment allowing the contained muscle to expand. Once muscular necrosis occurs, the fibrous scar is irreversible. Fasciotomy performed early, that is, less than 12 hours after the onset of symptoms, results in the return to normal function in 68 percent of patients, whereas only 8 percent of those with fasciotomies done after 12 hours had completely normal

function.[11] Complications are also much higher when fasciotomy is delayed: a complication rate of 4.5 percent with early fasciotomy, and 54 percent with late fasciotomy.[11] When all four compartments are involved in the syndrome, a double incision fasciotomy or fibulectomy has been advocated.[7]

☐ Deep Posterior Compartment Syndrome
The deep posterior compartment encloses the flexor digitorum longus, the tibialis posterior, and the flexor hallucis longus as well as the posterior tibial artery and nerve. The transverse crucial septum forms the posterior wall of the compartment while the interosseous membrane forms the anterior wall. The clinical picture of this syndrome is usually complicated by involvement of other surrounding compartments. The most common cause of the syndrome appears to be fractures of the tibia and the fibula, usually in the middle or distal thirds.[6] Other causes have been implicated including contusions of the leg, arterial injuries, and even fractures of the calcaneous and the talus.[6]

Clinical Presentation
The patient often has few initial complaints. There is increased pain on passive extension of the toes and weakness of flexion as well as hypesthesia over the distribution of the posterior tibial nerve along the sole. The patient also has tenseness and tenderness along the medial distal part of the leg. All of these signs may become evident within 2 hours to as long as 6 days from the onset of the event that caused it.

Treatment
Once the diagnosis is suspected, all circumferential dressings should be removed and the extremity com-

pletely examined. Once the syndrome is established, fasciotomy is indicated. This is a somewhat more complex technique than for the anterior compartment syndrome and has been described by Paranen.[8]

☐ Chronic Exertional Compartment Syndrome of the Lower Leg

The clinical history of chronic exertional compartment syndrome (CECS) of the lower leg is typically that of an athletic person who describes recurrent pain in the area of the affected compartment during activity. The pain is usually depicted as achiness or tightness and occurs over the particular compartment with exercise. After a period of rest, the pain characteristically subsides only to recur with the onset of the same exercise again. In some patients, paresthesias may develop over an involved nerve.

Clinical Presentation

The patient has a scarcity of definitive findings on examination. Many of the patients demonstrate muscular hypertrophy; however, this finding is common in a population of well-trained athletes. In stress fracture patients, there is often probable tenderness and, in some cases, a sense of soft tissue fullness, swelling, and thickening. In a large number of patients with this syndrome, there appears to be some element of muscle herniation associated with the compartment syndrome. This syndrome should be suspected on clinical grounds and a bone scan should be ordered to rule out any occult fracture or periostitis. The patient should be referred for compartment pressure measurements in order to make a conclusive diagnosis.

Treatment

This condition is not as urgent in requiring treatment as an acute compartment pressure syndrome. The patient should be referred for compartment pressure measurements to an appropriate clinician. These measurements are usually taken postexercise to facilitate making distinctions and comparisons with the normal extremity.

Various treatment modalities such as physical therapy, orthotics, rest, and alternate activity have minimal or no effect. Once the diagnosis of CECS is established, surgical decompression of the involved compartment is recommended.

☐ RUPTURE OF THE POSTERIOR MUSCLES OF THE LEG

Rupture of the gastrocnemius or soleus can occur anywhere from the attachment on the femur or the belly of the muscles to their attachment on the calcaneus, which is the most common site of rupture (along the musculotendinous junction). Another muscle that is subject to

rupture is the plantaris muscle, which is described as a pencil-sized muscle that originates at the lateral condyle of the femur and passes beneath the soleus to attach on the Achilles tendon.

With ruptures of the gastrocnemius or the soleus, the patient notes pain and swelling with diffuse tenderness over the calf. Both active contraction and passive stretching cause pain along the muscle that may bunch up on any attempt at contraction. Surgical repair is indicated for complete ruptures. In patients with partial ruptures, an equinus cast is used until healing is complete. To detect a complete rupture, the physician should place the patient in a prone position with the feet hanging over the end of the table. Squeeze the upper calf and look for plantar flexion spontaneously occurring. If this does not occur, suspect a complete rupture. In patients with plantaris rupture the pain is noted deep in the calf, and it may be disabling. Repair is not needed here; only symptomatic treatment is indicated. The patient may complain of a sudden sharp snap in the posterior part of the leg followed by a more dull deep ache.

☐ FASCIAL HERNIA

Fascial hernias are uncommon; however, patients with these hernias can present with symptoms to the emergency department. The usual site is at the attachment of the anterior fascia along the anterior border of the tibia. The patient complains of an ache here that may be diagnosed as a contusion or periostitis initially. Later, a well-localized mass appears lateral to the tibial crest, which may be tender. The mass bulges when the muscle is relaxed and the examiner may feel a defect on palpation. These patients usually are asymptomatic; however, if symptoms are noted, surgical repair may be indicated.

☐ STRESS FRACTURES

Stress fractures are common in the leg. The fibula is especially prone, being second only to the metatarsal in frequency. Often stress fractures are misdiagnosed as contusions or strains. They occur in young athletes, dancers, or military recruits early in their training period.[9] They can occur in the tibia but are more common along the neck of the fibula.

The patient complains of an insidious onset of soreness or a dull ache in the leg, which is increased with activity. Later the ache becomes continuous even at rest and at night. There is localized tenderness over the fracture site, which is usually at the upper third; and some swelling of the soft tissue. Radiographs taken early are

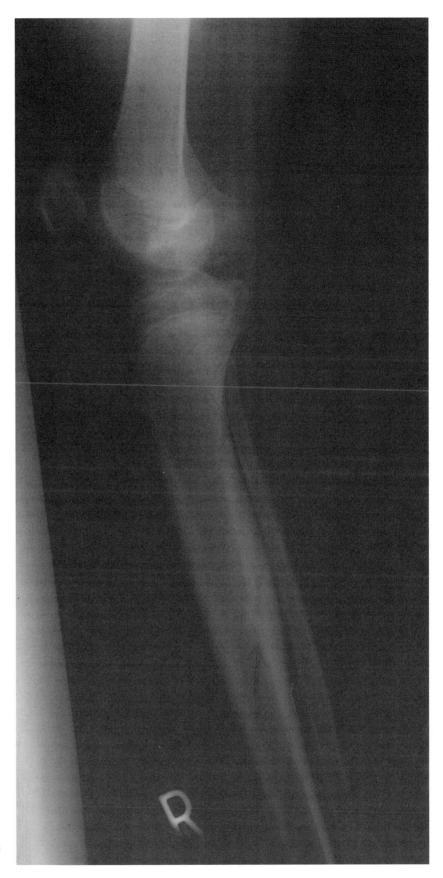

Figure 28–4. Tibial shaft stress fracture.

negative, and the condition may be diagnosed as shin splints. Ten to fourteen days later, however, the examiner will see a transverse fine line with periosteal reactivity along one or both cortices making the diagnosis (Fig. 28–4).

The treatment of a fibular stress fracture is symptomatic with local heat and restriction of activity. Although tibial fracture is less common, it is more disabling and may require casting to protect the tibia until union takes place.

REFERENCES

1. Andrish JT: A prospective study on the management of shin splints. *J Bone Joint Surg* **56**(8):1697, 1974.
2. Bouch RT: Chronic compartment syndromes of the lower leg. *Amer Pediatr Med Assoc* **80**(12):633, 1990.
3. Bourne RB, Rorabeck CH: Compartment syndromes of the lower leg. *Clin Orthop* **3**:97, 1989.
4. Detmer DE, Sharpe K, Sufit RL, Girdley FM: Chronic compartment syndrome: Diagnosis, management and outcomes. *Am J Sports Med* **13**:162, 1985.
5. Kirby NG: Exercise ischaemia in the facial compartment of the soleus. *J Bone Joint Surg* [Br] **52**(4):738, 1970.
6. Matsen FA, Clawson DK: The deep posterior compartmental syndrome of the leg. *J Bone Joint Surg* **57**(1):34, 1975.
7. Murbarak SJ, Owen CA: Double incision fasciotomy of the leg for decompression in compartment syndromes. *J Bone Joint Surg* **59**(2):184, 1977.
8. Paranen J: The medial tibial syndrome. *J Bone Joint Surg* [Br] **56**(4):712, 1974.
9. Protzman RR, Griffis CG: Stress fractures in men and women undergoing military training. *J Bone Joint Surg* **59**(6):825, 1977.
10. Rorabeck CHI, Macnab I: The pathophysiology of the anterior tibial compartmental syndrome. *Clin Orthop* **113**:52, 1975.
11. Sheridan GW, Matsen FA: Fasciotomy in the treatment of acute compartment syndrome. *J Bone Joint Surg* **58**(1):112, 1976.

29
CHAPTER

FRACTURES OF THE ANKLE

The ankle bears more weight per unit area than any other joint in the body. Injuries that are not anatomically reduced often result in the development of traumatic arthritis. It is essential for the physician to realize that ankle fractures and ligamentous injuries frequently coexist. Any treatment plan must include both types of injuries.

Sir Percivall Pott in 1768 was one of the first investigators of ankle fractures.[11] He described a fibular fracture located 3 inches proximal to the malleolus associated with a tear of the deltoid ligament. To this day the term *Pott's fracture* is still used to describe (although inaccurately) a bimalleolar fracture. Since that time several investigators have studied ankle injuries and attempted to develop classification systems. In 1922, Ashurst and Bromer developed a system based on the mechanism of injury.[1] Unfortunately, the progression of injury forces and the associated ligamentous injuries were not properly emphasized, and the system is of little use. In 1949, Niels Lauge-Hansen developed a classification system that took into consideration the position of the foot and the ankle at the time of injury.[11-13] In this classification system the first word refers to the position of the foot at the time the injuring force is applied; the second word pertains to the direction of the injuring force. Unfortunately, this system does not include direct injuries such as impaction or axial compression. In addition, combination forces that account for most injuries are not included in this system. Wilson[18] developed a classification system that included combination forces.

Unfortunately, the system is redundant and places too little emphasis on the position of the foot at the time of injury.

After a brief discussion of functional anatomy, the University of Chicago Emergency Medicine Classification System of ankle injuries will be described in detail. As with any classification system, its worth is measured by its practical applicability and use. This classification system enables the physician to study the x rays of a patient with a fractured ankle and determine the mechanism by which the injury and the associated ligamentous injuries occurred. The physician will know the total extent of the injury and will be able to determine whether the fracture is stable or unstable and thus develop a rational treatment program. Because the classification system emphasizes the mechanism of injury as well as the significant associated injuries, a separate section on each of these topics will not be included.

Functional Anatomy

The ankle has been described in the past as a hinge joint but it more accurately resembles a saddle joint.[9] The talar dome or saddle is wider anteriorly than it is posteriorly (Fig. 29–1). With dorsiflexion, the talar dome fits snugly into the ankle mortis yielding greater stability when compared with plantar flexion. The only "pure" motion occurring at the ankle joint is plantar and dorsiflexion. Inversion and eversion take place at the subtalar joint formed by the talus and calcaneus. This subtalar joint is very strong; the talus should always be thought of as moving with and in the same direction as the calcaneus. Ankle injuries typically follow forces that are directed perpendicular to the normal motion of the joint.

Note: Classification drawings can be found in the tables.

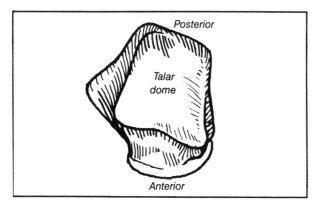

Figure 29–1. Note that the talar dome is wider anteriorly than it is posteriorly.

In ankle injuries, inversion and eversion forces are common and are directed perpendicular to the usual motion of plantar or dorsiflexion.

The ligaments surrounding the lateral portion of the ankle are shown in Figure 29–2 and include the anterior and posterior talofibular and the calcaneofibular ligaments. The strong deltoid ligament as shown in Figure 29–3 is located on the medial surface of the joint and consists of the tibionavicular, tibiocalcaneal, and the tibiotalar components. The deltoid ligament is the only ligament of the ankle containing elastic fibers.

The tibia and the fibula are joined distally by the anterior and posterior tibiofibular ligaments (see Fig. 29–2). These ligaments serve to strengthen the ankle mortise and join proximally to form the interosseous membrane.

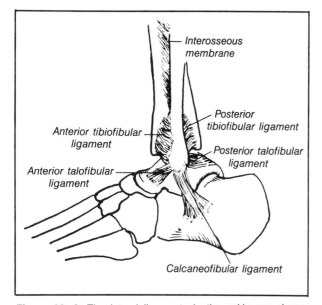

Figure 29–2. The lateral ligaments in the ankle are shown. Note the anterior and posterior tibiofibular ligaments.

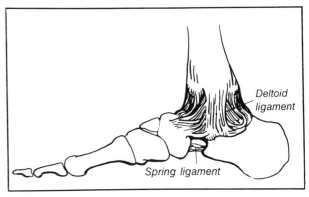

Figure 29–3. Deltoid Ligament.

The motions of the ankle and the foot are described by a number of interchangeable terms.

1. *Eversion*: External rotation
2. *Inversion*: Internal rotation
3. *Dorsiflexion*: Extension
4. *Plantar flexion*: Flexion
5. *Abduction*: Lateral deviation of the forepart of the foot on a longitudinal axis through the tibia
6. *Adduction*: Medial deviation of the forepart of the foot on a longitudinal axis through the tibia
7. *Supination*: Adduction and inversion
8. *Pronation*: Abduction and eversion

These motions must be understood before any further discussion of fractures occurring at this joint. The authors will use the terms listed above in discussing joint fractures throughout this chapter. Inversion is shown in Figure 29–4A. Eversion is shown in Figure 29–4B. Abduction and adduction are demonstrated in Figures 29–4C and 29–4D, respectively. Supination (Fig. 29–4E) is a combined motion involving a combination of adduction and inversion whereas pronation (Fig. 29–4F) involves a combination of abduction and eversion. Note that those motions that displace the talus and the foot in a medial direction are inversion and adduction. Those motions that displace the talus and the foot in a lateral direction are eversion and abduction. This concept must be clearly understood for comprehension of the classification system that follows.

Classification

Multiple classification systems exist for ankle fractures and sprains. The classification system that follows permits a number of axioms that gives the emergency specialist a great deal of information about associated injuries. It is based on an increasing injury with increased force applied in a specified direction. The injury that results depends on:

1. The position of the foot at the moment of injury
2. The direction in which the injuring force displaces the talus

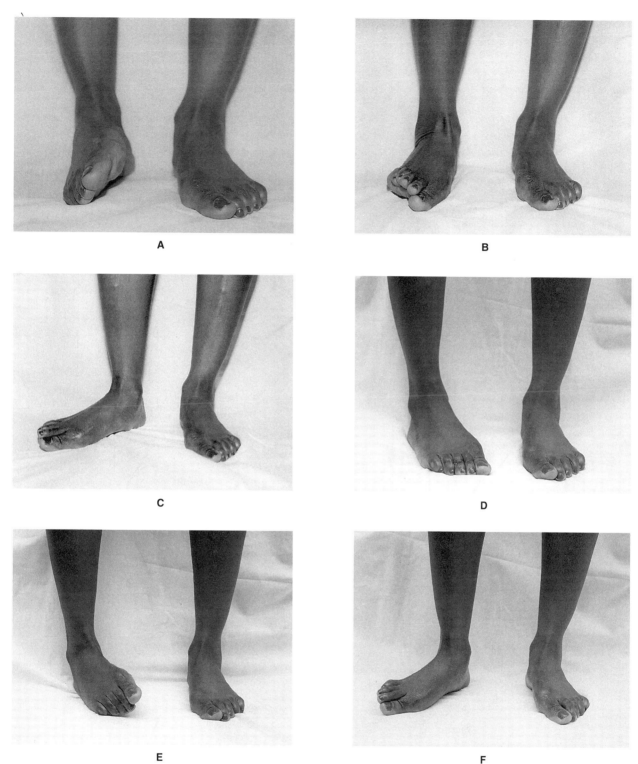

Figure 29–4. **A.** Inversion. **B.** Eversion. **C.** Abduction. **D.** Adduction. **E.** Supination. **F.** Pronation.

3. The intensity of the force and the resistance of the supporting structures

There are three primary forces that act on the ankle. Using the talus as the "reference point," forces may be

directed *medially*, *laterally*, or may result in axial *compression*. Each of these "primary injury forces" may be combined later with secondary injury forces (added to the primary force in parenthesis in the tables). Forces that displace the talus laterally are abduction or eversion forces (class A). The force displacing the talus medially is an adduction force (class B). Class C fractures are the result of axial compression. The position of the foot at the time the force is applied is a determinant of the type and sequence of structures injured and is included in the classification system.[3,6,9,14,16]

Many classification systems exist for ankle fractures. The following discussion enables a number of axioms to be derived and also facilitates an understanding of the mechanism of these fractures. However, the emergency physician is best served by the Neer classification. In this classification system, the ankle is thought of as a closed ring of bone and ligaments surrounding the talus (see below).

The ring in this conceptualization is composed of tibia, tibiofibular ligament, fibula, lateral ligaments of the ankle, calcaneous, and, finally, the deltoid ligament.

A single disruption of the ring, whether osseous or ligamentous, results in a *stable injury*.

If the ring is disrupted in two places, an *unstable injury* results. Unstable injuries can involve two bones such as a bimalleolar fracture or a ligament and a bone (see below).

Stable injuries require no reduction, can be treated in a walking cast (although initially the patient may be placed in a nonwalking cast until the swelling goes down), and have an excellent prognosis. *Unstable injuries* require reduction and are treated surgically. If they are treated conservatively in cases where the patient refuses surgery, they always require a nonwalking cast. In addition, unstable injuries have a guarded prognosis.

This simple classification system enables the emergency physician to determine everything he or she needs to know about ankle fractures.

ANKLE FRACTURES

☐ Class A: Forces that displace the talus laterally (Table 29–1)

☐ Class B: Forces that displace the talus medially (Table 29–2)

☐ Class C: Forces that apply axial compression to the talus (Table 29–3)

TABLE 29–1. CLASS A: FORCES THAT DISPLACE THE TALUS LATERALLY

Type I: Eversion Force

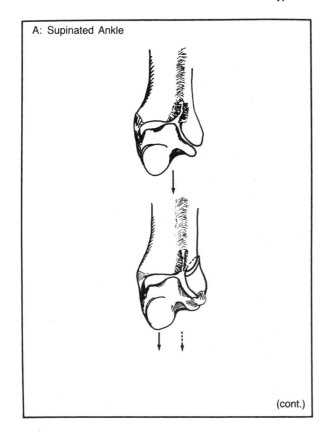

A: Supinated Ankle

(cont.)

1: Rupture of anterior inferior tibiofibular ligament (eversion force)

2: Spiral oblique fracture of the lateral malleolus (eversion force). Dashed arrow represents transition from a spiral oblique fracture to a fracture of the medial malleolus.

TABLE 29-1. CLASS A: FORCES THAT DISPLACE THE TALUS LATERALLY

Type I: Eversion Force

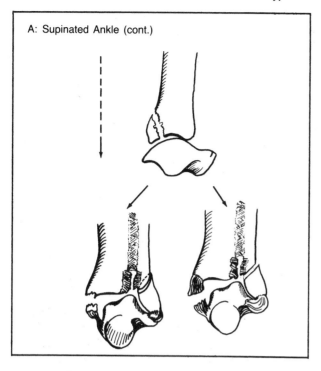

3: Fracture of the posterior lip of the tibia (posterior malleolus) (eversion force and axial pressure)

4: Fracture of the medial malleolus or rupture of the deltoid ligament (eversion force and pronation)

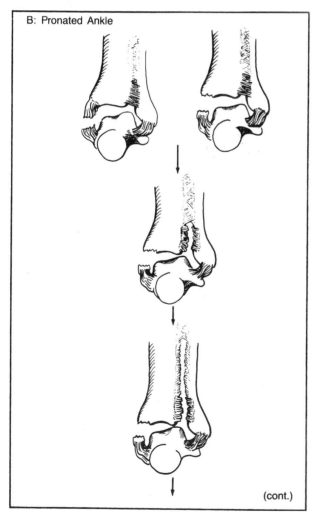

1: Rupture of the deltoid ligament or fracture of the medial malleolus (eversion force)

2: Rupture of the anterior inferior tibiofibular ligament (eversion force)

3: Tear of the interosseous membrane (eversion force)

(cont.)

TABLE 29-1. CLASS A: FORCES THAT DISPLACE THE TALUS LATERALLY

Type I: Eversion Force (cont.)

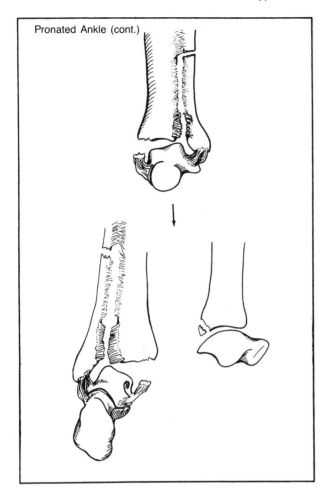

Pronated Ankle (cont.)

4: Spiral fracture of the fibula 7 to 8 cm proximal to the tip of the lateral malleolus (eversion force)

5: Rupture of the posterior inferior tibiofibular ligament or avulsion fracture of the posterior lip of the tibia, or up to 50 percent of articular surface of the tibia included in fracture (eversion force and axial pressure)

Type II: Abduction Force

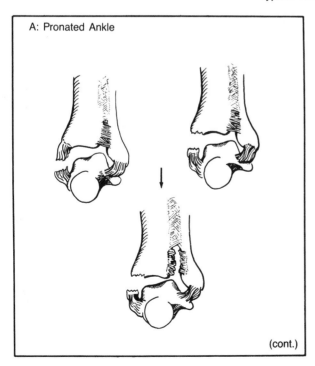

A: Pronated Ankle

(cont.)

1: Fracture of the medial malleolus or rupture of the deltoid ligament (abduction force)

2: Rupture of the anterior inferior tibiofibular ligament and the transverse ligament (abduction force)

TABLE 29–1. CLASS A: FORCES THAT DISPLACE THE TALUS LATERALLY

Type II: Abduction Force (cont.)

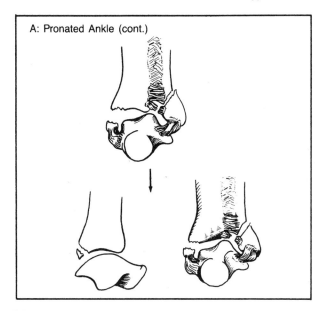

A: Pronated Ankle (cont.)

3: Oblique supramalleolar fracture of the fibula (abduction force)

4: Fracture of the posterior tibial tubercle or an impaction fracture of the lateral tibial plafond (abduction force and axial compression)

☐ CLASS A: FORCES THAT DISPLACE THE TALUS LATERALLY

☐ Class A: Type IA (Eversion Force Applied to the Supinated Ankle, Table 29–1)

This force usually ruptures the anterior inferior tibiofibular ligament or results in a fracture at its insertion on the anterior lateral surface of the distal tibia (Tillaux fracture).[7] This is followed by a spiral fracture of the lateral malleolus at the joint line extending from the anteroinferior direction to the posterosuperior region (Fig. 29–5). If the eversion force persists, an avulsion fracture of the posterior lip of the tibia may occur. There must be a degree of axial compression for this fracture to occur.[6] If the eversion force continues the ankle may be displaced from supination to a pronated position and a deltoid ligament injury or medial malleolar fracture will result.[6]

☐ Class A: Type IB (Eversion Force Applied to the Pronated Ankle, Table 29–1)

This force typically results in a rupture of the deltoid ligament or an avulsion fracture of the medial malleolus. A continuation of the force will result in a rupture of the anterior inferior tibiofibular ligament. If the force persists, the interosseous membrane will rupture proximally followed by a short spiral fracture of the fibula 7 to 8 cm proximal to the ankle mortise. If an axial compression force is added, an avulsion fracture of the posterior lip of the tibia or a rupture of the posteroinferior tibiofibular ligament will follow.

Axiom: *A spiral fracture of the fibula 2 to 3 inches proximal to the ankle mortise is associated with a rupture of the deltoid ligament or a medial malleolar fracture and with rupture of the anterior inferior tibiofibular ligament.*

☐ Class A: Type II (Abduction Force Applied to the Pronated Ankle, Table 29–1)

With a significant force there will be a rupture of the deltoid ligament or an avulsion fracture of the medial malleolus. If the force persists, the anterior inferior tibiofibular and transverse ligaments will rupture. After this an oblique fibular fracture will occur (Fig. 29–6). If an axial compressive force is added there may be a fracture of the posterior tibial tubercle or an impaction fracture of the tibial plafond.

TABLE 29–2. CLASS B: FORCES THAT DISPLACE THE TALUS MEDIALLY

Type I: Adduction Force

A: Supinated Ankle	1: Avulsion of the lateral malleolus or rupture of the talofibular ligament (adduction force)
	2a: Vertical fracture of the medial malleolus (adduction force)
A₁: Dorsiflexed Ankle	2b: Medial malleolar fragment contains part of the anterior articular margin of the tibia (adduction force and axial pressure)
A₂: Plantar-flexed Ankle	2c: Medial malleolar fragment contains part of the posterior articular margin of the tibia (adduction force and axial pressure)

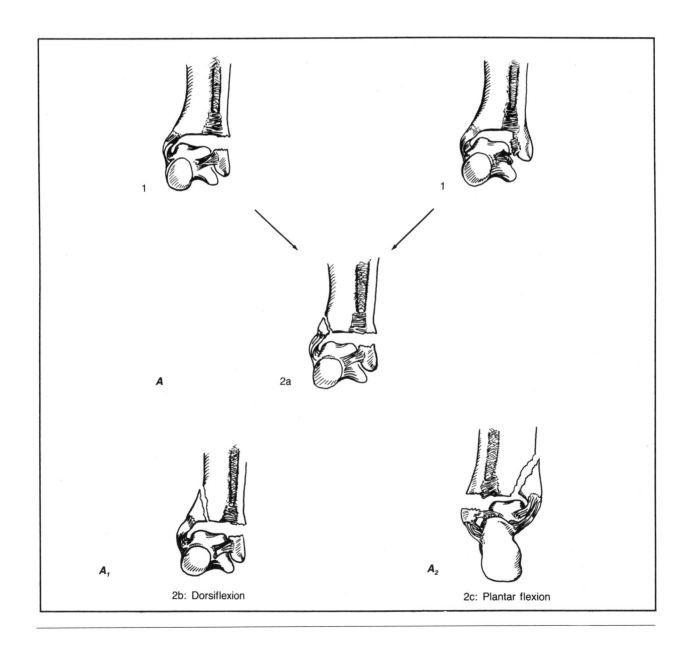

A

1

1

2a

A₁

2b: Dorsiflexion

A₂

2c: Plantar flexion

TABLE 29–3. CLASS C: FORCES THAT APPLY AXIAL COMPRESSION TO THE TALUS

Type I: Axial Compression Forces

A: Dorsiflexed Ankle
B: Plantar-flexed Ankle

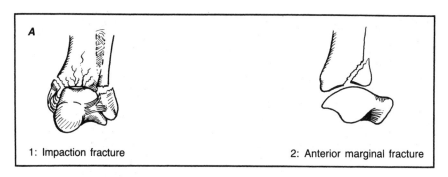

1: Impaction fracture (axial pressure)
2: Anterior marginal fracture (axial pressure)

A

1: Impaction fracture   2: Anterior marginal fracture

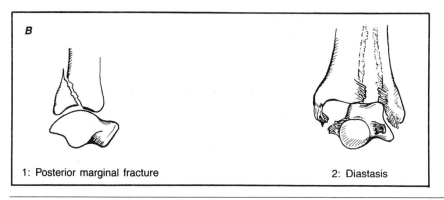

1: Posterior marginal fracture (axial pressure)
2: Diastasis of tibia and fibula (axial pressure)

B

1: Posterior marginal fracture   2: Diastasis

☐ CLASS B: FORCES THAT DISPLACE THE TALUS MEDIALLY (TABLE 29–2)

The first structures to be injured with this mechanism include either the anterior talofibular ligament or an avulsion fracture of the lateral malleolus. If the mechanism continues, the talus pushes against the medial malleolus resulting in a "push-off" or vertical fracture of the medial malleolus.

Axiom: *A vertical medial malleolar fracture is associated with either a lateral malleolar fracture or rupture of the lateral ligaments.*

If there is a component of dorsiflexion, the medial malleolar fracture may include a portion of the anterior articular margin of the tibia. With plantar flexion, the medial fragment may include a portion of the posterior tibial margin.

☐ CLASS C: FORCES THAT APPLY AXIAL COMPRESSION TO THE TALUS

☐ Class C: Type IA (Axial Compression Force Applied to the Dorsiflexed Ankle, Table 29–3)

This mechanism typically results in injuries that occur alone or in combination with other injuries rather than in a series. The impaction fracture and the anterior marginal fracture may be seen after this mechanism of injury.

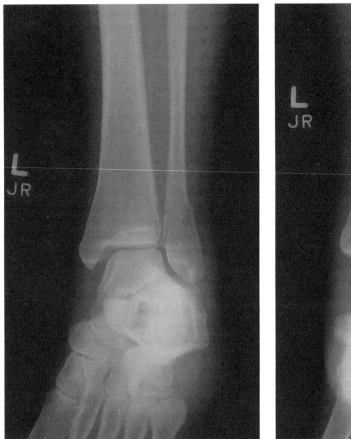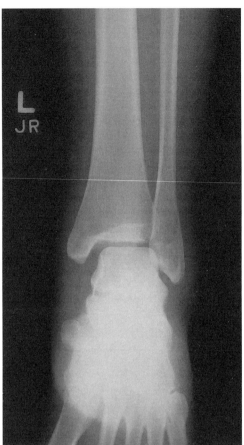

Figure 29–5. Nondisplaced lateral malleolus fracture without widening of the joint space. This is a stable fracture.

□ Class C: Type IB   (Axial Compression Force Applied to the Plantar-flexed Ankle, Table 29–3)

An axial force on the plantar-flexed foot may result in a posterior marginal fracture of the talus or a tibiofibular diastasis (rupture of the tibiofibular ligaments). If the diastasis is severe medial and lateral ligament injuries may be seen.

Examination

The patient will present with pain and swelling that is localized early but may diffusely involve the ankle later. The examiner should attempt to elicit an exact mechanism of injury and to carefully examine the ankle for focal tenderness or swelling. The dorsalis pedis and posterior tibial pulses should be palpated and compared with the uninvolved extremity. Swelling or ecchymosis surrounding the Achilles tendon may indicate a posterior malleolar fracture.

Axiom: *Any distal fibular fracture at the joint line should raise the suspicion of a deltoid ligament injury. A displaced lateral malleolar fracture is usually accompanied by a medial malleolar fracture or a deltoid ligament rupture.*

Axiom: *Medial malleolar "inversion fractures" must be accompanied by a lateral fracture or a ligament rupture. Medial malleolar "eversion fractures" are usually accompanied by a lateral malleolar fracture or a tibiofibular ligament rupture.*

X Ray (Fig. 29–7)

Routine views including anteroposterior (AP), lateral, and mortis views are usually adequate. Fractures secondary to ligamentous avulsion are transverse; those

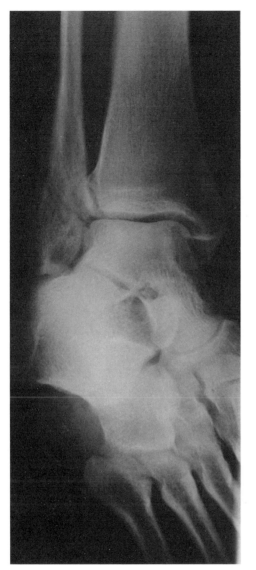 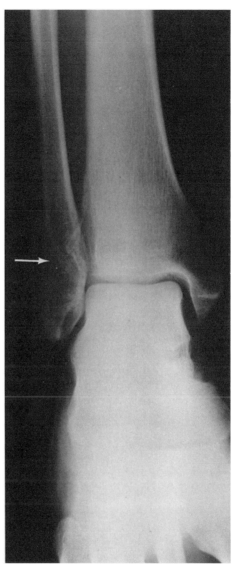

Figure 29–6. Ankle fracture with medial joint widening.

secondary to talar impaction are usually vertical, spiral, or comminuted. The AP view should be examined carefully for medial or lateral talar shift as well as for malleolar fractures. The mortise view (AP view with 20 degrees of internal rotation) should be examined carefully for the normal clear zone between the medial malleolus and the talus; ligamentous rupture may result in widening of this space. Complex fractures or those with uncertainty may require tomograms, computed tomography (CT) scan or magnetic resonance imaging (MRI) for clarification.[5,15]

Axiom: *Displaced malleolar fractures are always accompanied by a ligamentous injury.*

Axiom: *Transverse malleolar fractures are avulsion injuries. Vertical malleolar fractures are secondary to talar impaction.*

Associated Injuries
After an axial compression injury, calcaneal and spinal compression fractures may be seen and must be carefully looked for.

Treatment
The therapeutic goal is to anatomically restore the ankle mortise. Conceptually, the ankle should be thought of as a closed ring surrounding the talus.[1] As shown in Figure 29–8, the ring is composed of the tibial plafond, medial

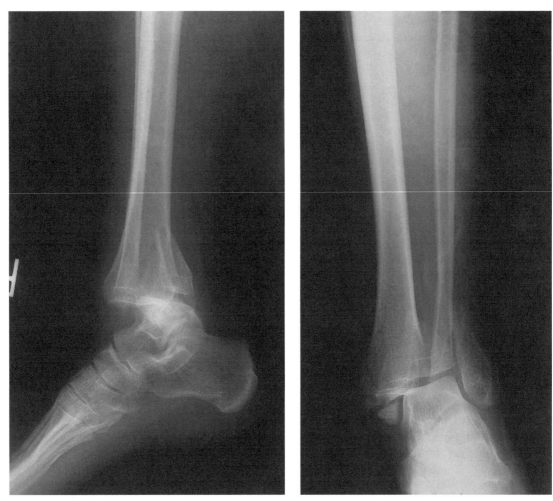

Figure 29-7. Ankle trimalleolar fracture.

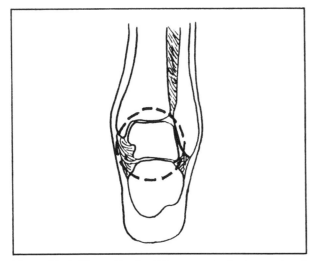

Figure 29-8. The ankle should be conceptualized as a closed ring surrounding the talus. The ring is composed of the tibial plafond, medial malleolus, deltoid ligament, calcaneus, lateral ligaments, lateral malleolus, and interosseous membrane.

malleolus, deltoid ligament, calcaneus, lateral ligaments, lateral malleolus, and interosseous membrane. As with pelvic fractures a single disruption in the ring (osseous or ligamentous) results in a stable injury. An example of a stable injury is a fibular malleolar fracture (Fig. 29–9). Two or more disruptions in the ring, however, will result in an unstable injury. Stable injuries by definition require no reduction and may be treated with a posterior splint, elevation, ice, and non–weight bearing. As the swelling diminishes, a walking cast with the foot in a neutral position should be used for approximately 4 to 6 weeks. Unstable injuries usually require reduction. An example of an unstable injury is a bimalleolar fracture, a fracture of the fibular malleolus that is displaced. Just as with a pelvic ring fracture, a significantly displaced fracture in the ring of structures indicated above would mean a second injury and would be classified as an unstable injury. Closed manipulative reduction is usually attempted first; however, open reduction is often required. The emergency manage-

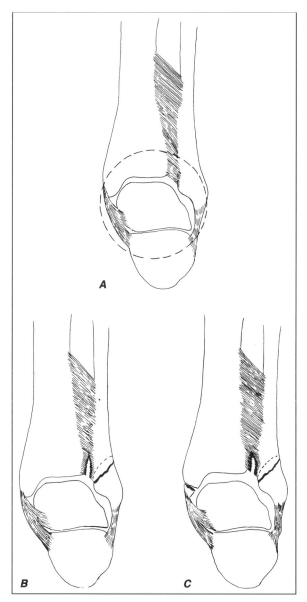

Figure 29–9. As noted in **A,** the ring includes both bone and soft tissue. **B.** A stable fracture is a fracture through the distal fibula or tibia without displacement. **C.** An unstable fracture involves displacement of the fibular or tibial fracture. Alternatively, an unstable fracture may involve a displaced fracture of the fibula with a ligamentous tear in the deltoid demonstrated by stress x rays to open up and be classified as unstable.

ment of these injuries should include ice, elevation, immobilization, and emergent referral. The management of these injuries varies from closed reduction with casting to open reduction with internal fixation (more commonly used), and more recently, the combination of internal and external fixation.[2,8] Delayed management of acute complex ankle injuries treated surgically has been shown to be associated with a higher incidence of complications.[4] In addition, these injuries are followed by a high incidence of complications.

Complications

Ankle fractures are often complicated by the development of several significant complications.

1. Traumatic arthritis of the talar mortise occurs in 20 to 40 percent of ankle fractures.[10,17,19] Comminuted tibial plafond fractures or those involving elderly patients are particularly predisposed to develop arthritis.
2. Persistent talar instability frequently follows sprains secondary to elongation of the lateral ligaments. These patients are predisposed to the development of recurrent sprains.
3. Subluxation of the peroneal tendons may follow sprains secondary to a rupture of the superior peroneal retinaculum.
4. Sudeck's atrophy is a form of sympathetic dystrophy with a rapidly developing osteoporosis distal to the injury. Patients may complain of a distal burning pain. The restoration of normal ankle function is usually curative.
5. Ossification of the interosseous membrane commonly occurs and patients may complain of a weakening or aching sensation in the ankle.
6. Osteochondral fractures of the talar dome may present with chronic pain, locking, or swelling.

REFERENCES

1. Ashurst A, Bromer RS: Classification and mechanism of fractures of the leg bone involving the ankle. *Arch Surg* **4:**51, 1922.
2. Brumback RJ, McGarvey WC: Fractures of the tibial plafond. *Orthop Clin North Am* **26**(2):273–285, 1995.
3. Burnwell HN, Charnley AD: The treatment of displaced fractures of the ankle by rigid internal fixation and early joint movement. *J Bone Joint Surg* **47**(13):634, 1965.
4. Carragee EJ, Csongradi JJ, Bleck EE: Early complications in the operative treatment of ankle fractures. *J Bone Joint Surg* **73B**(1):79–82, 1991.
5. Daffner RH: Ankle trauma. *Sem Roentgogr* **XXXIX**(2):134–151, 1994.
6. Diaz LC, Foerster TP: Traumatic lesions of the ankle joint. *Clin Orthop* **100:**219, 1974.
7. Duchesneau S, Fallat LM: The tillaux fracture. *J Foot Ankle Surg* **35**(2):127–133, 1996.
8. Karas EH, Weiner LS: Displaced pilon fractures. *Orthop Clin North Am* **25**(4):651–663, 1994.
9. Kleiger B: Mechanisms of ankle injury. *Orthop Clin North Am* **5**(1):78, 1974.
10. Klossner O: Late results of operative and nonoperative treatment of severe ankle fractures. *Acta Chir Scand* (suppl) **293:**1, 1962.
11. Lauge-Hansen N: Fractures of the ankle. Analytic historic survey as the basis of new experimental roentgenologic and clinical investigations. *Arch Surg* **56:**259, 1948.

12. Lauge-Hansen N: Fractures of the ankle II. Combined experimental surgical and experimental roentgenologic investigations. *Arch Surg* **60:**957, 1950.

13. Lauge-Hansen N: Ligamentous ankle fractures. *Acta Chir Scand* **97:**544, 1949.

14. Malka JS, Tailland W: Results of nonoperative and operative treatment of fractures of the ankle. *Clin Orthop* **67:**159, 1969.

15. Mitchess MJ, Ho C, Howard BA, et al: Diagnostic imaging of trauma to the ankle and foot. II. *J Foot Surg* **May-June:**266–271, 1989.

16. Pankovich AM: Maisonneuve fracture of the fibula. *J Bone Joint Surg* **58**(3):337, 1976.

17. Vasli S: Operative treatment of ankle fractures. *Acta Chir Scand* (suppl) **226:**1, 1957.

18. Wilson FC: Ankle fractures. In Rockwood C, Green D (eds): *Fractures*. Philadelphial: Lippincott, 1975.

19. Wilson FC, Skilbred LA: Long-term results in the treatment of displaced bimalleolar fractures. *J Bone Joint Surg* **48:**1065–1078, 1966.

BIBLIOGRAPHY

Anderson LD: *Fractures. Campbell's Operative Orthopaedics*, 5th ed. St. Louis: Mosby, 1971, pp. 509.

Bonnin JG: *Injuries to the Ankle*. Philadelphia: Hafner, 1970.

Childress HM: Vertical transarticular pain fixation for unstable ankle fractures. *J Bone Joint Surg* **47:**1323, 1965.

Dias LC, Tachdjian MO: Physeal injuries of the ankle in children. *Clin Orthop* **136:**230, 1978.

Eventov I, et al: An evaluation of surgical and conservative treatment of fractures of the ankle in 200 patients. *Trauma* **18**(4):271, 1978.

Hughes JL, et al: Evaluation of ankle fractures. *Clin Orthop* **138:**111, 1979.

Joy G, Patzakis MJ, Harvey JP: Precise evaluations of the reduction of severe ankle fractures. *J Bone Joint Surg* **56**(5):979, 1974.

Lauge-Hansen N: Fractures of the ankle. IV. Clinical use of genetic roentgen diagnosis and genetic reduction. *Arch Surg* **64:**488, 1952.

Lauge-Hansen N: Fractures of the ankle. V. Pronation-dorsiflexion fracture. *Arch Surg* **67:**813, 1953.

Lauge-Hansen N: Fractures of the ankle. III. Genetic roentgenologic diagnosis of fractures of the ankle. *AJR* **71:**456, 1954.

Maisonneuve MJG: Recherches sur la fracture du perone. *Arch Gen Med* **7:**165, 1840.

Malks JS, Taillard W: Results of nonoperative and operative treatment of fractures of the ankle. *Clin Orthop* **67:**159, 1969.

Neer CS II: Injuries of the ankle joint evaluation. *Conn State Med J* **17:**580, 1953.

Rockwood C, Green D: *Fractures*. Philadelphia: Lippincott, 1975.

Salter RB: Injuries of the ankle in children. *Orthop Clin North Am* **5**(1):147, 1974.

Solonen KA, Lauttamus L: Operative treatment of ankle fractures. *Acta Orthop Scand* **39:**223, 1968.

30
CHAPTER

SOFT TISSUE INJURIES, DISLOCATIONS, AND DISORDERS OF THE ANKLE

Essential Functional Anatomy

The ankle is a hinge joint in which the only motions are flexion and extension. Inversion and eversion take place at the calcaneotalar articulation, which is a gliding joint. The calcaneotalar joint is a very strong articulation with firm ligamentous support, and most inversion–eversion stresses injure the ankle joint rather than the subtalar joint. The ankle is composed of the distal ends of the tibia and the fibula which form a mortise into which the talus fits. The talar dome is wedge-shaped, wider in front than behind, and is the portion of the talus that articulates with the tibia and fibula (Fig. 30–1). In dorsiflexion, the wider anterior part of the "wedge" fits solidly into the mortise and the joint is very stable; however, in plantar flexion the narrow posterior portion of the talar wedge engages the mortise and fits loosely thus permitting significant play in the joint (Fig. 30–2). With this in mind it is easy to see why most ankle injuries occur when the ankle and the foot are in *plantar flexion*.

To understand the disorders that occur around this crucial joint the emergency physician must have a good

knowledge of the fundamental soft tissue structures that surround it. These structures are best divided into three "layers" surrounding the joint (each superficial to the previous layer). The first layer is the *capsule*, which contains the ligaments of the ankle; the second includes the

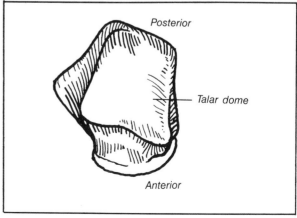

Figure 30–1. The talar dome is wider anteriorly than posteriorly.

511

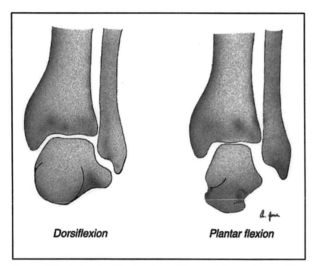

Figure 30–2. In dorsiflexion the wider anterior portion of the talar dome engages the ankle mortise and little motion is permitted. With the ankle in plantar flexion the narrow posterior part of the talar dome lies within the mortise, permitting a significant degree of inversion–eversion "play" to occur in the joint.

tendons, which traverse the joint to reach the foot; and the third are the *fibrous bands* (retinaculi), which hold the tendons in place as they act on the foot.

The Capsular Layer

The capsule that surrounds the ankle is divided into four parts (ligaments): anterior, posterior, lateral, and medial. The capsule is weaker anteriorly and posteriorly but is strengthened laterally and medially by ligaments. The

anterior ligament is thin, connects from the anterior tibia to the neck of the talus, and is commonly involved in extensive tears of the lateral ligament. The *posterior ligament* is shorter than its anterior counterpart and extends from the posterior tibia to the posterior talus. The *lateral ligament* is divided into three important components, which are the most commonly injured ligaments of the body. Extending from the lateral malleolus to the neck of the talus is the *anterior talofibular ligament*, the most commonly injured ligament in the ankle. From the lateral malleolus to the posterior tubercle of the talus (if separate called the *os trigonum*) is the *posterior talofibular ligament*, and from the lateral malleolus to the calcaneus extends the *calcaneofibular ligament* (Fig. 30–3). Proximal to the lateral ligaments the fibula is connected to the tibia by a series of tough fibrous structures together forming what is called the *tibiofibular syndesmosis*. This syndesmosis is composed of the interosseous ligament that connects the tibia and the fibula throughout their entire length. This ligament is strengthened inferiorly by two thickened fibrous bands: the *anterior inferior tibiofibular ligament* and the *posterior inferior tibiofibular ligament* (see Fig. 30–3).

The medial ligament is called the *deltoid ligament* and is a quadrangular structure that has the distinction of being the only ligament in the ankle to contain elastic tissue, giving it the ability to stretch rather than tear. The deltoid ligament is composed of four bands intermingled with each other and extending from the medial malleolus to the navicular, talus, and calcaneus. Two bands of the deltoid extend to the talus, one called the *anterior tibiotalar ligament* inserting to the neck of the talus and

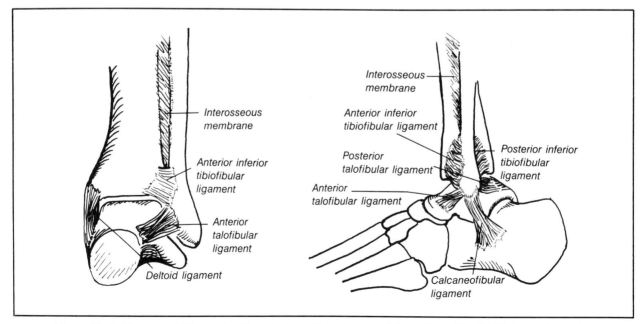

Figure 30–3. The essential ligaments of the anterior and lateral aspect of the ankle and the tibiofibular syndesmosis.

the other the *posterior tibiotalar ligament*, which is the deepest of the four structures. The portion of the deltoid that connects from the medial malleolus to the calcaneus is called the *tibiocalcaneal ligament* and attaches to the sustentaculum tali (Fig. 30–4).

The talus, supported by these ligaments, moves with the *foot* in pure dorsiflexion or plantar flexion and moves with the leg in pure inversion and eversion. A ligament of importance that is not included in the capsule of the ankle but is involved in injuries of the ankle and the midpart of the foot is the *spring ligament*. This ligament extends from the sustentaculum tali to the navicular and bridges the gap between the calcaneus and the navicular bones. It functions to give added support to the head of the talus against the weight of the body and is composed of dense fibrous tissue, portions of which resemble articular cartilage (see Fig. 30–4).

The Tendon Layer

Superficial to the capsule of the ankle are a series of tendons, none of which attach to the ankle per se but all of which traverse this joint and are important in considering associated injuries to the ankle. These tendons are subdivided into two groups, the *extensors* and the *flexors* of the foot. The extensors pass anterior to the ankle joint and the flexors pass posterior to the medial malleolus. A third group are the *peroneals*, which pass posterior to the lateral malleolus (Fig. 30–5). These tendons are surrounded by synovial sheaths, some up to 8 cm long.

The Retinacular Layer

Superficial to the tendons are three divisions of thick fibrous bands that hold the tendons in place. These divisions follow the same categorization as the tendons and are similarly termed the *extensor retinaculum*, the *flexor retinaculum*, and the *peroneal retinaculum*. The extensor retinaculum is divided into the *superior extensor reti-*

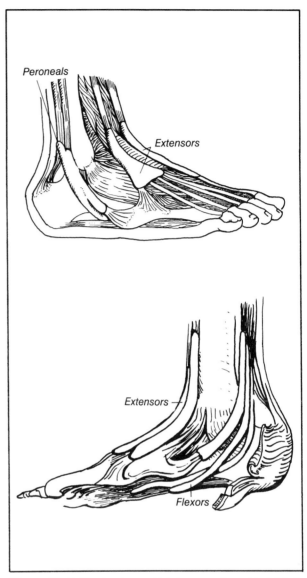

Figure 30–5. The tendons, which traverse the ankle joint, lie superficial to the capsular layer. Note the synovial sheaths on the tendons.

naculum (Fig. 30–6) and the *inferior extensor retinaculum*. The flexor retinaculum consists of one fibrous band that courses posterior to the medial malleolus called the *flexor retinaculum*. The peroneal retinaculum has two divisions, the *superior peroneal retinaculum* and the *inferior peroneal retinaculum* (see Fig. 30–6).

□ SPRAINS

Sprains of the ankle are the most common injury to this joint presenting to the emergency department, and perhaps the most commonly mistreated injury confronting the emergency physician. It is an irony that most

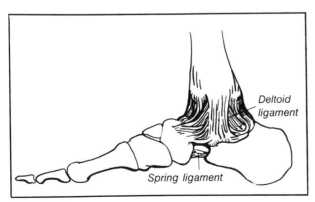

Figure 30–4. The deltoid ligament. Note the spring ligament connecting the sustentaculum tali of the calcaneous to the navicular.

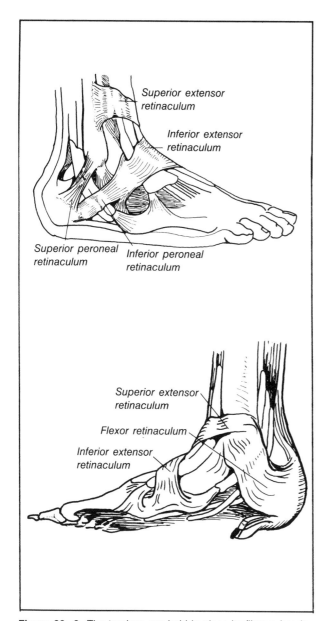

Figure 30–6. The tendons are held in place by fibrous bands.

TABLE 30–1. SEQUENCE OF STRUCTURES INJURED WITH INVERSION AND EVERSION ANKLE SPRAINS

Inversion Stress	Eversion Stress
Lateral joint capsule ↓	Avulsion of medial malleolus or deltoid ligament rupture ↓
Anterior talofibular ligament ↓	Anterior inferior tibiofibular ligament ↓
Calcaneofibular ligament ↓	
Posterior talofibular ligament[5]	Interosseous membrane

↓ = next structure to be injured.

ligament. In plantar flexion, the anterior talofibular ligament becomes perpendicular to the direction of force when an inversion stress is applied to the ankle.

Eversion injuries to the ankle are much less common and usually result in avulsion of the medial malleolus rather than rupture of the strong and elastic deltoid ligament. With either of these injuries as the force continues the anterior tibiofibular ligament or the interosseous membrane will tear as shown in Table 30–1.

The most common inversion injury to the ankle is a sprain and the most common eversion injury is a fracture of the *lateral malleolus* due to the strength of the deltoid ligament.[26] Thus, the most common injury with either an inversion or eversion stress involves the lateral portion of the ankle.

Classification

Sprains of the ankle are classified by two separate methods. The first method categorizes sprains as either first-, second-, or third-degree injuries according to the clinical presentation (Table 30–2) and the instability

TABLE 30–2. CLASSIFICATION OF SPRAINS

First-degree sprain
    Little or no functional loss
    Able to bear weight
    Little or no swelling noted
    Mildly tender to palpation over injured ligament
    No abnormal motion
    Mild pain on stress
Second-degree sprain
    Moderate degree of functional loss
    Swelling and local hemorrhage noted
    Pain noted immediately after injury
    May see sprain—fracture on x ray
    Moderate to severe pain on stress
    Pain on normal motion
Third-degree sprain
    Positive stress test
    Significant functional loss
    Resists motion of the foot
    Diffuse swelling and tenderness
    May be painless with complete rupture
    Egg-shaped swelling within 2 hours of injury

emergency physicians have a limited understanding of the "simple sprain" yet this disorder confronts them more commonly than any other single entity involving the extremities! Ankle sprains occur most often in athletes between 15 and 35 years of age involved in basketball, football, and women's cross country.[3,5] Sprains are due to either inversion or eversion of the ankle, usually occurring while the ankle is plantar flexed. *Inversion stresses* account for 85 percent of all sprains to the ankle and follow a specific sequence of structures injured with increa-sing force as shown in Table 30–1.[14] The first structures injured are the lateral joint capsule and the anterior talofibular ligament when an inversion stress is applied to the ankle; this is followed by a tear of the calcaneofibular ligament and finally the posterior talofibular

demonstrated by stress testing. The diagnosis of the degree of tear a ligament has undergone is crucial to the adequate treatment of the simple sprain." First-degree injuries are easy to diagnose, while difficulty exists in distinguishing the second- and third-degree injuries.

In a *first-degree sprain*, there is no functional loss in the ankle and these patients rarely seek care, usually treating themselves at home. These patients demonstrate little or no swelling of the ankle, no pain on normal motion of the ankle, and only mild pain on stressing the joint in the direction of the insulting force, usually inversion.

Patients with a *second-degree sprain* are more difficult to diagnose because second-degree sprains mean that the ligament is partially torn. This can run the gamut of anything from more than a few fibers being torn to tears involving almost the entire ligament with only a few fibers remaining intact. The patients present with moderate swelling and admit to immediate pain on injuring the ankle as compared with the first-degree injury where the patient may not know he or she had a sprain until the next day or after a period of rest. The second-degree sprain is fraught with many complications including the chance of ligamentous laxity with recurrent sprains due to instability.

Third-degree sprains are easily defined as there is a complete tear of the ligament. It is often difficult to differentiate a severe second-degree sprain from a third-degree injury without adequate stress testing and possibly arthrography.[10,22,27,30,32] There may also be little or no pain, but the patients are often incapacitated during the injury and there is usually swelling and tenderness of the ankle.

The second method of classification deals with the number of ligaments involved in the injury. A *single sprain* shows injury to the anterior talofibular ligament and the capsule. A *double sprain* is identical to a single sprain with the addition of calcaneofibular ligament injury. Finally, *triple sprains* display injuries to all three major ligaments in the ankle: The anterior talofibular ligament, the calcaneofibular ligament, and the posterior talofibular ligament.[13]

Clinical Presentation

Much of the clinical picture of the ankle sprain has been discussed in the presentation of the classification of these injuries. The distinction must be made between second-degree sprains and third-degree injuries. Stress testing aids in differentiating these two entities.

Stress tests described in the literature deal primarily with determining complete rupture of the lateral ligaments of the ankle as these are the ones most commonly involved in sprains.[16,18] Two tests are described: the *inversion stress test* and the *anterior drawer sign* of the ankle. These can be supplemented with radiographs of the ankle and comparison views may be necessary.

Injection of the ankle may be necessary to adequately perform stress tests of the acutely injured ankle. This is done by injecting the joint opposite to the side of the injury (usually medially) and infiltrating 5 to 10 mL of lidocaine. An additional infiltration of the ligaments around the lateral malleolus may be necessary. However, when dealing with an inversion stress test, diagnostic accuracy is only 68 percent with anesthesia compared to 92 percent without anesthesia.[28]

The anterior drawer sign is the first stress test to be performed because it examines for rupture of the anterior talofibular ligament. If this test is negative then there is no need to go to the inversion stress test because it requires both the anterior talofibular and the calcanofibular ligament to be ruptured to be positive.

The anterior drawer sign of the ankle can be done with the patient either sitting or supine. The anterior and posterior muscles must be relaxed surrounding the ankle. The knee should be flexed somewhat to relax the gastrocnemius muscle, and the ankle must be positioned at 90 degrees to the leg because it is often impossible to demonstrate even a markedly positive sign in the plantar flexed ankle (Fig. 30–7).[18] The examiner places the base of the hand over the anterior aspect of the tibia, extending the fingers around the medial side of the tibia. The other hand cups the heel and displaces the foot anteriorly, which stresses the anterior talofibular ligament.[18] Rupture of the anterior talofibular ligament is indicated by anterior displacement of the talus or the tibia. One should always compare this with the normal side and radiographs can be taken to confirm if necessary. Besides stress tests, a *talar tilt test* could be implicated to reveal an incompetent calcaneofibular ligament. This test measures the angle produced by the tibial plafond and the

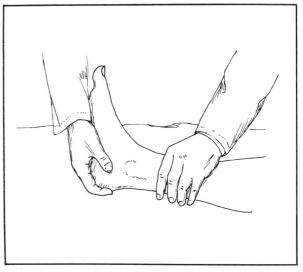

Figure 30–7. Technique for performing anterior drawer test of the ankle.

dome of the talus in response to forced inversion. Several diagnostic conclusions are revealed such as

1. If the lateral malleolus swelling increases the ankle circumference by 4 cm, then the probability of ligament rupture within the ankle is 70 percent.
2. If palpation of the calcaneofibular ligament produces pain, the chance of rupture of this ligament is 72 percent.
3. Tenderness of the anterior talofibular ligament reveals a 52 percent chance of rupture.
4. If all three symptoms are present, then there is a 91 percent chance of major ligament damage.[5]

One often notes tenderness along the medial joint line of the ankle over the deltoid ligament with inversion sprains of the ankle. Partial rupture of the anterior deep fibers of the deltoid ligament can occur in extreme degrees of inversion stresses or plantar flexion of the ankle.

An "egg-shaped" swelling over the lateral ligaments of the ankle occurring within 2 hours of injury indicates a third-degree injury of the ankle in most cases.

Although most of the discussion has been limited to the inversion sprain, the same applies to the deltoid ligament injured by an eversion stress.

Arthrography

Arthrography of the ankle has proponents for[22,32] and those against[30] it with regard to detailing the extent of injury in ankle sprains. There is a good correlation between arthrography and tears of the anterior inferior tibiofibular ligament, and the literature states that arthrography aids in distinguishing those lesions that need early surgery from those that will heal with time. Mehrez[32] states that arthrography provided unequivocal evidence of complete tears whereas stress tests and stress radiographs were uncertain due to accompanying muscle spasm. Fordyce,[16] in a study of 21 cases that went to surgery, stated that stress views differed with different examiners and that arthrograms were unreliable in showing the extent of tear because the fluid tended to seek the path of least resistance. He agreed that arthrograms were helpful in telling if there was a tear of the anterior inferior tibiofibular ligament. He also stated that the concept of greater than 6 degrees talar tilt being abnormal is erroneous because some patients with normal ankles have a talar tilt of as much as 23 degrees. The authors of this text agree with this concept and believe that comparison views and comparative examinations are essential in determining whether or not laxity really does exist.

In the authors' experience, arthrograms are of value when they show extensive extravasation, but of limited usefulness when they are negative or show only a small leak. In performing an arthrogram they recommend the technique published previously in which the ankle is thoroughly prepped and a 22-gauge needle, attached to a 10-mL syringe, is inserted into the side opposite the injury and about 6 mL of the solution is injected. The solution consists of 50 percent diatrizoate meglumine and diatrizoate sodium (Hypaque) and is diluted to 25 percent with sterile water. Radiographs are then taken of the ankle. Extravasation will be seen laterally outside of the ankle joint along the lateral malleolus with rupture.

X Ray

Radiographs of the ankle should be taken in all but definite first-degree injuries. The routine views can be supplemented with stress views taken during an inversion stress or during the anterior drawer sign of the ankle. In some patients with a second-degree sprain one will note a small flake of bone off of the lateral malleolus. This indicates an incomplete tear and is usually associated with a second-degree injury to the lateral ligaments called a *sprain-fracture.*

Treatment

The "simple sprain" is associated with a high degree of morbidity. Only 20 to 60 percent of patients are symptom-free 1 to 4 years after a sprain to the ankle. The average disability from sprains of the ankle is from 4.5 to 26 weeks. There is a high incidence of recurrent sprains in patients who sustain second- and third-degree injury to the ankle, with patients complaining of chronic instability of the ankle and "giving way" on running, leading to the old adage "once a sprain, always a sprain." Although controversy exists about the treatment of second- and third-degree injuries to the ankle, suffice it to say that most sprains of the ankle are inadequately treated, leading to prolonged disability.

The treatment goals are twofold: the complete reestablishment of weight bearing on the tibia and the fibula, and the maintenance of the integrity of the mortise. Many physicians believe that surgery offers the best modality of achieving these goals with a third-degree injury involving two ligaments; however, it can be argued that if only one side is injured (lateral) and the deltoid is intact one can cast because this is a stable injury, whereas if both are injured surgical intervention is needed.

The following is the authors' approach to the injured ankle where ligamentous injury is diagnosed based on a review of the literature and their current experience.[12,16,40] For the first-degree sprain they recommend ice packs, elevation, and an elastic bandage with early mobilization because the integrity of the ligament is not in question. Patients with second- or third-degree sprains are divided into two groups: those in which the diagnosis is certain and those where one cannot establish the diagnosis. In patients with definite mild second-degree sprains the authors prefer to apply ice packs and elevation for 72 hours followed with an ankle support which provides much more stability than an elastic bandage until healing is complete.

In patients with a definite third-degree injury as established by either stress testing or arthrogram or both, one of three approaches have been recommended and there remains considerable controversy. If, in the lateral ligament complex, the tear includes both the calcaneofibular and anterior talofibular ligaments and where there is talar instability surgical repair is recommended by some authors, particularly in the young athletic patient. Because the literature remains controversial in the treatment of patients with two-ligament ruptures, the authors of this text advocate immobilization in a splint for 72 hours with ice, elevation, and referral. Early mobilization and physical therapy is recommended by some authors whereas others believe that surgical intervention should be done.[2,7-9,20,23,31,33,38] Early mobilization with physiotherapy is recommended by some authors.[20,30,40] Orthopedic consultation for these injuries, as with any serious injury fraught with complications, is recommended. In patients with either severe second-degree or possibly a third-degree sprain in which the examiner cannot be certain, the authors recommend applying a posterior splint for 72 hours, ice packs and elevation, and reexamination after the swelling and the pain have subsided at which time differentiation may be easier, and it remains early enough for repair should this course be selected. In patients found to have severe second-degree sprains or patients with rupture of only the anterior talofibular ligament, the authors recommend immobilization in any one of a number of commercially available ankle supports that fit into the patient's shoe or an Unna Boot (Glenwood Inc., Tenafly, NJ) for 2 to 3 weeks with physical therapy. If the pain continues, an additional 3 weeks of immobilization is advised. When applying a cast or a splint, it is vitally important to keep the ankle out of equinus and in the neutral position.

All athletes with a history of recurrent inversion injuries to the ankle should be advised to wear a felt-trimmed outer heel wedge of approximately $1/4$-inch inserted in the heel when engaging in vigorous activities. Prophylactic ankle stabilizers (PAS) have recently been used to reduce the frequency and severity of ankle injuries.[39] These have been shown to be quite effective. They range from cloth lace on braces to semirigid bimalleolar orthoses made of thermal plastics and plastic polymers.[39] Also, in all types of ankle sprains proprioception may be decreased due to prior stretch of the ligaments. This disability can be treated with tilting board exercises.[14]

Complications
Ankle sprains are fraught with complications, the most common being instability,[35,40] which even Freeman (an advocate of early mobilization) concedes surgical repair

more surely eliminates.[17] Patients complain of a feeling of insecurity and weakness in the ankle. Recurrent sprains[35] are another common complication, and these can be prevented to a large extent by adequate immobilization for a sufficient length of time while the ligaments are healing. Some patients complain of persistent pain, stiffness, recurrent swelling of the ankle joint, and of giving way on running. *Peroneal tendon dislocation* or subluxation is an infrequent complication of lateral ligament sprains which may tear the peroneal retinaculum and requires surgical repair. Many patients with ligamentous injuries of the ankle have peroneal nerve injury. In one series, 17 percent of patients with second-degree sprains had mild peroneal nerve injuries. Eighty-six percent of patients with third-degree sprains injured either the peroneal[34] or the posterior tibial nerve. Thus, many patients with impaired ability to walk 5 to 6 weeks after a sprain may have this because of peroneal nerve injury. This injury is probably caused by mild nerve traction or hematoma in the epineural sheath. The most common complication, lateral talar instability, can be treated by isometric peroneal exercises to improve stability, and $1/2$-inch lateral based heel. In severe cases surgical intervention to stabilize the joint may be warranted.

Syndromes Related to Inversion Injuries
A subtalar stress injury has been described as caused by an inversion stress. Patients present with chronic midfoot pain and a limp and unlimited subtalar motion. This injury occurs in the preadolescent athlete. The injury produces a positive bone scan. The subtalar motion usually returns to normal but this may take anywhere from 6 months to 2 years.

The sinus tarsi syndrome is a well-defined post-traumatic foot syndrome characterized by pain over the lateral opening of the sinus tarsi and a feeling of ankle instability. Most of these patients have a history of repeated ankle sprains. The findings include pain at the lateral side of the foot, which is increased by firm pressure over the lateral opening of the sinus tarsi and a feeling of hind foot instability on uneven ground.[42] One can diagnose this syndrome by injecting a local anesthetic into the sinus tarsi and seeing whether the patient has relief of symptoms. The treatment may require repeated injections of a steroid and analgesic mixture. In some patients, surgical intervention has offered excellent results.

☐ CHONDRAL FRACTURE

"Ankle sprain followed by traumatic arthritis" and "adolescent with nonhealing ankle sprain" are two common situations that should make the emergency physician consider the possibility of a chondral fracture in a patient presenting with an old ankle injury.[41] There are two locations where chondral fractures commonly occur in the ankle, both being on the dome of the talus, one at the superolateral margin and the other at the superomedial margin of the dome. Chondral fractures of the superolateral margin occur secondary to dorsiflexion and inversion and the ligaments may or may not rupture. This is seen more commonly in the child with elastic ligamentous tissue. in superomedial chondral fractures they occur with plantar flexion where the narrow talus engages the mortise with a "direct blow" such as would occur when a jumper comes down hard on the toes with the foot inverted. Other less common sites for chondral fractures are the fibular edge and the posterior articular surface of the navicular. Figure 30–8 shows the mechanism of chondral fractures of the talus. (See also Fig. 30–9).

Clinical Presentation

Patients complain of a painful ankle resistant to all modes of treatment with symptoms persisting longer than the sprain. There is usually no tenderness at the malleoli or over the ligaments during palpation. The patients' symptoms are aggravated by activity and completely relieved with rest, although there may be slight swelling with a dull ache after excessive walking. The entire examination may be negative except when the examiner *palpates the talar dome* with the ankle *plantar flexed* and point tenderness is elicited. A synovitis may occur in the ankle joint with recurrent swelling.

Radiographs of the ankle may show a crater or a particle of bone that appears opaque surrounded by radiolucency in some cases. The best views to demonstrate

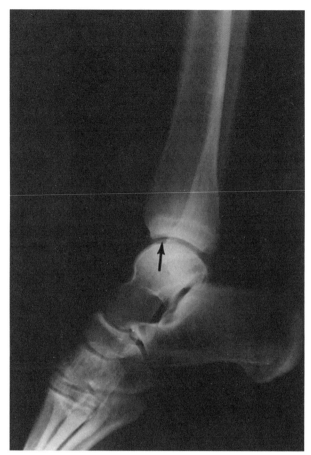

Figure 30–9. Osteochondral fracture of the talar dome.

the lesion are the anteroposterior (AP) with dorsiflexion of the ankle and 10 degrees of internal rotation when the lesion is lateral and the AP view in plantar flexion when the lesion is medial.

Treatment

Patients in whom one suspects this diagnosis should be referred for orthopedic consultation because traumatic arthritis is the sequel to delayed care. Surgical therapy offers the best results although conservative treatment is attempted in some cases with 6 months of absolute non–weight bearing in a cast. If the fragment dislodges, it grinds into the joint, resulting in irreversible chronic arthritis.

□ TALOTIBIAL EXOSTOSIS

Exostosis is the filling up of bone at the site of an irritative lesion in response to direct trauma. In the normal ankle the distal anterior aspect of the tibia is round (Fig. 30–10) and there is a sulcus at the neck of the talus. As one hyperextends the ankle, the anterior border of the tibia comes in contact with the sulcus and an irritative lesion may lead to exostosis at that site (Fig. 30–10).

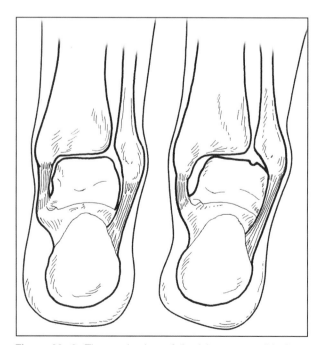

Figure 30–8. The mechanism of the injury responsible for a chondral fracture of the superolateral talar dome.

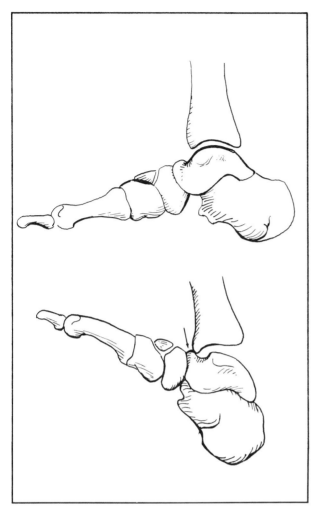

Figure 30–10. The mechanism by which a talotibial exostosis forms.

This condition occurs at two sites, the sulcus of the talus and the anterior low margin of the tibia. A third less common site is at the medial and lateral malleolus because of direct trauma from the talus in sprains. A large number of athletes and nonathletes have exostosis that is asymptomatic. Some of these patients, however, will present to the emergency department with complaints related to the anterior aspect of the ankle and the only finding is exostosis.

Clinical Presentation and Differential Diagnosis

The patient's primary complaint is usually that he or she cannot run or play as hard as before. The patient complains of pain only on extreme dorsiflexion of the ankle. On examination the physician will note some swelling of the anterior aspect of the joint with tenderness to palpation and increasing pain on hyperextension of the foot.

One must differentiate this condition from osteophytes that are a response to degenerative processes in the joint. In exostosis there is no degeneration of the joint or chronic changes noted. The joint line is normal on x ray with this condition.

☐ TENOSYNOVITIS

The most common tendons involved in tenosynovitis around the ankle are the posterior tibial, peroneal longus, anterior tibial, and extensor digitorum longus. There are two types of tenosynovitis: stenosing and rheumatoid. Stenosing tenosynovitis is common at the inferior retinaculum of the peroneus tendon with thickening of the sheath noted on examination. Rheumatoid tenosynovitis more commonly presents medially, involving the posterior tibial and flexor hallucis longus tendons; laterally the peronei are involved; and anteriorly the most common site is the anterior tibial tendon.

Clinical Presentation

The tibialis posterior muscle is the main inverter of the subtalar joint. Dysfunction of the posterior tibial tendon can be acute or chronic.[19] Most commonly, the condition consists of an acute tenosynovitis secondary to overuse, without any structural change in the hind foot. Chronic tenosynovitis, which is usually found in nonathletic patients, is associated with tendinosis and structural changes in the hind foot.[43] Patients who have tenosynovitis of the tibialis posterior tendon report pain along the posterior medial aspect of the foot and ankle. A patient who has tibialis posterior tendon dysfunction may have an increased valgus posture of the calcaneus and a fullness that is seen just distal to the medial malleolus. Lack of heel inversion usually indicates dysfunction or weakness of the tibialis posterior tendon.[21] Frequently, patients with this condition are unable to stand on the tiptoe at all because of pain.[43]

On examination of patients with stenosing tenosynovitis the examiner often can palpate the thickened sheath along its course. These patients are usually more than 40 years old and have some predisposing occupational trauma. The tendon is tender to palpation and motion increases the pain with either form. Spontaneous rupture can occur, particularly in patients with flat foot or rheumatoid arthritis or those with some unusual activity.

Treatment

Acute tenosynovitis, when it is mild, can be treated with a decrease in the level of activity. However, if the symptoms are moderate, the foot and ankle should be put at rest and anti-inflammatory medication and ice should be used. In some cases, immobilization and a weight-bearing, below-the-knee cast for 4 weeks may be necessary.[43] Rarely, if symptoms fail to respond after this initial treatment, surgical treatment may be necessary in acute tenosynovitis.[43]

☐ SYNOVITIS

This condition may present to the emergency department, and the physician must be aware to look for the inciting cause. Acute synovitis can follow an injury or infectious process or a metabolic problem such as gout. The patient presents with a painful, swollen, hot joint. Chronic synovitis usually follows osteochondral fractures of the talus, mild tibiofibular separation, or instability of the lateral collateral ligament. One should treat the cause if possible, but if it is unknown, then a period of rest is advisable and referral for follow-up is recommended.

☐ DISLOCATION OR SUBLUXATION OF THE PERONEAL TENDON

This condition is common and occurs after injuries that disrupt the peroneal retinaculum permitting subluxation or actual dislocation of the tendons (Fig. 30–11). This condition could be caused by laxity of the retinaculum or the retinaculum could be congenitally absent. Some factors may contribute to the frequency of dislocations, such as convex or flat posterior surface of the distal fibula and a bifid peroneal brevis muscle. During injury, the peroneal muscles contract reflexively and overcome their fibro- osseous sheath causing the tendons to pass anteriorly.[6] The condition may be acute or chronic in its presentation.[15]

Classification

Peroneal tendon dislocations are categorized into three separate entities:[11]

- **Grade 1:** The retinaculum with the periosteum is stripped off the lateral malleolus and collagenous lip by the dissecting tendons.
- **Grade 2:** The distal 1 to 2 cm of the dense fibrous lip are elevated along with the retinaculum.
- **Grade 3:** The retinaculum avulses a thin fragment of bone along the fibrous lip.[6]

Clinical Presentation

The patient with acute subluxation will give a history of having sustained a blow to the back of the lateral malleolus while the foot was taut in dorsiflexion and eversion.[15] On examination there is tenderness directly over the peroneal tendons, which can be confused with tenosynovitis if a history is not obtained.

In patients with chronic subluxation there is a history of slipping of the tendon with eversion of the foot. There is less pain than in the acute form and the patient usually complains of a dull ache and the sensation of the tendon subluxating as it slips out of its normal position.

Treatment

Most physicians recommend surgical treatment for this condition. There is a debate as to whether it is best to treat patients surgically or conservatively. In one large study, 74 percent of patients treated conservatively had to return for surgical correction at a later date. Because only grade III injuries can be seen on x ray, it is felt that these are the only ones that should be treated conservatively, with the remainder being treated surgically.[11] In an acute injury, the physician must incise, plicate, and suture the lax peroneal retinaculum to the fibrocartil-agenous ridge, or through

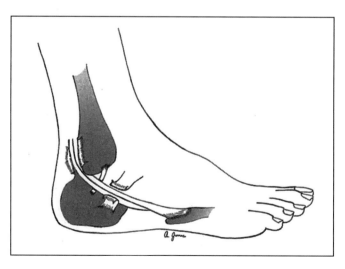

Figure 30–11. Dislocation of the peroneal tendon caused by rupture of the retinaculum is shown.

drill holes in the posterior malleolus if the lip is not intact. A different procedure is required for chronic injury. This includes rerouting of the tendons, deepening of the peroneal groove via bony procedures, repairing the soft tissue of the retinaculum, reconstructions, and reinforcements.[6]

☐ DISLOCATION OF THE ANKLE (FIG. 30–12)

Posterior (Fig. 30–13)

These are one of the most common types of dislocation of the ankle. Even this type is relatively rare, however. Most are accompanied by a fracture of one or both malleoli. The mechanism causing posterior dislocations is a strong forward-thrust of the posterior tibia usually secondary to a blow. The patient is usually in plantar flexion when this occurs.

The patient presents with the foot plantar flexed and with a shortened appearance.

The treatment involves plantar flexion of the foot and pulling the foot forward. (Fig. 30–14) The vascular integrity must always be assessed and x rays should be taken before reduction. A posterior splint is applied and the patient referred as capsular tears and fractures are often surgically repaired.

Anterior

Anterior dislocations are less common than posterior and are almost always associated with a fracture of the anterior lip of the tibia. The mechanism causing this type of dislocation is usually a force that causes posterior displacement of the tibia on the fixed foot or forcible dorsiflexion of the foot such as occurs during a fall on the heel with the foot dorsiflexed.

The patient presents with the foot in dorsiflexion and elongated. On examination the supporting ligaments and capsule are disrupted. This injury is also commonly associated with fracture of the malleoli.

The treatment is to dorsiflex the foot slightly to disengage the talus and apply downward traction and push the foot directly posteriorly back into its normal position.

Lateral

These are perhaps the most common form of dislocations seen in the emergency department and are *always* associated with fractures of the malleoli or distal fibula. These fractures are discussed in the section on the fractures of the ankle and we will only concern ourselves here with the relevant part of the examination and treatment of this injury.

Clinically there is usually obvious deformity with the foot laterally displaced (Fig. 30–15) and the skin on the medial aspect of the ankle joint is very taut. These

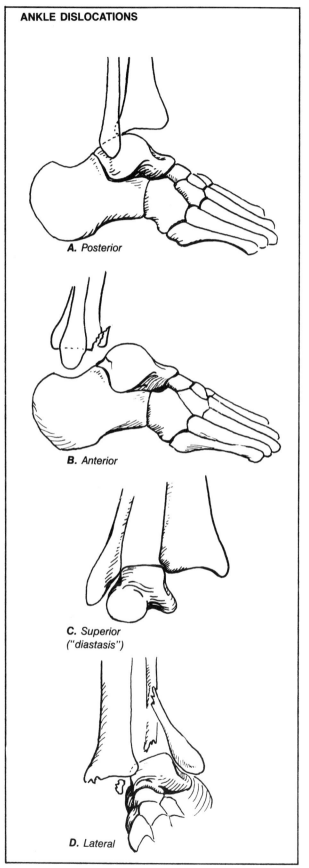

ANKLE DISLOCATIONS

A. Posterior

B. Anterior

C. Superior ("diastasis")

D. Lateral

Figure 30–12.

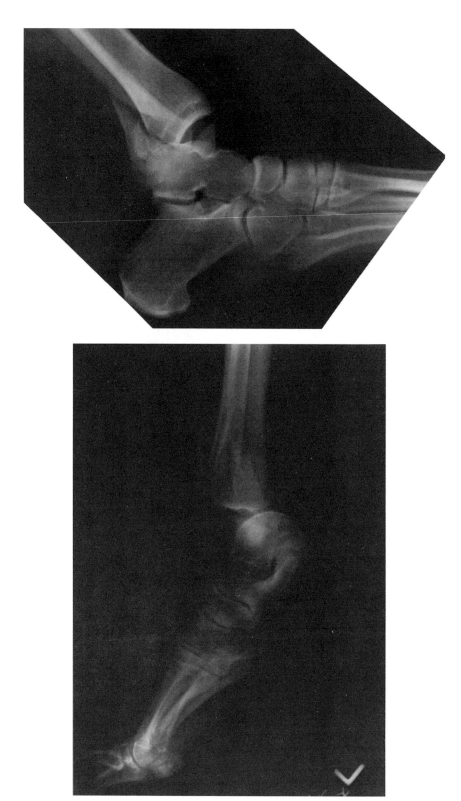

Figure 30–13. Posterior dislocation of the ankle with trimalleolar fracture of the ankle.

injuries are not usually open and are associated with either a fracture of the medial malleolus or, less commonly, rupture of the deltoid ligament. One should assess the vascular integrity before engaging in any

treatment regimen and obtain appropriate x rays unless there is vascular compromise.

The reduction of this dislocation is relatively simple and involves longitudinal traction on the foot with

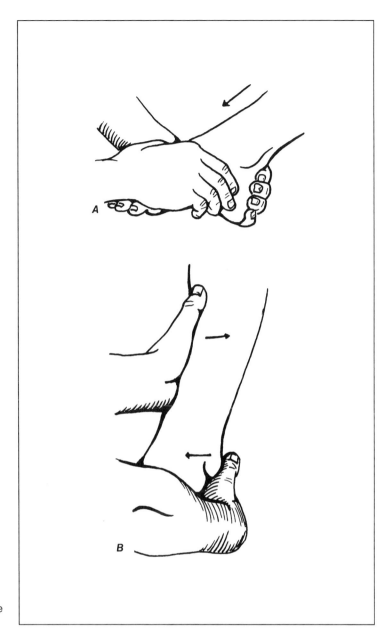

Figure 30–14. Reduction technique for posterior dislocation.

one hand on the heel and the other on the dorsum of the foot while a partner applies countertraction on the leg and simple manipulation medially back into its normal position. Usually the talus will go into position with little difficulty (Fig. 30–16).

Anesthesia for all of these dislocations should be either a Bier block, which is preferred by the authors, or by IV narcotics and muscle relaxants or general anesthesia. Posterior splints should be applied after reduction and the patient referred for surgical repair, which is almost always indicated in these injuries.

Superior

Superior dislocations (diastasis) are uncommon injuries often associated with articular damage. These cases should be splinted and emergent consultation obtained.

☐ REFLEX SYMPATHETIC DYSTROPHY

The source of consistent pain following any injury or surgical procedure is often difficult to diagnose and treat. When pain persist beyond an expected time of healing and physical signs and symptoms are attributed to psychological influences, one must consider sympathetic nervous system involvement and the diagnosis of reflex sympathetic dystrophy (RSD) or causalgia. This is a complex disorder or group of disorders that is an all-inclusive term encompassing disorders such as

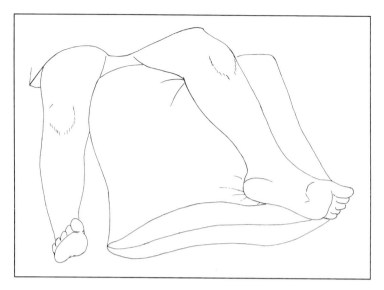

Figure 30–15. Lateral ankle dislocation classic position.

causalgia, posttraumatic pain syndrome, chronic traumatic edema, and Sudeck's atrophy.[1,4,29,37,44] It has been associated with a number of etiologies or precipitating events, including gunshot wounds, reticulopathy, arthroscopy, surgery, fractures, tendonitis, arthritis, diabetes, and myocardial infarction. The most common cause of RSD is accidental trauma.[36]

Clinical Presentation
Untreated, RSD passes through three stages:

- **Stage 1:** In the acute phase, which usually begins within days to weeks or sometimes months after an injury. The patient experiences constant burning or aching pain. Hyperalgesia, hyperaesthesia, localized edema, and muscle spasm as well as tenderness throughout the limb may be present.[24,25] Pain is aggravated by movement or emotional stress. Initially, the skin is warm, red, and dry in this stage. It may progress by the end of the stage to become cyanotic, cold, and sweaty. A bone scan, if done, would show increased uptake in the small joints. Stage 1 can last as long as 6 months.
- **Stage 2** (dystrophic): This stage is characterized by continuous burning, aching, throbbing pain, marked allodynia, hyperalgesia, and hyperaesthesia. The skin is cool, pale gray, and cyanotic. Hair growth is decreased and the nails are brittle or cracked in this stage. X rays would show a spotty osteoporosis.
- **Stage 3** (atrophic): At this stage, the patient has irreversible marked tissue changes. The pain,

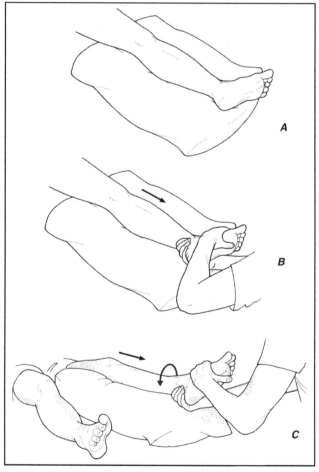

Figure 30–16. Lateral dislocation of the ankle. **A.** The typical position of a lateral ankle dislocation. **B.** The application of distal traction to the plantar-flexed foot. **C.** To reduce the dislocation, return the foot to its proper anatomic position while maintaining distal traction of the foot. This maneuver usually produces a palpable "thud."

allodynia, and hyperalgesia may be less severe. The skin appears smooth, glossy, and pale, or cyanotic. Skin temperature is decreased. The digits are thin and pointed. There is marked atrophy of the muscles at this stage, particularly the interosseous of the foot. Interphalangeal joints and other joints of the foot are weakened with limited motion and eventually become stiff. Bone atrophy becomes diffuse.

The mechanism of RSD is entirely unknown. The diagnosis is based on a history of trauma or disease and the presence of this persistent burning, aching, and throbbing pain beyond the expected time period.

Treatment

The mainstay of treatment for RSD is interruption of sympathetic outflow to the affected extremity.[36] The treatment initiated in stage 1, sympathetic blockade, has been reported to result in complete or total remission in 80 percent of patients. If patients present in stage 2 or 3, in addition to sympathetic blockade they should undergo intensive physical therapy, exercise programs, as well as psychotherapy, if appropriate. Further discussion of treatment of this condition is beyond the scope of this book. The patient should be referred to an appropriate clinician.

REFERENCES

1. Abramowitz AJ: Chronic exertional compartment syndrome of the lower leg. *Orthop Rev* **23**(3):219–226, 1994.
2. Balduini FC, Tetzlzff J: Historical perspectives on injuries of the ligaments of the ankle. *Clin Sports Med* **1**:3, 1982.
3. Barry NN, Mcguire JL: Acute injuries and specific problem in adult athletes. *Rheum Dis Clin North Am* **22**:3, 1996.
4. Black KP, Taylor DE: Current concepts in treatment of compartment syndromes in athletes. *Sports Med* **15**(6):408–418, 1993.
5. Borota PM, Biship JO, Braly WG, Tullos HS: Acute lateral ankle ligament injuries: A literature review. *Foot Ankle* **11**(2):107, 1990.
6. Brage ME, Hansen ST: Traumatic subluxation/dislocation of the peroneal tendons. *Foot Ankle* **13**(7):423, 1992.
7. Brand RL, Collins MDF, Tempelton T: Surgical repair of ruptured lateral ankle ligaments. *Am J Sports Med* **9**:40, 1981.
8. Brooks SC, Potter BT, Rainey JB: Treatment for partial tears of the lateral ligament of the ankle. A prospective trial. *Br Med J* **282**:606, 1981.
9. Broston L: Sprained ankles. I. Anatomic lesions in recent sprains. *Acta Chir Scand* **128**:483, 1964.
10. Broston L: Sprained ankles. III. Clinical observations in recent ligament ruptures. *Acta Chir Scand* **130**:560, 1965.
11. Butler BW, et al: Subluxing peroneals: A review of the literature and case report. *J Foot Ankle Surg* **32**:2, 1992.
12. Charnley J: Sprains and dislocations. *Practitioner* **164**:314, 1950.
13. Demaio M, Paine R, Drez D: Chronic lateral ankle instability-inversion sprains: Part I. *Orthopedics* **15**(1):87, 1992.
14. Diamond JE: Rehabilitation of ankle sprains. *Clin Sports Med* **8**(4):877, 1989.
15. Eckert WR, et al: Acute rupture of the peroneal retinaculum. *J Bone Joint Surg* **58**(5):670, 1976.
16. Fordyce AJ: Arthrography in recent injuries of the ligaments of the ankle. *J Bone Joint Surg* [Br] **54**:116, 1972.
17. Freeman MAR: Instability of the foot after injuries to the lateral ligament of the ankle. *J Bone Joint Surg* [Br] **47**:669, 1965.
18. Frost HM: Technique for testing the drawer sign in the ankle. *Clin Orthop* **123**:49, 1977.
19. Garrett WE: Muscle strain injuries. *Am J Sports Med* **24**:6, 1996.
20. Garrick JG: When can I . . . ? A practical approach to rehabilitation illustrated by treatment of an ankle injury. *Am J Sports Med* **9**:67, 1981.
21. Gerow G, et al: Compartment syndrome and shin splints of the lower leg. *J Manipulative Physiol Therap* **16**:4, 1993.
22. Gillies H, Chalmers J: The management of fresh ruptures of the tendoachillis. *J Bone Joint Surg* **52**(2):337, 1970.
23. Glick JM, Gordon RB, Nishimoto O: The prevention and treatment of ankle injuries. *Am J Sports Med* **4**:136, 1976.
24. Gulli B, Templeman D: Compartment syndrome of the lower extremity. *Orthop Clin North Am* **25**(4):677–684, 1994.
25. Hutchinson MR, Ireland ML: Common compartment syndromes in athletes. Treatment and rehabilitation. *Sports Med* **17**(3):200–208, 1994.
26. Johnson KA, Teasdall RD: Sprained ankles as they relate to the basketball player. *Clin Sports Med* **12**:2, 1993.
27. Lamy C, Stienstra JJ: Complications in ankle arthroscopy. *Clin Podiatr Med Surg* **11**:3, 1994.
28. Lassiter TE, Malone TR, Garrett WE: Injury to the lateral ligaments of the ankle. *Orthop Clin North Am* **20**(4):629, 1989.
29. Mabee JR, Bostwick TL: Pathophysiology and mechanisms of compartment syndrome. *Orthop Rev* **22**(2):175–181, 1993.
30. Mann RA: Tarsal tunnel syndrome. *Orthop Clin North Am* **5**(1):109, 1974.
31. Mann RA, Baxter DE, Lutter LD: Running symposium. *Foot Ankle* **1**:190, 1981.
32. Mehrez M: Arthrography of the ankle. *J Bone Joint Surg* [Br] **52**:308, 1970.
33. Niedermann B, et al: Rupture of the lateral ligaments of the ankle: Operation or plaster cast? *Acta Orthop Scand* **52**:279, 1981.
34. Nitz AJ, Dobner JJ, Kersey D: Nerve injury and grades II and III ankle sprains. *Am J Sports Med* **13**:177, 1985.
35. Percy EC, et al: The "sprained" ankle. *J Trauma* **9**:12, 1969.
36. Rogers JN, Valley MA: Reflex sympathetic dystrophy. *Clin Podiatr Med Surg* **11**:1, 1994.

37. Ross DG: Chronic Compartment syndrome. *Orthop Nurs* **15:**3, 1996.

38. Seligson D, Gassman J, Pope M: Ankle instability: Evaluation of the lateral ligaments. *Am J Sports Med* **8:**39, 1980.

39. Sitler MR, Horodyski M: Effectiveness of prophylactic ankle stabilisers for prevention of ankle injuries. *Sports Med* **20**(1):53–57, 1995.

40. Staples SO : Ruptures of the fibular collateral ligaments of the ankle. *J Bone Joint Surg* **57**(1):101, 1975.

41. Swain RA, Holt WS: Ankle injuries. *Post Grad Med* **93:**3, 1993.

42. Taillard W, Meyer J-M, Garcia J, Blanc Y: The sinus trasi syndrome. *Int Orthop* **5:**117, 1981.

43. Teitz CC, et al: Tendon problems in athletic individuals, chap 55. *Instruc Course Lect* **46:**569–582, 1997.

44. Tornetta P III, Templeman D: Compartment syndrome associated with tibial fracture, chap 30. Tibial fractures. *Instruc Course Lect* **46:**303, 308, 1997.

31
CHAPTER
FRACTURES AND DISLOCATIONS OF THE FOOT

CALCANEAL FRACTURES

CLASS A: CALCANEAL PROCESS OR TUBEROSITY FRACTURES
(p. 536)

Type I: Medial or lateral tuberosity fractures

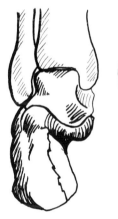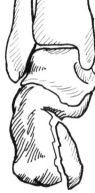

A: Nondisplaced   *B:* Displaced

Type II: Fractures of the sustentaculum tali

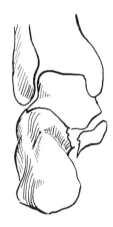

Type III: Fractures of the calcaneocuboid or calcaneonavicular processes

Type IV: Displaced and nondisplaced fractures of the posterior tuberosity

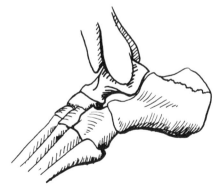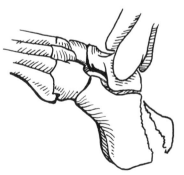

A: Nondisplaced   *B:* Displaced

CALCANEAL FRACTURES (cont.)

CLASS B: CALCANEAL BODY FRACTURES
(p. 537)

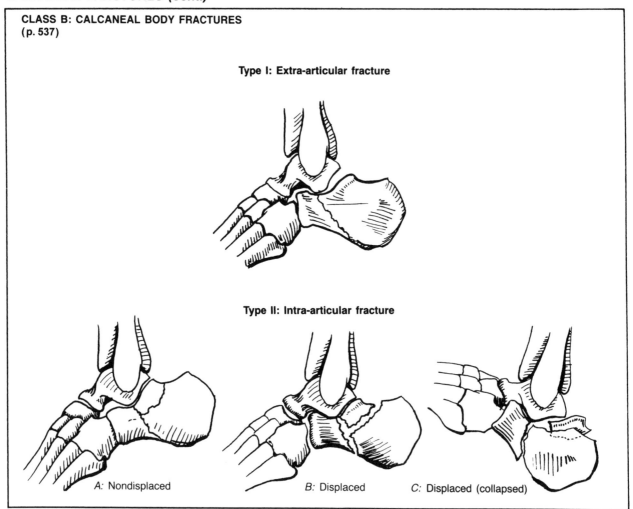

Type I: Extra-articular fracture

Type II: Intra-articular fracture

A: Nondisplaced   B: Displaced   C: Displaced (collapsed)

TALAR FRACTURES

CLASS A: MINOR FRACTURES
(p. 541)

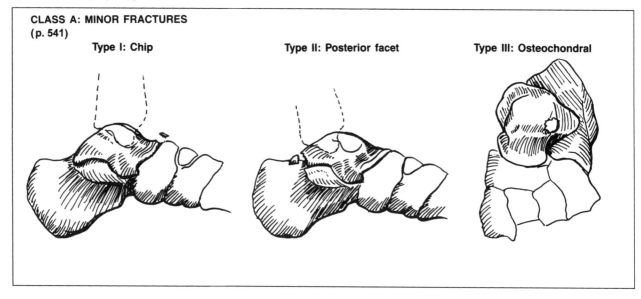

Type I: Chip   Type II: Posterior facet   Type III: Osteochondral

TALAR FRACTURES (cont.)

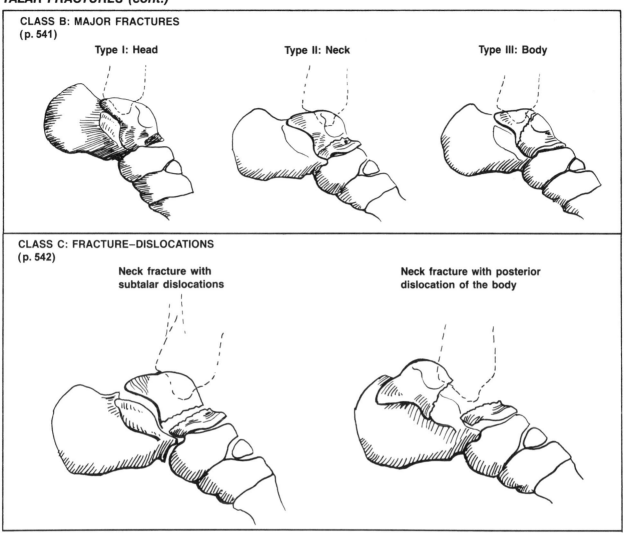

CLASS B: MAJOR FRACTURES
(p. 541)

Type I: Head   **Type II: Neck**   **Type III: Body**

CLASS C: FRACTURE–DISLOCATIONS
(p. 542)

Neck fracture with subtalar dislocations

Neck fracture with posterior dislocation of the body

TALAR DISLOCATIONS

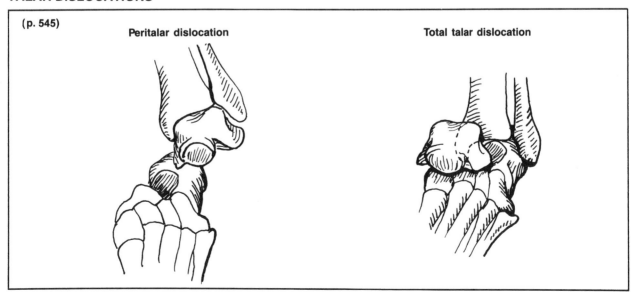

(p. 545)

Peritalar dislocation   **Total talar dislocation**

MIDFOOT FRACTURES AND DISLOCATIONS

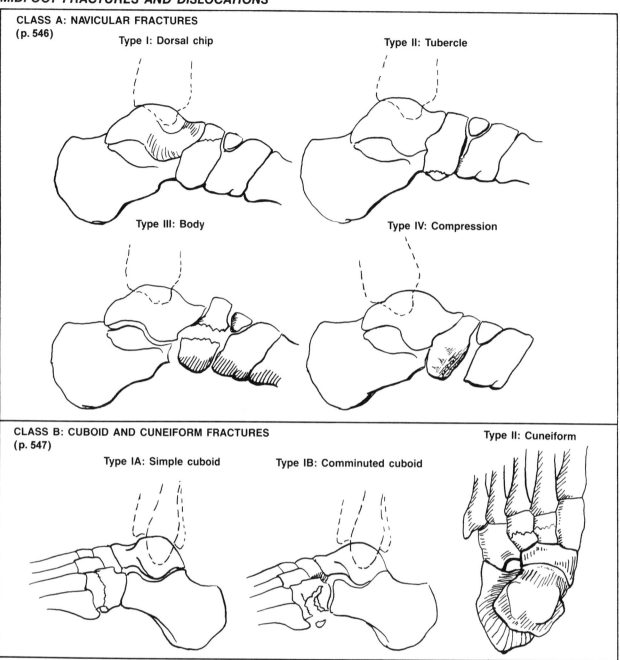

CLASS A: NAVICULAR FRACTURES
(p. 546)

Type I: Dorsal chip

Type II: Tubercle

Type III: Body

Type IV: Compression

CLASS B: CUBOID AND CUNEIFORM FRACTURES
(p. 547)

Type IA: Simple cuboid

Type IB: Comminuted cuboid

Type II: Cuneiform

TARSOMETATARSAL FRACTURE–DISLOCATIONS

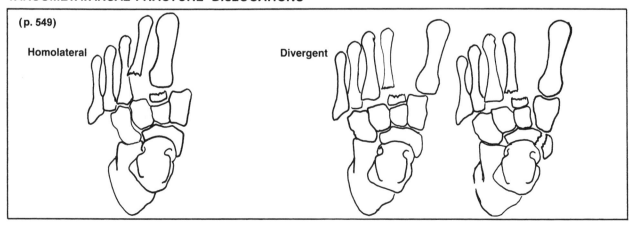

(p. 549)

Homolateral

Divergent

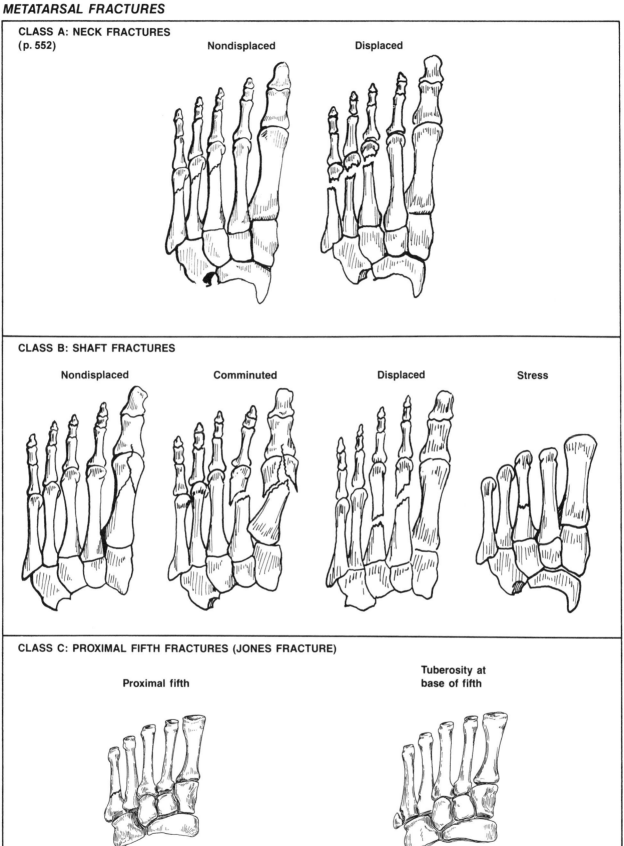

CLASS A: NECK FRACTURES
(p. 552)

Nondisplaced   Displaced

CLASS B: SHAFT FRACTURES

Nondisplaced   Comminuted   Displaced   Stress

CLASS C: PROXIMAL FIFTH FRACTURES (JONES FRACTURE)

Proximal fifth

Tuberosity at
base of fifth

SESAMOID AND PHALANGEAL FRACTURES

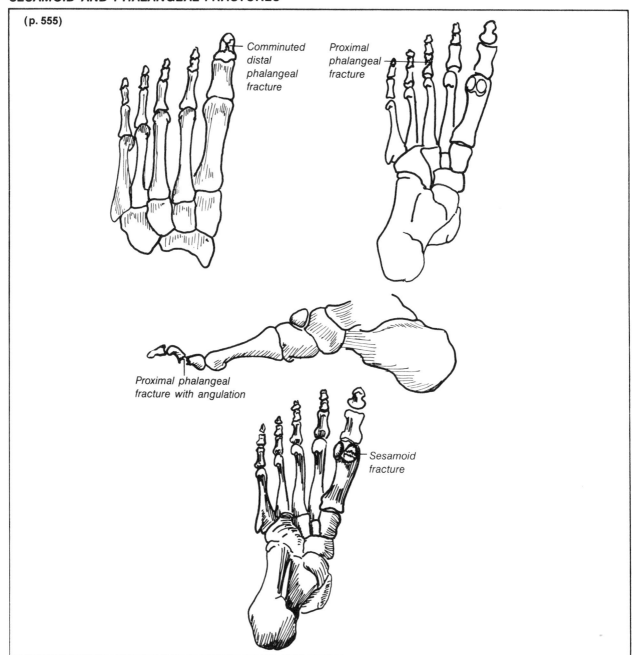

(p. 555)

Comminuted distal phalangeal fracture

Proximal phalangeal fracture

Proximal phalangeal fracture with angulation

Sesamoid fracture

INTERPHALANGEAL DISLOCATIONS

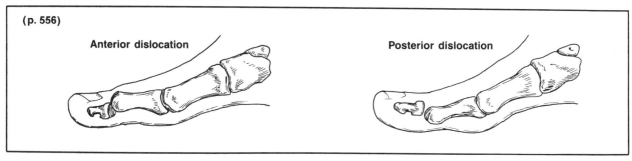

(p. 556)

Anterior dislocation

Posterior dislocation

METATARSOPHALANGEAL DISLOCATIONS

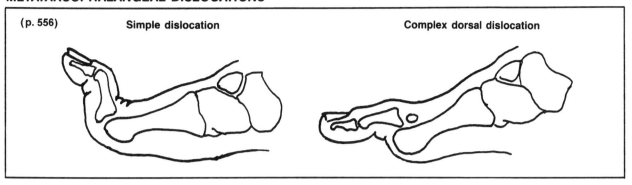

(p. 556) Simple dislocation   Complex dorsal dislocation

The foot contains 28 bones and 57 articulations. Foot fractures are common and account for 10 percent of all fractures. Conceptually, the foot can be divided into three regions: the hindfoot (talus and calcaneus), the mid foot (navicular, cuneiforms, and cuboid), and the forefoot (metatarsals and phalanges). The bones of the foot including common sesamoids seen in medial and lateral projections are shown in Figures 31–1 and 31–2.

The foot has a wide range of normal motion including flexion, extension, inversion, and eversion. In addition, supination or the combination of adduction and inversion as well as pronation representing abduction and eversion are part of the normal range of foot motion. The foot contains two arches: a longitudinal arch (midpart of foot) and a transverse arch (forepart of foot). Weight is normally borne equally on the forefoot and the heel. Weight is not equitably distributed on the metatarsal heads as the first bears twice as much weight

as the remaining four. The maximum weight applied to the foot occurs during the pushoff phase of walking and running.

Foot fractures are generally the result of one of three basic mechanisms of injury including direct trauma, indirect trauma, and overuse. The radiologic diagnosis of foot fractures is frequently complicated by the secondary ossification centers and sesaoids. Commonly seen sesamoids include os trigonum, os tibiale externum, os peroneum, and os vesalianum. These centers can often be distinguished from fractures by their smooth sclerotic bony margins.

The classification system used in this chapter is modified from that used in the remainder of the text. Because dislocations of the foot (with the exception of interphalangeal dislocations) are nearly always associated with fractures, the authors have included them in this chapter rather than in Chapter 32.

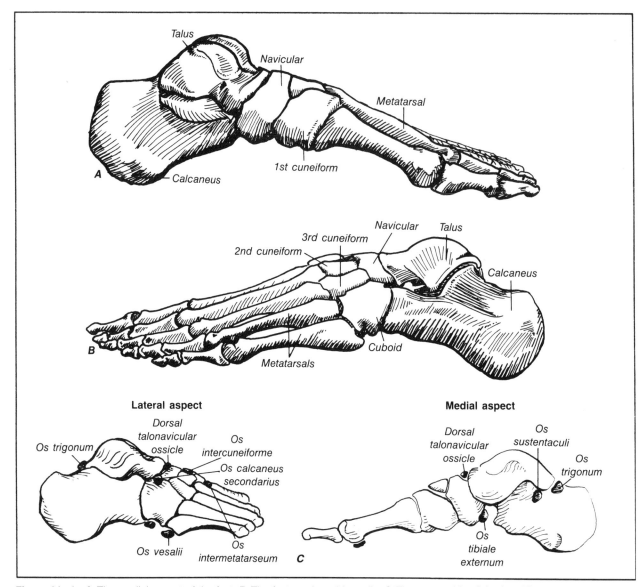

Figure 31–1. **A.** The medial aspect of the foot. **B.** The foot as viewed laterally. **C.** The sesamoids of the foot. These are commonly confused for fractures.

CALCANEAL FRACTURES

The calcaneus is the largest of the tarsal bones and serves as a springboard for locomotion and as an elastic support for the weight of the body. The calcaneus is the most frequently fractured tarsal bone representing 60 percent of all tarsal fractures (Figs. 31–3 and 31–4). On the plantar surface of the foot are the medial and lateral processes serving as points of insertion for the plantar fascia and muscles. The principal articulation of the calcaneus is with the talus forming the subtalar joint. Of the

nonavulsion calcaneal fractures, 75 percent involve the subtalar joint and 75 percent of these are depressed.[18]

Classification

The classification system used is a simplification of the Rowe system, which is based on treatment and prog- nosis.[25]

- **Class A:** Calcaneal process or tuberosity fractures
- **Class B:** Calcaneal body fractures

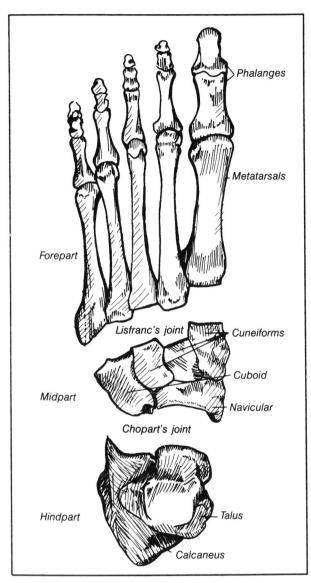

Figure 31–2. Note the foot is divided into a hindpart, a midpart, and a forepart. The Chopart's joint separates the hindpart from the midpart and the Lisfranc's joint separates the midpart from the forepart.

☐ CLASS A: CALCANEAL PROCESS OR TUBEROSITY FRACTURES

☐ Class A: Type I (Medial or Lateral Tuberosity Fractures) (Fig. 31–3)

These fractures may be divided into nondisplaced or displaced injuries and generally have an excellent prognosis.

Mechanism of Injury

These fractures are usually secondary to an abduction or adduction force as the heel strikes the ground while the foot is in eversion or inversion. With eversion, a medial process fracture is likely, whereas with inversion, a lateral fracture is more likely. Typically, the patient will relate a history of jumping from a height and landing on an inverted or everted ankle.

Examination

The patient will complain of pain, swelling, and tenderness over the posterolateral or posteromedial heel. The ankle may have a full range of motion; however, acute hyperextension will usually be painful.

X Ray

Calcaneal radiographs must include posteroanterior (PA), lateral, and axial views. If clinically indicated, ankle views should be obtained. Computed tomography (CT) analysis may be helpful in delineating the anatomy of injuries that are unclear on plain radiographs.[5]

Associated Injuries

Twenty-six percent of calcaneal fractures are associated with other injuries to the lower extremities.[3] Ten percent of calcaneal fractures are bilateral.[32] Compression fractures of the dorsolumbar spine are associated with 10 percent of calcaneal fractures.[3] Stress fractures of the calcaneus are typically posterior and may be difficult to see on plain films despite months of symptoms. Bone scanning may be helpful in delineating these injuries.[27]

Treatment

Nondisplaced medial or lateral calcaneal tuberosity or process fractures can be treated with ice, elevation, and bulky compressive dressing. Within 1 to 2 weeks, a well-molded walking cast should be applied and left in place until the bones are united. Partial weight bearing using crutches should be continued for at least 8 weeks. Displaced fractures require reduction, which is usually adequate after closed manipulation. This should be followed by a well-molded cast until the bones are united. Some authors recommend open reduction with internal fixation primarily; thus, early consultation is strongly recommended.[5,12,26,33]

Complications

Calcaneal fractures can be associated with a 10 percent incidence of the development of a compartment syndrome of the foot. Symptoms include tense swelling and severe pain and may be associated with long-term problems, including clawing of the lesser toes, stiffness, chronic pain, weakness, sensory changes, atrophy, and forefoot deformities. The diagnosis can be made in the acute phase utilizing pressure measurements within the compartment. Fasciotomy is the recommended treatment.

The long-term consequences of these fractures may be disabling. Typically, nonarticular fractures of the calcaneus heal without significant morbidity. Unfortunately,

CALCANEAL FRACTURES

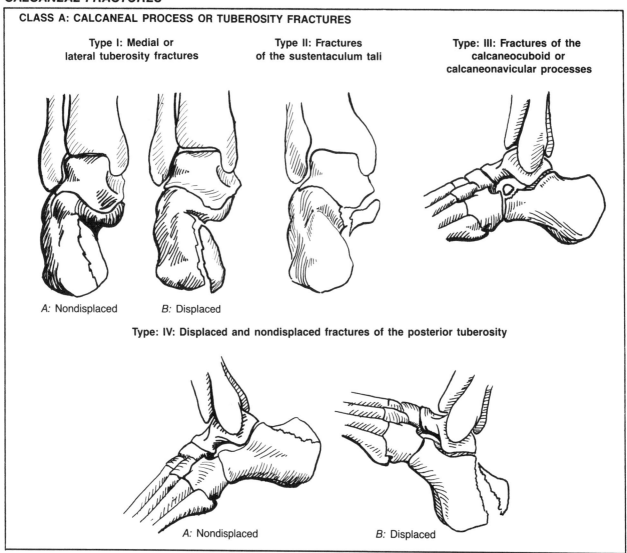

CLASS A: CALCANEAL PROCESS OR TUBEROSITY FRACTURES

Type I: Medial or lateral tuberosity fractures

Type II: Fractures of the sustentaculum tali

Type: III: Fractures of the calcaneocuboid or calcaneonavicular processes

A: Nondisplaced   *B:* Displaced

Type: IV: Displaced and nondisplaced fractures of the posterior tuberosity

A: Nondisplaced   *B:* Displaced

Figure 31–3.

up to 75 percent of calcaneal fractures include a disruption of the subtalar joint and are associated with significant long-term complications.[5]

Posttraumatic arthritis with stiffness and chronic pain is the most frequent complication. Spur formation with chronic pain or nerve entrapment may complicate the long-term management of these fractures.

☐ Class A: Type II   (Fractures of the Sustentaculum Tali) (Fig. 31–3)

Mechanism of Injury
This is uncommon as an isolated injury. The most common mechanism of injury is axial compression on the heel with marked inversion of the foot.[21]

Examination
The patient will present with pain, tenderness, and swelling just distal to the medial malleolus and over the medial heel. The pain will be exacerbated by inversion of the foot or hyperextension of the great toe as this will pull on the flexor hallucis longus which passes beneath the sustentaculum tali.[21]

X Ray
Routine radiographs including comparison axial views may be necessary to diagnose these fractures. CT analysis may be helpful in delineating the anatomy of injuries that are unclear on plain radiographs.[5]

Associated Injuries
The reader is referred to the discussion included under class A, type I fractures.

CALCANEAL FRACTURES

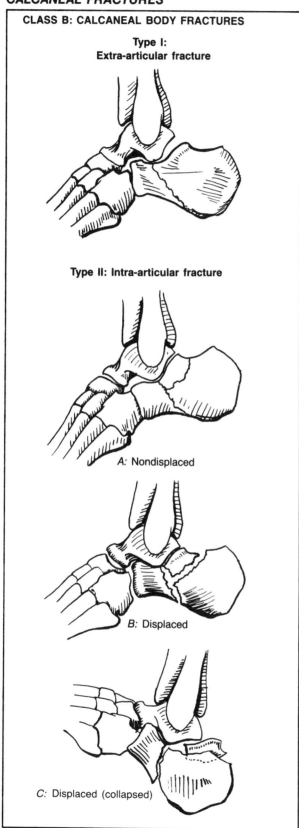

CLASS B: CALCANEAL BODY FRACTURES

Type I:
Extra-articular fracture

Type II: Intra-articular fracture

A: Nondisplaced

B: Displaced

C: Displaced (collapsed)

Figure 31–4.

Treatment

The management of these fractures includes ice, elevation, and immobilization in a compression dressing for 24 to 36 hours.[21] Nondisplaced fractures should then be casted and remain non–weight bearing for 8 weeks. Orthopedic referral is strongly recommended as many of these fractures may be followed by long-term pain. Displaced fractures require emergent orthopedic referral for consideration of open reduction. Accurate analysis of fragment position by CT may be very helpful. It is recommended that surgery be performed within 3 weeks (optimally 10 days or less) after foot and ankle swelling has been reduced.[26]

Complications

The reader is referred to the discussion included under class A, type I fractures.

☐ Class A: Type III   (Fractures of the Calcaneocuboid or Calcaneonavicular Processes) (Fig. 31–3)

Mechanism of Injury

This is an uncommon avulsion fracture secondary to abduction with the foot in plantar flexion.[24] This position stresses the bifurcate ligament which inserts on the calcaneus as well as both the cuboid and the navicular. Severe stress results in a ligamentous rupture or an avulsion fracture of the calcaneus at its articulation with the cuboid or the navicular.

Examination

The patient will usually present with a history of "twisting" the foot and will complain of pain, swelling, and tenderness just distal to the lateral malleolus.

X Ray

Routine views are usually adequate for defining the fracture fragments. The lateral projection of the hindfoot is especially helpful in visualizing subtle fractures. CT analysis may be helpful in delineating the anatomy of injuries that are unclear on plain radiographs.[5]

Associated Injury

The reader is referred to the discussion included under class A, type I fractures.

Treatment

The recommended management of these injuries includes ice, elevation, and weight bearing as tolerated.[21] Casting is usually avoided as chronic stiffness is a common complication. Orthopedic referral for follow-up is recommended.

Complications
The reader is referred to the discussion included under class A, type I fractures.

☐ Class A: Type IV   (Displaced and Nondisplaced Fractures of the Posterior Tuberosity) (Fig. 31–3)

Mechanism of Injury
The most common mechanism of injury for this avulsion fracture is stress on the tendocalcaneus as occurs during a fall or a jump landing on the dorsiflexed foot with the knee extended.[18]

Examination
The patient will present with pain, swelling, and tenderness over the fracture; inability to walk; and weak plantar flexion of the foot.[18,21]

X Ray
Routine views and, in particular, the lateral radiograph are usually adequate in defining these fractures.[21] CT analysis may be helpful in delineating the anatomy of injuries that are unclear on plain radiographs.[5]

Associated Injuries
The reader is referred to the discussion included under class A, type I injuries.

Treatment
Nondisplaced fractures should be treated in a non–weight-bearing cast with the foot in equinus for 6 to 8 weeks. Early consultation and referral is strongly recommended. Displaced fractures require emergent orthopedic referral for consideration of open reduction. Accurate analysis of fragment position by CT may be very helpful.[5,21] It is recommended that surgery be performed within 3 weeks (optimally 10 days or less) after foot and ankle swelling has been reduced.[26]

Complications
The reader is referred to the discussion included under class A, type I fractures.

☐ CLASS B: CALCANEAL BODY FRACTURES

☐ Class B: Type I   (Extra-articular Fractures) (Fig. 31–4)

Mechanism of Injury
This an uncommon fracture that does not involve the subtalar joint. The most common mechanism is a fall which results in the patient landing on the inverted or everted heel.

Examination
The patient will present with pain, swelling, and an inability to bear weight. If the medial and lateral swelling remains untreated for 8 or more hours, these patients may develop superficial skin blistering. The pain is exacerbated with inversion, eversion, flexion, or extension.

X Ray
Routine calcaneal views are generally adequate in demonstrating these fractures. CT analysis may be helpful in delineating the anatomy of injuries which are unclear on plain radiographs.[5]

Associated Injuries
These fractures may be associated with sural nerve entrapment in addition to the other complications as discussed under class A, type I injuries.

Treatment
The emergency management of these fractures should include ice, elevation, immobilization in a bulky dressing, and early referral. Nondisplaced fractures may be treated with non–weight bearing, hydrotherapy, and active exercise for a minimum of 8 to 12 weeks before ambulation. A Jones compression dressing has been used in the treatment of these fractures and weight bearing has been permitted after the first couple of days. Weight bearing of 10 to 20 percent of total body weight and eventually 100 percent of body weight over a 2- to 4- week period has been advocated by some orthopedic surgeons.[16] Excellent results have been reported in 75 percent of patients, which is comparable to most other methods of therapy.[16] For a discussion of displaced fractures the reader is referred to the class B, type II treatment section. Early ice and elevation are important in preventing the formation of skin blisters.

Complications
In addition to those discussed under class A, type I injuries, these fractures may be complicated by the development of fracture blisters with subsequent skin loss or infection.[20]

☐ Class B: Type II   (Intra-articular Displaced and Nondisplaced Fractures) (Fig. 31–4)

Mechanism of Injury
The most common mechanism is a fall where the weight of the body is absorbed by the heel.

Examination

The patient will present with pain, swelling, and ecchymosis on the sole of the foot with loss of the normal depressions along both sides of the Achilles tendon.

X Ray (Fig. 31–5)

Routine radiographic views are generally adequate in defining this fracture. Böhler's angle should be calculated whenever a class B, type II fracture is diagnosed. The angle can be calculated by measuring the intersection of two lines, one drawn from the superior margin of the posterior tuberosity of the calcaneus through the superior tip of the posterior facet and another from this same point through the superior tip of the anterior process (Fig. 31–6).

Normally, this angle measures 20 to 40 degrees. If the angle measures less than 20 degrees, a depressed fracture can be diagnosed. This may alter the treatment as some orthopedic physicians will elevate the depressed segment whereas others will treat this in a similar manner as other calcaneal body fractures. (See Fig. 31–7). CT analysis may be helpful in delineating the anatomy of injuries which are unclear on plain radiographs.[5]

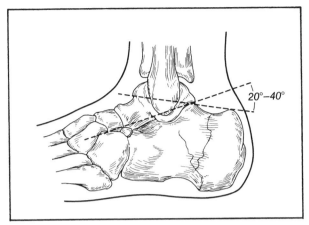

Figure 31–6. Böhler's angle. This should be calculated whenever a class B, type II fracture is diagnosed. The angle is calculated by measuring the intersection of two lines, one drawn from the superior margin of the posterior tuberosity of the calcaneus, extending through the superior tip of the posterior facet and another line from this later point extending through the superior tip of the anterior process. The normal angle measures approximately 20 to 40 degrees. If the angle measures less than 20 degrees, a depressed fracture can be diagnosed.

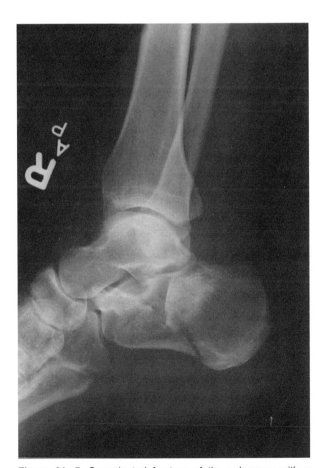

Figure 31–5. Comminuted fracture of the calcaneus with a Böhlers angle of 15 degrees.

Associated Injuries

Nearly one half of these patients have associated fractures of the spine or extremities thus mandating a thorough examination. Additional associated injuries are discussed under class A, type I fractures.

Treatment

The emergency management of these fractures includes ice, elevation, and immobilization in a bulky compressive dressing. Nondisplaced fractures may be treated with non–weight bearing, hydrotherapy, and gradual exercises for a minimum of 8 to 12 weeks. The treatment of displaced fractures is controversial and varies from a conservative approach through surgical repair. Early consultation and referral is strongly recommended in the management of these injuries. In patients with comminuted and displaced intra-articular fractures, a good outcome requires the reestablishment of joint congruity and the elevation of depressed fragments.[15] Surgical management including open reduction with internal fixation is recommended.[26]

Complications

In addition to the complications discussed under class A, type I fractures, these fractures are often followed by the development of severe degenerative changes. Joint widening may develop resulting in fibular pressure and peroneal tendon entrapment. These fractures have a very poor prognosis.

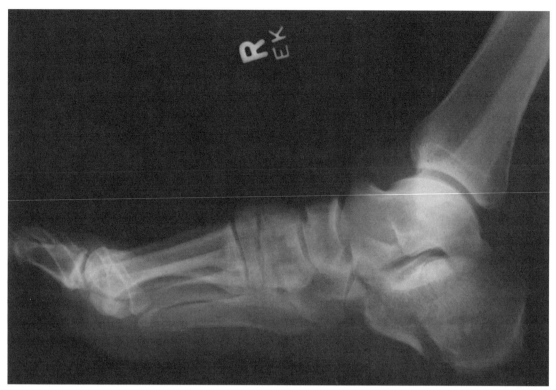

Figure 31–7. Comminuted displaced calcaneal fracture.

TALAR FRACTURES

The talus is the second most frequently fractured tarsal bone[21] (Figs. 31–8 through 31–10). The talus is held in place by ligaments and has no muscles inserting on it. In addition, 60 percent of its surface is covered by articular cartilage. The vascular supply to the bone does not penetrate the articular cartilage but enters by way of the deltoid ligament, the talocalcaneal ligament, the anterior capsule, and the sinus tarsi. The blood supply is, therefore, somewhat tenuous and avascular necrosis is not uncommon after displaced fractures. Proximal talar fractures are particularly predisposed to develop avascular necrosis of the proximal fragment.[21]

The most common fractures of the talus are chip or avulsion fractures followed by talar neck, body, and finally talar head fractures.[18,21] Osteochondral talar fractures are common injuries that typically present after an inversion or eversion ankle injury.[2,7] The talus thus impacts against the medial or lateral malleolus resulting in a cartilage fracture. These injuries are discussed in more detail in Chapter 30.

Classification
The following classification system is based on radiographic and clinical findings and is a modification of the system developed by Coltart.[4]

☐ **Class A (Minor Talar Fractures [Fig. 31–8])**
- Type I: Talar chip fractures
- Type II: Posterior facet fractures
- Type III: Osteochondral fractures
              (discussed in Chap. 30)

☐ **Class B (Major Talar Fractures [Fig. 31–9])**
- Type I: Talar head fractures
- Type II: Talar neck fractures
- Type III: Talar body fractures

TALAR FRACTURES

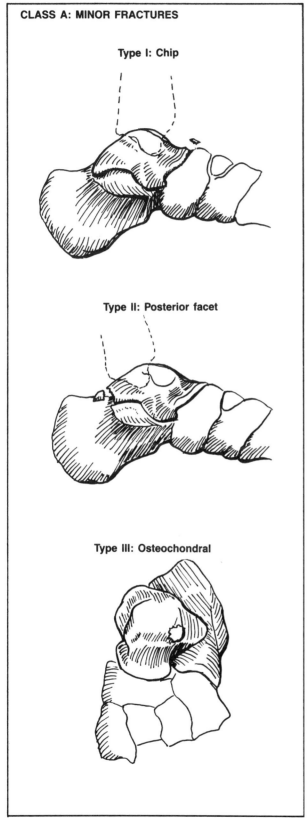

Figure 31–8.

TALAR FRACTURES

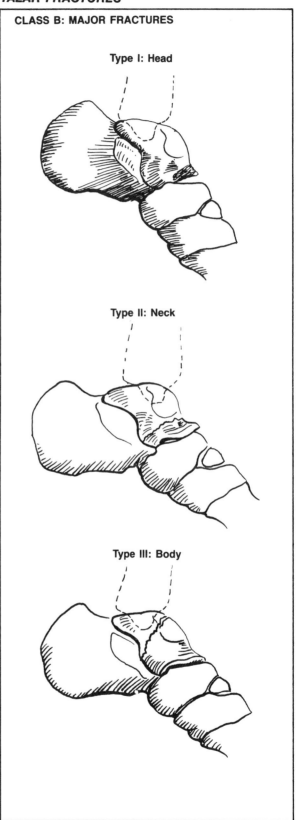

Figure 31–9.

TALAR FRACTURES

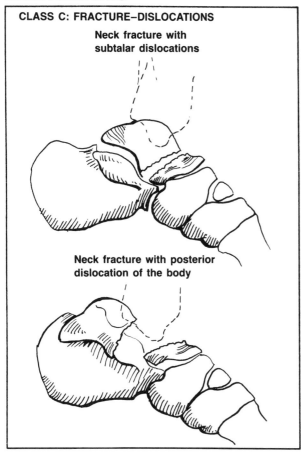

CLASS C: FRACTURE–DISLOCATIONS

**Neck fracture with
subtalar dislocations**

**Neck fracture with posterior
dislocation of the body**

Figure 31–10.

□ *Class C (Fracture–Dislocation
of the Talus [Fig. 31–10])*

□ CLASS A: MINOR FRACTURES
(FIG. 31–8)

Chip fractures are the most common type of talar fracture. Osteochondral fractures will not be discussed in this section as they are included in the discussion of ankle injuries in Chapter 30.

Mechanism of Injury

Chip or avulsion fractures commonly follow excessive flexion or extension combined with a rotational force. A type II posterior facet fracture is often the result of extreme flexion with impingement of the facet against the posterior tibia and calcaneus.

Examination

Patients with type I fractures typically present with a history of a severe twisting injury often followed by an audible pop. The patient will present with swelling, tenderness, and deep pain, which is poorly localized. The pain is exacerbated with motion, and joint locking secondary to a displaced fragment may occur. Tenderness is maximal over the dorsum of the foot along the talus. Type II fractures typically present with posterior lateral pain, tenderness, and swelling.

X Ray (Fig. 31–11)

Class A fractures typically present with only minimal radiographic findings. The abnormalities may be limited to a tiny avulsion fragment of bone over the involved area. Special oblique views may be necessary to demonstrate the fracture fragment. Tomography or CT may be necessary to adequately evaluate these fractures. The smoothly rounded os trigonum may at times be confused with a fracture, but knowledge of its typical location and shape will aid in avoiding this confusion.

Treatment

Class A, type I avulsion or chip fractures should be treated with ice, elevation, and immobilization in a short leg walking cast with the ankle in a neutral position and referral for follow-up. Fragments greater than 0.5 cm in diameter may require excision or internal fixation to prevent migration with subsequent joint locking. Type II posterior facet fractures should be treated as previously discussed except the foot should be casted in 15 degrees of equinus.[21] Type III injuries require surgical excision of the fragment.

Complications

Type I and II injuries are generally not complicated by any long-term disorders. If the fragments are large, nonunion with migration may result in joint locking and eventually traumatic arthritis. Type III osteochondral fractures frequently result in the development of traumatic arthritis if untreated.

□ CLASS B: MAJOR FRACTURES

□ Class B: Type I (Head) (Fig. 31–9)

Mechanism of Injury

These injuries are usually the result of direct impact such as falling on the fully extended foot. The force is transmitted from the forefoot to the talus, which impacts against the anterior edge of the tibia.[21]

Examination

The patient will usually present with pain, swelling, ecchymosis, and tenderness over the talar head and the talonavicular joint.[21] Ankle motion will be normal although inversion of the foot will exacerbate the pain over the talonavicular joint.

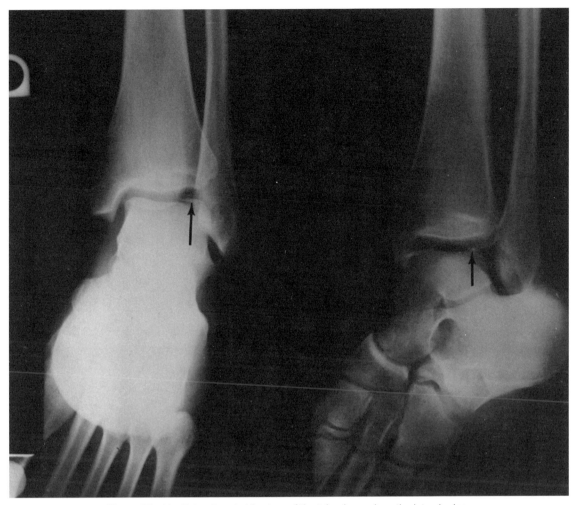

Figure 31–11. Osteochondral fracture of the talar dome along the lateral edge.

X Ray

Routine views often do not adequately demonstrate these fractures. Oblique radiographs, tomography, or CT may be necessary to adequately evaluate these fractures.[1]

Treatment

The emergency management of this fracture should include ice, elevation, immobilization in a bulky compression dressing, and early consultation. Some orthopedic surgeons prefer early weight bearing as tolerated whereas others recommend a short leg walking cast for 6 to 8 weeks followed by arch support for 12 weeks.[23] Some surgeons recommend a non–weight-bearing cast for 6 to 8 weeks as the preferred mode of treatment. Open reduction with internal fixation is recommended if the fragment:

1. Causes instability of the talonavicular joint
2. Is displaced resulting in an articular step off
3. Is larger than 50 percent of the articular surface.[1]

Complications

Talar head fractures may be complicated by the development of talonavicular osteoarthritis or chondromalacia.

☐ Class B: Type II (Neck) (Fig. 31–9)

Mechanism of Injury

These injuries typically follow acute hyperextension of the foot and the ankle and are frequently seen after automobile accidents or falls from heights. With hyperextension the neck of the talus impacts against the anterior edge of the tibia. Continuation of the force may result in ligamentous tearing, fragment displacement, or subtalar and talar body dislocation.

Examination

The patient will present with a history of acute hyperextension followed by pain, swelling, and extreme tenderness to light palpation or motion.

X Ray

The fracture is best visualized on the routine lateral view. The oblique view may be helpful in the presence of subtle subluxations or dislocations.

Associated Injuries

Talar neck fractures are frequently associated with dislocations of the peroneal tendons.

Treatment

The emergency management of these fractures includes ice, elevation, analgesics, immobilization, and early consultation. Nondisplaced fractures may be treated with a short leg nonwalking cast for 6 weeks followed by 3 weeks of partial weight bearing. Displaced fractures or those associated with dislocations require a neurovascular assessment followed by an emergent referral for an anatomic reduction by either open or closed means.

Complications

The management of talar neck fractures may be complicated by the development of several disorders.

1. Peroneal tendon dislocations often follow these fractures.
2. Avascular necrosis of the talus may be seen after these injuries. Fracture–dislocations are particularly predisposed to the development of this complication.
3. Delayed union may complicate the management of these injuries.

☐ Class B: Type III (Body) (Fig. 31–9)

Mechanism of Injury

Nondisplaced talar body fractures may be the result of an acute hyperextension injury. Comminuted or displaced fractures typically are the result of axial compression with hyperextension.

Examination

The patient will present with a history of hyperextension and intense but diffuse ankle pain, tenderness, and swelling.

Treatment

The emergency management of nondisplaced talar body fractures should include ice, elevation, analgesics, and a short leg nonwalking cast for 6 to 8 weeks. The prognosis for these injuries is very good. Displaced or comminuted fractures require an anatomic reduction, and early consultation and referral is strongly recommended.

Complications

Displaced or comminuted body fractures are often complicated by the development of avascular necrosis.

☐ CLASS C: FRACTURE–DISLOCATIONS (FIG. 31–10)

Mechanism of Injury

Continued hyperextension after a talar neck fracture will result in locking the talus in the ankle mortise. The foot will be locked into hyperextension with the continuation of this mechanism. Posterior fracture–dislocations require a more severe hyperextension injury force.

Examination

These patients will present with a history of hyperextension and the foot locked into a hyperextended position. Pain, tenderness, and swelling are typically marked.

X Ray

Routine views are generally adequate in demonstrating the abnormality.

Treatment

The emergency management of these injuries includes analgesics, elevation, and emergent referral for reduction. Delayed reductions are associated with an increased incidence of skin necrosis and avascular necrosis.

Complications

These injuries are complicated by the development of avascular necrosis, skin necrosis, traumatic arthritis, and delayed union.

TALAR DISLOCATIONS

Talar dislocations may be classified into two types: *total talar dislocations* and *peritalar dislocations* (Fig. 31–12). With total talar dislocations, the talus is completely dislocated out of the ankle mortise and rotated such that the in-ferior articular surface points posteriorly and the talar head points medially. Shepard coined the term *peritalar dislocations* to more accurately describe the dislocation of the talus from its surrounding joints (talonavicular, etc.) and

DISLOCATIONS

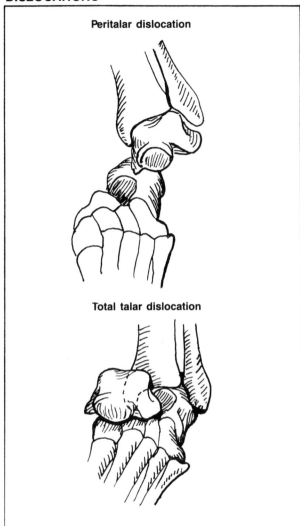

Peritalar dislocation

Total talar dislocation

Figure 31–12.

the subtalar joint.[28] Peritalar dislocations may be classified as medial or lateral depending on the position of the foot relative to the distal tibia.[34] The more common medial type presents with the talar head palpable laterally.[17,21] Lateral peritalar dislocations are less common, and the talar head is directed medially and usually palpable.

Mechanism of Injury

Peritalar dislocations typically follow an inversion and plantar flexion injury.[17,21] The talocalcaneal and talonavicular ligaments rupture as the bones of the foot are displaced medially. This injury has been reported in basketball players who land on the inverted plantar-flexed foot. Severe plantar flexion and inversion may result in rupture of the anterior, medial, and lateral ligaments with talar detachment. The talus remains in the anterolateral position whereas the remainder of the foot recoils into medial displacement.

Examination

The patient will present with a history of severe trauma followed by the development of marked pain, swelling, and tenderness. With medial dislocations, the foot will be displaced medially and the talus palpable laterally. The vascular supply to the skin is often compromised due to talar pressure.

X Ray

Routine views including anteroposterior (AP), lateral, and oblique are usually adequate in demonstrating these injuries. Postreduction films are required for documentation as well as to exclude the presence of occult fractures.

Associated Injuries

Total talar and peritalar dislocations may be associated with the following injuries:

1. Tarsal fractures
2. Malleolar fractures
3. Talar neck fractures
4. Rupture of the ankle and metatarsal supporting ligaments[17]

Treatment

The emergency management of closed injuries includes analgesics and prompt reduction to avoid the complication of skin necrosis. If prompt consultation is not available an attempt at closed reduction should be made. For medial dislocations, firm but gentle traction in plantar flexion and adduction should be applied initially followed by pressure over the talar head and an abduction force concomitantly applied to the forefoot. If this is unsuccessful, open reduction is indicated. Lateral dislocations may be reduced by firm traction followed by adduction over the forefoot. Open talar dislocations are quite common. These injuries should not be reduced in the emergency department. The lacerations should be shaved and cleansed with sterile saline and antibiotics started early along with tetanus immunization if indicated. As with all open fractures or dislocations, reduction should be performed in the operating suite.

Complications

Talar dislocations may be complicated by the development of several significant disorders.

1. Avascular necrosis of the talus frequently complicates the long-term management of these disorders.
2. Loss of ankle motion and traumatic arthritis are commonly noted after talar dislocations.
3. Ischemic skin loss secondary to underlying talar pressure may be seen after these injuries.[9,12,13]

MIDFOOT FRACTURES AND DISLOCATIONS

The midfoot is the least mobile portion of the foot and includes the navicular, the cuboid, and the three cuneiforms. Typically midfoot injuries involve multiple fractures or fracture–dislocations (Figs. 31–13 and 31–14). The most frequent navicular fracture involves the dorsal lip. Tubercle fractures are second in frequency and are followed by navicular body fractures, which may be transverse or horizontal. Cuboid and cuneiform fractures usually occur in combination and typically are the result of crush injuries.

Classification
Midfoot fractures are classified on the basis of anatomy.

☐ Class A: (Navicular Fractures
                     [Fig. 31–13])
• Type I: Dorsal chip fractures
• Type II: Tubercle fractures

• Type III: Body fractures
• Type IV: Compression fractures
• Type V: Stress fractures (not visualized on x-rays)

☐ Class B: (Cuboid and Cuneiform Fractures
                     [Fig. 31–14])
• Type I: Cuboid fractures
• Type II: Cuneiform fractures

☐ CLASS A: NAVICULAR FRACTURES (FIG. 31–13)

Mechanism of Injury
Type I chip fractures are usually the result of acute flexion with inversion of the foot. The talonavicular joint capsule is stressed and may avulse the proximal dorsal aspect of the navicular. Type II tuberosity fractures

MIDFOOT FRACTURES AND DISLOCATIONS

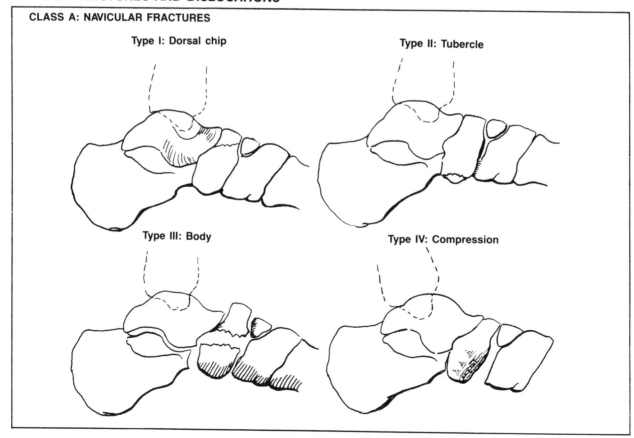

CLASS A: NAVICULAR FRACTURES

Type I: Dorsal chip   **Type II: Tubercle**

Type III: Body   **Type IV: Compression**

Figure 31–13.

MIDFOOT FRACTURES AND DISLOCATIONS

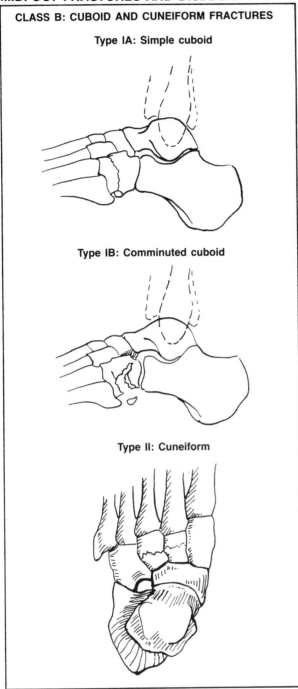

CLASS B: CUBOID AND CUNEIFORM FRACTURES

Type IA: Simple cuboid

Type IB: Comminuted cuboid

Type II: Cuneiform

Figure 31–14.

typically follow an acute eversion force on the foot. Eversion of the foot results in increased tension on the tibialis posterior tendon and it may avulse a portion of the navicular tuberosity. Type III body fractures and type IV compression fractures of the navicular are rare injuries. Previously reported mechanisms of injury include acute hyperextension with compression, direct trauma, or extreme flexion with rotation.[19]

Examination

The patient will present with pain, swelling, and tenderness over the involved area. For chip fractures, the dorsal and medial aspect of the midfoot will be tender. Tubercle fractures present with pain localized to the overlying area, which is exacerbated with eversion of the foot. (See Fig. 31–15.)

X Ray

AP, lateral, and oblique views are generally adequate in demonstrating these injuries. Subtle, nondisplaced fractures may be difficult to diagnose and may require comparison views or follow-up films for adequate visualization. An accessory bone, the os tibiale externum, is often confused with an avulsion fracture of the navicular. Stress fractures of the navicular may require bone scanning and CT evaluation to demonstrate the fracture.[30]

Associated Injuries

Dorsal chip fractures are often associated with lateral malleolar ligament injuries. Tuberosity fractures are often accompanied by cuboid fractures.

Treatment

☐ Class A: Type I   (Dorsal Chip)

Small chip fractures are treated symptomatically with ice, elevation, and elastoplast compressive dressing with crutch walking for about 2 weeks or until the pain subsides. The compressive dressing should be applied from the midtarsal region to above the ankle joint including the heel. Large chip fragments require a short leg walking cast for 3 to 4 weeks.

☐ Class A: Type II   (Tubercle)

Small, nondisplaced avulsion fractures can be treated with a compression dressing and a short leg splint. With the reduction in swelling, a well-molded short leg cast with the foot in inversion resulting in a slack posterior tibial tendon should be utilized for 6 weeks.[30] Significant displacement of the avulsed fragment will require emergent orthopedic referral for consideration of surgical reattachment.[8,30]

☐ Class A: Type III   (Body)
Type IV   (Compression)

Nondisplaced body fractures should be treated with a well-molded, below-the-knee walking cast for 6 to 8 weeks. After this, longitudinal arch support should be employed. Displaced navicular body fractures require open reduction with internal fixation in the active ambulatory patient. Nonambulatory patients may be treated symptomatically with a compressive elastoplast dressing. Navicular fracture–dislocations require open reduction with internal fixation.

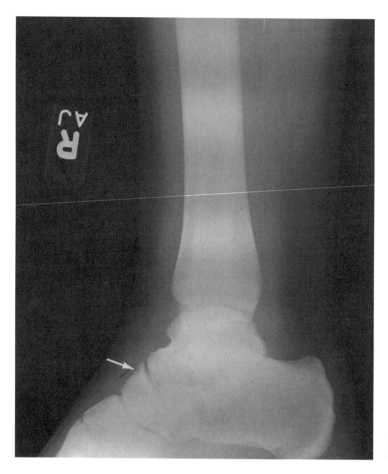

Figure 31–15. Dorsal chip fracture of the navicular.

☐ Class A: Type V (Stress)

This fracture rather is now more recognized, particularly in the serious athlete. Symptoms may have been present for months in many instances. Plain radiographs often do not demonstrate the fracture. Bone scanning and CT typically demonstrate the fracture. Orthopedic referral is indicated as delayed union, nonunion, cyst formation and chronic pain are complications of this fracture.[32]

Complications

Navicular tuberosity fractures are often complicated by nonunion. Body fractures may develop aseptic necrosis or traumatic arthritis.

☐ CLASS B: CUBOID AND CUNEIFORM FRACTURES (FIG. 31–14)

Mechanism of Injury

Cuboid and cuneiform fractures are usually the result of direct crush injuries to the foot. Cuboid and cuneiform dislocations are rare injuries and may be the result of acute inversion or eversion of the foot.[19]

Examination

The patient will usually present with severe pain, tenderness, and swelling over the involved area. Midfoot motion will exacerbate the pain. Dislocations usually present with a palpable deformity and severe pain.

X Ray

AP, lateral, and oblique views are usually adequate for visualizing these fractures. Comparison views may be necessary for subtle fractures or for those involving the articular surfaces to exclude displacement. Suspected dislocations often require comparison views for a definitive diagnosis. Occult fractures including stress fractures of the cuboid and cuneiform may benefit from a bone scan with a CT scan.[32]

Associated Injuries

Cuboid and cuneiform fractures are usually the result of crush injuries and are often associated with significant soft tissue injuries. Cuboid fractures are often associated with calcaneal fractures. Cuneiform fractures may be seen with metatarsal fractures or tarsometatarsal dislocations.

Axiom: *A distal cuboid or cuneiform fracture is associated with a tarsometatarsal dislocation that may have spontaneously reduced until proven otherwise.*

Treatment

Noncomplicated cuboid or cuneiform fractures should be treated with a well-molded short leg cast for 6 to 8 weeks.[21] After cast removal a longitudinal arch support should be used for 5 to 6 months. Dislocations or fracture–dislocations of the cuboid or cuneiforms are frequently unstable after reduction and thus early referral is strongly recommended.

TARSOMETATARSAL FRACTURE–DISLOCATIONS

With the exception of the first, all five metatarsal bones are interconnected by a transverse ligament. The second metatarsal is recessed and firmly bound by ligaments between the medial and lateral cuneiforms and acts as the primary stabilizing force of the metatarsal–tarsal complex. A tarsometatarsal dislocation commonly results in a fracture of the base of the second metatarsal (Fig. 31–16). Usually all the metatarsals dislocate from the tarsals.

Axiom: *A fracture of the base of the second metatarsal is pathognomonic of further tarsometatarsal joint disruption.*

Classification

Tarsometatarsal fracture–dislocations have been referred to as *Lisfranc's fractures*. For emergency department purposes these dislocations may be divided into two groups: *homolateral* and *divergent dislocations*. Homolateral dislocations involve displacement of 4 or all 5 metatarsals in the same direction (see Fig. 31–16). Divergent dislocations involve a split usually between the first and second metatarsals.

Mechanisms of Injury

Homolateral dislocations may follow a fall with the foot landing in plantar flexion.[31] Compressive forces such as those which occur during an automobile accident or

TARSOMETATARSAL FRACTURE–DISLOCATIONS

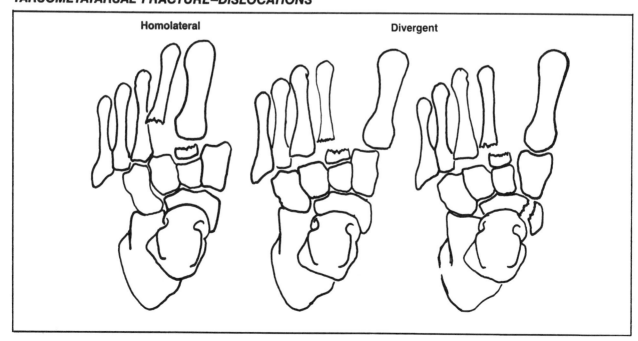

Figure 31–16.

rotational stress may also produce this type of dislocation. Divergent dislocations typically follow a compressive injury force that splits the groove between the first and second metatarsals. Divergent dislocations are frequently associated with avulsion chip fractures of the tarsometatarsal joints.

Examination

The patient will usually present with extreme midfoot pain, swelling, and on occasion paresthesias. On examination there may be a prominence of the base of the first metatarsal or an apparent shortening of the forefoot. The neurovascular status of the foot should be carefully examined and documented. (See Fig. 31–17.)

X Ray

AP, lateral, and oblique views are usually adequate. These injuries are often subtle and may require comparison views for a definitive diagnosis. CT scanning has proven to be a valuable diagnostic tool for delineating occult injuries.[11]

Axiom: *Normally, the medial aspect of the middle cuneiform is directly in line with the medial aspect of the second metatarsal. Any disruption of this alignment is indicative of a dislocation, which may have spontaneously reduced.*

Axiom: *Cuboid chip or compression fractures are frequently associated with tarsometatarsal dislocations.*

Associated Injuries

Tarsometatarsal dislocations may be associated with the following injuries:

1. Fractures of the base of the second metatarsal
2. Chip fractures of adjacent tarsals or metatarsals
3. Cuboid chip or compression fractures
4. Spasm or thrombosis of pedal arteries
5. Cuneiform or navicular fracture–dislocations

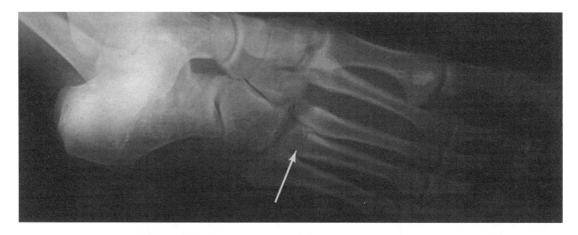

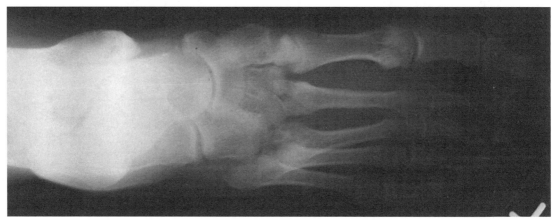

Figure 31–17. A Lisfranc dislocation is noted.

Treatment

The emergency department management of these injuries includes analgesics, ice, elevation, and emergent referral for an attempt at closed reduction under general anesthesia.[25] Typically, Chinese finger traps applied to the toes, and when combined with countertraction on the ankle will usually result in reduction. Pinning after reduction is often necessary to produce stability. An anatomic reduction is necessary and may necessitate an open reduction with internal fixation. After reduction, a short leg cast should be applied for 6 to 12 weeks.[34] A custom arch support may be utilized for the following 12 months.

Complications

Tarsometatarsal dislocations are frequently complicated by the development of degenerative arthritis or impaired circulation to the distal foot.[31]

METATARSAL FRACTURES

As with the hand, the first, fourth, and fifth metatarsals are mobile whereas the second and third are relatively fixed. Maximum weight bearing during the push-off phase of walking is applied to the second and third metatarsals and as a result this is where most stress fractures are seen. Chronic excessive stress results in the development of microfractures that over a prolonged time will result in bone remodeling. Acute episodes of repeated stress over short time intervals may result in the development of stress fractures. Direct trauma or crush injuries may also be responsible for the development of metatarsal fractures. Frequently, this mechanism results in the development of multiple metatarsal fractures.

Classification

Metatarsal fractures are classified on the basis of anatomy and therapy (Fig. 31–18).

- **Class A:** Metatarsal neck fractures
- **Class B:** Metatarsal shaft fractures
- **Class C:** Proximal fifth metatarsal fractures (Jones fracture)

Mechanism of Injury

The majority of metatarsal fractures are the result of a direct crush injury as when a heavy object is dropped on the foot. An indirect mechanism as with twisting of the forefoot often results in a fracture of the base of the fifth metatarsal. Plantar flexion and inversion stresses the peroneus brevis tendon and may result in an avulsion of the styloid process or tuberosity at the base of the fifth metatarsal. If the mechanism is primarily inversion, a nondisplaced transverse styloid process fracture is common.[6]

Examination

Class A and B fractures usually present with pain, swelling, and tenderness localized over the dorsal mid-part of the foot. Axial compression along the involved metatarsal will exacerbate the pain. The strength and quality of the dorsalis pedis pulse should be documented in all patients with suspected metatarsal shaft or neck fractures. Class C fractures usually present with tenderness localized to the involved area and only minimal swelling. The typical history is one of a sprained ankle. Patients with stress fractures often present with a history of an increase in activity with the insidious onset of chronic pain. The pain will usually be poorly localized and accompanied by mild swelling and ecchymosis. (See Fig. 31–19.)

X Ray

AP, lateral, and oblique views are usually adequate in demonstrating these fractures. Often these fractures are accompanied by dorsal angulation secondary to the pull of the intrinsics. The presence of the *os vesalianum* (a secondary center of ossification) at the base of the fifth metatarsal may be confused with a fracture (see Fig. 31–1C). Secondary ossification centers are typically smooth, rounded, bilateral, and often have sclerotic margins. Stress fractures may be radiographically nondetectable initially. After 2 to 3 weeks, however, a fracture line is usually visible and by 4 weeks callus formation is usually evident.

Associated Injuries

Metatarsal fractures are frequently accompanied by phalangeal fractures.

Treatment

Class A nondisplaced neck fractures require ice, elevation, analgesics, and a 24-hour observation period for severe swelling. After this, a short leg walking cast should be applied for 4 to 6 weeks. Displaced neck fractures require ice, elevation, analgesics, and early referral

METATARSAL FRACTURES

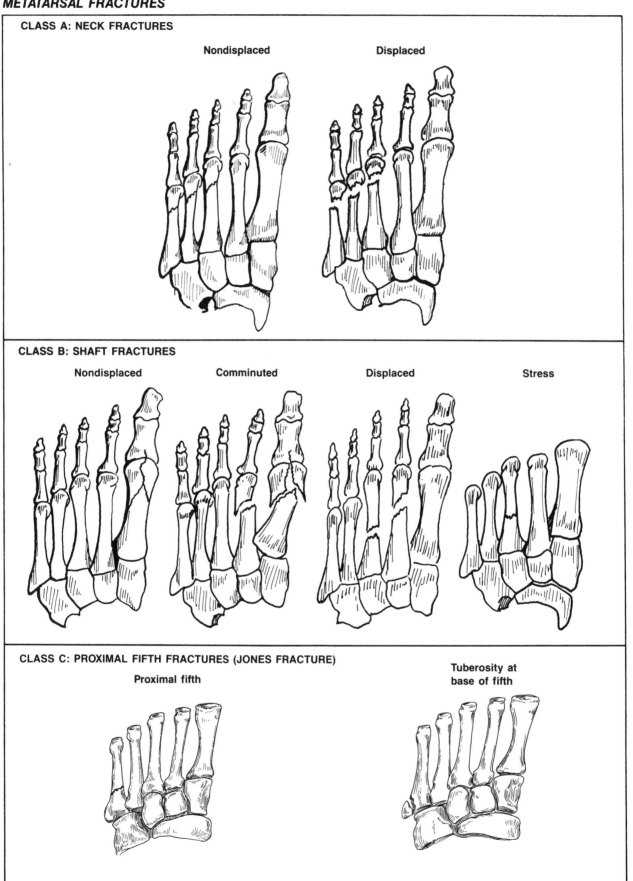

CLASS A: NECK FRACTURES

Nondisplaced   Displaced

CLASS B: SHAFT FRACTURES

Nondisplaced Comminuted Displaced Stress

CLASS C: PROXIMAL FIFTH FRACTURES (JONES FRACTURE)

Proximal fifth   Tuberosity at base of fifth

Figure 31–18.

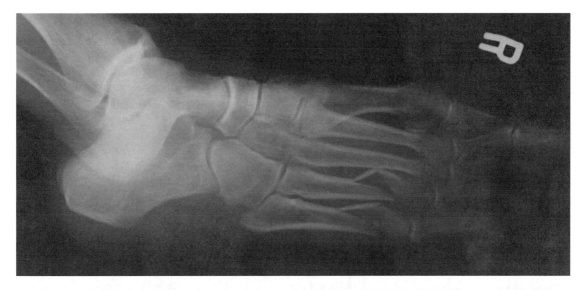

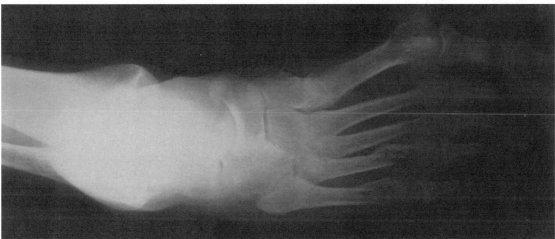

Figure 31–19. Comminuted and displaced fractures of the fourth and fifth metatarsal bones.

for reduction. Nondisplaced shaft fractures of meta-carpals 2 through 5 may be treated with elevation, ice, analgesics, and bulky compression dressing for the first 24 hours. After this a Thomas-shaped metatarsal pad beneath the forefoot with crutches is recommended. Full weight bearing is allowed as tolerated. Nondisplaced first metatarsal shaft fractures require a non–weight-bearing short leg cast for 2 to 3 weeks followed by a short leg walking cast for an additional 2 weeks. Displaced metatarsal shaft fractures involving the second through the fifth metatarsals require reduction. If orthopedic referral is not available, local anesthesia and Chinese finger traps to the toes should be applied. Countertraction should then be applied to the distal tibia by a sling with weights. After reduction, a well-padded non–weight-bearing plaster cast should be applied from the tips of the toes to the hindfoot. At this point the distal tibial countertraction should be removed, and the cast extended to the tibial tuberosity. Postreduction x rays are strongly recom-

mended. After 4 weeks a weight-bearing walking cast for an additional 3 to 4 weeks is recommended. Displaced first metatarsal fractures require referral for reduction. If unavailable, closed reduction as previously described should be attempted. If successful, a non–weight-bearing cast for 6 weeks should be applied. Open reduction may be required for those resistant to closed attempts.

Class C nondisplaced avulsion fractures at the base of the fifth metatarsal require a compression dressing with weight bearing as tolerated. For those patients with severe pain, a short leg walking cast for 3 weeks may be of benefit. This may be followed by a plantar metatarsal pad for arch support. One should be careful not to confuse a transverse fracture of the proximal shaft of the fifth metatarsal with a Jones fracture, which involves the tuberosity. Fractures that are above the tuberosity and transversely across the shaft have an entirely different prognosis and treatment. These fractures have a high incidence of delayed union or nonunion.

Transverse fractures of the proximal shaft of the fifth metatarsal are treated with a short leg, non–weight-bearing cast for 6 to 8 weeks. Displaced fractures should be referred for operative fixation.[22] The prognosis is guarded and there is a high incidence of delayed and nonunion.[23]

Complications

Displaced or angulated metatarsal neck or shaft fractures frequently develop plantar keratitis and thus early referral is recommended. Transverse proximal fifth or meta-tarsal shaft fractures may develop nonunion and require referral due to the high incidence of nonunion.[6]

SESAMOID AND PHALANGEAL FRACTURES, INTERPHALANGEAL DISLOCATIONS, AND METATARSOPHALANGEAL DISLOCATIONS

Phalangeal fractures are common injuries and usually the result of direct trauma (Fig. 31–20). Metatarsophalangeal (MP) or proximal interphalangeal (PIP) dislocations are also common injuries and typically present with inferior displacement of the phalangeal segment (Figs. 31–21 and 31–22). Two sesamoids are commonly found within the tendon of the *flexor hallucis brevis* and are only infrequently fractured.

Mechanism of Injury

The majority of phalangeal fractures are the result of a direct blow such as when a heavy object is dropped on the foot. Hyperextension of the toe, an indirect mechanism, may result in a spiral or an avulsion fracture. Sesamoid fractures are usually the result of acute or chronic direct trauma. Medial sesamoid fractures are more common than are lateral. Dislocations of the MP joint are secondary to compression with dorsiflexion of the proximal phalanx. This results in avulsion of the plantar capsule and a dorsal dislocation of the proximal phalanx on the metatarsal.[14] Medial or lateral MP dislocations are the result of injury forces splitting the gap between the toes forcing the MP joint to dislocate. With a complex dislocation, the volar plate of the great toe along with the sesamoid entrap the phalanx on the dorsal surface of the metatarsal (see Fig. 31–22).[14]

Examination

Phalangeal fractures present with pain, swelling, and ecchymosis within the first 2 to 3 hours. Subungual hematomas may develop within the first 12 hours. Dislocations of the MP joints present with pain, swelling, inability to walk, and visible deformity. Typically, the toe is hyperextended resting on the dorsum of the metatarsal. With complex dislocations, the sesamoids may be palpable dorsal to the metatarsal. Sesamoid fractures present with localized pain to palpation over the plantar aspect of the first metatarsal head. Extension of the first phalanx results in an exacerbation of pain referred to the plantar aspect of the MP joint.

X Ray

Phalangeal fractures are usually best seen on AP and oblique views. Sesamoid fractures require oblique tangential views for adequate visualization. Bipartite sesamoids are smooth rounded structures not frequently confused with acute fractures. MP dislocations may be diagnosed on the AP view as there is generally an overlap between the distal metatarsal and proximal phalanx. Interphalangeal dislocations are best seen on the AP and oblique views and are frequently associated with fractures.

Treatment

Nondisplaced phalangeal fractures involving the second through the fifth digits may be treated by dynamic splinting. Dynamic splinting involves the use of cotton padding and then securely taping the injured toe to its adjacent uninjured toe (Fig. 31–23). The splint should be changed every few days and used for a period of 2 to 3 weeks. An open shoe may be of benefit. Displaced phalangeal fractures require reduction as shown in

SESAMOID AND PHALANGEAL FRACTURES

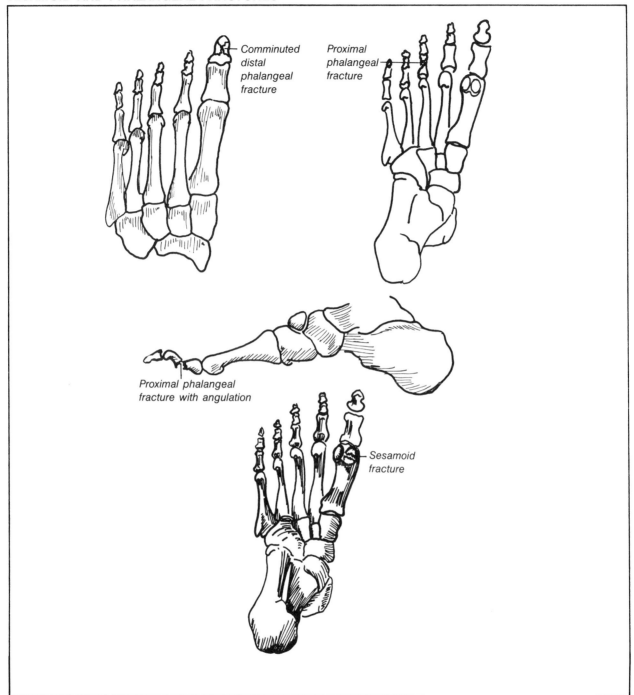

Comminuted distal phalangeal fracture

Proximal phalangeal fracture

Proximal phalangeal fracture with angulation

Sesamoid fracture

Figure 31–20.

Figure 31–24. Postreduction films are indicated, and, if unstable, early referral for internal fixation is strongly recommended. Distal phalangeal fractures with a subungual hematoma of greater than 50 percent of the nail bed will require nail plate avulsion and exploration of the nail bed.[29] Nail bed lacerations should be repaired using interrupted absorbable suture. All open phalangeal fractures require thorough irrigation, debridement, and appropriate suturing. A sterile dressing and antibiotics, typically a broad-spectrum cephalosporin, for 7 to 10 days along with early referral are recommended. Heavily contaminated fractures or those with extensive soft tissue injuries require emergent referral for repair. Comminuted fractures of the great toe require a walking cast

INTERPHALANGEAL DISLOCATIONS

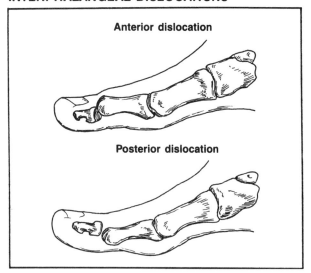

Figure 31–21.

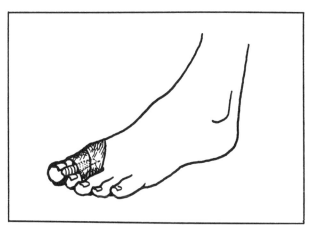

Figure 31–23. Treatment of fractures of the phalanges of the toes. A piece of Webril is placed between the toes and the fractured toe is taped to the adjacent toe. A hard soled shoe should be worn.

METATARSOPHALANGEAL DISLOCATIONS

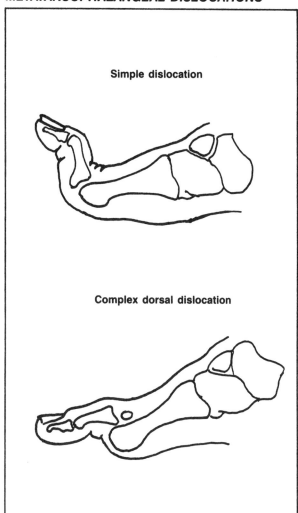

Figure 31–22.

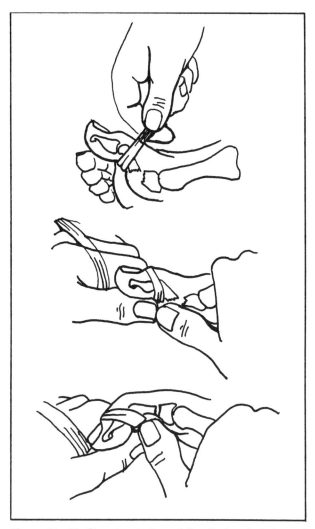

Figure 31–24. Closed reduction of the displaced phalangeal fracture.

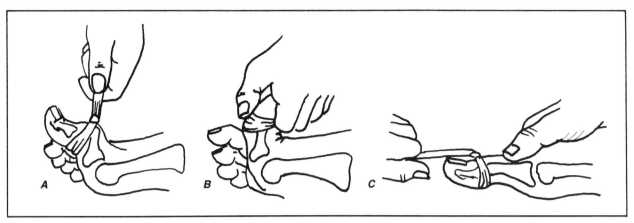

Figure 31–25. Reduction of dislocation of the metatarsophalangeal joint. **A.** Traction is applied in the line of deformity. **B.** Hyperextension is used to reproduce the injuring force. **C.** With traction maintained, reduction is accomplished.

as dynamic splinting offers insufficient immobilization. Sesamoid fractures may be treated with arch supports for 8 weeks; however, if the symptoms are severe, a short leg walking cast may be indicated.

PIP dislocations may be treated with a closed reduction followed by splinting to the adjacent toe. Unstable reductions require early referral for internal fixation. MP dislocations require parenteral analgesics as well as local anesthesia prior to the attempted reduction. As shown in Figure 31–25, hyperextension with distal traction is usually adequate in reducing these dorsal dislocations. Stable reductions require a metallic splint for 2 to 5 weeks whereas unstable reductions require early referral for casting or internal fixation. Those injuries resistant to a single attempt at closed reduction require early referral for open reduction.

REFERENCES

1. Adelaar R: The treatment of complex fractures of the talus. *Orthop Clin North Am* **20**(4):691, 1989.
2. Berndt A, Harty M: Transchondral fractures of the talus. *J Bone Joint Surg* **41**:988, 1959.
3. Cave EF: Fracture of the os calcis: The problem in general. *Clin Orthop* **30**:116, 1963.
4. Coltart WD: Aviators astragalus. *J Bone Joint Surg* [Br] **34**:545, 1952.
5. Crosby LA, Kamins P: The history of the calcaneal fractures. *Orthop Rev* **20**:(6), 1991.
6. Dameron TB: Fractures and anatomical variations of the proximal portion of the fifth metatarsal. *J Bone Joint Surg* **57**(6):788, 1975.
7. Davidson AM, et al: A review of twenty-one cases of transchondral fracture of the talus. *J Trauma* **7**:378, 1967.
8. Davis CA, Lubowitz J, Thordarson DB: Midtarsal fracture-sublaxation. *Clin Orthop Rel Res* **292**:265–268, 1993.
9. Day AJ: The treatment of injuries to the tarsal navicular. *J Bone Joint Surg* **29**:359, 1947.
10. Felder-Johnson KL, Murdoch DP, McGainty P: Lisfranc's fracture-dislocation. *Clin Podiatr Med Surg* **12**(4): 565–602, 1995.
11. Fox IM, Collier D: Imaging of injuries to the tarsometatarsal joint complex. *Clin Podiatr Med Surg* **14**(2): 357–368, 1997.
12. Garcia A, Parkes JC: Fractures of the foot. In Giannestras NJ (ed): *Foot Disorders, Medical and Surgical Management*. Philadelphia: Lea & Febiger 1973, pp. 522–563.
13. Giannestras NJ: *Foot Disorders, Medical and Surgical Management*, 2nd ed. Philadelphia: Lea & Febiger, 1973.
14. Giannikas AC, et al: Dorsal dislocation of the first metatarsophalangeal joint. *J Bone Joint Surg* [Br] **57**(3): 1975.
15. Hammesfahr R, Fleming LL: Calcaneal fractures: A good prognosis. *Foot Ankle* **2**:161, 1981.
16. Hanam SR, Dale SJ: Conservative treatment of calcaneal fractures: A preliminary report. *J Foot Surg* **24**:127, 1985.
17. Kenwright J, Taylor RG: Major injuries of the talus. *J Bone Joint Surg* [Br] **52**(1):36, 1970.
18. Lee WE: Fractures of the foot. *Surg Clin North Am* **20**:1815, 1940.
19. Main BJ, Lowett RL: Injuries of the midtarsal joint. *J Bone Joint Surg* [Br] **57**(1):89, 1975.
20. Myerson M, Manoli A: Compartment syndromes of the foot after calcaneal fractures. *Clin Orthop Rel Res* **20**:142–150, 1993.
21. Parker JC: Injuries of the hindfoot. *Clin Orthop* **132**:28, 1977.
22. Quill Jr, GE: Fractures of the proximal fifth metatarsal. *Orthop Clin North Am* **26**(2):353–361, 1995.
23. Rockwood CA, Green DA: *Fractures*. Philadelphia: Lippincott, 1975.
24. Rowe CR, et al: Fractures of the os calcis. *JAMA* **184**:98, 1963.
25. Rowe CR, et al: Fractures of the os calcis: A long-term follow-up study of 146 patients. *JAMA* **184**:920, 1963.
26. Sanders R: Intra-articular fractures of the calcaneus: Present state of the art. *J Orthop Trauma* **6**(2):252, 1992.
27. Sartoris DJ: Diagnosis of foot trauma: The essentials. *J Foot Ankle Surg* **32**(5):539–550, 1993.
28. Shepard E: Tarsal movements. *J Bone Joint Surg* [Br] **33**:258, 1951.

29. Tucker, Jules KT, Raymond F: Nailbed injuries with hallucal phalangeal fractures: Evaluation and treatment. *J Am Podiatr Med Assoc* **86**(4):170–173, 1996.

30. Valkosky GJ, Pachuda NM, Brown W: Midfoot fractures. *Clin Podiatr Med Surg* **12**(4):773–789, 1995.

31. Wilson DW: Injuries of the tarso-metatarsal joints. *J Bone Joint Surg* [Br] **54**(4):677, 1972.

32. Wilson NJ: *Watson-Jones Fracture and Joint Injuries*, 5th ed, vol 2. London: Churchill Livingston, 1976, pp. 1091–1211.

33. Wilson PD: Treatment of fractures of the os calcis by arthrodesis of the subastragalar joint. *JAMA* **89**:1676, 1927.

34. Zatzkin HR: Trauma to the foot. *Semin Roentgenol* **5**:419, 1970.

BIBLIOGRAPHY

Aitken AP, Poulson D: Dislocations of the tarsometatarsal joints. *J Bone Joint Surg* **45**:246, 1963.

Allan JH: The open reduction of fractures of the os calcis. *Ann Surg* **141**:890, 1955.

Anderson LD: Injuries of the forefoot. *Clin Orthop* **122**:18, 1977.

Barnard L, Odegard JK: Conservative approach in the treatment of fractures of the calcaneus. *J Bone Joint Surg* **52**:1689, 1970.

Böhler L: *Treatment of Fractures*, 5th ed. New York: Grune & Stratton, 1956.

Bonnin JG: *Injuries to the Ankle*. London: Heinemann, 1950.

Bremer AE, Warrick CK: Les fractures du calcaneum. *Acta Orthop Belg* **17**:217, 1951.

Buckingham WW, LeFlore I: Subtalar dislocation of the foot. *J Trauma* **13**:753, 1973.

Essex-Lopresti P: Results of reduction in fractures of the calcaneum. *J Bone Joint Surg* [Br] **33**:284, 1951.

Haliburton RA, et al: The extraosseous and intraosseous blood supply of the talus. *J Bone Joint Surg* **40**:1115, 1958.

Harris RI: Fractures of the os calcis: Their treatment by tri radiate traction and subastragalar fusion. *Ann Surg* **124**:1082, 1946.

Harty M: Anatomic considerations in injuries of the calcaneus. *Orthop Clin North Am* **4**:179, 1973.

Lance EM, et al: Fractures of the os calcis: Treatment by early mobilization. *Clin Orthop* **30**:79, 1963.

Larson RL, et al: Trauma, surgery, and circulation of the talus. What are the risks of vascular necrosis? *J Trauma* **1**:13, 1961.

Lenormant C, Wilmoth P: Les fractures sousthalamiques du calcaneum. *J Chir* **40**:1, 1932.

Lindsay WRN, Dewar FP: Fractures of the os calcis. *Am J Surg* **95**:555, 1958.

Maxfield JE: Treatment of calcaneal fractures by open reduction. *J Bone Joint Surg* **45**:868, 1963.

McLaughlin HL: *Trauma*. Philadelphia: Saunders, 1959.

Mindell ER, et al: Late results of injuries to the talus. *J Bone Joint Surg* **45**:221, 1963.

Nelson GE, et al: Blood supply of the human tibia. *J Bone Joint Surg* **42**:625, 1960.

O'Connell F, et al: Evaluation of modern management of fractures of the os calcis. *Clin Orthop* **83**:214, 1972.

Palmer I: The mechanism and treatment of fractures of the calcaneus. Open reduction with the use of cancellous grafts. *J Bone Joint Surg* **30**:12, 1948.

Pennal GF: Fractures of the talus. *Clin Orthop* **30**:53, 1963.

Pennal GF, Yadav MP: Operations treatment of comminuted fractures of the os calcis. *Orthop Clin North Am* **4**:197, 1971.

Schottstaedt ER: Symposium: Treatment of fractures of the calcaneus introduction. *J Bone Joint Surg* **45**:863, 1963.

Sneed WL: The astragalus: A case of dislocation, excision and replacement. *J Bone Joint Surg* [Br] **7**:384, 1925.

Thompson KR: Treatment of comminuted fractures of the calcaneus by triple arthrodesis. *Orthop Clin North Am* **4**:189, 1973.

Watson-Jones R: *Fractures and Joint Injuries*, 4th ed, vol II. Edinburgh, London: E & S. Livingstone, Ltd, 1962, p. 878.

Wiley JJ: The mechanism of tarsometatarsal joint injuries. *J Bone Joint Surg* [Br] **53**:475, 1971.

32
CHAPTER

SOFT TISSUE INJURIES AND DISORDERS OF THE FOOT

GENERAL DISORDERS OF THE FOOT

Foot disorders usually present to the emergency department with the patient complaining of pain. The disorders of the foot will be considered in four groups: painful conditions about the heel, pain about the midpart and forepart of the foot, pain about the dorsum of the foot, and disorders of the toes. In this first section the authors will consider those disorders that are not easily classified under the other headings, both traumatic and nontraumatic.

☐ CONTUSIONS

Contusions of the foot are common and usually caused by direct trauma such as dropping an object on the foot. Many tendons, nerves, and vessels course subcutaneously on the dorsum of the foot, the region most commonly involved by contusive injuries. The physician must be aware of possible nerve damage leading to intractable pain, vessel injury with phlebitis or hemorrhage, and damage to tendons with resulting tenosynovitis or traumatic periostitis of the bones or joints. The

treatment is directed at alleviating swelling with ice packs, elevation, and analgesics for pain. A tenosynovitis diagnosed when patients present several days after a contusion can be treated with local injection of long-acting anesthetics and steroid preparations.

☐ STRAINS

Strains of various tendons occur commonly at several sites in the foot, the most common being at the insertion of the Achilles tendon to the calcaneus. The patient will have pain on walking and tenderness over the Achilles accentuated by stress. The attachment of the anterior tibial tendon on the medial side of the foot is posterior to the lateral malleolus and extending proximally over the peroneal tendons. Within a few hours the entire lateral surface of the ankle is swollen and palpation reveals tenderness at the posterior lip of the lateral malleolus. This is often misdiagnosed as a sprain of the lateral ligament unless two important clues are recognized: the history of a *click* or *snap* over the lateral malleolus on walking, and local tenderness along the *posterior lip* of the lateral malleolus.[21] Radiographs may show a fragment of bone avulsed from the lateral or distal end of the lateral malleolus. The treatment is surgical repair.[21]

☐ ENTRAPMENT NEUROPATHIES

Of the entrapment neuropathies, tarsal tunnel syndrome is, perhaps, the best known. Other entrapment syndromes are also be discussed.

☐ Tarsal Tunnel Syndrome

The tarsal tunnel syndrome is a syndrome that results from compression of the posterior tibial nerve within the fibroosseous tunnel formed by the flexor retinaculum behind and below the medial malleolus of the ankle.[65] Patients complain of an insidious onset of pain described as burning in nature that is well localized to the plantar aspect of the foot. The pain, which is increased activity and decreased with rest, originates at the medial malleolus and radiates to the sole and heel. Also, paresthesia, dysaesthesia, and hypesthesia could be noticed in the distribution of the posterior tibial nerve.[65] However, the presentation varies, with some patients complaining of pain only in the metatarsal area whereas others note pain along the lateral aspect of the foot, and about one half of the patients state that the pain radiates superiorly along the medial side of the calf.[48] Rubbing of the foot seems to offer temporary relief. The one feature that clinches the diagnosis is a *positive Tinel sign*, which was present in all patients studied,[3,48] with pain radiating down the medial or lateral plantar nerve distribution on percussion of the nerve within the canal. This can be confirmed by nerve conduction times. Surgical release of the flexor retinaculum is the treatment of choice for this condition, and patients should be appropriately referred when the diagnosis is suspected. Also, during surgery, one can notice that ganglia development within the tarsal tunnel is relatively common.[65]

☐ Lateral Plantar (Calcaneal) Nerve Entrapment

Approximately 10 to 15 percent of athletes with chronic unresolved heel pain have entrapment of the lateralplantar nerve between the deep fascia of the abductor hallucis muscle and the medial caudal margin of the quadratus plantar muscle.[72] Running and jogging are major causes as well as soccer, tennis, and track. The patient presents with chronic heel pain of 1 to 2 years' duration that is a dull, aching, and sharp in character. The pain may radiate into the ankle and is intensified by walking or running. There is point tenderness over the first branch of the lateral plantar

nerve deep to the abductor hallucis muscle. The Tinel sign is infrequently positive and a hypermobile foot may be noted. Orthotics should be tried with the patient referred for fitting, although these devices have variable success. Often, these patients require surgical neurolysis.

☐ Peroneal Nerve Entrapment

The deep peroneal nerve can be entrapped most commonly under the inferior extensor retinaculum. The superficial peroneal nerve can be entrapped at its exit from the deep fascia. Both of these neuropathies can be caused by recurrent ankle sprains or repetitive trauma from running. Clinically, the patient with deep peroneal involvement presents with dorsal medial foot pain that is dull, aching, sharp, or spasmodic in nature and may radiate to the first toe web. There is reduced sensation in the first toe web and reproduction of the pain with either dorsiflexion or plantar flexion. Superficial neuropathy is suggested by pain, parethesis, or numbness over the outer border of the distal cath, dorsum of the foot, and ankle, but sparing the first web space. There may be point tenderness and a fascial defect where the nerve emerges from the deep fascia. There is usually a history of recurrent sprains in this problem. Treatment includes conservative modalities such as nonsteroidal anti-inflammatory drugs (NSAIDs), orthotics, or injection therapy. In this situation, neurolysis is reserved for cases of intractable pain or atrophy.

☐ Sural Nerve Entrapment

The leading cause of this is running. Another cause is recurrent ankle sprains. The patient presents with a shooting pain and parathesis, typically extending to the lateral foot border, which is confirmed by local tenderness, a positive Tinel sign, and occasionally an area of hyperesthesis. A trial of NSAIDs is useful; however, injection therapy should be tried and orthotics may be necessary. If all of this fails, surgical release usually is definitive.

☐ Medial Calcaneal Nerve Entrapment

This condition is most commonly known as jogger or runner's foot. Entrapment of the medial calcaneal branch of the posterior tibial nerve causes acute irritation and inflammation and chronic fibrosis and neuroma formation. The patient usually is a runner. The patient complains of aching pain along the medial border of the heel that is more severe on weight bearing but does not radiate further into the foot. If the foot is in hyperpronation, this tends to aggravate the condition further. Anti-inflammatory agents and a custom molded orthotic are good, conservative therapies. If the patient does not respond after several months, then he or she should be referred for operative neuralysis.

☐ PUNCTURE WOUNDS

Puncture wounds of the foot are a difficult problem. They are usually treated superficially and must be managed more aggressively. If the wound is *tender*, generally there is a greater likelihood of a retained foreign body. Remember that lacerations are generally not tender to palpation or only minimally so. Thus, a tender wound in our judgment indicates a greater likelihood of a retained foreign body. The most common bacterial pathogens are staphylococci and streptococci. Staphylococcal infections usually form an abscess with a characteristic creamy or yellow discharge, while streptococcal infections usually are painful, tender, and erythematous. Epidermal inclusion cysts have occurred after a foreign body retention in a puncture wound.[45]

Classification

Puncture wounds of the foot can be separated into five types depending on the degree of penetration, infection, and the presence of the foreign body. *Type I*, which is named *superficial cutaneous penetration*, involves the epidermis and/or the dermis with no signs or symptoms of infection.[7] *Type II* wounds are the most common of all puncture wounds and have subcutaneous or articular joint involvement without signs or symptoms of infection. *Type IIIA* is characterized by established soft tissue infection including pyarthrosis and a retained foreign body. Wounds classified as *type IIIB* involve penetration of the foreign body into the bone. Finally, *type IV* puncture wounds are characterized by osteomyelitis secondary to a puncture wound injury. This type will be discussed later in this section.[60]

X Ray

The authors advocate the probing of all wound sites.[59] Wooden particles can be seen as filling defects in patients with puncture wounds.[55] Paint or increased water content in the wood produces a negative shadow of the wood and results in less visibility.[55] Glass, foreign bodies, and metal are usually easily seen on radiographs. To localize a metal foreign body, use multiview radiographs, radiopaque grid system, surgical magnets, computed tomography sonography, and fluoroscopy.[60] Thus, the authors believe that x rays should be taken whenever a patient presents with a puncture wound, and in whenever the examiner is uncertain a retained foreign body is present.

Treatment

For the proper management of all puncture wounds of the foot, particularly those in which a nail punctures the sole of a sneaker or other similar such material, one must irrigate the puncture wound under pressure and cleanse it with iodine daily. *Pseudomonas* and *Staphylo-*

coccus aureus are common offending organisms that may lead to infection or osteomyelitis.[53] The patient should be encouraged to cleanse the wound twice daily with idophor. Unfortunately, prophylactic antibiotics have not been shown to be useful in these wounds.[53]

The treatment of type I puncture wounds includes cleaning of the area of the injury twice daily and wearing a protective covering. If there is discomfort when walking, non–weight-bearing activities are recommended.

Type II wounds require a local anesthetic so that the physician can explore the wound with a blunt probe and splinter forceps. However, one must avoid anesthetizing through the wound or close to it in order to prevent the inoculation of healthy tissues with possible pathogens. After the removal of the foreign body, the patient should avoid bathing or showering the affected area until the wound has healed.

Puncture wounds in the type IIIA category require aggressive treatment and surgical intervention. It must be noted, however, that it is not necessary to remove a foreign body if the body is inert, asymptomatic, not a threat to function, and not within a joint.

Type IIIB injuries are very serious and the treatment must be very aggressive. The foreign body must be surgically removed with curettage of the osseous defect, debridement of soft tissue, copious lavage, and open packing. Intravenous antimicrobial prophylaxis is also implemented, pending intraoperative cultures and sensitivities.

It is necessary that type IV wounds receive prompt, aggressive treatment. This will be discussed later in this section.[60]

☐ VENOUS STASUS ULCERS

These ulcers commonly occur around the medial malleolus and are due to chronic venous pulling secondary to venous insufficiency. The skin is usually darkened because of hemosiderin deposits and there is skin atrophy that ultimately leads to ulceration in the elderly. The optimal treatment here is a Una boot, and debridement only if necessary.

☐ DIABETIC ULCERATION OF THE FOOT

Diabetic foot ulcers are common conditions seen in the emergency department. They are usually a result of small vessel disease associated with diabetes.[56] One of the most important aspects in treating patients is to make certain that they are referred to an appropriate clinic where preventive care at 2- to 3-month intervals can be done.[6] This preventive care includes nail care and removal of any calluses as well as fitting the patient with appropriate shoes.

Diet regulating the patients' blood sugar, bed rest, antibiotics when appropriate, debridement, and local antisepsis are critical measures.[32,58] The pain associated with polyneuropathy can be managed initially with simple analgesics. Ischemic ulcers and diabetes should be recognized by clinical examination and evaluated for the possible need of revascularization. Neuropathic ulcers can be subdivided into mild, moderate, or severe, depending on the depth of the ulcer and the presence or absence of bone involvement. Essential guidelines that should be adhered to in the treatment of neuropathic ulcers are as follows: non–weight bearing; soaking of the wound macerates the tissue but does not debride the necrotic tissue and should be avoided. Enzymatic chemical debridement and whirlpool soaks are not useful. Although dextran may help in cleansing the wound, a wet or moist dressing of dilute iodine, changed twice daily, combined with a thorough wound debridement, is the safest and most effective method of wound care.[26,27] A fine, mesh, dry, sterile nonadherent gauze dressing is preferred to either plain gauze or occlusive or semiocclusive dressing. Topical antibiotic solutions or ointments are effective against methicillin-resistant strains of staphylococci species. Surgical treatment is indicated for severe claudication, intractable rest pain, necrosis, or nonresponding ulcers.[29]

□ OSTEOMYELITIS AFTER PUNCTURE WOUNDS

Puncture wounds of the foot resulting in osteomyelitis or even clinically significant infection are unusual. The condition does occur, however, and wider recognition of the entity will help in prevention and early diagnosis.[52,61] Puncture wounds of the foot may have serious sequelae. Johaanson described 11 patients with osteomyelitis after puncture wounds from various causes,[37] and Houston and co-workers,[33] investigating 2583 patients who presented to the emergency department with puncture wounds of the body, found that 10 percent experienced late infection. In a study by Fitzgerald and co-workers[25] 132 of 774 children examined with puncture wounds experienced cellulitis and 16 had osteomyelitis.

The penetrating agents include needles, nails, wood splinters, thorns, and toothpicks (often with pieces of clothing) that have been broken off below the skin level before the patients present to the emergency department.[61] The infections seen have been caused by *Pseudomonas* species in most cases or a mixed flora.[52,61] Other organisms that could cause osteomyelitis include *Escherichia coli* and *S aureus*.[60]

The clinical presentation is that of a patient who has stepped on a nail 2 to 3 weeks before admission and was treated well, showing initial improvement, to be followed later by worsening of pain at the puncture site with no systemic manifestations. Local swelling, erythema, and pain over the puncture site are noted. The patient usually has either no fever or a low-grade temperature and the sedimentation rate is slightly elevated with a white blood count within normal limits. Radiographs are consistent with an osteomyelitis.

The treatment of these patients includes the injection of saline into the site and aspiration to retrieve the organism. Gentamicin is the drug of choice in most cases because it is effective against *Pseudomonas* species. Once infection develops in a puncture wound one must be aggressive, including surgical exploration of the wound, debridement, irrigation, and removal of all foreign material as well as the use of antibiotics.[67] Table 32–1 suggests key points that should be followed in dealing with puncture wounds of the foot.

□ TINEA PEDIS

This is one of the most common conditions affecting the foot. The condition may be a quite disabling form of dermatitis with blisters, fissures, thickening of the sole, and infections secondarily. The most common causes are *Trichophyton rubrum* and *Trichophyton mentagrophytes*.[20,50]

Patients may present with a *wet type* affecting either the sole of the foot or the web spaces. The *dry type* usually affects the web spaces or the sole and heel of the foot. This is associated with scaling, pruritus, erythemia, and fissuring. This condition can be confusing in that a contact dermatitis of the dry form or a dyshidrosis in the wet form can be mistaken for tinea pedis. A microscopic examination of the material

---

TABLE 32–1. KEY FACTORS IN THE APPROACH TO PUNCTURE WOUNDS OF THE FOOT

1. All puncture wounds where a foreign body is suspected require an x ray.
2. Iodophor should be used in cleaning puncture wounds as opposed to hexachlorophene, which is bacteriostatic.[61]
3. Tetanus prophylaxis when indicated should be done.
4. If the wound is deep and the examiner suspects bone or joint contact or possible retained foreign body, exploration of the wound is indicated or excision of the puncture tract.
5. A grossly contaminated wound should not be closed.
6. Cultures should be taken from deep wounds and broad-spectrum antibiotics begun when indicated.
7. Non–weight bearing should be recommended in deep puncture wounds; elevation and close observation for infection.

scraped from the margin of a diseased area or a vesicle wall with a number 11 or 15 scalpel blade will clinch the diagnosis. The material is heated with a few drops of 10 percent potassium hydroxide solution and a cover slip. Hyphae and myceliae, which are branching, are diagnostic of a superficial fungal infection. If one sees budding cells along with pseudohyphae this suggests a monilia.

In the dry form the infection responds usually quite well to antifungal solutions and creams applied at bedtime and also in the morning. A mild keratolytic agent such as Whitefield Ointment (salicylic acid) or a cold tar preparation is a good supplement for the dry defuse planter type which is often associated with keratosis.

Griseofulvin in a dosage of 500 to 1000 mg per day is useful in patients who are refractory to topical treatment. There are few side effects with the ultramicrosize form of griseofulvin. If one has an infection which does not respond to this agent, oral ketoconazole in a dosage of 200 mg per day can be used. When using this agent, however, liver function must be monitored because of hepatotoxicity. The present research points toward oral terbinafine (Lamisil) as the drug of choice in the future. There seem to be limited side effects and sustained clearing for months after completion of the treatment.[8]

In the wet form, wet soaks such as Burow's solution 1:20 can be applied until the skin returns to normal. Systemic antibiotics including erythromycin or tetracycline may be necessary if secondary bacterial infection appears. Oral griseofulvin in combination with a steroid cream can be used as effective therapy. One must encourage good aeration of the feet. Recurrences are common and the patient should be referred for follow-up therapy. Patients who have this problem should be encouraged to wear socks and shoe gear with natural fibers, such as wool, cotton, and so on.[9]

□ WARTS

Verruca vulgaris are common and occur on the plantar surface of the feet. These lesions present as a firm white growth which can appear as a flat lesion on the sole or be raised. Spontaneous regression is quite common in that the clone of virus usually survives for 4 to 6 months. Mosaic warts can occur when small warts coalesce.[22,42]

Large plantar warts are treated conservatively with weekly paring and the application of a keratolytic agent such as 40 percent salicylic acid plaster. Painful lesions are treated with more invasive techniques including cryotherapy and electrosurgery after a local lidocaine anesthetic block with 1 to 10,000 epinephrine. These patients should be referred for therapy.

□ SESAMOIDITIS

The first metatarsal sesamoids can become inflamed following trauma or spontaneously. Examination demonstrates a trigger point beneath the metatarsal head that increases with dorsiflexion of the metatarsophalangeal joint. On x ray a fractured sesamoid may be demonstrated. However, one must not confuse this with bipartite sesamoids. Low-heeled shoes and a metatarsal bar proximal to the metatarsal heads are usually satisfactory to alleviate the symptoms. Taping of the great toe, slight plantar flexion, and anti-inflammatory drugs are also useful.

□ SUBTALAR DISLOCATIONS

Subtalar dislocation is a rare condition accounting for only 1 to 2 percent of all dislocations.[18] This is most often caused by falls from heights but can be a result of sports accidents. There are two types of dislocations of the subtalar joint: *medial dislocation* and *lateral dislocation*. In medial dislocation there is a severe inversion of the foot causing the talus to use the sustenaculum as a fulcrum to dislocate out of the joint. First, the talonavicular joint dislocates which is then followed by a subtalar dislocation. In lateral dislocations there is a forcible eversion of the foot. The talar head is forced through the capsule of the talonavicular joint and the calcaneus. The remainder of the forefoot displaces laterally from the talus.

To reduce a medial dislocation, traction is applied to the foot and heel in line with the deformity. Countertraction is then applied to the leg that is held with the knee in flexion in order to relax the gastrocnemius, and the reduction is achieved by pressing down at the end of the talus while the foot is plantar flexed. In lateral dislocation reduction is achieved with the foot in adduction and dorsiflexion of the ankle. This often has a poor result due to the frequency of both open injuries and associated fractures.

□ REFLEX SYMPATHETIC DYSTROPHY

This condition is characterized by disproportionate pain with unusual intensity and duration from what would appear to be a minor trauma to an extremity. The critical feature in treating these patients is early detection. Mild local edema is seen in virtually all cases.[69] Dyshydrosis is a relatively common sign and temperature changes to the skin are also common. Use of a sympathetic and sensory epidural nerve block can also help in the differential diagnosis. Frequent sympathetic blocks over a 4-month period have been used in treating these patients. Physical therapy is recommended when pain is not present. Clonazepam is continued throughout the treatment, primarily as an anxiolytic and not as an analgesic.

Heel Pain

☐ PLANTAR FASCIITIS AND PLANTAR CALCANEAL SPURS

Plantar fasciitis and heel spurs are thought of as separate entities but some authors believe heel spurs are a further evolution of plantar fasciitis.[11] This condition occurs in occupations that involve excessive walking or standing. Heel spurs occur on the plantar aspect of the calcaneus at the attachment of the plantar aponeurosis where a bony prominence develops and extends across the plantar surface of the bone.[12] It is more common in patients with flattened arches and occurs most often in men. If the condition is bilateral one must think of rheumatoid arthritis, systemic lupus erythematosus, and gout.[43]

The mechanism by which these conditions develop is thought to be from friction on the periosteum with subperiosteal ossification secondarily. Strain of the fascial fibers occurs and a periostitis may develop.

The patient presents with pain on the undersurface of the heel on standing or walking and relief with rest. Frequently patients note pain after a period of bedrest. *Local tenderness* is noted to palpation at the attachment of the plantar fascia to the calcaneus. *Passive dorsiflexion* of the toes accentuates the pain.[15] The pain and tenderness are always anterior to the heel with radiation to the sole being a frequent accompaniment. Radiographs may or may not demonstrate a spur (Fig. 32–1). Indeed many patients with a calcaneal spur are asymptomatic.

The treatment is to relax the plantar fascia[11,68] which is done by raising the heel with a $^1/_2$-inch heel support that relieves the tension of the fascia. If there is one painful spot a sponge rubber heel pad with the center cut out affords relief of the discomfort. Phenylbutazone should be given; the dosage regimen recommended is four times per day for 7 days followed by a three times per day regimen for 7 days.[43] Ibuprofen (Motrin) is currently being used for this condition with good results. In resistant cases injection with hydrocortisone or needling with a local anesthetic often gives relief. Adjuncts to treatment include bed rest and hot soaks. Plantar fascial release, including the first layer of intrinsic muscles, has been shown to be effective in recalcitrant cases.[70]

☐ PAINFUL HEEL PAD

Elastic adipose tissue covers the heel of the calcaneus and similar tissue exists in other areas subject to pressure such as over the ischial tuberosity, fingertips, and infrapatellar region. The calcaneal fat pad is composed of fibroelastic tissue with fat cells impacted between septa that take on the shape of small sacs with the open end to the bone and the closed end in the plantar heel. This condition is common especially in the elderly. It is due to atrophy of the subcalcaneal fat pad and repetitive heel loading during walking. Obesity and prolonged ambulatory activity particularly on hard floors, aggravates the condition.[38] Furthermore, acute stress on the pad may rupture or strain the compartments, causing temporary loss of compressibility.

On examination, pain is generalized over the whole heel that is especially prominent on standing and less so on walking. Relief is gained by rest, which is in contrast to calcaneal spurs where the pain is more localized. Most of these patients are obese. Radiographs may demonstrate a smooth undersurface of the calcaneus in some patients; otherwise they are normal. Conservative treatment includes rest, NSAIDs, and a dispersion padding (U pad). A flexible heel protector, or MF heel protector, is a tight-fitting plastic that cups the heel and squeezes all of the fat under the calcaneous providing more cushioning. Over-the-counter silicone-based heel cushions are also available. If this treatment is ineffective after 5 days, the calcaneal bursa should be injected with triamcinalone and bupivicane. Up to four injections may be necessary to relieve the symptoms. They should

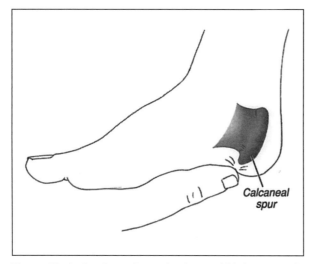

Figure 32–1. A calcaneal spur is shown which is commonly associated with plantar fasciitis.

be given weekly until the symptoms subside; thus, the patient should be referred. To prevent recurrence, shoe modification with heel dispersion padding or a foot orthotic should be used and the patient should be referred to an appropriate clinician.

☐ CALCANEAL EPIPHYSITIS (SEVER'S DISEASE)

This is an uncommon condition occurring in children, usually boys, between the ages of 9 and 14 years.[39] The condition is a low-grade inflammatory reaction in the posterior calcaneal epiphysis that has a separate center of ossification from the remainder of the calcaneus. This center appears at the age of 10 years and fuses to the calcaneus proper at the age of 15 years. Sever's disease becomes present at a time of rapid growth when muscles and tendons become tighter as bones become longer.[18] Thus, the epiphysis is subject to traction by pull of the calf muscles and the disorder can be classified as the second most common osteochondrosis seen in the younger athlete after Osgood-Schlatter disease.[18]

The patient presents with complaints of pain and tenderness in the back of the heel below the Achilles insertion, which is aggravated by standing on the tip toes or running. The onset is gradual, and the patient notes relief when the calf muscles are relaxed with the knee in flexion and the foot in equinus. The tenderness is most pronounced over the medial and lateral sides where the epiphyseal plate is more subcutaneous.

Early radiographs are usually of no help. Later fragmentation of the epiphysis, however, may be noted when compared with the normal side.

The condition is self-limited and treatment is symptomatic with recurrence until the epiphysis closes. Relieve tension from the epiphysis by building up the heel with a $1/4$-inch heel paid to place the foot in equinus, and rest as well as analgesics are advocated. Also, the child's activity should be modified, the calf muscles should be stretched, any biomechanical abnormalities should be corrected, and orthotics may be required.[18] In severe cases casting the foot in equinus may be necessary.

☐ RETROCALCANEAL AND POSTERIOR CALCANEAL BURSITIS

Two bursae are involved in inflammatory processes around the heel, one being between the calcaneus and the Achilles tendon called the *retrocalcaneal bursa* and the other located between the Achilles tendon and the skin called the *posterior calcaneal bursa* (Fig. 32–2).[10] In the latter form of bursitis, the inflamed bursa is usually secondary to friction from ill-fitting shoes and is especially common in women with high heels. The bursa is usually distended with fluid and visibly inflamed. In chronic cases, the bursa is thickened as well as the overlying skin with tenderness noted and swelling in the back of the heel where the shoes rub. In retrocalcaneal bursitis the patient complains of pain on motion and localized tenderness is noted to palpation just anterior to the Achilles tendon.

The treatment of retrocalcaneal bursitis is rest, heat, and elevation. In patients with posterior calcaneal bursitis proper-fitting shoes with low heels are essential. The back of the shoe may have to be cut out in acute cases. Puncture of the bursa and injection of hydrocortisone provide prompt relief of symptoms.

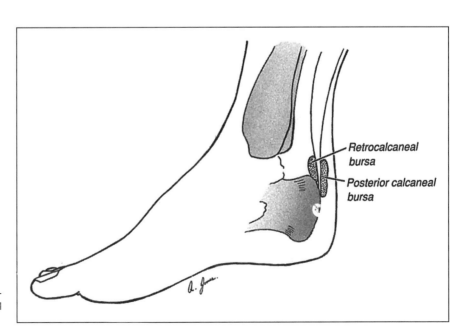

Retrocalcaneal bursa

Posterior calcaneal bursa

Figure 32–2. The posterior calcaneal bursa and the retrocalcaneal bursa are shown.

☐ TENOSYNOVITIS OF THE ACHILLES TENDON

This condition is secondary to excessive use of the calf muscles.[63] Improper muscle flexibility and improper exercise routines are other predisposing factors for this condition. Tensile load contraction plus the gravitational elongation produces microtears of tendon fascicles and a secondary inflammation reaction.[24] Patients present with swelling around the Achilles; tenderness and fine crepitus is perceived on motion of the foot.[41] The tender region is well localized, and the patient holds the foot in equinus to relieve the discomfort. Passive dorsiflexion will aggravate the pain. Also, morning stiffness is a typical symptom of tenosynovitis of the Achilles tendon.[4]

Achilles tendonitis is the third most common problem in distance runners and is the most frequent lesion in ballet dancers.[24] Heel pain can be caused by inflammation of the Achilles tendon itself, the tendon sheath, or the mesotendon. One must be certain to differentiate this condition from retrocalcaneal or posterior calcaneal bursitis. The pain is increased by running and is decreased by rest. There often is a palpable thickening over the tendon or periotendinous tissues as previously described. Conservative management includes decreasing the amount of running and elevating the heel inside the shoe with a small felt pad.[13] This often provides symptomatic relief.[64] The runner should be encouraged to perform sustained stretching exercises of the Achilles complex. Oral anti-inflammatory agents may be used, while intratendon injections of steroids should be avoided as they may lead to rupture.[4] Ice should be used for 10 to 12 minutes after running.[2] If the pain is acute and other measures have not helped, then a short leg walking cast can be used for 10 days.[2] In some patients, surgical intervention to release the thickened tenosynovium has been helpful.[9]

☐ RUPTURE OF THE ACHILLES TENDON

Rupture of the Achilles tendon occurs most commonly at the narrowest portion of the tendon, approximately 2 inches above its point of attachment to the calcaneus. This is more common in men between the ages of 40 and 50 years old who lead a sedentary life, but it also occurs in athletes.[14]

The mechanism of injury varies but basically three have been described: an extra stretch applied to a taut tendon, forceful dorsiflexion with the ankle in a relaxed state, and direct trauma to a taut tendon.

On examination the patient complains of acute agonizing pain in the lower calf that makes walking almost impossible. A partial tear may be difficult to diagnose and is often misdiagnosed as a strained muscle. The *Simmonds test* is performed by squeezing the calves of both

sides and noting that in the patient with a complete tear, plantar flexion of the injured side will not occur as it does on the normal side (Fig. 32–3). This condition is misdiagnosed in 20 to 30 percent of cases[35] because of insignificant pain occurring in some patients. Examination may show that the patient can plantar flex because of the action of the posterior tibial muscle, and a poor history of injury is presented. Mammography has been done to detect partial ruptures or complete ruptures of the Achilles tendon. It is also useful to differentiate this from a tendonitis. Its accuracy is approximately 75 percent in one study. Therefore, in the emergency department when one cannot distinguish between these injuries, consider mammography to help make the diagnosis.

The treatment until recently was operative repair and this is still the most commonly recommended.[28,51] Nonsurgical treatment has been advocated by some who report excellent results with cast immobilization.[28,44,51] These authors state that the Achilles tendon is able to regenerate when sectioned, and they recommend treatment with an equinus walking boot cast for 8 weeks followed by a 2.5-cm heel for an additional 4 weeks. A recent study dealing with younger athletes shows that surgical treatment is

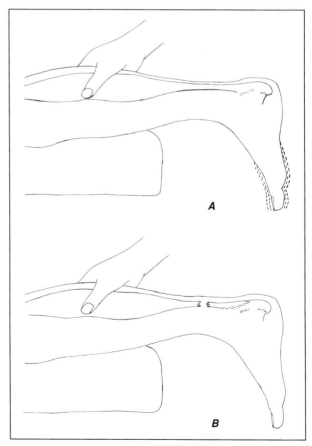

Figure 32–3. The Simmonds test is performed by squeezing the calf. In patients with a ruptured Achilles tendon there is no plantar flexion which normally occurs.

better when objectively compared with nonsurgical treatment.[35] The emergency physician should in this case consult with the orthopedist who will be caring for the patient.

□ SIMPLE BONE CYST OF THE CALCANEOUS

A simple bone cyst is a relatively common bone tumor and accounts for about 3 percent of all bone tumors.[62]

Males are more commonly affected in their first and second decades of life. A simple bone cyst can be asymptomatic or it may produce localized pain and swelling with tenderness and stiffness to adjacent joints. The findings may be similar to those seen in heel spur syndrome. The x ray shows a bone cyst. Steroid injection therapy has been shown to be successful and is preferable to surgical curettage.[62]

MIDPART AND FOREPART FOOT PAIN

□ FOOT STRAIN

The normal static foot has no muscle action that stabilizes it in the position it assumes. This position is maintained by the bones and the ligaments of the foot and the muscles act to protect it from excessive stresses applied to the bones and the ligaments. Foot pain on standing, therefore, is not muscular in etiology but mechanical, osseous, or ligamentous; whereas pain on walking may be muscular or from other soft tissues. The foot has two arches, a *longitudinal arch*, which extends from the calcaneus to the metatarsal heads with its apex medially being the navicular, and the *transverse arch*, which runs across the metatarsals. The arches are maintained by skeletal components held in place by ligaments. The longitudinal arch is maintained by the relationship of the talus and the calcaneus and the ligamentous support of the interosseous, the long and short plantars, and the spring ligament. The function of this arch is to provide a springboard for weight bearing and forward motion. The ligaments are stretched by excessive weight, pressure, or poor muscle tone leading to the condition of foot strain that can be acute, subacute, or chronic. Acute foot strain subsides with simple rest and gradual return to activity and is seen most often in patients who have just taken on a new job such as a teacher. Chronic foot strain is secondary to excessive stresses on normal structures or normal stresses on abnormal structures. All these patients should be referred for podiatric consultation as they may undergo a process of ligamentous elongation with strain followed by joint inflammation, degeneration, and arthrosis.

Clinical Presentation

As mentioned, most of these patients have recently changed life-styles to a more ambulatory role that they may not be used to. In other cases, excessive weight and exercise or incorrectly fitting shoes may be the causative factors. The patient complains of pain over the inner border of the foot with standing or walking and relief with rest. The patient has tenderness over the strained ligament that is often well *localized* under the *navicular* and anterior and posterior arches. Passive dorsiflexion of the foot intensifies the pain and plantar flexion is usually painless. The patient may have such significant strain that he or she may be unable to bear weight and complains of pain radiating to the calf. The feet feel tight and swollen and often a history of change in occupation or weight gain is elicited.

Treatment

The treatment of the acute form seen in the emergency department is rest and hot soaks to the foot. Support for the longitudinal arch can be provided with a sponge rubber pad fitted into the shoe. These patients should be referred if pain continues.

□ SINUS TARSI SYNDROME

Sinus tarsi syndrome is due to inflammation in the sinus tarsi which occurs after trauma or due to overuse. The chronic inversion ankle sprains are also a common etiology. Diffuse pain on the lateral side of the foot associated with a feeling of hindfoot instability, and a history of supination trauma are common complaints. One can elicit pain directly by palpating the sinus tarsi on the lateral aspect of the hindfoot. Pain will also occur upon inversion and eversion of the joint. Patients with sinus tarsi syndrome have regularly shown weakness of the peroneal muscles. One may have difficulty differentiating this condition from a sprain of the anterior tibiofibular ligament.[40] Routine radiographic examination of the ankle and subtalar joint, even with stress radiographs, usually does not show any pathology.

The treatment of this condition includes NSAIDs, and the patient is fitted with an orthotic. Conservative treatment is the treatment of choice and usually includes one to three injections of a local anesthetic and steroids into the sinus tarsi. The surgical treatment of sinus tarsi syndrome, when conservative treatment is unable to relieve the pain, can be done and the patient referred. Subtalar arthrodesis is used if conservative and surgical treatments are not successful.

☐ METATARSALGIA

Metatarsalgia is seen in the equinus foot with cavus deformity and in patients who wear high-heeled shoes. Most of the patients are middle-aged females.

This condition is characterized by pain and tenderness of the plantar heads of the metatarsals that occur when the transverse arch becomes depressed and the middle metatarsal heads bear a disproportionate amount of the weight. In normal weight bearing, the first meta-tarsal head and the two sesamoids bear one third of the body's weight. In the flattened or splayed foot, the second, third, and fourth metatarsal heads bear greater weight. This condition is most common after excessive weight gain and is seen most often in middle-aged women. There are many common factors that cause the syndrome of metatarsalgia, which should be considered in the follow-up clinical visit by the podiatrist. These include ligamentous stretching that permits the transverse arch to become more relaxed and subject to strain, muscle weakness of the intrinsics, and traumatic factors. Metatarsalgia in the adolescent may be due to osteochondrosis of the metatarsal head in which case the patient presents with painful swelling of the foot around the metatarsophalangeal joint that is aggravated by motion and weight bearing. One must remember that metatarsalgia is a symptom, not a disease, and refers only to pain around the metatarsal heads.[54]

Clinical Presentation

The patient presents with pain in the forefoot and decreased weight bearing on the forefoot. He or she, therefore, walks more on the heels.[54] The dorsum of the foot may be edematous and tenderness is noted at the middle of the shafts with flexion or extension of the toes, subsiding with rest and non–weight bearing but recurring with any exertion. The site of initial tenderness is over the metatarsal heads where later a callous may form to "protect." This callous actually aggravates the condition by increasing the pain.

Treatment

The treatment must be directed at the causative factor and is symptomatic initially, which may include anti-inflammatory agents. In order to have successful therapy, one must use a low-heeled shoe. These patients should be referred for work-up.

☐ MORTON'S NEUROMA

This is entrapment neuropathy of the interdigital nerve usually occurring proximal to its bifurcation (Fig. 32–4). The nerve most commonly involved is the one that supplies the second and third toes and the neuroma is found between the second and third metatarsals. This condition most commonly affects middle-aged women and is usually unilateral. Morton's neuroma is a type of metatarsalgia characterized by sudden attacks of sharp pain that radiates to the toes.[5] The cutaneous branches of the digital nerves divide on the plantar aspect of the transverse metatarsal ligament and supply the nerves to the sides of the toes. Pathologically the neuroma is a

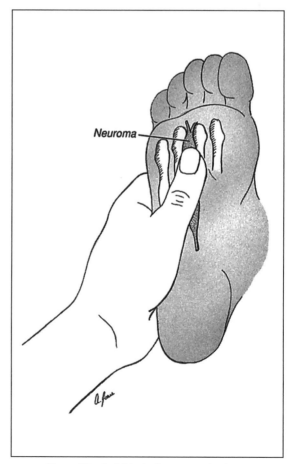

Figure 32–4. A Morton's neuroma is shown.

fusiform swelling occurring proximal to the bifurcation of the nerve that consists primarily of proliferative connective tissue and an amorphous eosinophilic material which may be the result of a nonspecific inflammatory neuritis or some type of localized arteritis.[54] The deposition of these materials are followed by slow degeneration of the nerve fiber.[5]

Clinical Presentation

The patient usually complains of a *burning pain* localized to the plantar aspect of the metatarsal heads, which is neuritic in nature and *radiates* to the toes and may be accompanied by paresthesias and numbness. The most common site is between the second and third metatarsals.[36] The pain is usually described as a lancinating, sharp pain that feels "like walking on a stone."[54] Initially, the pain occurs only with walking or standing but later persists even at rest. The patient obtains relief by removing the shoe and massaging the foot, which relieves the pressure between the metatarsal heads.[54] After these sudden attacks the tenderness may persist for days. The foot appears normal; however, on palpation one finds a small area of exquisite tenderness located in the third web space by firm palpation. In late cases, one may elicit crepitation and palpate a small tumor in the web space. Pressure between the metatarsal heads reproduces the pain whereas with metatarsalgia from other causes the pain is at the metatarsal heads[54] and this aids in the differentiation. Compression of the metatarsal heads together also causes pain in neuroma.[54] If the toes are hyperextended at the metatarsophalangeal joint the nerve is angulated over the transverse metatarsal ligament, and this evokes a throbbing type of pain in the involved toes. The most useful clinical test for the diagnosis of Morton's neuroma is to perform a web space compression test that produces severe pain by squeezing the metatarsal heads together with one hand and simultaneously compressing the involved web space with the thumb and the index finger of the opposite hand.[71] This compression test can also produce a painful and palpable click called a Mulder's sign.[71]

The differential diagnosis must include a foreign body, an epithelial cyst, and a traumatic bursitis.

Treatment

There are several steps in the treatment of Morton's neuroma. First, the patient's footwear must be examined to make sure that the forefoot and the toe box are large enough. Also, one must not lace the shoes too tight. Next, the physician could inject the affected area with corticosteroids followed by ultrasound, forefoot mobilization, and a temporary metatarsal pad. If all else fails, the physician must use a surgical treatment which consists of division of the transverse ligament with or without the excision of the neuroma.[5]

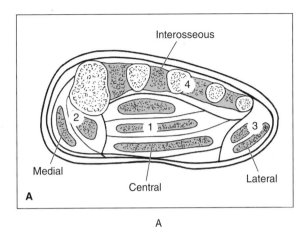
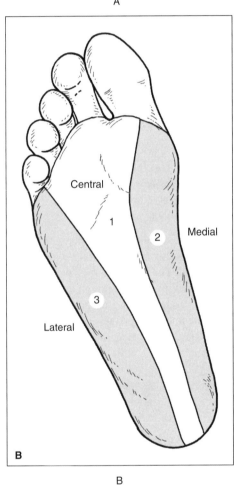

Figure 32–5. The anatomical compartments of the foot. **A.** A cross section of the forefoot showing the four compartments. **B.** The compartments of the sole of the foot.

☐ MARCH FRACTURE

No discussion of painful disorders of the forefoot would be complete without mention of stress fractures of the metatarsals called *March fractures*. This is discussed in Chapter 31, fractures of the foot. The patient usually gives a history of having gone on a long "march" or walk with no clear history of preceding trauma. On examination the patient has tenderness at the middle of the shaft of the third metatarsal, which is the one most commonly involved. The pain is worsened with flexion or extension of the toes and subsides with rest only to recur with exertion. Initial radiographs are negative but with-in 2 weeks a callous is seen in the midshaft of the metatarsal. The treatment is symptomatic with crutches in mild cases but if pain is significant and the patient's occupation requires prolonged standing or ambulation a walking cast is desirable for 3 or 4 weeks. Cardiovascular fitness could be maintained by pool running, the hydraulic hip flexor-extensor machine, cycling, and a rowing machine.[23]

□ BURSITIS OF THE FOREFOOT

Most of the bursitidies in this area are "adventitial bursa" and are abnormal bursa. These are due to overuse or trauma and are found in the joints of the foot that are exposed to pressure often from a shoe. The most common sites include the following:

- Dorsal interphalangeal joints of the toes
- Navicular tuberosity
- Medial first metatarsophalangeal joint
- Lateral fifth metatarsophalangeal joint

In acute bursitis, the patient presents with tenderness to palpation of the involved site along with erythema and edema localized. The treatment of these forms of bursitis include elimination of the inciting cause. One must protect the area from further irritation using ice therapy, NSAIDs, and injection therapy to relieve swelling and acute pain. These patients should be referred for follow-up care.

□ COMPARTMENT SYNDROME OF THE FOOT

This is a little known entity that commonly occurs and involves the interspace between the metatarsals. (Fig. 32–5A) The pain is out of proportion to what the injury would suggest and is not relieved by immobilization or with pain medication.[30] An early indicator is pain with passive dorsiflexion of the toes. After several hours signs of neurologic compromise may appear including numbness, burning, and paresthesias. The pain caused by compartment syndrome in the foot may be *exacerbated* by elevation. Decompression is recommended including either a medial longitudinal incision or a dorsal incision approach.

There are actually four compartments in the foot: medial, central, lateral, and interosseous, as previously discussed (Fig. 32–5B).[46] The medial compartment contains the muscles associated with the great toe, including the abductor hallucis, the flexor hallucis brevis, and flexor hallucis longus. The central compartment contains the flexor digitorum brevis, the quadratus plantae, the flexor hallucis longus, and peroneus longus tendons. In addition, the posterior tibial tendon, lumbricals, and adductor hallucis pass through this compartment. The lateral compartment contains the intrinsic muscles of the fifth digit. The interosseous compartment, discussed earlier, contains the seven interosseous muscles. As with all compartment syndromes elsewhere, the degree of pain in any of the compartments is out of proportion to the injury. Pain with passive dorsiflexion of the toes is an important sign. It is important to recognize that compartment syndrome may occur as a complication of infections in the feet of diabetic patients. These problems are extremely difficult to treat.[46] Compartment syndromes may also be seen in patients with calcaneal fractures.

DORSUM FOOT PAIN

□ ANTERIOR TIBIAL NEURITIS

In this condition pain is felt when the deep peroneal nerve is injured usually by a contusion on the dorsum of the foot. The nerve is superficial dorsally and lies under the cruciate crural ligament where it is essentially unprotected from the trauma of a poorly designed shoe or contusions. This nerve supplies sensation to the area between the first and second toes and the patient has a neuritic type of pain radiating to this region.

□ SKI BOOT COMPRESSION SYNDROME

With the increasing popularity of skiing one new complication has been described that is secondary to the ski boot tongue compressing anteriorly at the ankle causing a neuritis of the *deep peroneal nerve* and a *synovitis* of the extensor tendons.[47] On examination, the patient has induration and light palpation evokes severe pain over the dorsum of the foot. Sensation in the web space between the first and second toes is almost absent and the sensation over the remainder of the dorsum of the foot is decreased. Dorsiflexion of the toes is decreased markedly due to the tenosynovitis of the extensors; however, the dorsalis pedis pulse is normal.

The treatment includes elevation of the extremity, ice packs, and mild analgesics, with resolution usually occurring in 36 hours; however, sensation may not return to normal for up to 4 weeks. In refractory cases injection of steroids is recommended.[47]

☐ OSTEOCHONDROSIS OF THE NAVICULAR

The navicular is the last tarsal bone to ossify and is subject to aseptic necrosis, which usually occurs between the ages of 4 to 6 years and is often bilateral, causing a painful limp in a child with the disorder.[49] The etiology of this disorder is unclear, but the condition is usually self-limited and tends to spontaneous recovery.

On examination the patient is most often a boy between the ages of 4 and 10 years who complains of pain over the region of the navicular, usually accompanied by a limp. Palpation elicits tenderness over the navicular and there is usually no history of trauma.

Radiographs of the foot should be obtained with comparison views that demonstrate an increased density and loss of the trabicular pattern of the navicular, which is irregular in outline and often has a crush appearance.

The treatment consists of protecting the bone in the acute stage with restricted activity and casting for 6 to 8 weeks in more severe cases. Complete ossification occurs in 2 to 3 years and no permanent disability is expected.

☐ SYNOVIAL GANGLION

This is not common in the ankle but occurs in the foot with enough frequency to be considered here. The synovial herniation occurs after a chronic sprain that is accompanied by weakness of the capsules of one of the many joints of the foot. A frequent site is near the peroneal tendon insertion distal to the lateral malleolus where it may be quite large. Another site is at the dorsum of the foot along the long extensor tendons to the toes where the ganglion may come off the tendon sheath or from the tarsal joints.

The treatment is surgical removal; however, in some patients aspiration followed by a pressure dressing may yield good results.

DISORDERS OF THE TOES

☐ INGROWN TOENAIL

The lateral margins of the nail at its corner dig into the surrounding nail fold and cause discomfort that may lead to a paronychial infection. The causes of this condition are either a tightly fitting shoe that compresses the toes together leading to maceration and infection of the nail fold, or trimming the nails in such a way that the corners can grow out into the skin, leading to granuloma formation and infections. The condition is very common, most often involving the great toe.

The treatment depends on the stage at which the condition is seen. Early, before the development of any infection or granuloma, the examiner will notice only erythema and some swelling of the nail fold where the nail is penetrating the skin. At this stage treatment should consist of warm soaks and elevation of the leading corner of the nail with a cotton pledget soaked in an

antiseptic solution placed under the corner. The patient should be advised on how to trim the nails properly and cautioned against wearing shoes that are narrow or have a high heel. When the nail fold is acutely inflamed and there is a paronychial infection, warm soaks are used to localize the infection and the nail freed and elevated by a cotton pledget or a plastic insert that has recently been devised.[34]

☐ SUBUNGUAL EXOSTOSIS

This is a painful condition of the distal phalanx usually affecting the first toe. When it occurs the toe deviates laterally, causing difficulty with walking. The exostosis forms over the distal portion of the distal phalanx, and the patient presents with complaints of pain and swelling along with increased sensitivity of the toe over the exostosis. Subungual exostosis more commonly affects women than men by a ratio of 2 to 1.[19] Most lesions occur patients who are in the early twenties. This is an uncommon bony tumor that manifests as a painful, firm hyperkeratotic nodule at the free edge of the nail plate.[53] The treatment for the condition is surgical removal.

□ HALLUX VALGUS

Hallux valgus (bunion) is a deformity in which the large toe deviates laterally and a bony prominence develops over the medial aspect of the first metatarsal head and neck. When it occurs, the toe deviates laterally, causing difficulty with walking. The medial portion of the first metatarsal head enlarges and a bursa forms over the medial joint that may become inflamed and thickened. It is this bursitis that may bring the patient to the emergency department. The treatment here is the application of warm moist soaks to the region and, if an infectious bursitis is diagnosed, incision and drainage with the application of warm soaks and the institution of antibiotic therapy is indicated. These patients should be referred to a podiatrist for definitive care. In the adolescent, weight-bearing views of both anteroposterior and lateral x rays are necessary to access bunions.[17] Non-surgical treatment in adolescents is usually adequate to relieve symptoms but not to correct the deformity.[66] Treatment consists predominantly of shoe modifications.[66]

□ PARTIAL OR COMPLETE NAIL AVULSION

This can be due to direct or indirect trauma. Examination of the nail bed may demonstrate a badly lacerated nail bed which may need repair. There are two schools of thought as to how to treat patients with a partially avulsed nail. If there is no fracture, the nail can be removed and then put back in place and the patient's toe bandaged. However, some authors feel that a complete nail avulsion may cause more trauma to an already injured area. Leaving the nail on may allow the injured nail to act as a splint to guide new nail formation. Other authors, however, feel that this may block the new nail formation. It is probably best to assess the degree of trauma, particularly to the root and roof matrix. If there is no root or roof matrix involvement it is probably best that the nail be left on. If a nail bed repair is necessary, the nail should be uplifted as if one is lifting the hood of a car leaving the root and roof matrix intact. One must remember to give tetanus immunization if necessary.

Partial Nail Removal
Local anesthetic is first administered. To anesthetize the great toe, the anesthetic is injected using a 25-

gauge $1\frac{1}{4}$-inch needle. The initial puncture is at the base of the proximal phalanx laterally. (Fig. 32–6A) After aspiration, the wheel is raised at this site. The needle is advanced inferiorly. As the needle is slowly withdrawn, anesthesia is slowly injected. The needle is not removed completely from the first injection site. It is advanced toward the medial aspect of the digit where another wheel is raised. *Dorsal flexion of the toe allows the needle to pass underneath the extensor*

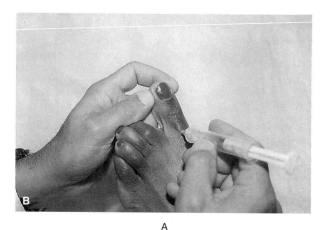

A

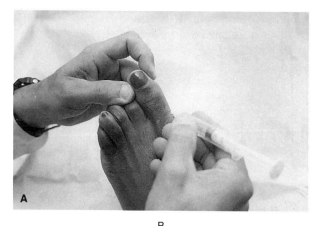

B

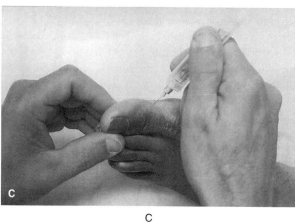

C

Figure 32–6. Blocking the large toe requires a stepwise procedure. See the text for discussion.

tendons. The needle is withdrawn slowly, injecting the anesthetic solution. A second puncture is made at the site of the medial wheel after the skin is numb. (Fig. 32–6B) The needle is advanced plantarly and the procedure repeated, injecting slowly while withdrawing. A third puncture is made at the plantar medial wheel (Fig. 32–6C). The needle is advanced laterally and the procedure is repeated for the last time. Following this, a rubber tourniquet is then applied, and a spatula is used to free the proximal nail fold on the affected side (Fig. 32–7). Ideally, a nail splitter is then inserted and positioned to remove the desired amount of nail, approximately one quarter to one third of the nail (see Fig. 32–7). Once this is complete, a hemostat is employed to grab the freed nail and remove it. Excessive granulation tissue can be further removed by trimming with scissors or cauterizing with a silver nitrate stick. The exposed nail can be destroyed or cauterized with *phenol* or surgically excised for permanent removal. In the authors' experience, phenol is the ideal agent to use in that it is difficult to excise the entire matrix (Fig. 32–8). Eighty percent phenol is administered with a sterile applicator stick to the exposed nail matrix for 1 to 2 minutes (see Fig. 32–8). Care must be taken not to get any phenol on the surrounding skin. After the applicator is removed, the area is flushed with alcohol to neutralize any remaining phenol. The phenol area should turn a grayish white. If this color is not observed, the procedure should be repeated. An aseptic dressing should be worn until the wound is dry. It is important that the toe box of the shoe be adequately sized. It may be necessary to prohibit both weight bearing and the wearing of the shoe for several days. The difficulty with phenol is that the wounds tend to drain for some time and there may be associated pain. Also, phenol that has touched the exposed skin causes painful burns and skin sluffing. Thus, some people may prefer excision of the nail bed rather than the phenol technique. However, cauterization with phenol has been shown to cause less frequent recurrences of this condition.[31,67] To complete this procedure, an elliptical segment of skin is removed and the edges left open or sutures can be placed with a compressive dressing. Basically, if one removes only the spicule of nail, one does not have to place sutures or remove an elliptical edge skin. If, however, the spicule is deep with a great deal of granulation tissue, it may be advantageous to remove the segment of skin and, as indicated above, one quarter to one third of the nail.[1,16]

□ GENERAL TREATMENT FOR FOOT DISORDERS

In this section, we discuss common modalities to treat foot problems described in this chapter. A description of common procedures performed by podiatry that are applicable to emergency medicine are discussed.

Padding
Padding is used to temporarily relieve the pain associated with a bursitis or a tendonitis or fasciitis presenting in the emergency department. Padding is also used to relieve pressure around areas that are painful such as bony prominences. Generally, adhesive felt foam which is approximately $1/4$-inch thick is used. Adhesive tape is preferred over other forms of tape. A number of prefabricated pads are available that have an adhesive backing.

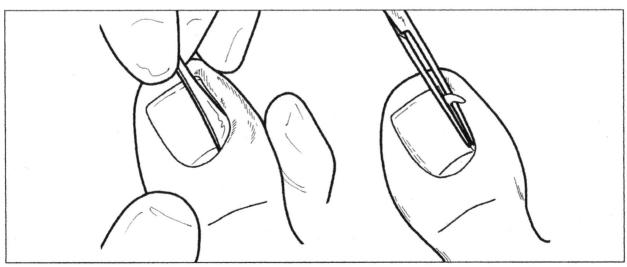

Figure 32–7. Free the proximal nail fold on the affected side using a blunt instrument.

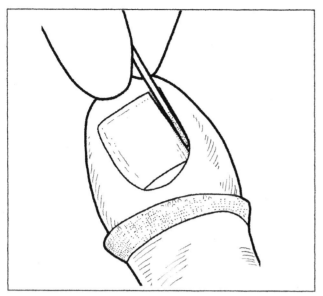

Figure 32–8. A contip applicator soaked in phenol is used to destroy the nail bed matrix of the toe so that this portion of the toenail does not grow back when treating an ingrown toenail.

A bunion pad can be shaped from felt (Fig. 32–9). This is a donut-shaped pad placed over the bunion and then covered with strips of adhesive tape to hold it in place for 3 to 4 days. A roll foam pad can be used to cover the large toe and the dorsomedial prominence which will also suffice. A digit should not be circumscribed with tape or any coverings since this may cause constriction later and circulatory impairment.

A pad can be used over a corn with a hole cut over the corn if necessary (Fig. 32–10). In patients with forefoot pain a $^1/_4$-inch-thick felt pad may be placed proximal to the metatarsal heads which disburses pressure away from the metatarsal heads and relieves discomfort there.

In patients with plantar fasciitis, one can obtain temporary relief by padding or strapping using a heel spur pad (see Fig. 32–11). A heel spur pad is made of a thicker felt padding and is fashioned in the shape of a U.

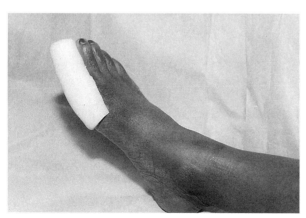

Figure 32–9. A pad is shown for a bunion.

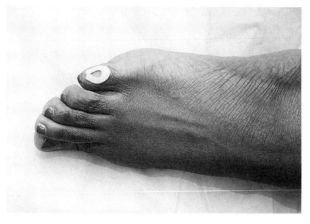

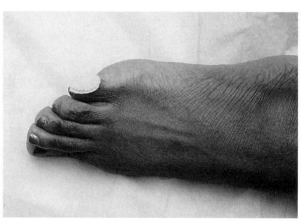

Figure 32–10. A pad for a corn is shown.

It is used directly over the affected heel and is covered with several strips of 2-inch tape. This pad disperses weight from the central and more painful part of the heel in patients with heel spurs and plantar fasciitis. Alternatively, a pad made of $^1/_4$-inch felt can be fashioned to fit in the longitudinal arch and taped into place, which relieves symptoms of plantar fasciitis by taking tension off of the plantar fasciia (Fig. 32–12A&B). A combination of the heel pad (U-shaped) described above and the longitudinal arch pad relieves the pain of plantar fasciitis until the patient can be seen by a podiatrist.

Paring

Paring is used for temporary relief of discomfort associated with corns or calluses. One can use a No. 15 or No. 10 blade. The nondominant hand supports the foot, which is elevated and at a comfortable height for the physician. The dominant hand debrides the corn or callus. The blade and scalpel handle should be held between the thumb and index finger and positioned so that it is almost parallel to the lesion. A thin slice is taken off using a semicircular motion from the corn or callus. This is then debrided repeatedly until healthy pink tissue is

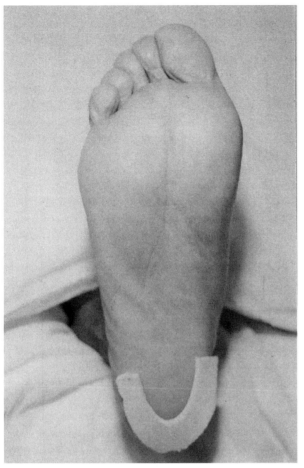

Figure 32–11. A heel spur pad is shown.

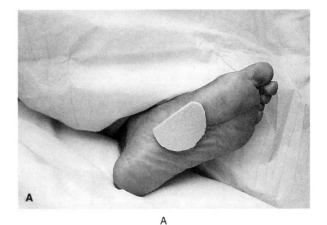

A

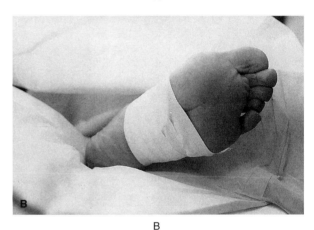

B

Figure 32–12. Planter fascia padding; see the text for discussion.

noted. Be certain that the cutting edge of the scalpel is always moving away from your hand to protect yourself. Inflamed bursae sometimes occur under a corn and these will require local injection with lidocaine prior to debridement. In addition, debridement of a callus in an unusual location may demonstrate a hidden foreign body or ulcerations. Figure 32–13 demonstrates an example of paring a planter callus. A corn or callus is debrided repeatedly until healthy, pink tissue is noted. One must remember that the cutting edge of the scalpel is always moved away from the practitioner. After the superficial debridement of the corn is complete, the central core must be removed to relieve symptoms. This deeper core is removed with the tip of the scalpel blade in a circular manner. One must be careful not to cut into the underlying healthy tissue. This procedure will offer 6 to 8 weeks of relief from the pain.

Strapping for Plantar Fasciitis

This technique is used to relieve the symptoms of fasciitis. This is an alternative to padding, as described earlier in the chapter. To apply this technique, the amount of tape is first measured. Using a role of 1-inch tape, the

end of the *non-adherent* side is applied against the skin, overlying the head of the first metatarsal. The tape is extended proximally around the heel along the lateral aspect of the foot to the head of the fifth metatarsal. The tape is torn at this point and stuck on or to the examination table so that it can hang freely. Two more pieces of the same length are measured. Next, using 2-inch tape and the same method of measuring, four pieces of tape are measured from the medial aspect of the metatarsal

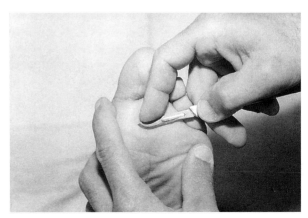

Figure 32–13. Paring of a callus is shown.

plantarly to the lateral. This tape placed nearby. Using the 1-inch strips and beginning medially at the first metatarsal head, the tape is applied all the way around the foot to the head of the fifth metatarsal. A second 1-inch strip is applied on top of the first, overlapping $1/4$-inch plantarly. The tape should be bow strung in the arch area. A 2-inch strip of tape is now applied from medial to lateral, starting just proximal to the metatarsal heads. The 2-inch tape should be based on both sides of the 1-inch tape from medial to lateral and overlapping by $1/2$-inch from distal to proximal. Once all of the 2-inch tape is in place the final piece of 1-inch tape is applied as a binder, exactly over the first two pieces of 1-inch tape. This strapping will last 3 to 5 days if it does not get wet (Fig. 32–14).

Injection Therapy

Injection therapy is used in any area of the foot where pain and inflammation are localized and are not relieved by NSAIDs. Conditions that typically require injection are bursitis, sesamoiditis, and most commonly heel spur syndrome. One must remember that injection therapy is contraindicated in diabetics and patients with peripheral vascular disease. The proce-

dure to use is to withdraw with an 18-gauge needle a 50/50 mixture of 1 percent lidocaine plain and 0.5 percent bupivacaine. A small amount of a long-lasting steroid is then added, such as dexamethasone. One must prepare the area to be injected with iodine and numb the area with ethyl chloride spray. Using a 25-gauge $1^1/_4$-needle, the agents withdrawn in the syringe are thoroughly mixed. The area of tenderness is determined by palpation prior to injecting. For example, at the medial tubercle of the calcaneous for a tender heel spur; the injection should be directed at the area of maximum tenderness. With a dart-like movement, the needle is inserted and advanced while simultaneously infiltrating the area with a combination steroid-anesthetic mixture. Tendons should never be injected. To determine if a sheath or area of tenderness is being infiltrated, simply ask the patient to move the muscle tendon unit. Movement of the syringe indicates that the needle is in the tendon. The area is massaged to ensure dispersion of the agent.[57]

REFERENCES

1. Adams SE: Conditions of the toenails. *Orthop Clin North Am* **25:**1, 1994.
2. Balduini FC, Tetzlaff J: Historical perspectives on injuries of the ligaments of the ankle. *Clin Sports Med* **1:**3, 1982.
3. Barry NN, McGuire JL: Acute injuries and specific problems in adult athletes. *Rheum Clin North Am* **22:**3, 1996.
4. Berkebile DE: Chronic achilles tendonitis. *South Dakota J Med* **44:**311, 1991.
5. Brantingham JW, et al: Morton's neuroma. *J Physiol Ther* **14:**317, 1991.
6. Bridges R, McIntire Jr, Deitch EA: Diabetic foot infections. *Surg Clin North Am* **74:**3, 1994.
7. Brook JW: Management of pedal puncture wounds. *Am Col Foot Ankle Surg* **33:**5, 1994.
8. Brooks KE, Bender JF: Tinea pedis: Diagnosis and treatment. *Clin Podiatr Med Surg* **13:**1, 1996.
9. Brooks SC, Potter BT, Rainey JB: Treatment for partial tears of the lateral ligament of the ankle: A prospective trial. *Br Med J* **282:**606, 1981.
10. Butcher JD, et al: Lower extremity bursitis. *Am Fam Phys* **53:**7, 1996.
11. Campbell JW, Inman VT: Treatment of plantar fascitis and calcaneal spurs with the UCBL shoe insert. *Clin Orthop* **103:**57, 1974.
12. Campbell P, Lawton JO: Heel pain: Diagnosis and management. *Br J Hosp Med* **52:**8, 1994.
13. Campbell P, Lawton JO: Spontaneous rupture of the Achilles tendon: Pathology and management. *Br J Hosp Med* **50:**6, 1993.
14. Cetti R, et al: Operative versus nonoperative treatment of Achilles tendon rupture. *Am J Sports Med* **21:**6, 1993.
15. Chandler TJ, Kibler WB: A biomechanical approach to the prevention treatment and rehabilitation of plantar fasciitis. *Sports Med* **15**(5):344–352, 1993.

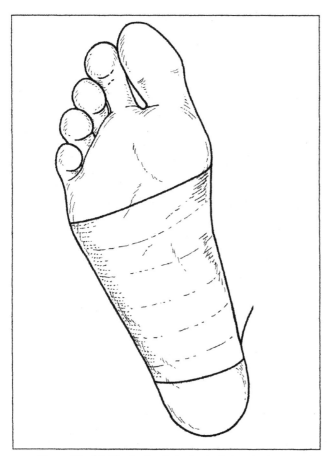

Figure 32–14. Planter fascia taping technique is shown.

16. Connolly AAP, et al: Local anaesthetis agents in surgery for ingrown toenail. *Br J Surg* **81:**425–426, 1994.

17. Coughlin MJ: Hallux valgus. *Instruc Course Lect* **46:**357–391, 1997.

18. Crenshaw AH (ed): *Campbell's Operative Orthopedics*, 8th ed. St Louis: Mosby, 1992.

19. Davis DA, Cohen PR: Subungual exostosis: Case report and review of the literature. *Pediatr Dermatol* **13**(3): 212–218, 1996.

20. DeGreef HJ, et al: Current therapy of dermatophytosis. *J Am Acad Dermatol* **31:**3, 1994.

21. Eckert WR, et al: Acute rupture of the peroneal retinaculum. *J Bone Joint Surg* **58**(5):670, 1976.

22. Esterowitz D, et al: Plantar warts in the athlete. *AJEM* **13:**4, 1995.

23. Evanski PM, Reinherz RP: Easing the pain of common foot problems. *Patient Care* **25:**38, 1991.

24. Fernandez-Palazzi F, Rivas S, Mojica P: Achilles tendonitis in ballet dancers. *Clin Orthop* **257:**257, 1990.

25. Fitzgerald RH, et al: Puncture wounds of the foot. *Orthop Clin North Am* **6:**965, 1975.

26. Giacalone VF, et al: The University of Texas health science center at San Antonio: Experience with foot surgery in diabetics. *J Foot Ankle Surg* **33:**6, 1994.

27. Gibbons GW, Habershaw GM: Diabetic foot infections. *Infec Dis Clin North Am* **9:**1, 1995.

28. Gillies H, Chalmers J: The management of fresh ruptures of the tendoachillis. *J Bone Joint Surg* **52**(2):337, 1979.

29. Giurini JM, Rosenblum BI: The role of foot surgery in patients with diabetes. *Clin Podiatr Med Surg* **12:**1, 1995.

30. Goldman FD, Dayton PD, Hanson CJ: Compartment syndrome of the foot. *J Foot Surg* **29**(1):37, 1990.

31. Greig JD, et al: The surgical treatment of ingrowing toenails. *J Bone Joint Surg* **73B:**131, 1991.

32. Griffiths GD, Wieman TJ: Meticulous attention to foot care improves the prognosis in diabetic ulceration of the foot. *Surg Gynecol Obstet* **174:**49, 1992.

33. Houston AN, et al: Tetnus prophylaxis in the treatment of puncture wounds of patients in the deep south. *J Trauma* **2:**439, 1962.

34. Ilfeld FW, August W: Treatment of ingrown toenail with plastic insert. *Orthop Clin North Am* **5**(1):94, 1974.

35. Inglis AE, et al: Ruptures of the tendoachillis. *J Bone Joint Surg* **58**(7):990, 1990.

36. Jahss MH: *Diseases of the foot*, vol I. Philadelphia: Saunders, 1986, pp 964–977.

37. Johaanson PH: *Pseudomonas* infections of the foot following puncture wound. *JAMA* **204:**262, 1962.

38. Karr SD: Subcalcaneal heel pain. *Orthop Clin North Am* **25:**1, 1994.

39. Katcherian DA: Treatment of Freiberg's disease. *Orthop Clin North Am* **25:**1, 1994.

40. Kjaersgaard-Anderson P, et al: Sinus tarsi syndrome: Presentation of seven cases and review of the literature. *J Foot Surg* **28**(1):3, 1989.

41. Kvist M: Achilles tendon injuries in athletes. *Sports Med* **18**(3):173–201, 1994.

42. Landsman MJ, et al: Diagnosis, pathophysiology, and treatment of plantar verruca. *Clin Podiatr Med Surg* **13:**1, 1996.

43. Lea RB, et al: Plantar fascitis. *J Bone Joint Surg* **57**(5):673, 1975.

44. Lea RB, et al: Rupture of the Achilles tendon, nonsurgical treatment. *Clin Orthop* **60:**115, 1968.

45. Leach RE, James S, Wasilewski S: Achilles tendonitis. *Am J Sports Med* **9:**93, 1981.

46. Lee BY, et al: Compartment syndrome in the diabetic foot. *Adv Wound Care* **8**(6):36,38,41,42,44–46, 1995.

47. Lindenbaum BA: Ski boot compression syndrome. *Clin Orthop* **140**(1):78, 1979.

48. Mann RA: Tarsal tunnel syndrome. *Orthop Clin North Am* **5**(1):109, 1974.

49. Manusov EG, et al: Evaluation of pediatric foot problems: part III. The hindfoot and the ankle. *Am Fam Phys* **54:**3, 1996.

50. Masri-Fridling D: Dermatophytosis of the feet. *Derm Clin* **14:**1, 1996.

51. Mehrez M: Arthropathy of the ankle. *J Bone Joint Surg* [Br] **52:**308, 1970.

52. Miller EH, Semian DW: Gram negative osteomyelitis following puncture wounds in the foot. *J Bone Joint Surg* **57**(4):535, 1975.

53. Miron D, et al: Infections following nail puncture wound of the foot: Case reports and review of the literature. *Isr J Med Sci* **29:**194–197, 1993.

54. Morris MA: Morton's metatarsalgia. *Clin Orthop* **127:**203, 1977.

55. Mucci B, Stenhouse G: Soft tissue radiography for wooden foreign bodies—a worthwhile exercise? *Injury* **16:**402, 1985.

56. Murray HJ, Boulton AM: The pathophysiology of diabetic foot ulceration. *Clin Podiatr Med Surg* **12:**1, 1995.

57. Nakano T, Aherne FX: The phatogenesis of osteochondrosis—a hypothesis. *Med Hypotheses* **43:**1–3, 1994.

58. Newsman L: Imaging techniques in the diabetic foot. *Clin Podiatr Med Surg* **12:**1, 1995.

59. Reinherz RP, Hong DT, Tisa LM, Winters GJ: Management of puncture wounds in the foot. *J Foot Surg* **24:**288, 1985.

60. Resnick CD, Fallat LM: Puncture wounds: Therapeutic considerations and a new classification. *J Foot Surg* **29**(2):147, 1990.

61. Riegler HF, Routson GW: Complications of the deep puncture wounds of the foot. *J Trauma* **19**(1):18, 1979.

62. Smith SB, Shane HS: Simple bone cyst of the calcaneus: A case report and literature review. *J Am Podiatr Med Assoc* **84:**3, 1994.

63. Soma CA, Mandelbaum BR: Achilles tendon disorders. *Clin Sports Med* **13:**4, 1994.

64. Taillard W, et al: The sinus tarsi syndrome. *Int Orthop* **5:**117, 1981.

65. Takakora Y, et al: Tarsal tunnel syndromes. *J Bone Joint Surg* **73B:**125, 1991.

66. Thompson GH: Bunions and deformities of the toes in children and adolescents. Chap 40, Foot and ankle. *Instruc Course Lect* **45:**355–367, 1996.

67. Van der Ham AC, Hackeng CA, Yo TI: The treatment of ingrowing toenails. *J Bone Joint Surg* **72B:**507, 1990.

68. Van Wyngarden TM: The painful foot, part III: Common rearfoot deformities. *Am Fam Phys* **55:**6, 1997.

69. Van Wyngarden TM, Bleuart AL: Reflex sympathetic dystrophy involving the foot. *J Foot Surg* **31**(1):75, 1992.
70. White DL: Plantar fascial release. *J Am Podiatr Med Assoc* **84**:12, 1994.
71. Wu KK: Morton's interdigital neuroma: A clinical review of its etiology, treatment, and results. *J Foot Ankle Surg* **35**:2, 1996.
72. Young G, Lindsey J: Etiology of symptomatic recurrent interdigital neuromas. *J Am Podiatr Med Assoc* **83**:5, 1993.

BIBLIOGRAPHY

Albert SF, Jahnigen DW: Treating common foot disorders in older patients. *Geriatrics* **38**:42, 1993.
Amis J, Jennings L, Graham D, et al: Painful heel syndrome: Radiographic and treatment assessment. *Foot Ankle* **9**:91, 1988.
Anderson KJ, Lecoc JF: Operative treatment of the injury to the fibular collateral ligament of the ankle. *J Bone Joint Surg* **36**:825, 1954.
Anderson KJ, et al: Athletic injury to the fibular collateral ligament of the ankle. *Clin Orthop* **23**:147, 1962.
Antoniou D, et al: Osteomyelitis of the calcaneus and talus. *J Bone Joint Surg* **56**(2):338, 1974.
Bonnin JG: Injury to the ligaments of the ankle (editorial). *J Bone Joint Surg* [Br] **47**:609, 1965.
Chisholm CD, Schlesser JF: Plantar puncture wounds: Controversies and treatment recommendations. *Am Emerg Med* **18**:1352, 1989.
Coltart WD: Sprained ankle. *Br Med Assoc J* **57**:957, 1957.
Cracehiolo A III: Office treatment of adult foot problems. *Orthop Clin North Am* **13**:511, 1982.
Dziob JM: Ligamentous injuries about the ankle joint. *Am J Surg* **91**:692, 1956.
Freeman MAR, et al: The etiology and prevention of functional instability of the foot. *J Bone Joint Surg* **47**:678, 1965.
Gleckman RA, Czachor JS: Managing diabetes-related infections in the elderly. *Geriatrics* **44**:37, 1989.
Grundy M, et al: An investigation of the centres of pressure under the foot while walking. *J Bone Joint Surg* [Br] **57**(1):98, 1975.
Helal B: Metatarsal osteotomy for metatarsalgia. *J Bone Joint Surg* [Br] **57**(2):187, 1975.
Kwong PK, Kay D, Voner RT, White MW: Plantar fasciitis mechanics and pathomechanics of treatment. *Clin Sports Med* **7**:119, 1988.
Meals RA: Peroneal nerve palsy complicating ankle sprain. *J Bone Joint Surg* **59**(7):966, 1977.
Miller PR, Levi JH: Hair strangulation. *J Bone Joint Surg* **59**(1):132, 1977.
Omer GE, Pomerantz GM: Initial management of severe injuries and traumatic amputations of the foot. *Arch Surg* **105**:696, 1972.
Parieser DM: Superficial fungal infections. *Postgrad Med* **87**:205, 1990.
Scranton PE: Metatarsalgia: A clinical review of diagnosis and management. *Foot Ankle* **1**:229, 1989.
Silferskjold JP: Common foot problems. *Postgrad Med* **89**:183, 1991.
Sutherland AD: Equinus deformity due to haemangioma of calf muscle. *J Bone Joint Surg* [Br] **57**(2):104, 1975.

PART III

APPENDIX

APPENDIX

SPLINTS, CASTS, AND OTHER TECHNIQUES

☐ DORSAL DISTAL PHALANX SPLINTS

Dorsal and volar splints are very useful in treating avulsion fractures of the distal phalanx as discussed in the text. The authors' preference is the dorsal splint, which provides more support because there is less "padding" on the dorsal aspect of the finger. The splint is in closer contact with the bone. When using these splints one should not hyperextend the distal interphalangeal joint as was previously recommended in older texts. Full extension is the position of choice when applying the splint.

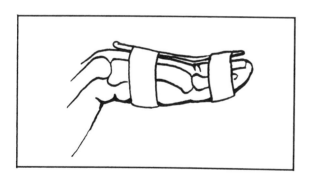

☐ HAIRPIN SPLINT

This splint is made from a thin metal strip. It provides protection for distal phalangeal fractures resulting from external injury. This splint provides no structural support.

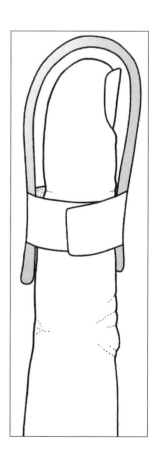

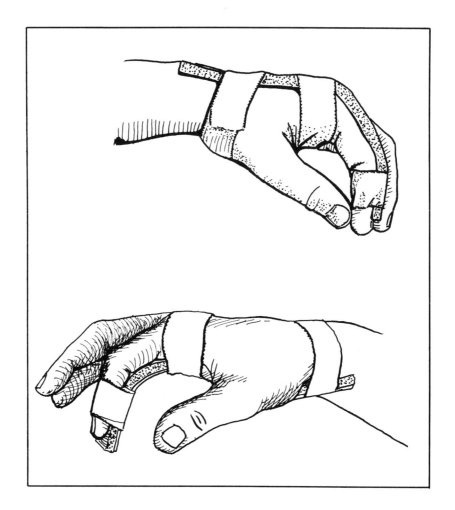

☐ DORSAL AND VOLAR FINGER SPLINTS

These splints are fashioned from commercially available metallic splints that have a sponge rubber padding on one side. The splint is cut to the proper size and shaped as desired.

The splints should be applied with the metacarpophalangeal joint at 50 degrees of flexion and the interphalangeal joints flexed approximately 15 to 20 degrees. This is better shown in the diagram of the dorsal splint.

☐ DYNAMIC FINGER SPLINTING

The injured finger is splinted to the adjacent normal finger. This provides for support of the injured digit while permitting motion of the metacarpophalangeal joint and some motion at the interphalangeal joint. This type of splinting is used commonly in sprains of the collateral ligaments of the interphalangeal joints and other injuries discussed in the text. A piece of felt cut to proper size is inserted between the fingers and the two digits taped together as shown.

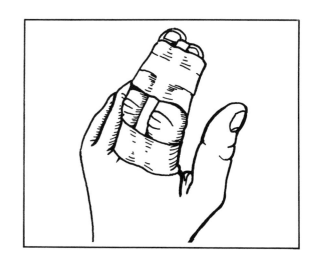

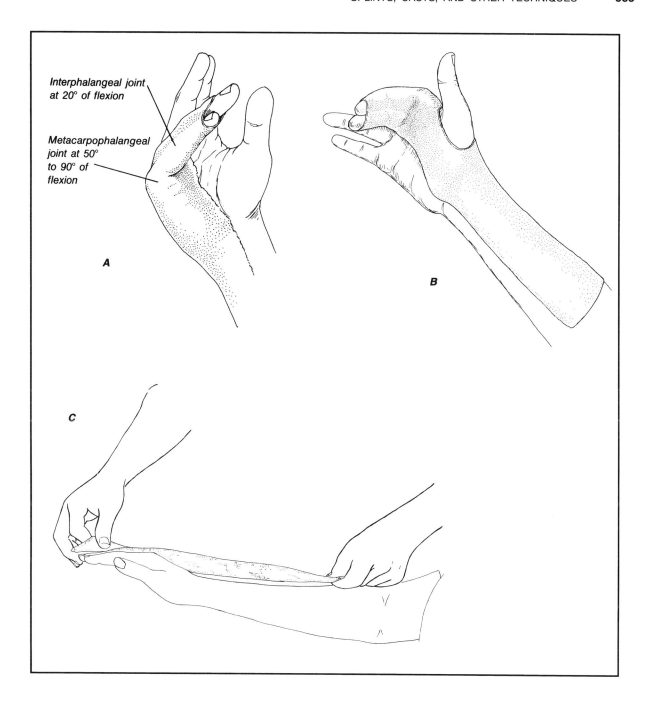

Interphalangeal joint
at 20° of flexion

Metacarpophalangeal
joint at 50°
to 90° of
flexion

A

B

C

☐ GUTTER SPLINTS

Gutter splints are used for the treatment of phalangeal and metacarpal fractures as discussed in the text. Fractures of the ring and little finger are immobilized in an ulnar gutter splint as shown in **A.** Fractures involving the index finger and the long finger are immobilized in a radial splint as shown in **B.** The splint is made by using plaster sheets cut to the proper size. The measurement should be from the tip of the finger to a point two thirds of the way down the forearm (**C**).

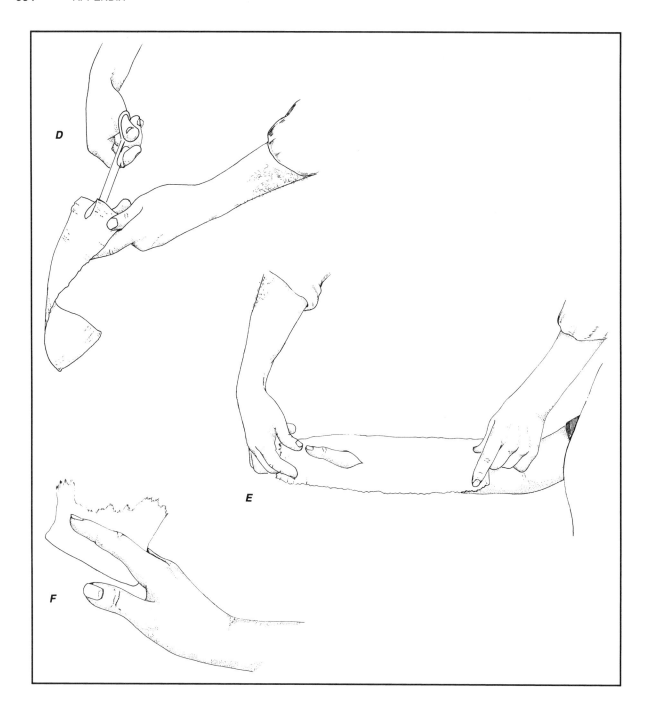

When applying a radial gutter splint cut out the hole for the thumb (***D***). Next, apply the plaster over the fingers to be immobilized making certain that the index and long fingers are incorporated into the splint (radial gutter splint) (***E***) or the little finger and ring finger are incorporated for the ulnar gutter splint. Remove the dry plaster which has now been measured to size and apply cotton roll (Webril) between the fingers to be immobilized (***F***).

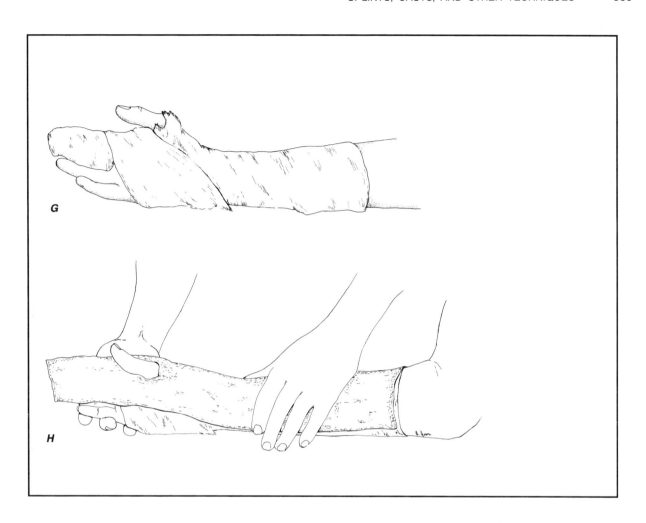

After doing this apply the cotton roll around the digits to be immobilized and apply this around the forearm (**G**). Next, immerse the plaster splint in water, remove the excess water and apply this over the cotton roll (**H**).

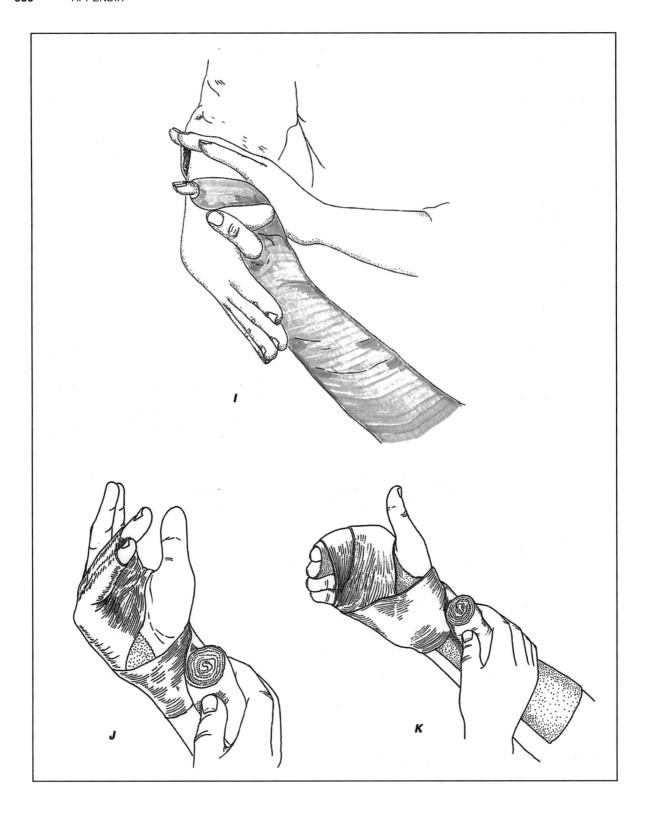

When holding the extremity splint in the proper position; 15 degrees of extension at the wrist and 50 to 90 degrees of flexion at the metacarpophalangeal joint, make certain that you use the palm of the hands (*I*) so as not to leave imprints in the plaster. The proper final position for the plaster splint is 50 to 90 degrees of flexion at the metacarpophalangeal joint and extension at the interphalangeal joints (*J*) and (*K*).

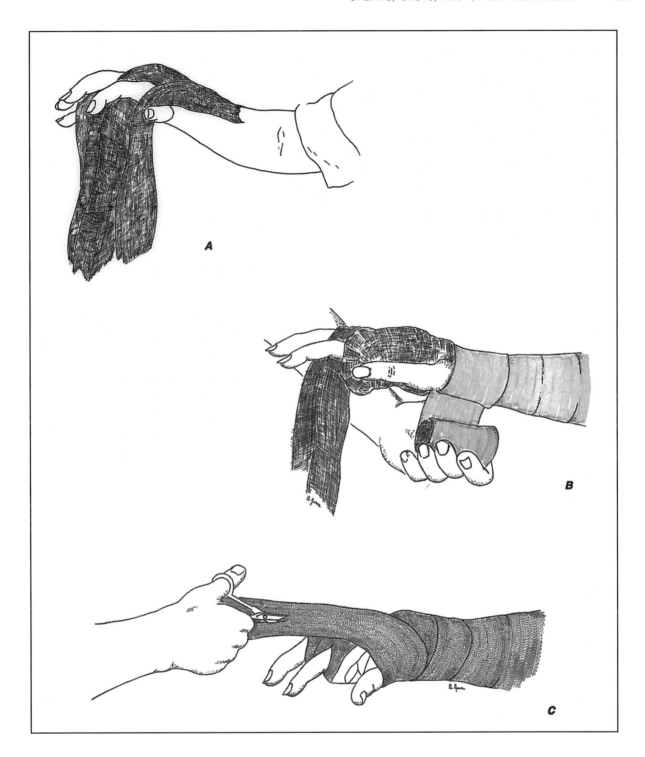

☐ A UNIVERSAL HAND DRESSING

The universal hand dressing is used when treating inflammatory conditions that affect the hand. This is a soft dressing that places the hand in a position which allows for maximal drainage. In applying this dressing, the fingers are separated by gauze fluffs as shown (*A*). An elastic bandage is then applied around the forearm and onto the hand (*B*). When encircling the fingers, the elastic bandage is cut so as to allow the fingers to go through the bandage (*C*).

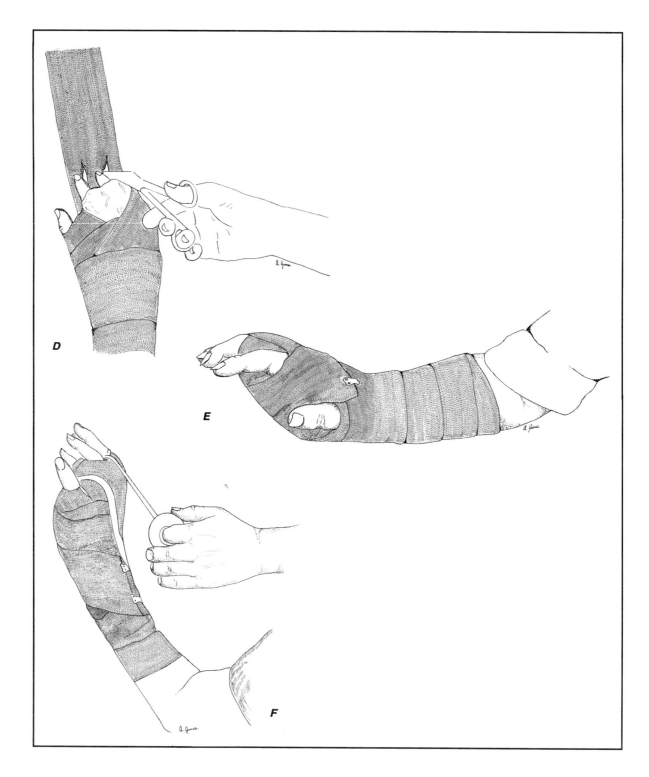

In the final stages of encircling the digits, the elastic bandage courses along the palmer aspect of the hand, holes are then cut through the elastic bandage to incorporate the fingers and the hand is pulled back so that the wrist is held in extension (*D, E*). To assist in maintaining the wrist at 15 degrees of extension with the fingers separated, 1/2-inch cloth tape is used between the fingers applied from the palmer aspect to the dorsum of the hand so as to pull the wrist back (*F*).

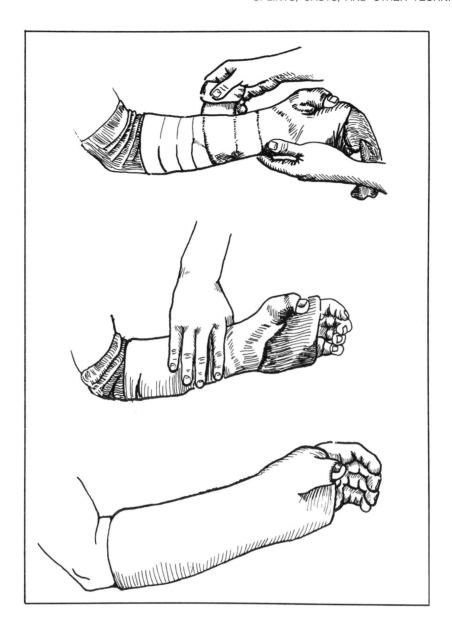

□ THUMB SPICA OR WRIST GAUNTLET CAST

(Wine Glass Position of the Thumb)*
The uses of this cast are discussed in Chapter 1. It is made by applying stockinette dressing to the arm extending from the hand to the midarm or more proximally when making a long arm spica cast. This is followed by application of cotton bandage (Webril), which is then followed by plaster rolls. The method of applying the plaster rolls is discussed in the introductory chapter on casting. Before application of the final roll, the stock-

inette is folded back over the cast and the final plaster roll is applied.

Note the position of the thumb that must be maintained in applying this cast. Although the interphalangeal joint is incorporated in the cast here, controversy exists as to the need to do this. The fingers are left free so there is full motion of the metacarpophalangeal joints. The position of the wrist shown here is the neutral position. In using this cast for fractures of the scaphoid the authors advocate extending it to above the elbow, making it a long arm cast.

*Long arm thumb spica not shown here.

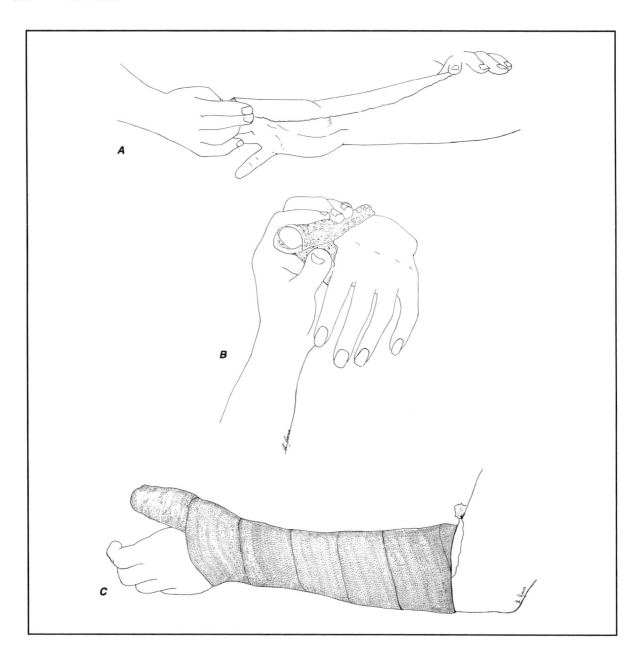

□ THUMB SPLINT

A. The thumb splint is made by applying a plaster slab from the tip of the thumb to approximately two thirds of the way along the forearm as shown. *B.* In applying the plaster be certain that the width is wide enough so that the two ends overlap at the distal tip of the thumb as shown. *C.* After applying cotton roll under the plaster slab, apply the plaster as shown in *A* above and then wrap with an elastic bandage.

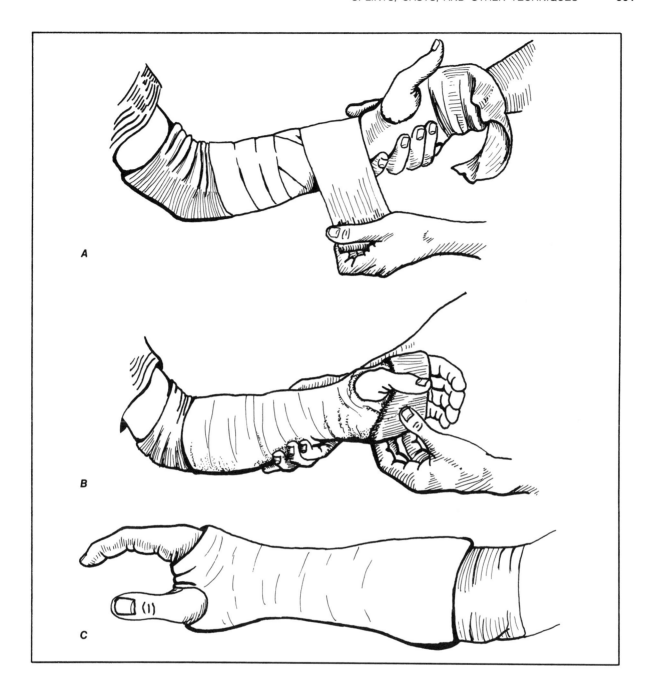

☐ SHORT ARM CAST

A short arm cast is used for immobilizing a number of fractures of the forearm. The cast is made by applying a stockinette from the fingers to above the elbow as shown in **A.** Cotton bandage (Webril) is then applied over the stockinette with the thumb remaining free at the meta-carpophalangeal joint and the fingers free at the same level. Plaster rolls are used while the hand is maintained in the position as shown in **B.** The stock-inette is then folded down over the cast and cut and the final roll of plaster bandage is applied (**C**). Note that the fingers and thumb are free and the patient is able to use the fingers without any impingement on normal motion.

A *long arm cast* is produced in a similar fashion except that it is extended above the elbow to approximately the midarm.

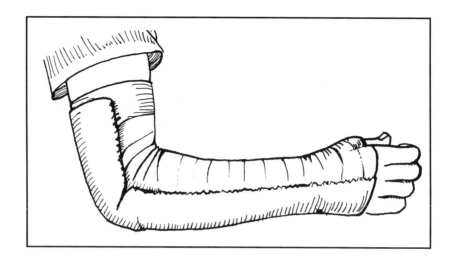

□ LONG ARM POSTERIOR SPLINT

A long arm posterior splint is used to immobilize a number of injuries around the elbow and forearm as discussed in the text. The splint is produced by wrapping a cotton bandage (Webril) around the forearm from the midpalmar region to the midarm. Next, a posterior plaster splint is applied to the arm held in a position of 90-degree flexion at the elbow and neutral position at the wrist. This is followed by an elastic bandage to hold the posterior slab in position. A sling should be applied after the splint is in position.

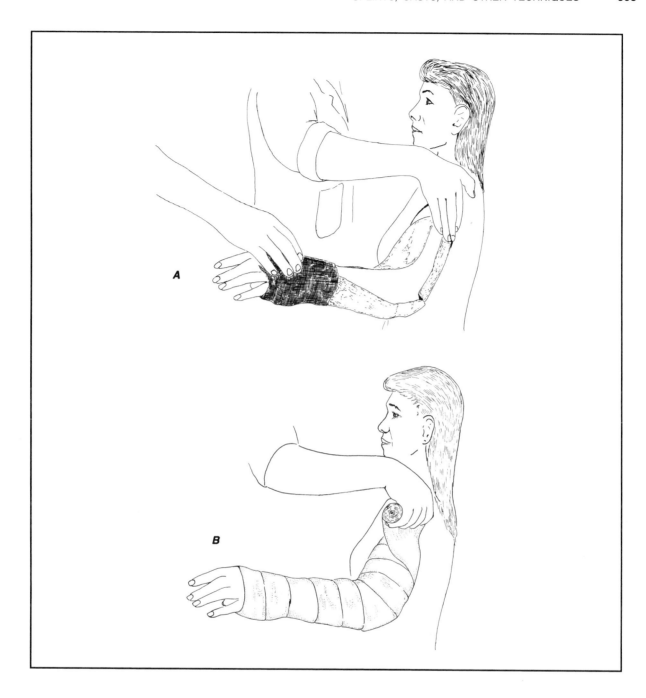

□ LONG ARM ANTERIOR–POSTERIOR SPLINT

The arm is positioned as dictated by the type of fracture. This splint is utilized for fractures of the distal humerus, combined fractures of the radius and ulna; and an unstable distal radius or proximal ulna fracture. Generally speaking the arm, forearm, and wrist are placed in a position most comfortable for the patient in that this position usually conforms to the most relaxed placement of the muscles. *A.* Apply a plaster slab over the volar and dorsal portion of the arm and forearm. The plaster slab should extend from the midarm to the dorsum of the hand, incorporating both the elbow and wrist joints. It is important that the volar (anterior) and dorsal (posterior) slabs do not meet so as to form a circumferential "cast." After measuring the slabs, place cotton roll on the undersurface and apply the plaster slab to the extremity. The authors use a small amount of gauze wrapping at the distal end of the splint as shown to keep the slab in place during application. An assistant can hold the upper end. *B.* Wrap the splint with an elastic bandage as shown.

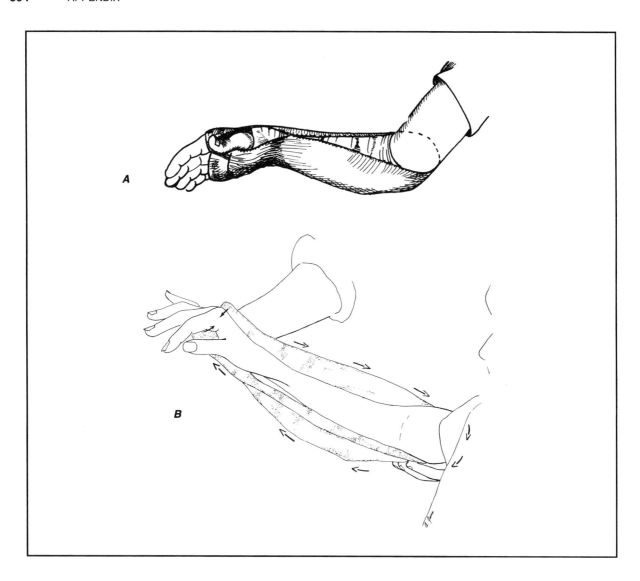

□ SUGAR TONG SPLINT

A. This splint is used in distal forearm fractures, especially fractures of the distal radius (Colles'). The forearm can be supinated or pronated during the application of the splint. A cotton bandage is first applied to the injured limb. After this a single long plaster splint is applied by encircling the elbow (**B**).

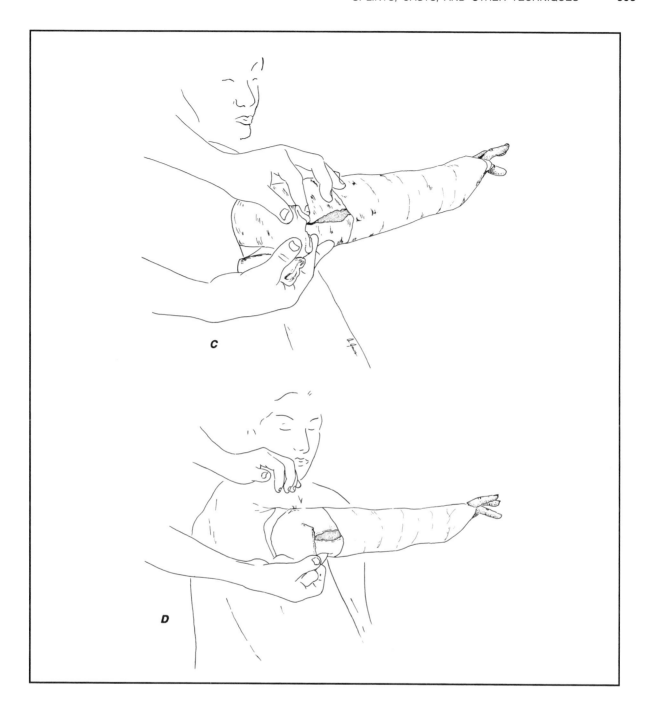

The splint should extend from the metacarpophalangeal joint palmarly around the elbow to the dorsal aspect of the hand just proximal to the metacarpophalangeal joint. The excess plaster, created by encircling the elbow, is tucked (*C, D*). An elastic bandage holds the splints in position.

The advantage of this splint is that it permits immobilization in a position of pronation or supination without a circumferential cast being applied to the extremity. A sling should be used with the splint.

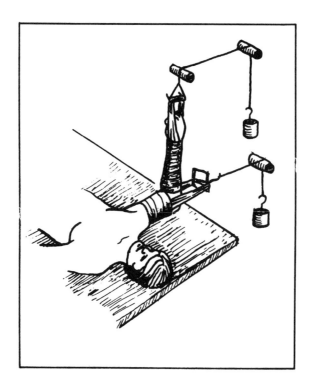

☐ DUNLOP'S TRACTION

Dunlop's skin traction is used in a number of fractures of the distal humerus where continuous traction is needed to maintain reduction. As with all forms of skin traction, its use should be temporary in the adult. The principles and manner in which it is applied is shown, with traction maintained by weights at two locations.

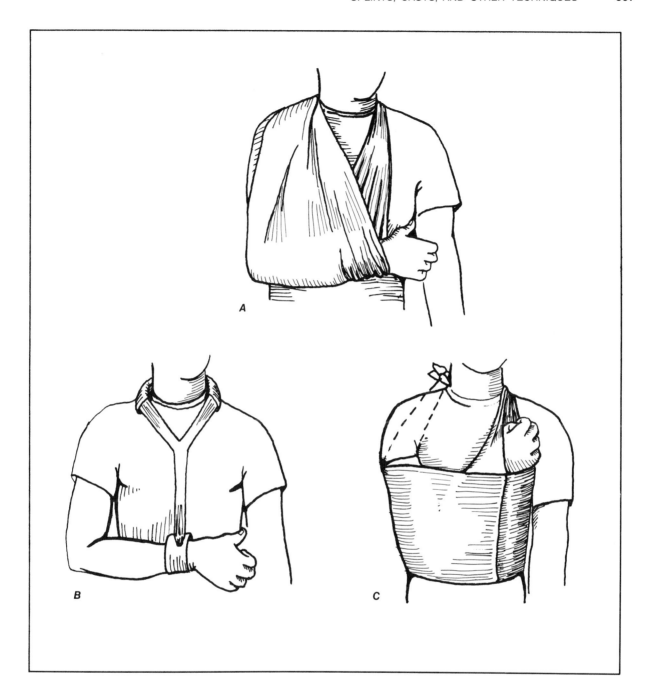

□ VARIOUS KINDS OF "SLINGS"

A. A commercial sling is used to support the arm for a number of injuries as discussed in the text. **B.** A *collar and cuff* is an alternate method used to support the forearm in patients with a humeral fracture treated with a coaptation splint. **C.** A *stockinette Valpeau* and swathe (the component encircles the patient's waist) is used in situations where there is an unstable fracture of the proximal humerus, which has a tendency to displace due to contraction of the pectoralis major muscle. This position relaxes the pectoralis major.

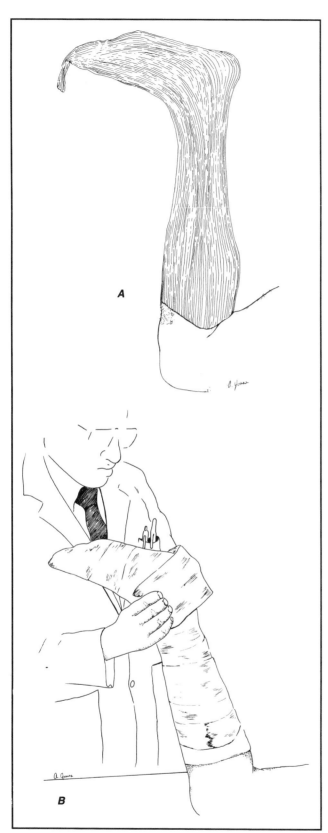

□ APPLICATION OF A POSTERIOR SPLINT TO THE ANKLE

Stockinette is applied over the foot and ankle with the patient lying in the prone position (*A*). Following this, cotton roll (Webril) is applied over the stockinette with extra padding applied over the malleoli and heel (*B*).

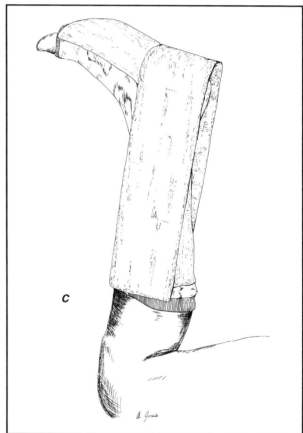

Plaster slabs which have been premeasured are then applied (*C*). The volar slab courses from the base of the toes just distal to the metatarsophalangeal joints to just below the knee and is applied over the cotton bandage. To add additional side-to-side support a U-shaped coaptation splint is applied over the heel.

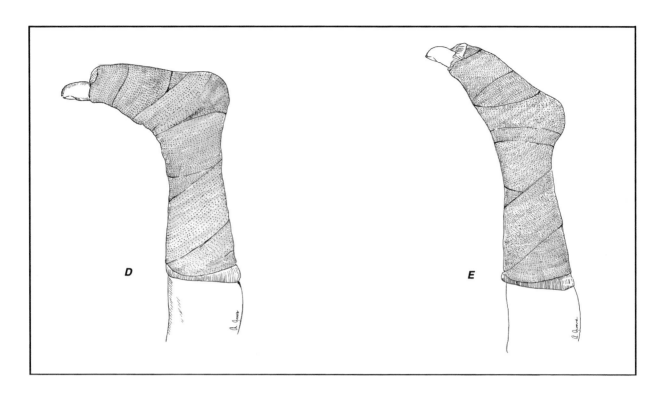

Finally, an elastic bandage is applied over the plaster splints. The ankle is then held in either neutral position (**D**) when treating ankle sprains or most foot fractures or in equinus (**E**) when treating Achilles tendon injuries or other conditions in which equinus is recommended. See text for discussion.

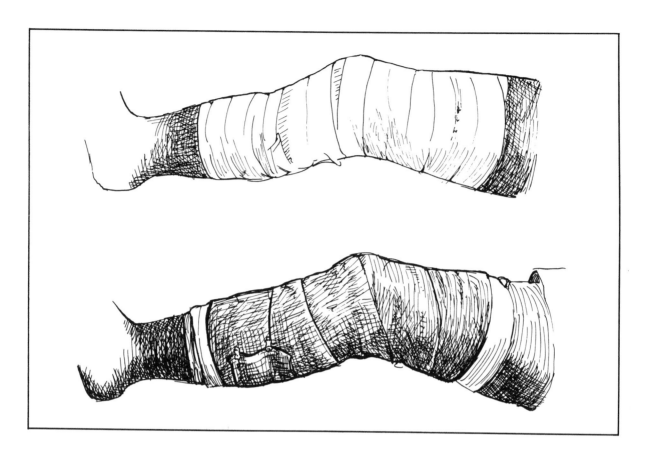

□ JONES' COMPRESSION DRESSING

A Jones' compression dressing is commonly used for soft tissue injuries of the knee. This dressing provides immobilization of the limb while permitting some flexion and extension and provides a compressive force that limits swelling at the knee. The dressing is made by applying a layer of cotton bandage (Webril) extending from the groin to just above the malleoli of the ankle. After this, an elastic wrap is applied circumferentially. A second layer of cotton bandage is then applied followed by another elastic wrap. This additional layer provides for added support that may or may not be necessary depending on the condition being treated.

INDEX

Page numbers followed by *t* and *f* indicate tables and figures, respectively.